HEALING SPACES

CHRIS VAN UFFELEN

HEALING SPACES

CONTEMPORARY HOSPITAL ARCHITECTURE

Therapy between High-tech, Wellness, Charity, and Economy

The development of hospital architecture reflects the ongoing transformation of medicine, society, and culture. Greek healing sanctuaries dedicated to Asclepius combined medicine, religion, and architecture into places of recovery. Roman valetudinaria, primarily built for soldiers and slaves, are early predecessors of modern hospitals. Even at that time, spatial organization, patient care, and the healing environment played an important role.
During the Middle Ages, Christian hospices and monasteries shaped hospital construction throughout Europe. Institutions such as the Hôtel-Dieu in Paris served the poor, pilgrims, and the sick alike. Large communal wards defined these early hospitals. Through the Crusades, European medicine also absorbed important knowledge from Islamic healthcare architecture. Islamic bimaristans already featured specialized departments, teaching facilities, and clearly separated functional areas, significantly influencing later European hospital design. The Renaissance marked the beginning of a more systematic approach to hospital planning. Large courtyard complexes such as the Ospedale Maggiore in Milan became models for future healthcare buildings. During the 17th and 18th centuries, new layouts with partly open courtyards and specialized facilities for mental health conditions emerged. At the same time, hygiene, ventilation, and organizational efficiency improved as architecture increasingly responded to medical knowledge and the need for better patient care.
The 19th century brought major medical and architectural innovations. Advances such as anesthesia, antisepsis, modern nursing, and new surgical techniques led to specialized clinics and university hospitals. The pavilion system, consisting of separate buildings to reduce infections, and comb-like floor plans emerged. At the same time, sanatoriums developed as therapeutic environments that used light, fresh air, and nature as healing elements. Large terraces, loggias, and outdoor spaces became central features. In the 20th century, technological progress resulted in more compact hospital forms and eventually the rise of the hospital high-rise. At the end of the 20. century, patient comfort and quality of stay gained importance. Beyond medical efficiency, architects increasingly focused on orientation, emotional well-being, and spatial quality.
This led to the concept of Healing Architecture, which uses daylight, ventilation, color, materials, and welcoming interiors to positively influence recovery. Today, hospitals are far more than functional healthcare facilities. Modern hospital architecture combines medical, economic, and social requirements with design, sustainability, and human-centered planning. Hospitals are intended to be places of healing, safety, and orientation that support patients, visitors, and staff alike. Architecture can reduce stress, strengthen identity, and create a positive healing environment. Hospital architecture now ranges from small healthcare centers to highly complex university medical campuses. Because hospitals remain in use for decades, they are among the most demanding building types.
Medical innovation, demographic change, new diseases, and shifting social expectations continuously reshape healthcare design. Hospitals are also increasingly expected to operate as competitive service providers, raising demands for flexibility, efficiency, and architectural quality. Sustainability has therefore become essential. Healthcare buildings must remain adaptable, technically flexible, and capable of future transformation. Modular systems support interdisciplinary collaboration and long-term usability. Hospitals are also recognized as important parts of the urban fabric, shaping cities, and contributing to public life.
Recent developments, especially the COVID-19 pandemic, have further influenced hospital planning. Flexible layouts, decentralized structures, digital healthcare, improved circulation systems, and single-patient rooms are becoming increasingly important. Hospital architecture continues to evolve as a reflection of medical progress, social change, and cultural values.

Chris van Uffelen

Martin-Pierre Gauthier: Hôpital Lariboisière, Paris, 1846–1854: comb layout around one courtyard.

Martin Gropius and Heino Schmieden: Klinikum in Friedrichshain, Berlin, 1866–1874: pavilion layout and floor plan.

Libéral Brutant and Jules Hardouin-Mansart: Hôtel des Invalides, Paris, 1670–1708: 15 closed courtyards.

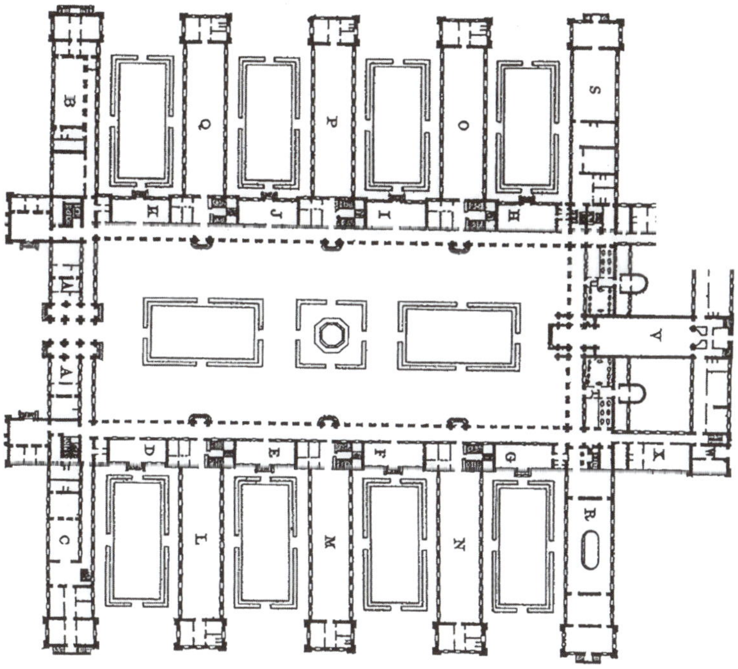

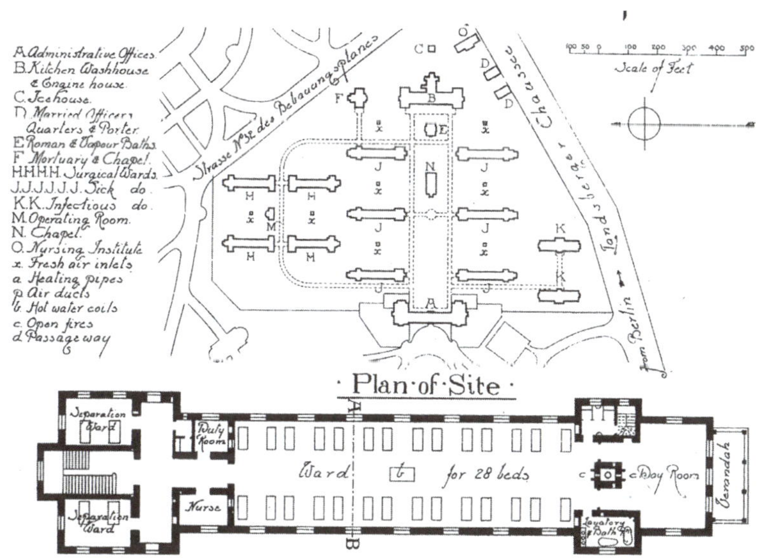
A. Administrative Offices
B. Kitchen Washhouse & Engine house
C. Icehouse
D. Married Officers Quarters & Porter
E. Roman & Vapour Baths
F. Mortuary & Chapel
HHHH. Surgical Wards
J.J.J.J.J. Sick do.
K.K. Infectious do.
M. Operating Room
N. Chapel
O. Nursing Institute
x. Fresh air inlets
a. Heating pipes
p. Air ducts
h. Hot water coils
c. Open fires
d. Passage way
Scale of Feet
Plan of Site
Separation Ward
Duty Room
Ward for 28 beds
Day Room
Verandah
Nurse
Separation Ward
Lavatory Bath

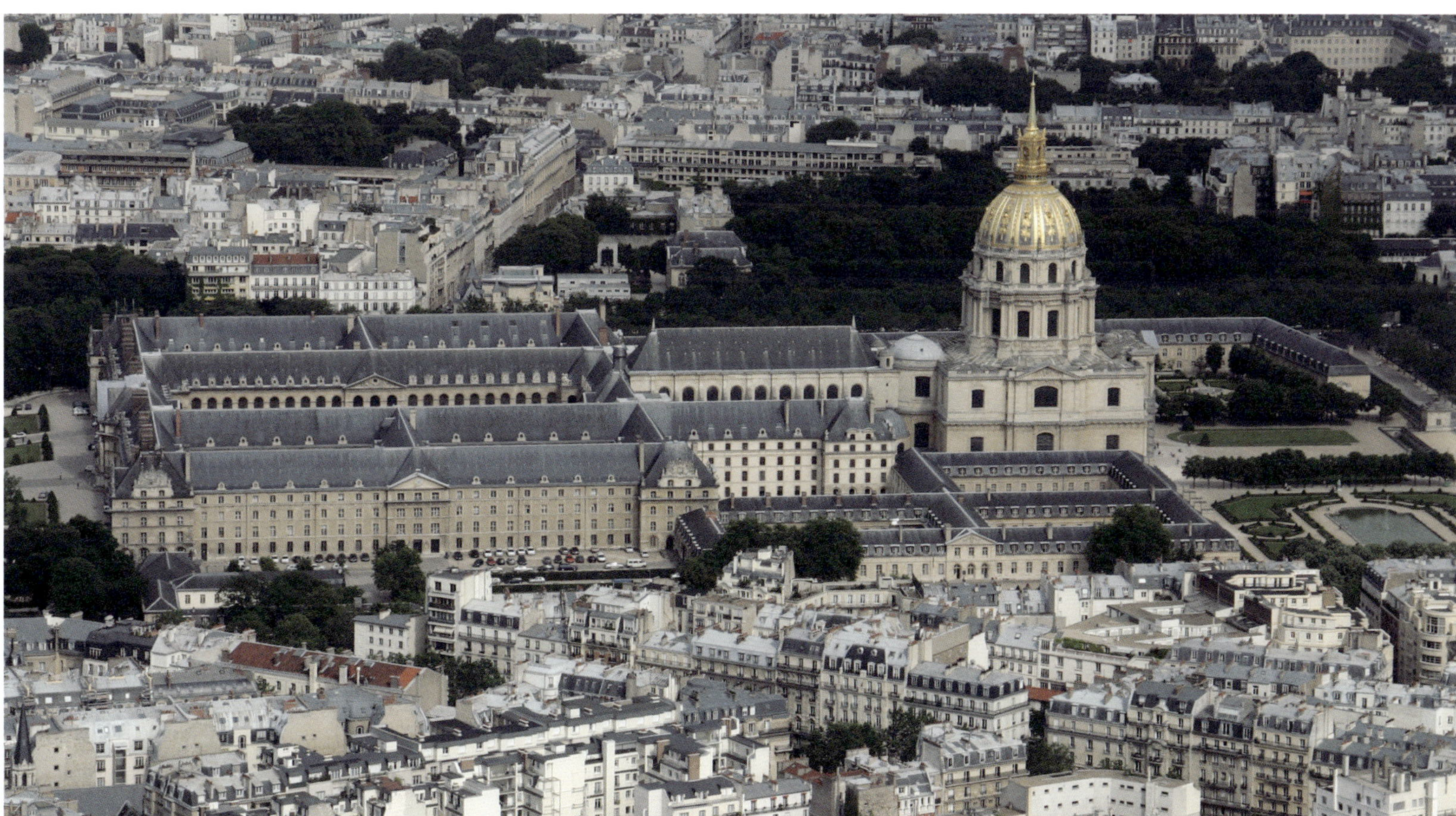

BBATS

Tarapaca
Chile

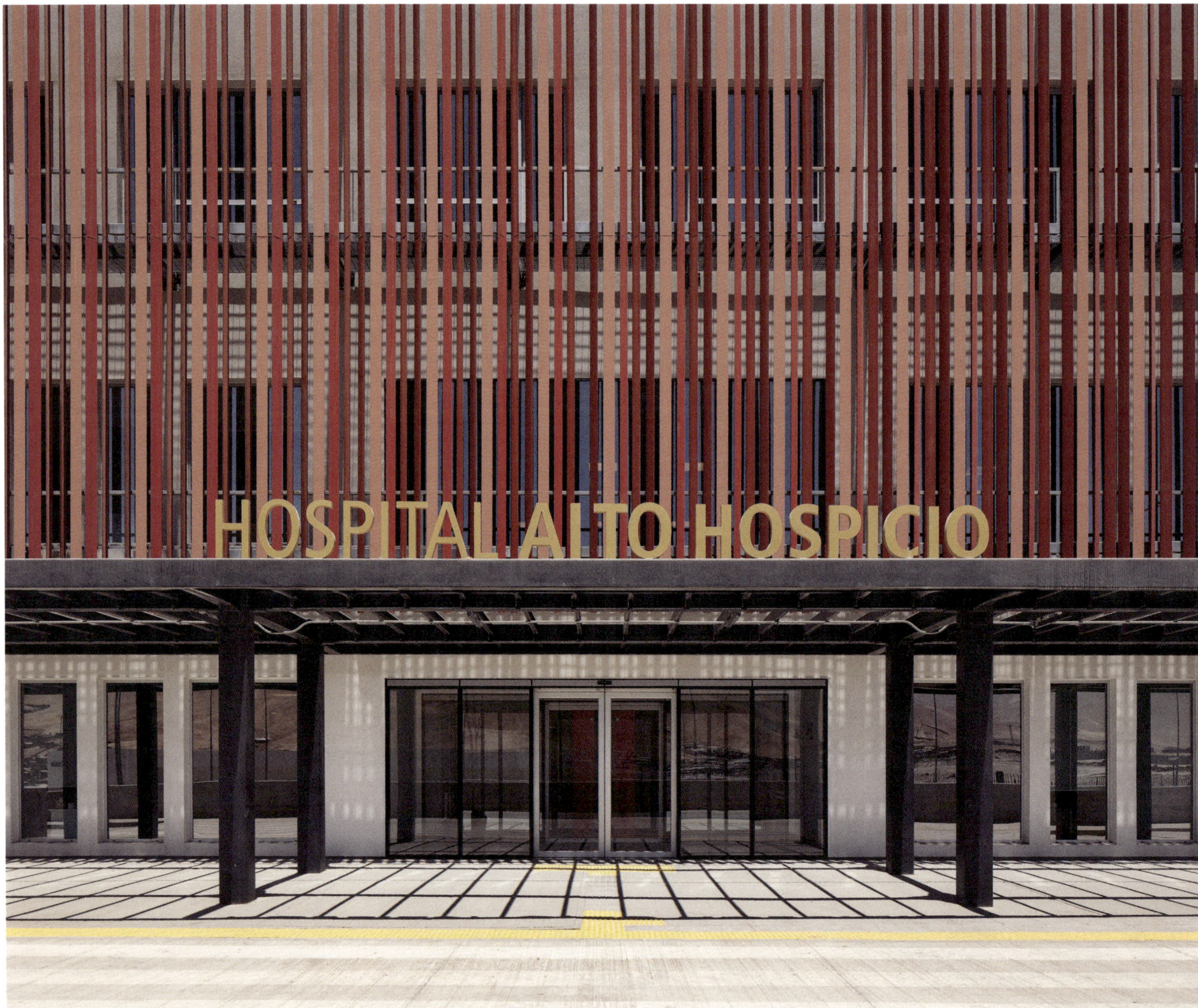

Hospital entrance marked by warm-toned surfaces and a recessed canopy.

Rectangular hospital building with a light-colored façade and vertical shading elements.

Hospital building set within an arid desert landscape, overlooking the surrounding city.

Hospital Alto Hospicio

Set in a remote desert context, the hospital is conceived as an isolated yet grounded healthcare facility, shaped by extreme climatic conditions, and Aymara references. A pure rectangular volume defines the form, wrapped in vertical louvers that reinterpret traditional ponchos, filtering intense sunlight into a softened veil of light. Large internal courtyards structure the spatial organization, introducing daylight and shadow to create calm, luminous environments for healing. The building follows the site's slope, distributing functions vertically with public services at entry level, critical care above, hospitalization at the top, and logistics below. Courtyards extend across levels, mediating between geometry and light while organizing circulation for public and technical flows. Through its presence, the hospital redefines the urban horizon, emerging as a civic landmark and catalyst for local activity.

Address: Alemania 3240, 1130724 Alto Hospicio, Tarapaca, Chile | **Client:** Alto Hospicio Hospital Consortium (Sacyr Infraestructure) | **Completion:** 2022 | **Size:** 42,624 m² | **Sector:** state | **Number of treatment rooms:** 33 | **Number of patient rooms:** 235

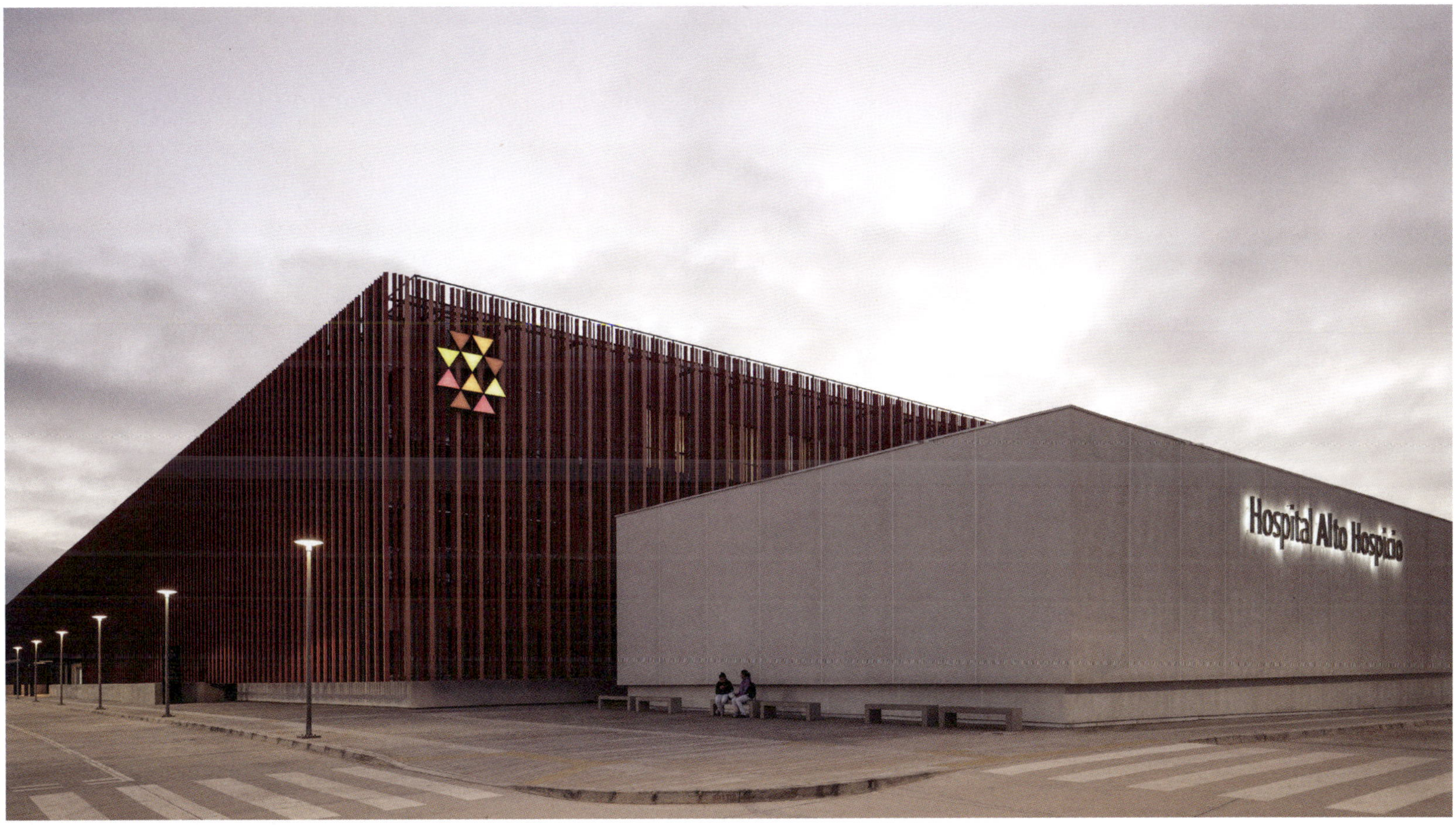

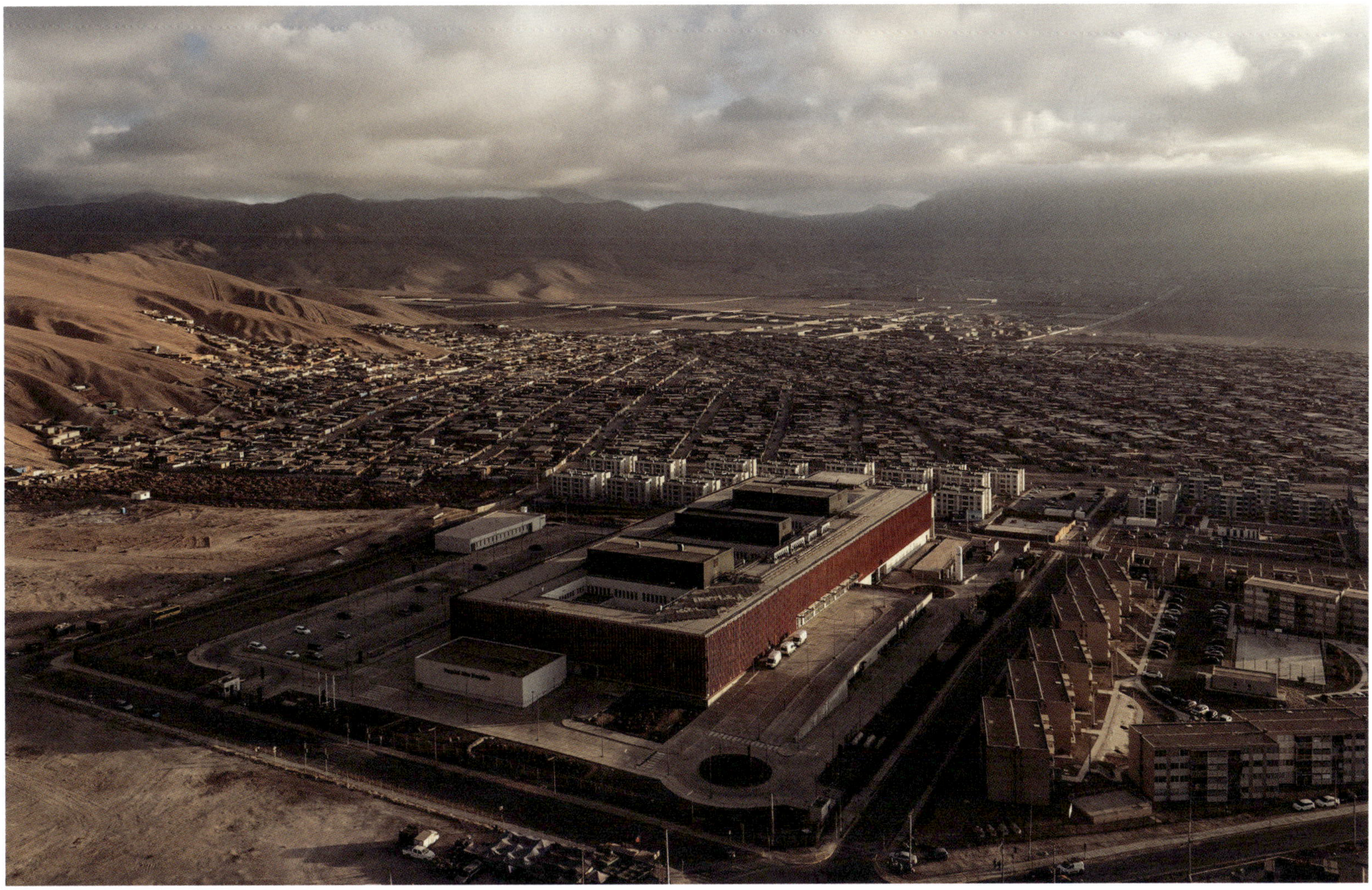

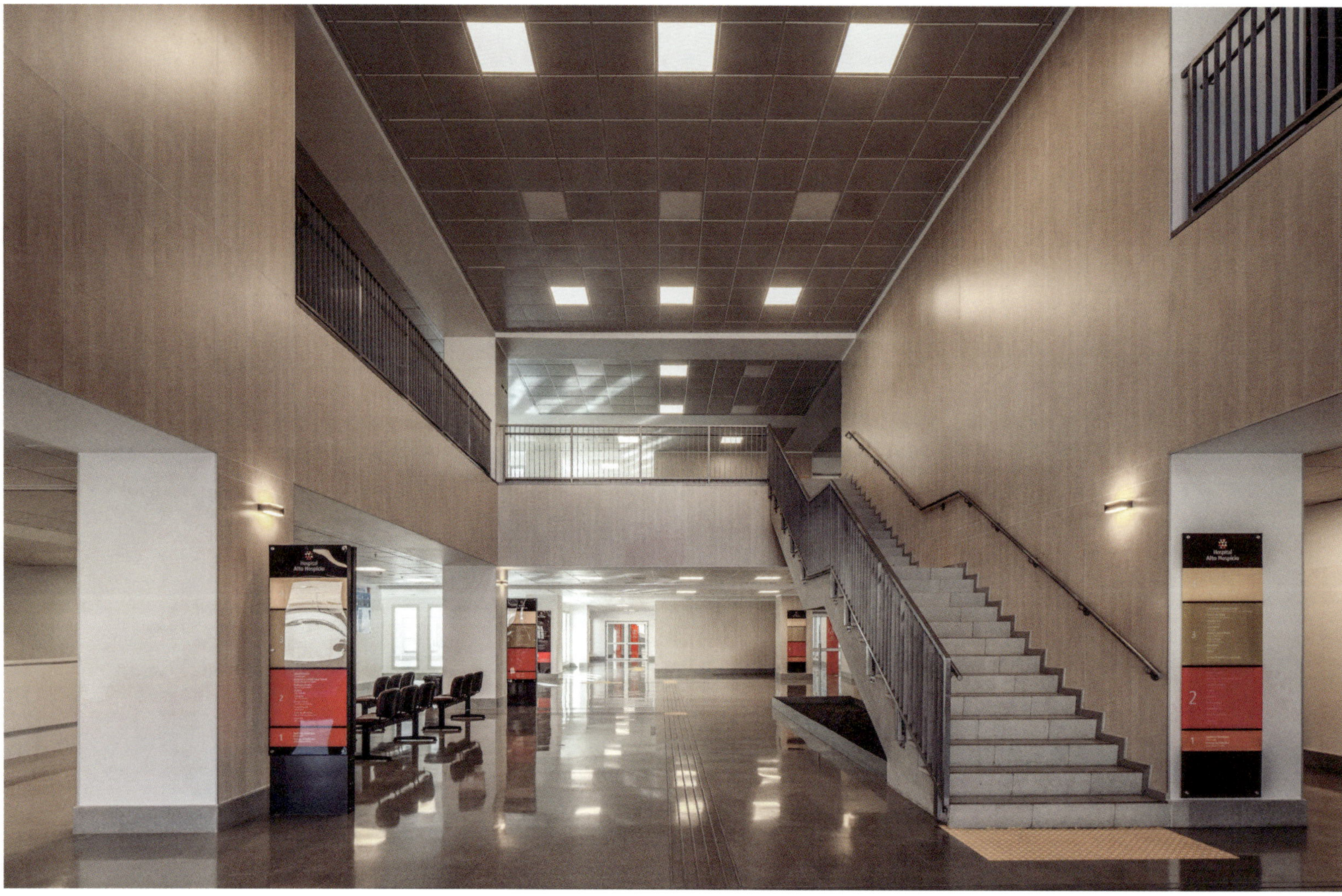

Main hall with an open spatial layout and a waiting area defined by large glazed surfaces and soft daylight.

Second floor plan.

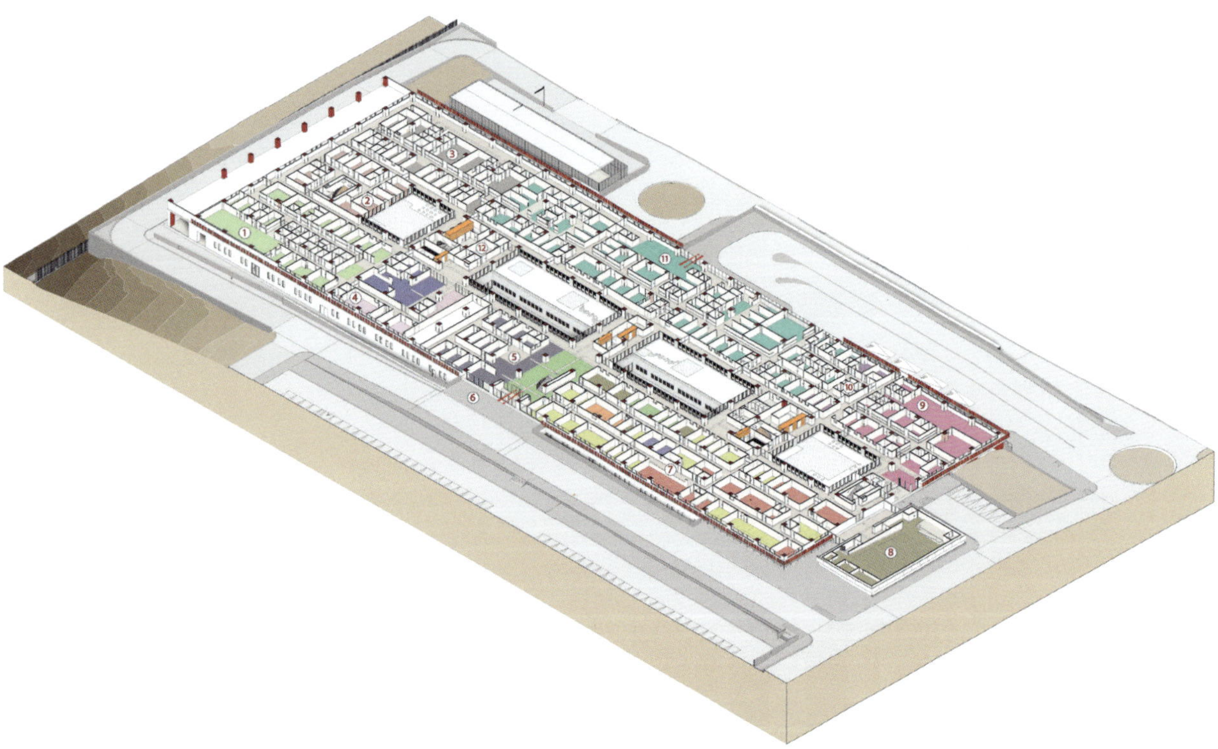

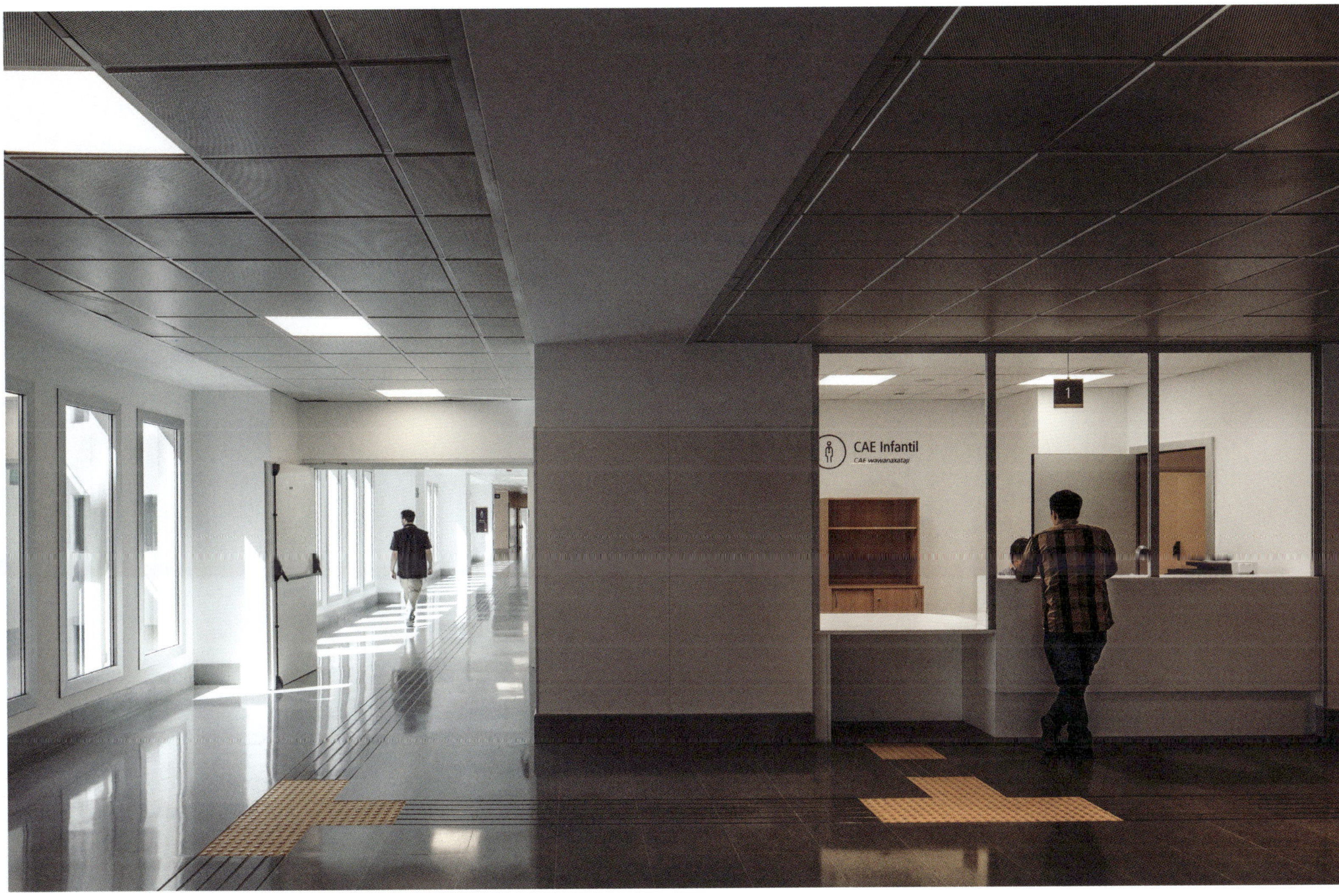

Hospital corridor with a reception desk, defined by clean surfaces and linear spatial organization.

Roof floor plan.

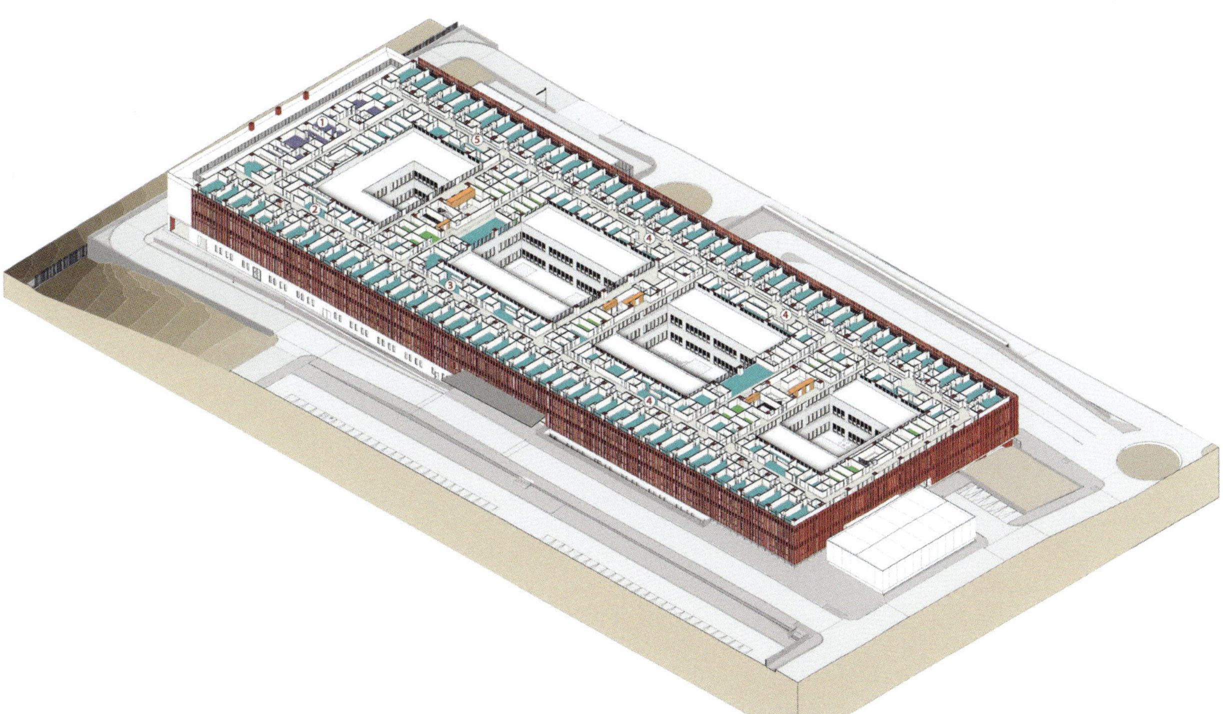

Davide Macullo Architects

Tirana
Albania

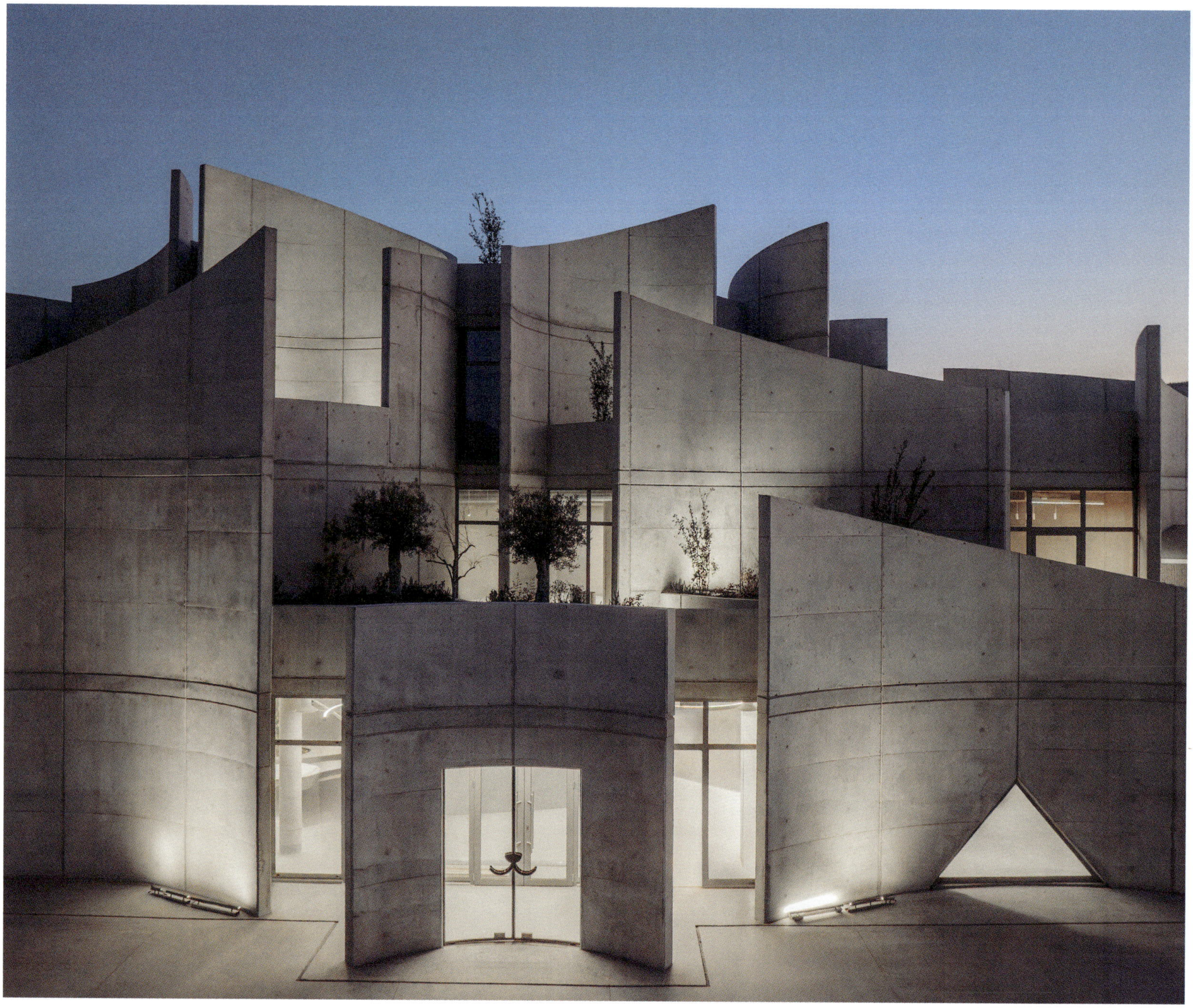

Detailed view of the entrance and greened terraces.

View of the sculptural façade at night.

Vet Hospital Tirana

This animal hospital underlines the importance of architecture creating not only simple building structures, but meaningful places. On the outside soft, organic, and flowing forms contrast with a sharp structured logic of the plan and the raw surface of brutalist concrete making the building appear like a living sculpture and creating a sense of wonder and harmony. The medical purpose remains almost hidden. Inside, the hospital is carefully planned to accommodate the psychological needs of its occupants. Just as in human healthcare, spatial psychology plays a critical role. Greened terraces serve as therapeutic spaces for the patients. The benefit of the treated animals in mind, the organization of spaces follows the same principles as those for humans: comfort, separation where necessary, and a thoughtful approach to coexistence is ensuring that the dogs and cats feel secure and at ease.

Address: Rruga Hiqmet Buzi, Pranë Liqenit të Thatë, Sauk Vjetër, Tirana, Sauk, Albania | **Client:** Vet Hospital | **Completion:** 2024 | **Size:** 2,243 m^2 | **Sector:** private | **Specialization:** veterinary | **Number of treatment rooms:** 103 | **Number of patient rooms:** 60 (for dogs and cats) | **Architects of record:** Orion Construction, S&L Studio

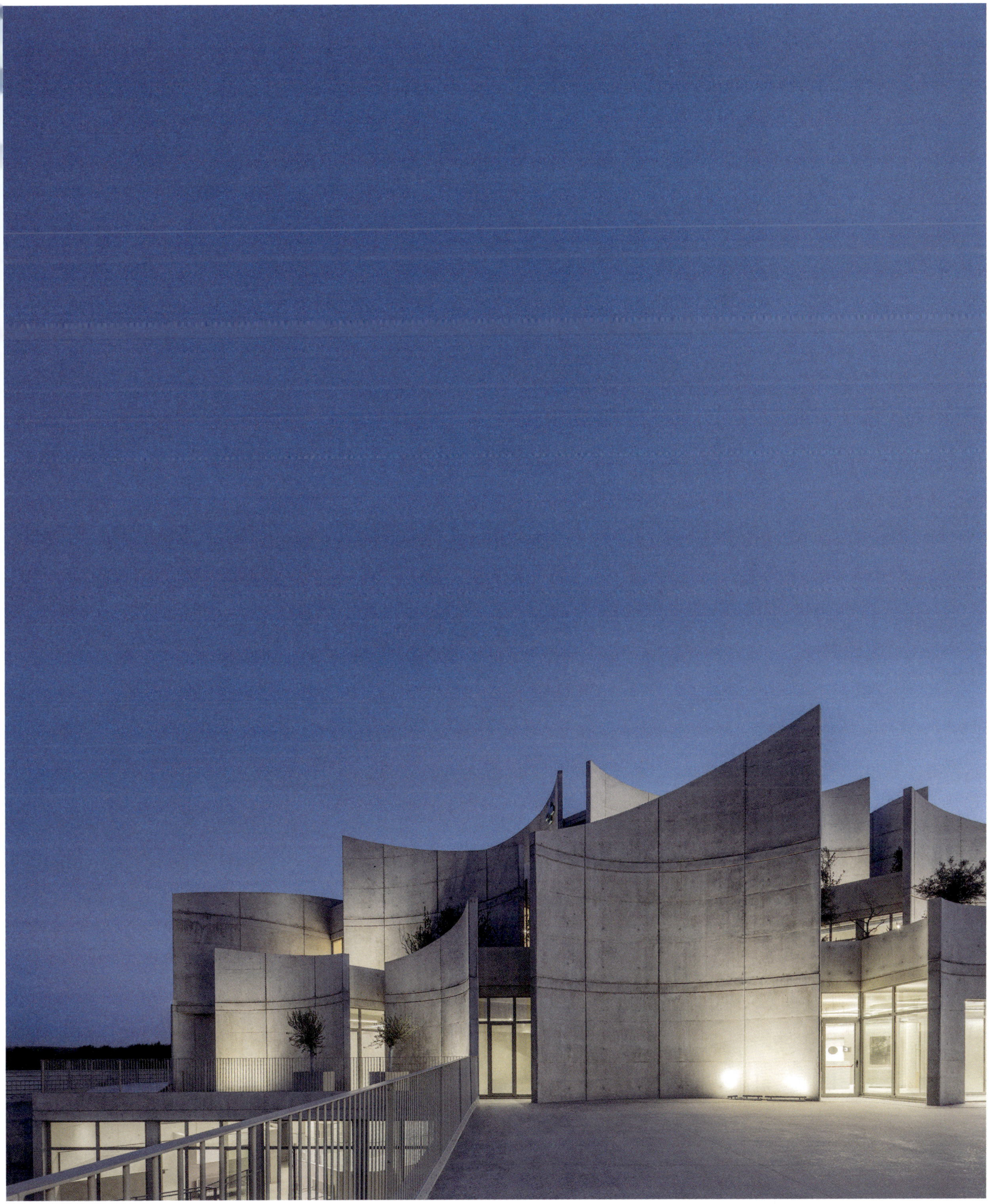

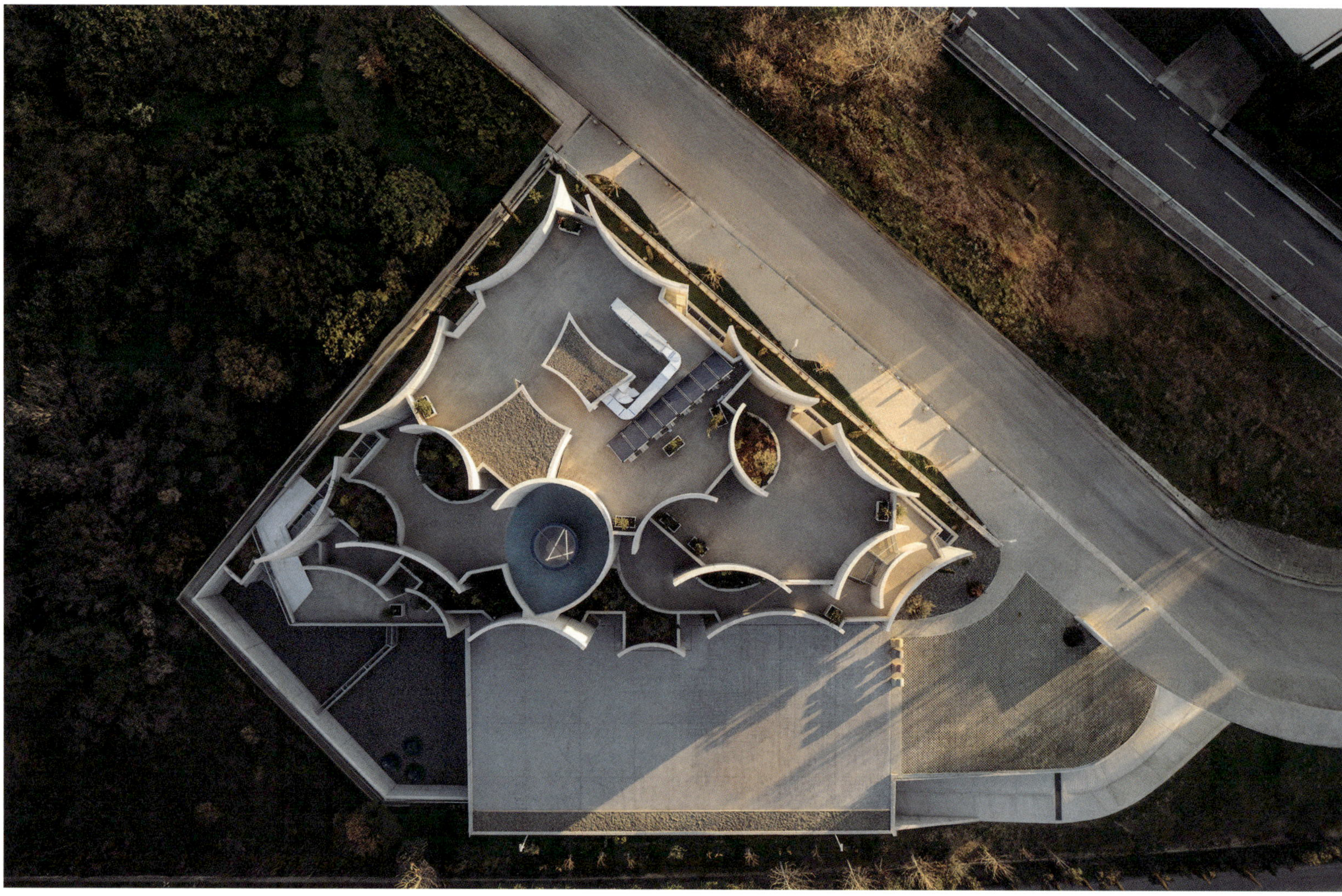

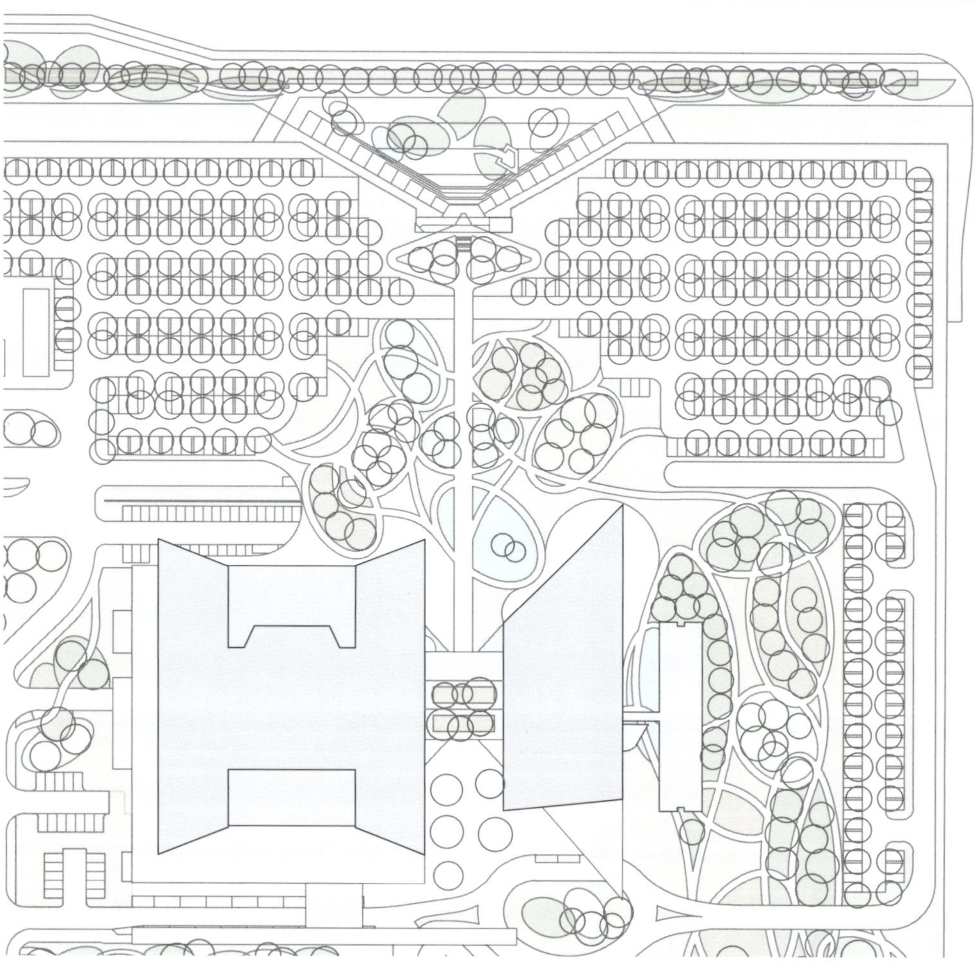

Top view of the Vet Hospital Tirana.

Ground floor plan.

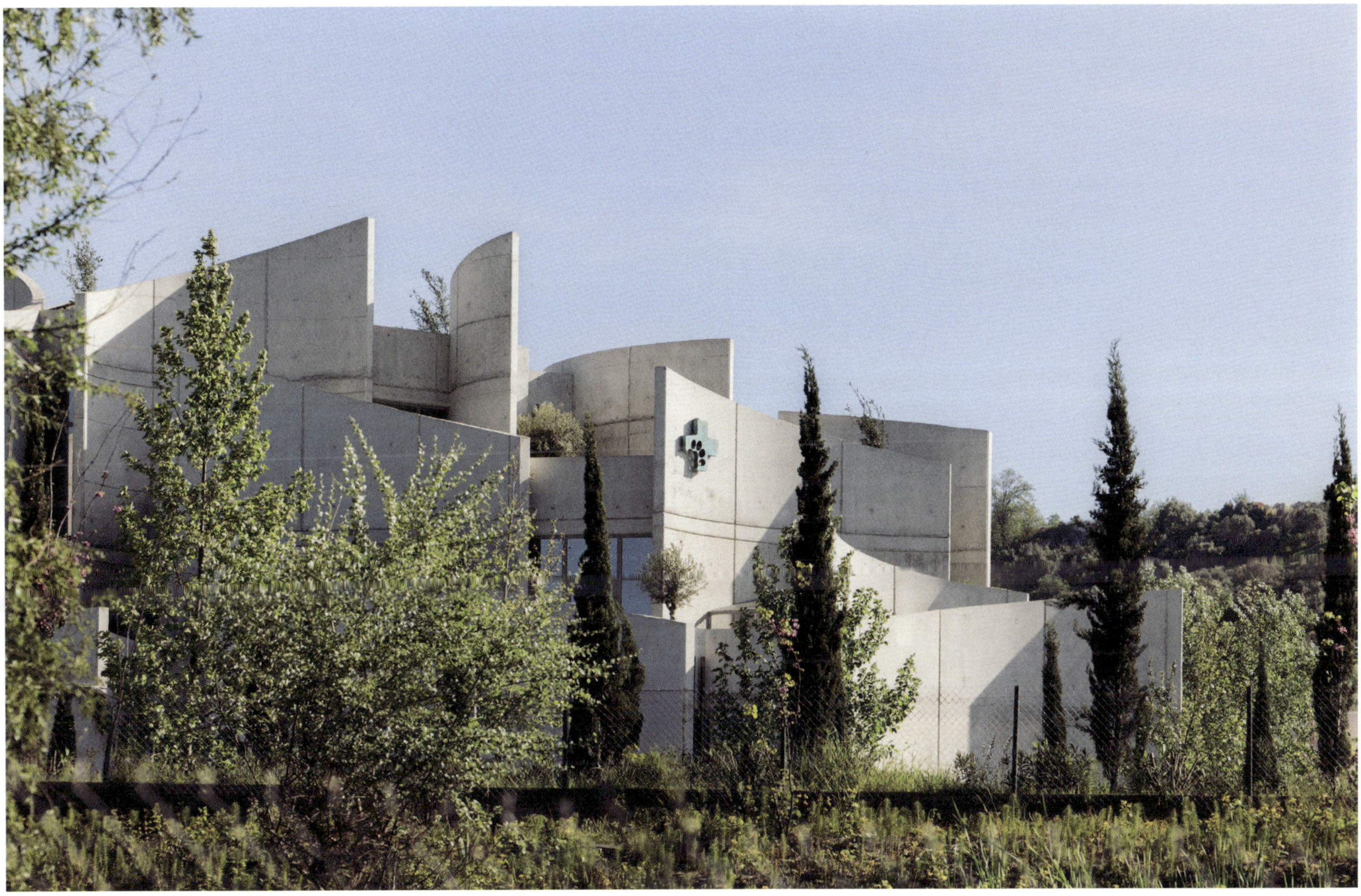

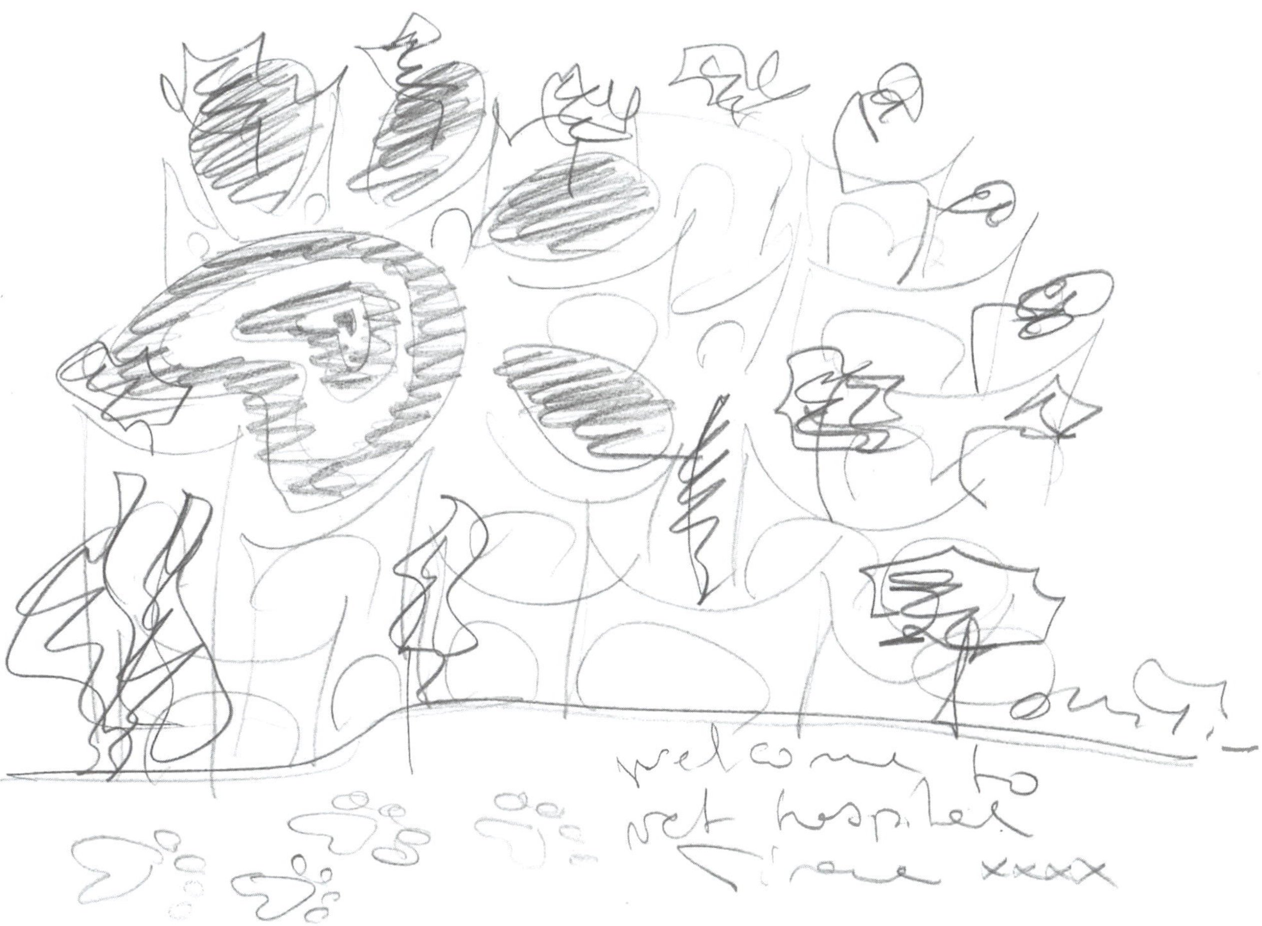

Detail of the façade within its green surroundings.

Original sketch.

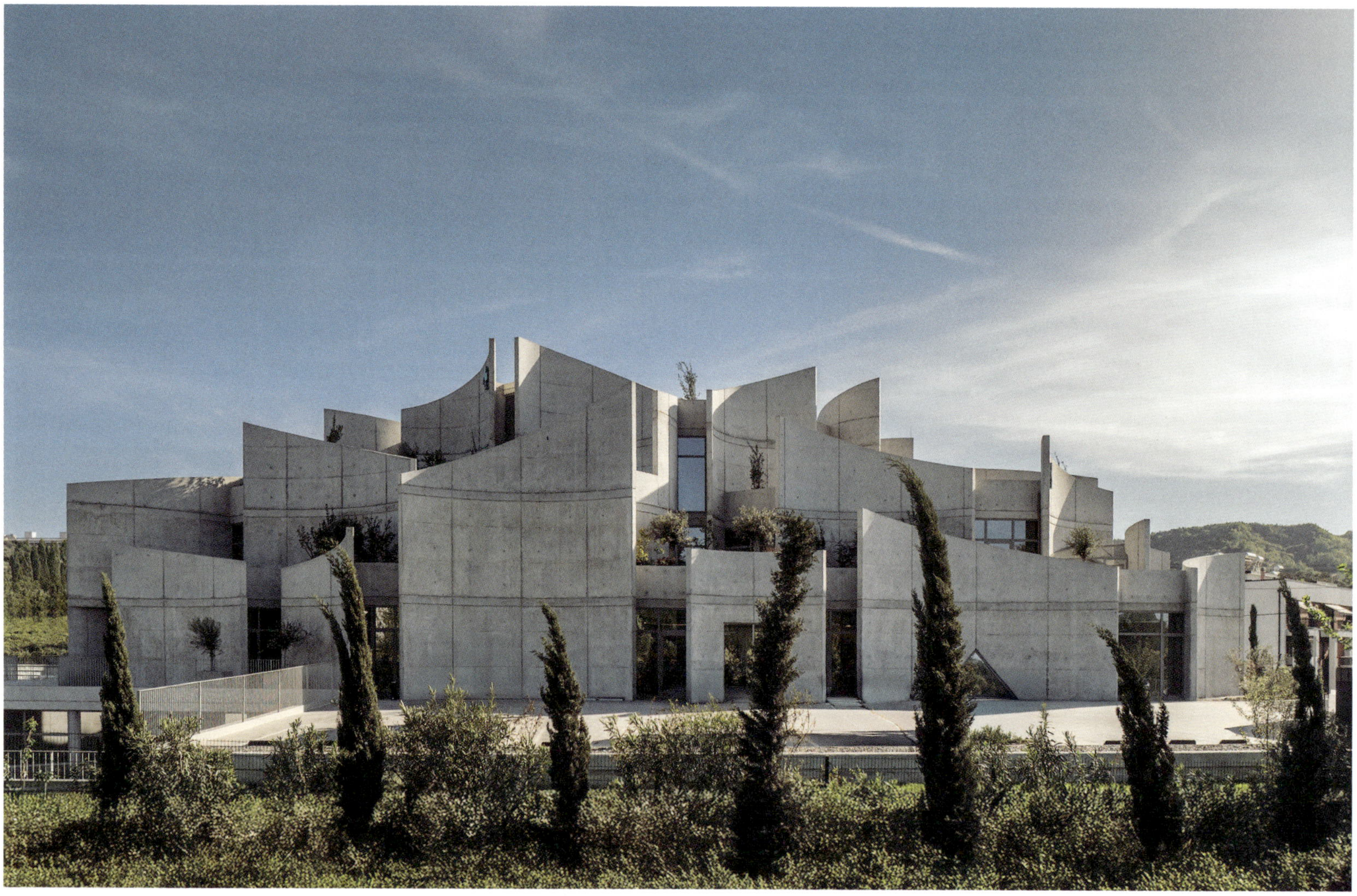

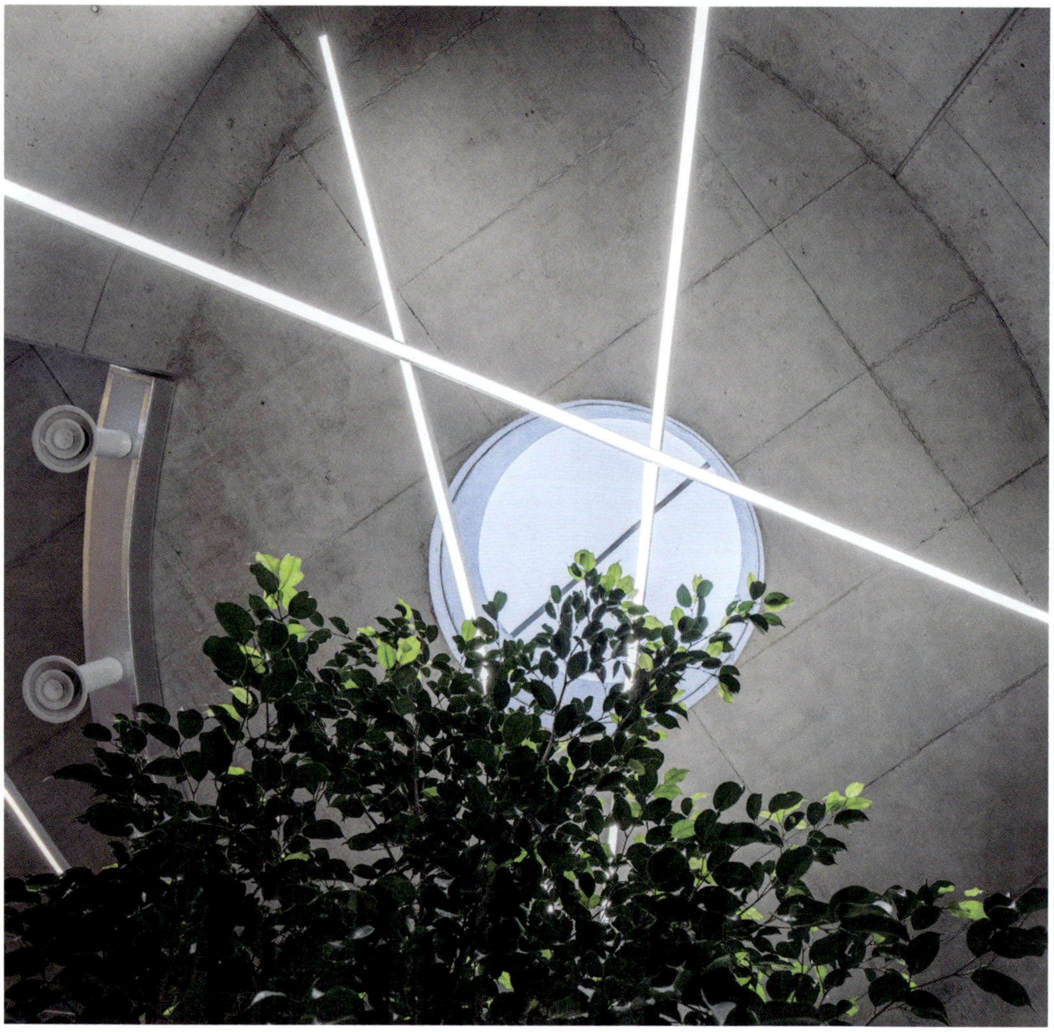

Building exterior during the day.

View of the interior ceiling with lighting and greening.

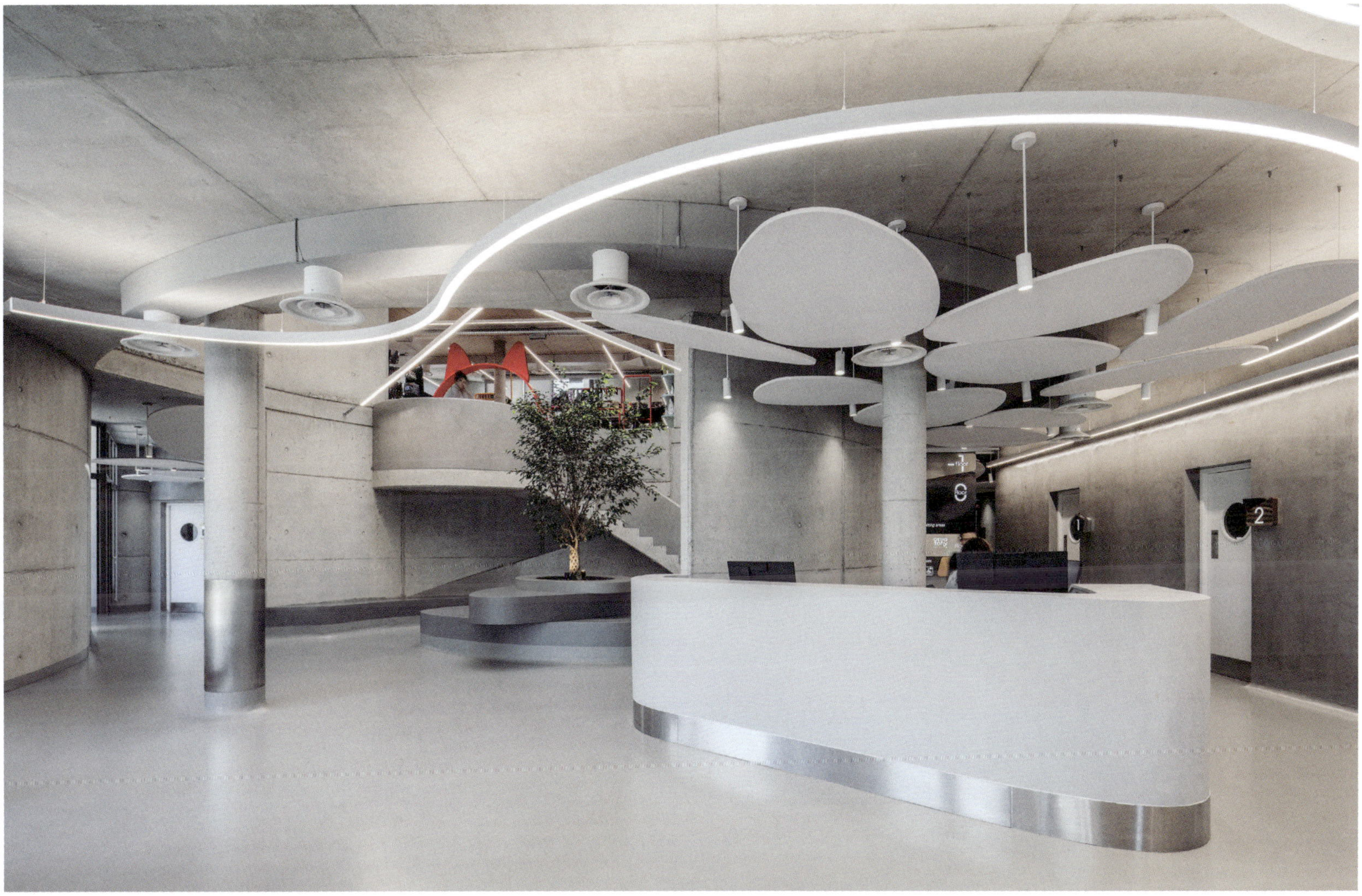

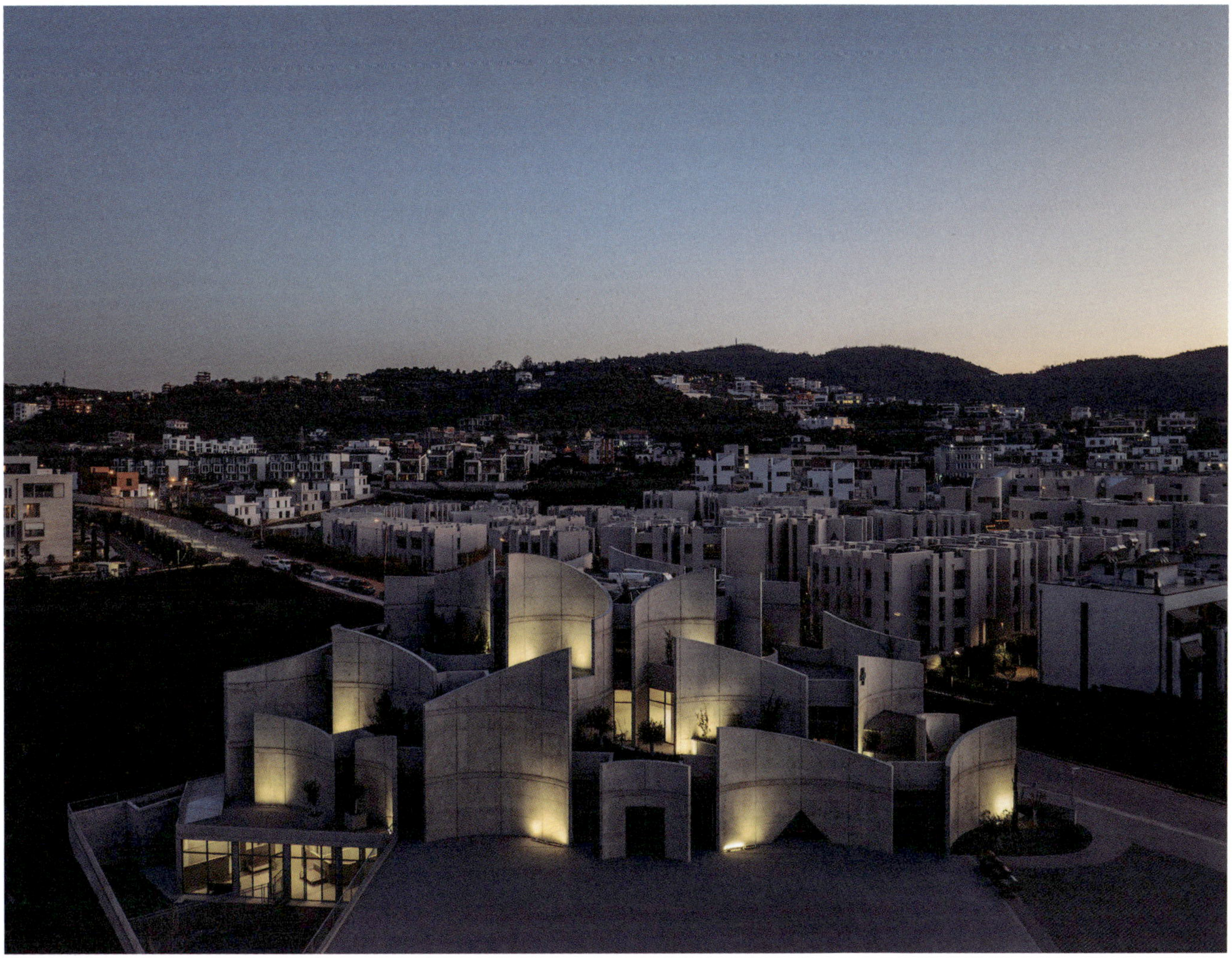

Interior view of the entrance hall

The building's location within the urban context.

NBBJ

Monterey
CA, USA

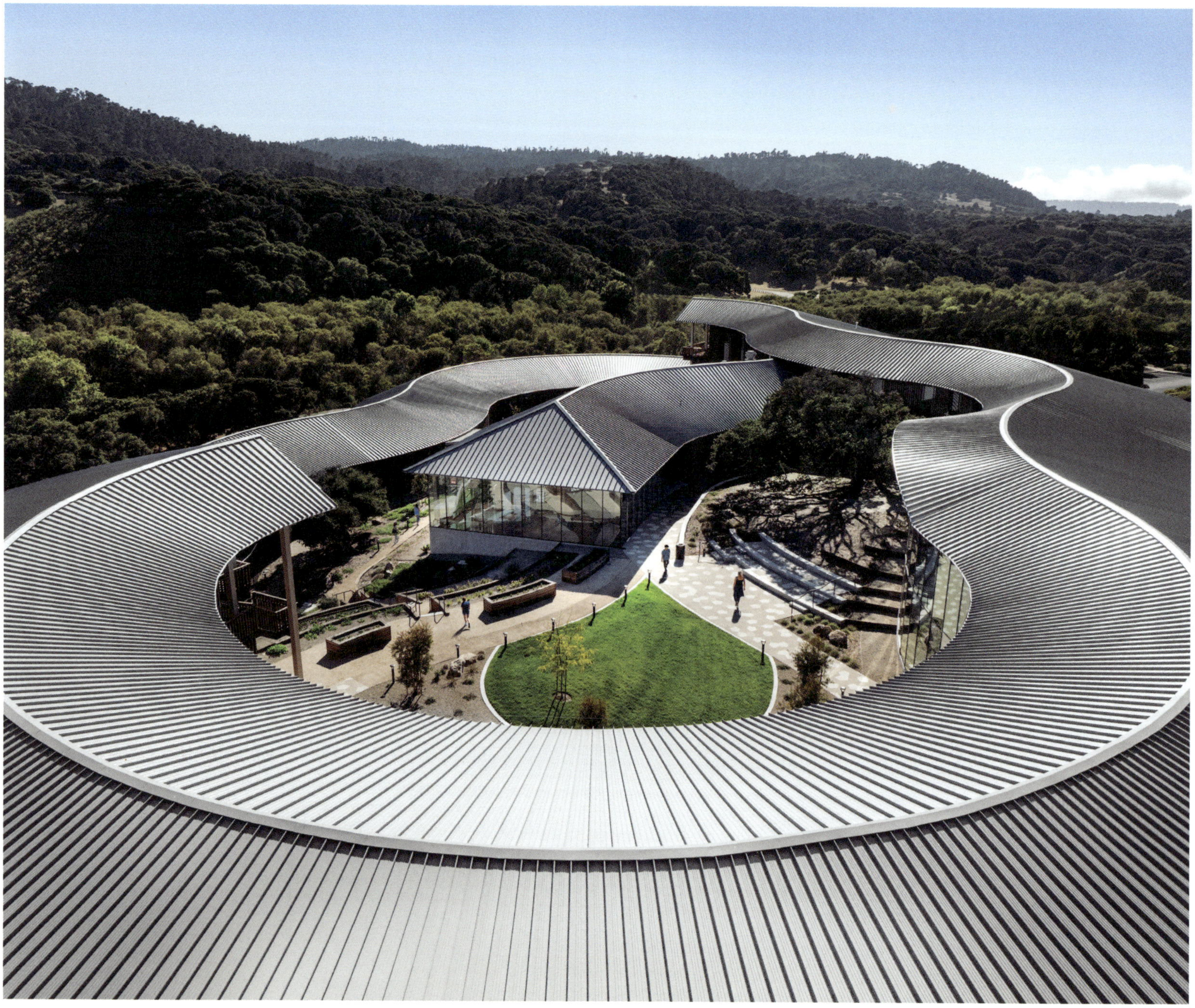

Courtyard surrounded by curving roof.

Rounded forms and natural materials shape the health-care environment.

The courtyard design enables informal meetings.

Montage Health Ohana Center for Behavioral Health

An increasing number of children are facing mental health challenges, yet treatment often occurs in facilities that isolate rather than heal. The Montage Health Ohana Center for Child and Adolescent Behavioral Health uses neuroscience-informed design to create an inclusive, restorative environment for pediatric patients, families, and caregivers. Designed by NBBJ in collaboration with neuroscientist Dr. John Medina and Montage Health, spatial strategies support executive function by enabling choice and individual control over environmental conditions. In addition, factors related to physical health and staff well-being are integrated, as these influence treatment processes. As a built example for child and adolescent behavioral healthcare, the project combines spatial organization, functional requirements, and health-related design criteria.

Address: 6 Lower Ragsdale Dr, Monterey, CA 93940, USA | **Client:** Montage Health | **Completion:** 2024 | **Size:** 5,166 m² | **Sector:** private | **Specialization:** behavioral health | **Number of patient rooms:** 16 | **Number of treatment rooms:** 29 | **Number of beds:** 16

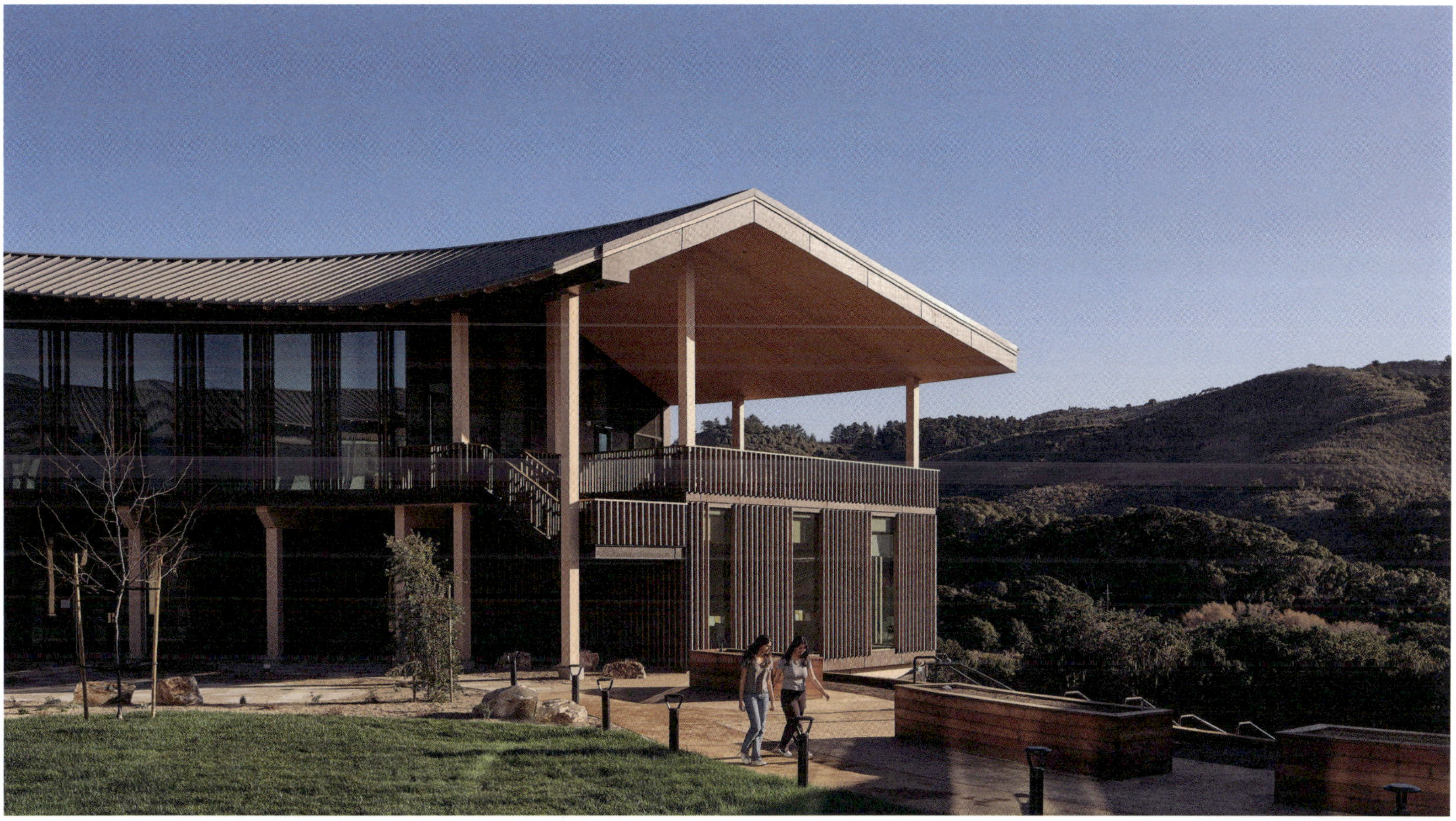

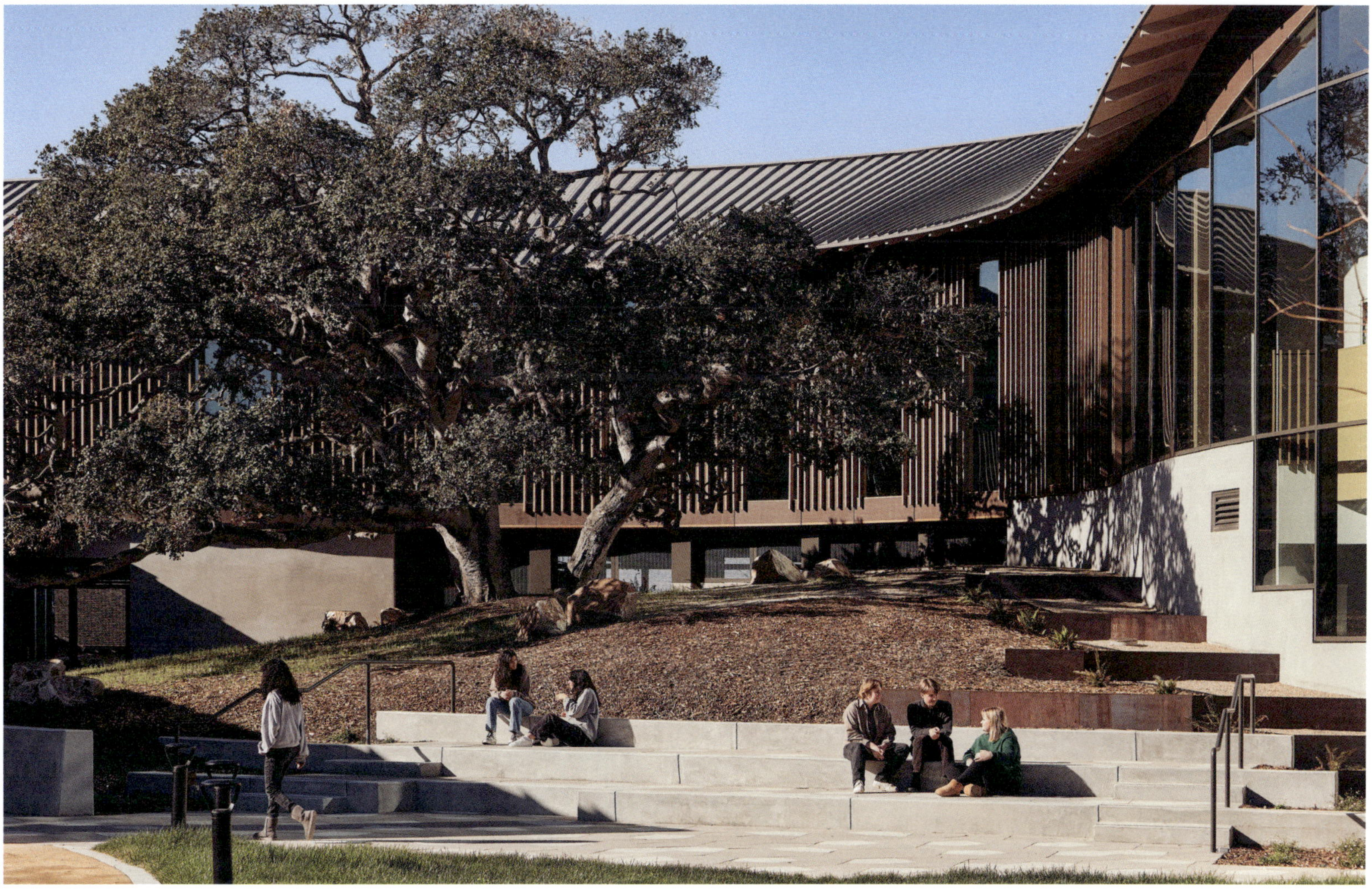

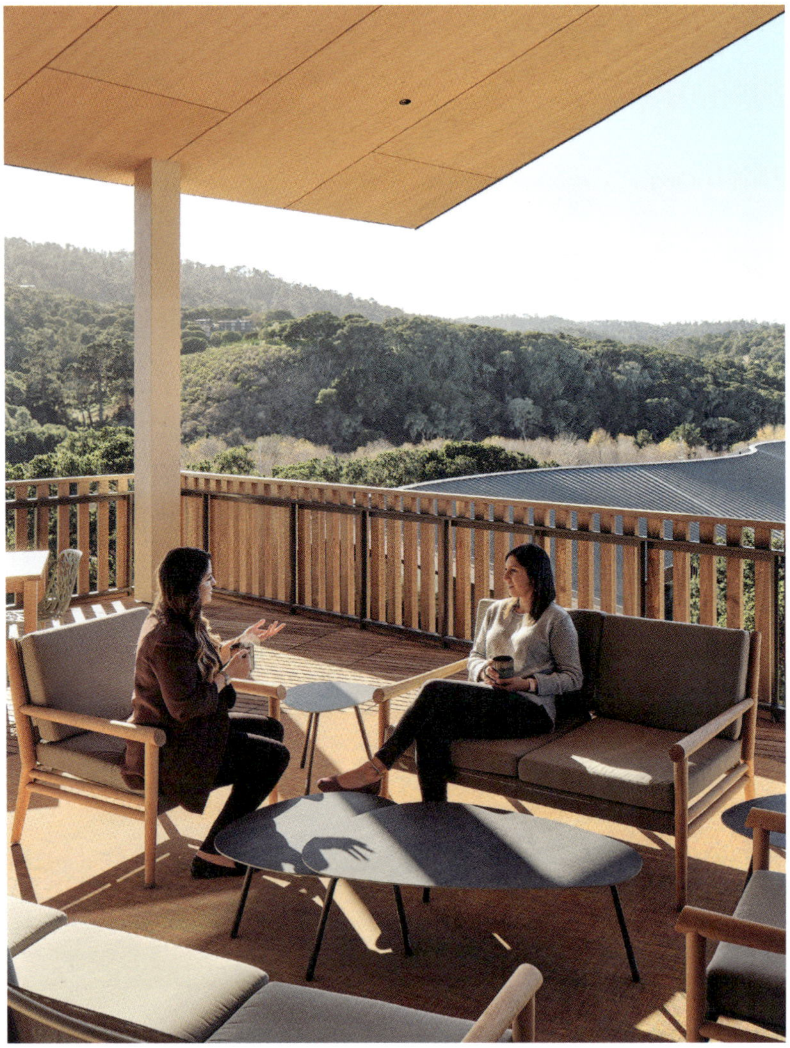

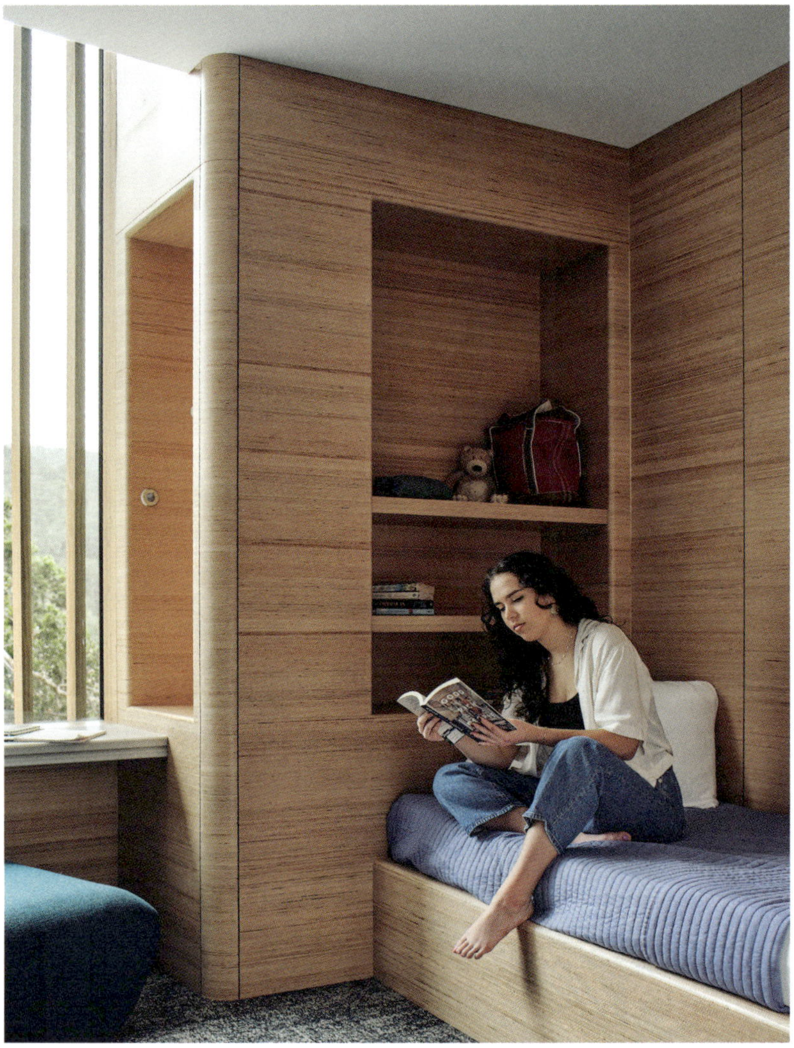

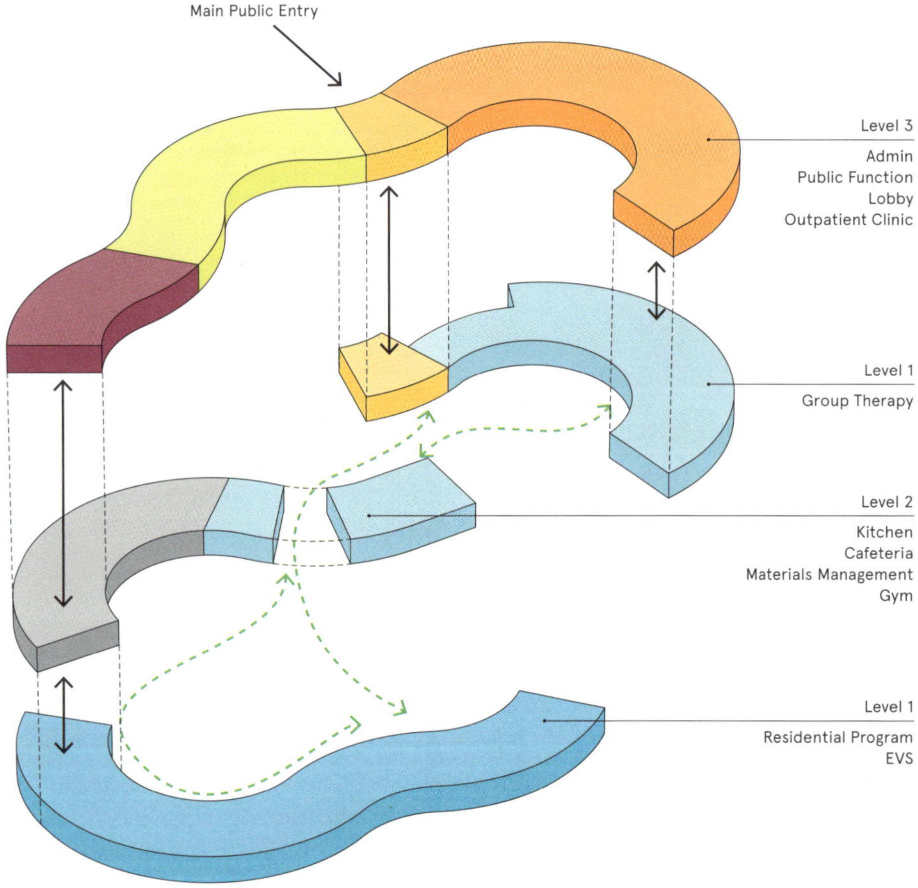

The project's garden-like environment is designed to reduce staff burnout.

The building's form creates an inward and outward sense of openness and comfort, reflecting the idea of 'Ohana'.

Floor plans of all three levels.

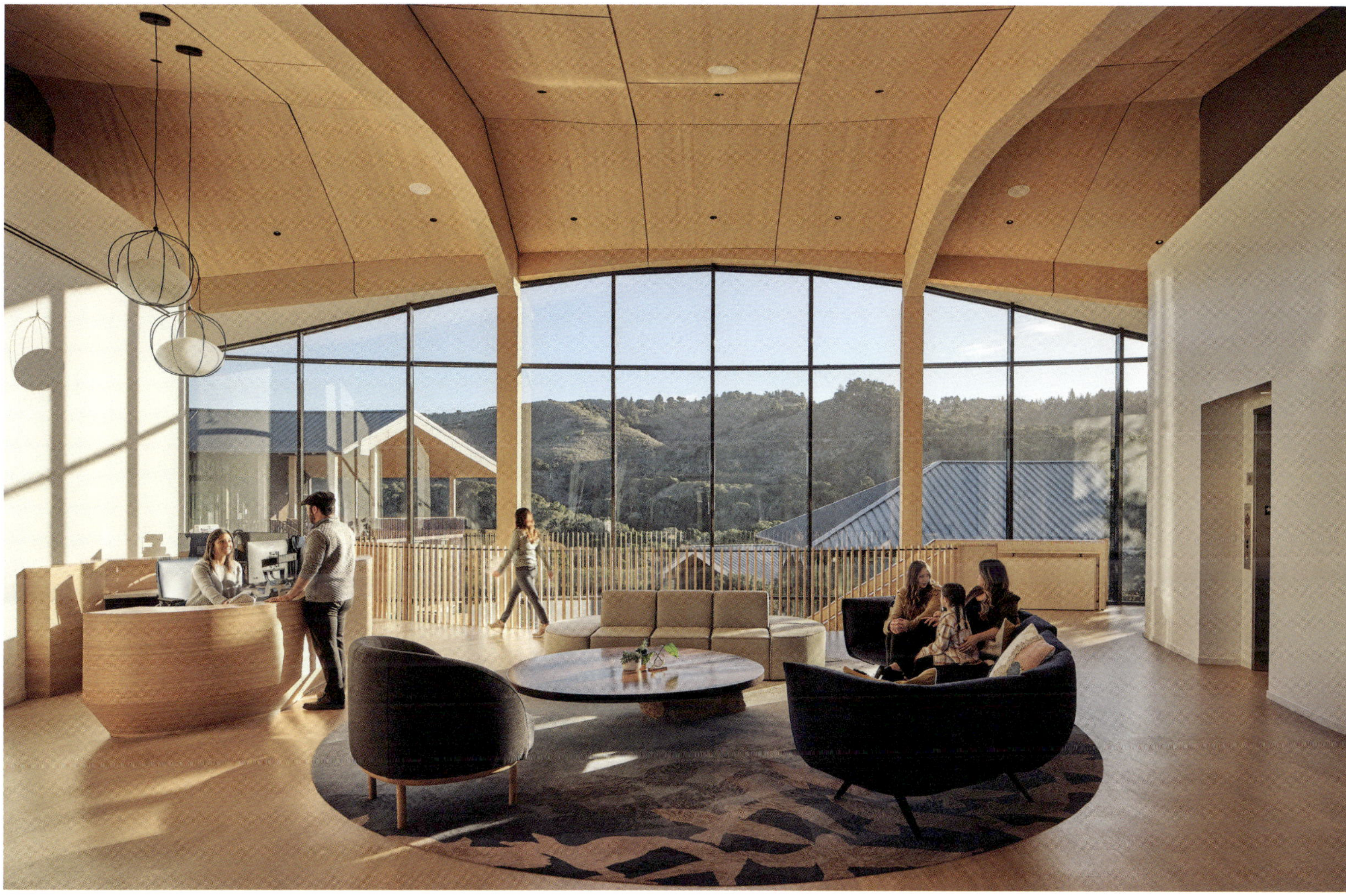

Mass timber construction and a prefabricated modular façade reduce material waste and minimize the building's on-site impact.

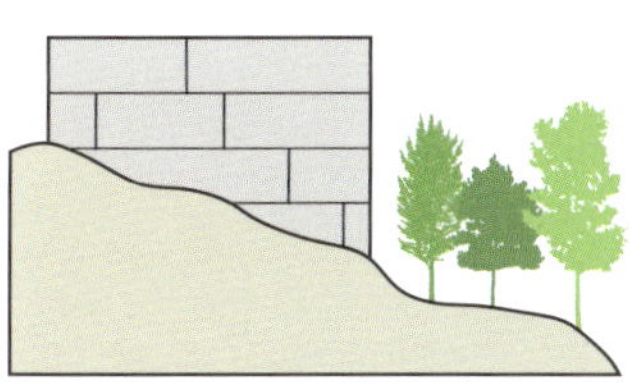

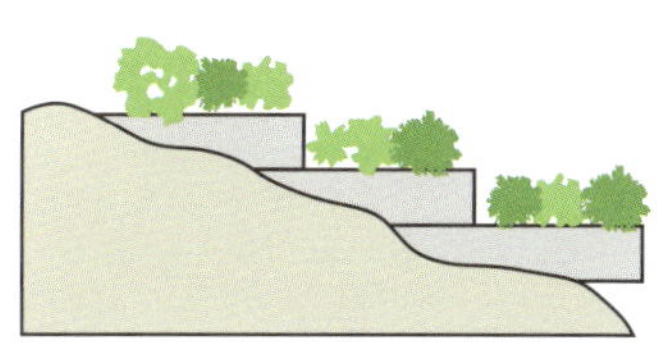

The architectural design integrates natural elements into the spatial concept.

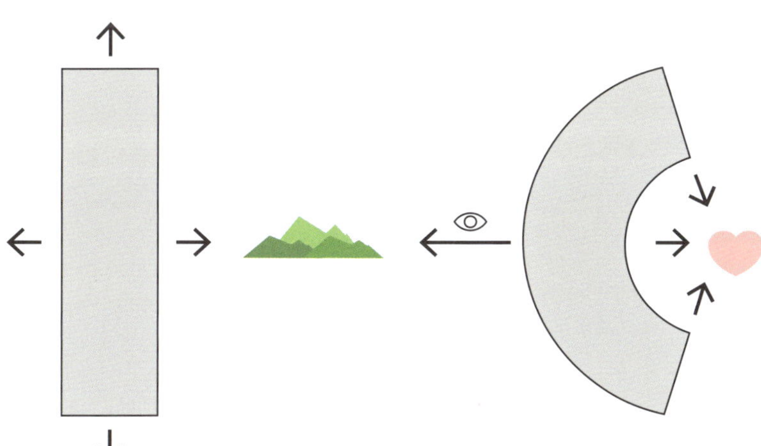

Nickl & Partner with Vamed + WWH and Pocket Hospital Switzerland AG

Worldwide

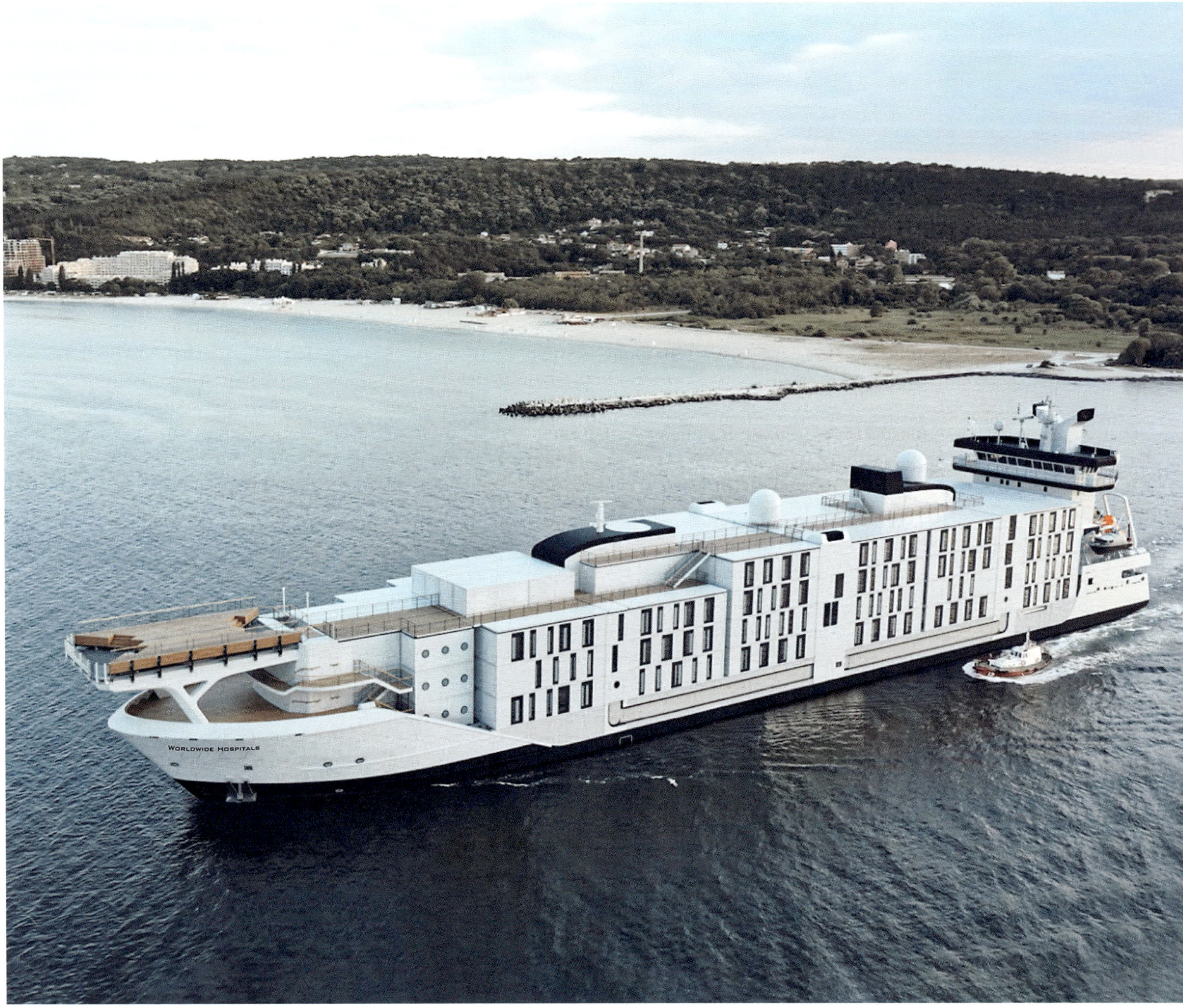

The ships enables fast, flexible, sustainable healthcare service.

Modular hospital units may be assembled on the ship.

Standardized, modular elements can be combined in many ways.

Hospital Ship

The modular hospital ship, designed by Nickl & Partner in collaboration with VAMED + World Wide Hospitals and Pocket Hospital Switzerland AG, marks a significant step forward in the development of global healthcare infrastructure. As a floating acute care hospital, it provides 9,300 m^2 of efficient clinical space across seven levels. Equipped with 111 inpatient beds, including 12 ICU beds, 32 outpatient examination rooms, three operating rooms, and three delivery rooms, it enables flexible, mobile, and high-performance medical care. Supported by around 214 clinical staff members, the ship can treat up to 28,000 outpatient and emergency cases, 1,200 inpatient admissions, and around 700 surgical procedures per month. Combining a maritime platform with prefabricated hospital modules, it represents a scalable and adaptive model for healthcare delivery in crisis regions and underserved areas.

Address: on the seven seas | **Client:** Sunshine X GmbH | **Completion:** 2025 | **Size:** 10,285 m² | **Sector:** non-profit / humanitarian organization | **Number of treatment rooms:** 35 | **Number of beds:** 111

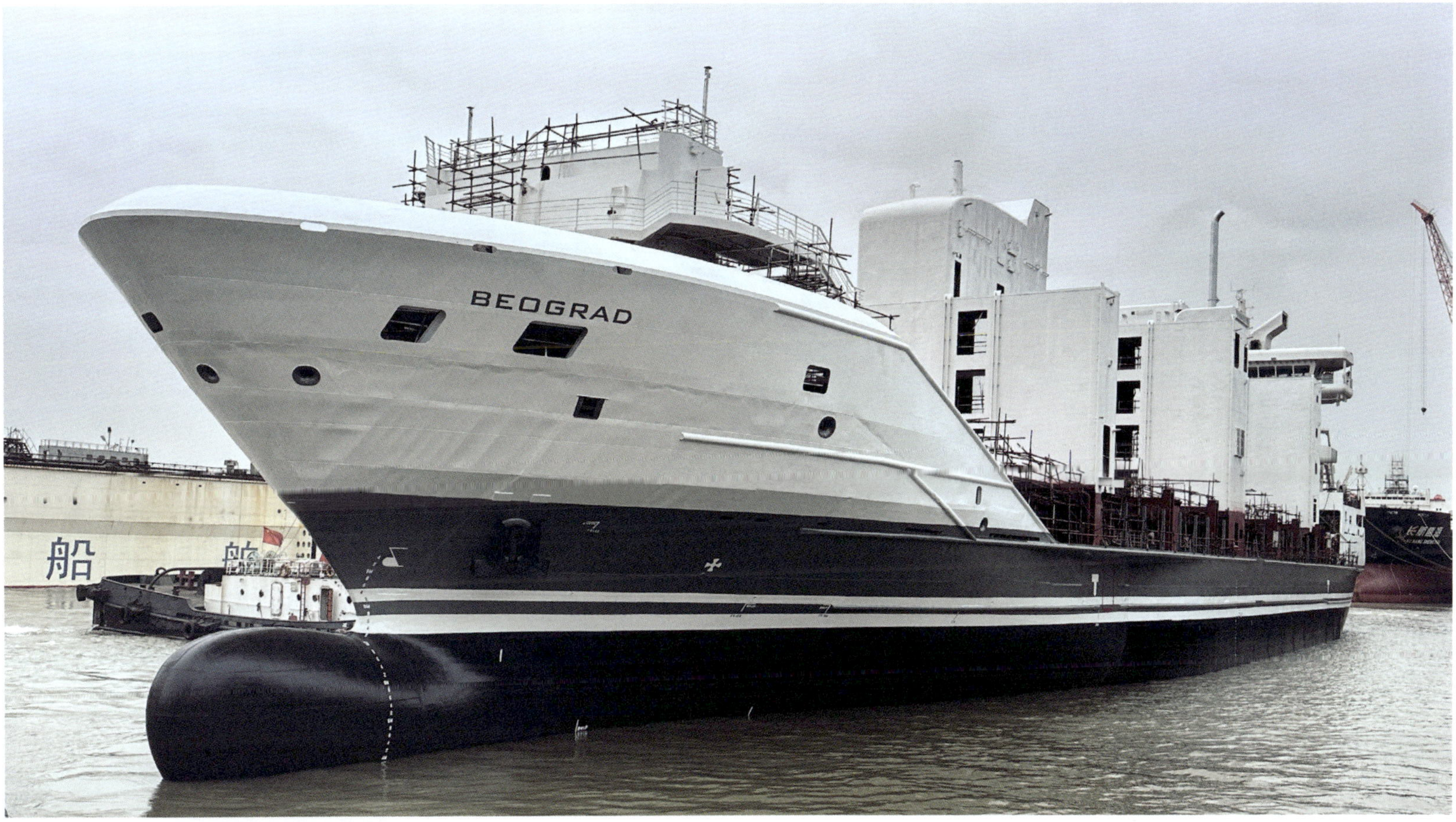

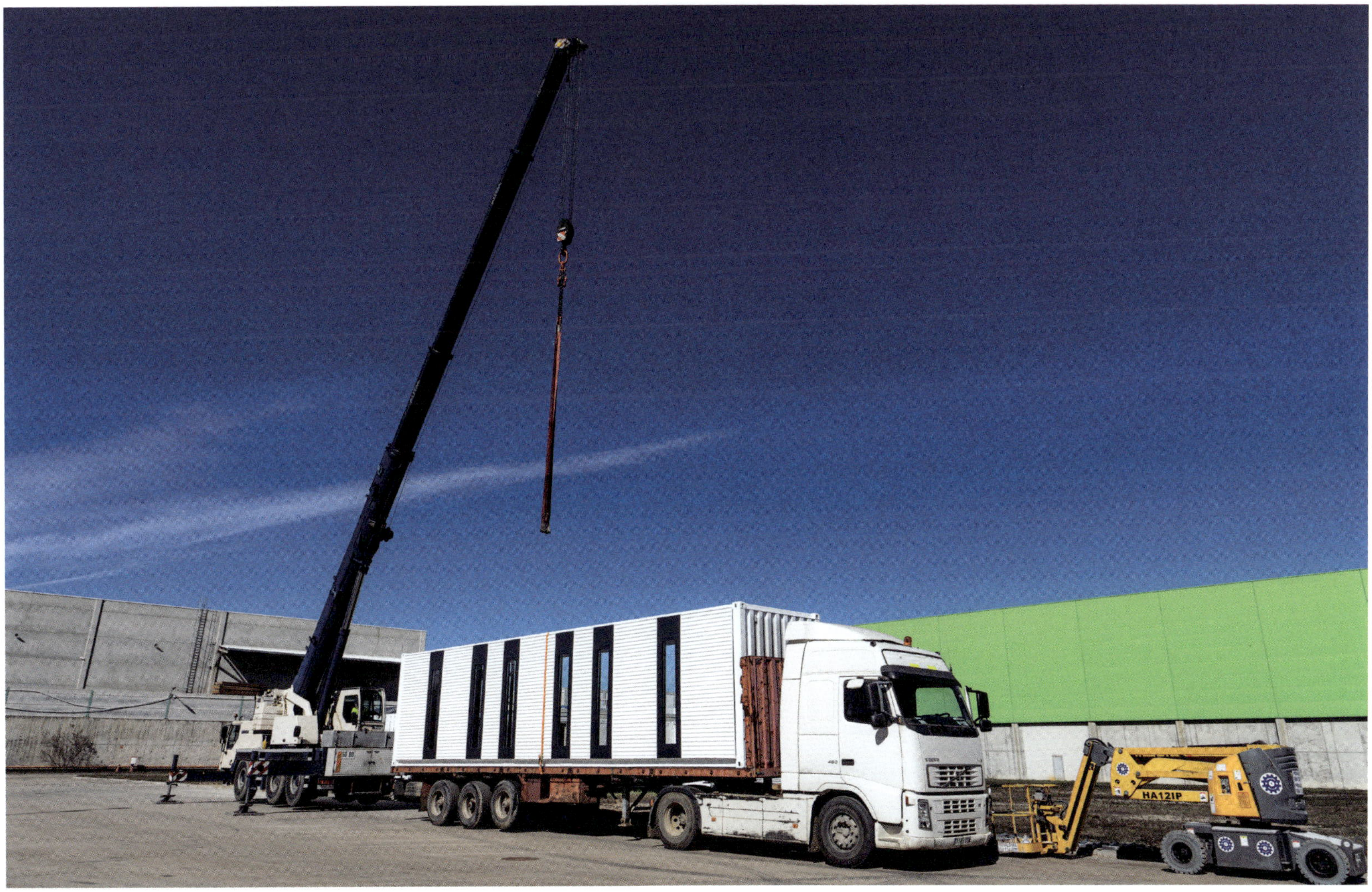

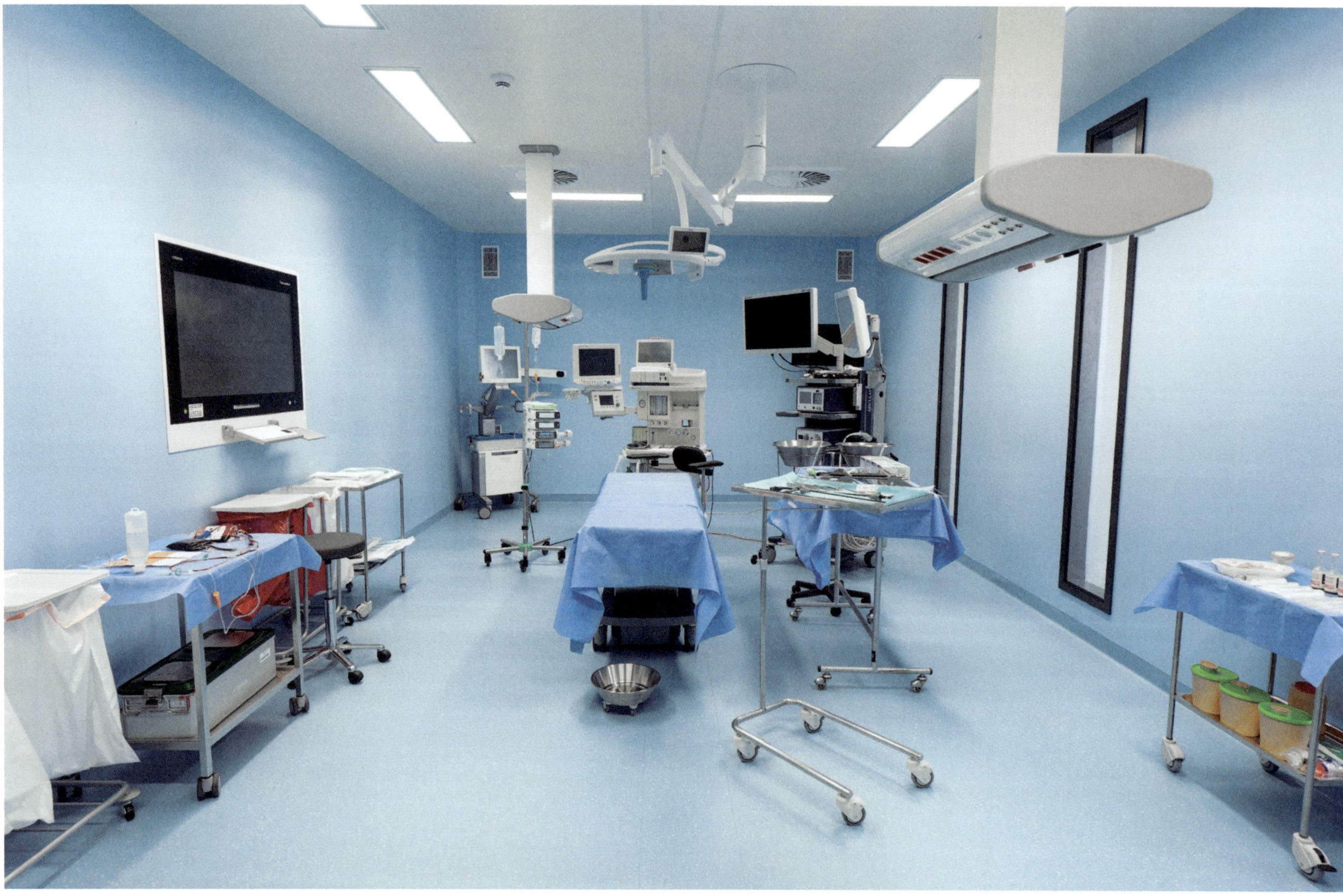

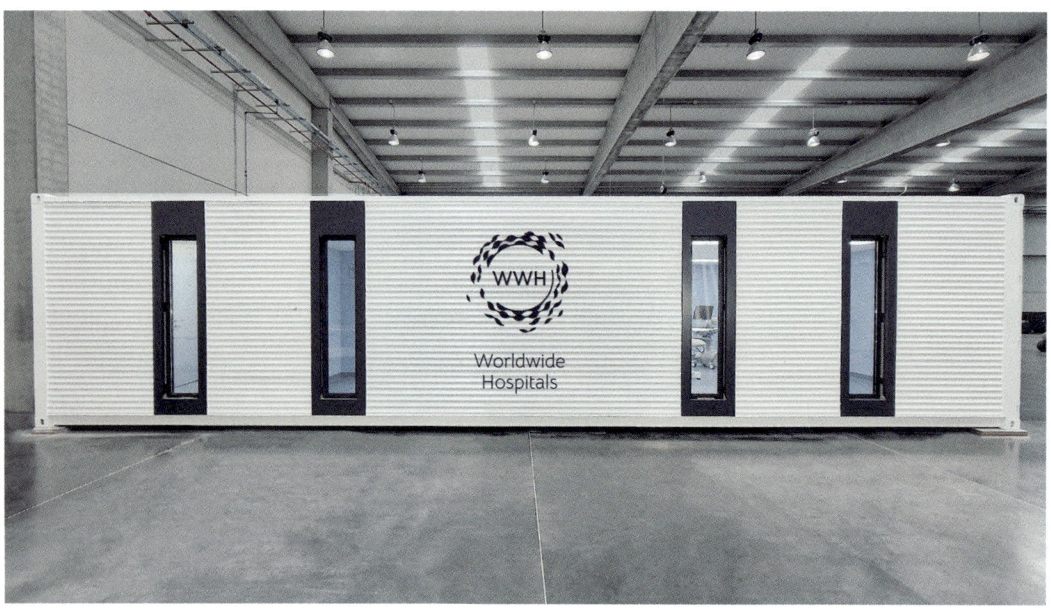

Standard facilities include two operating rooms, an ICU, an emergency room with CT and X-ray, and a full obstetrics unit with a C-section OR.

The construction is based on standardized, prefabricated modules.

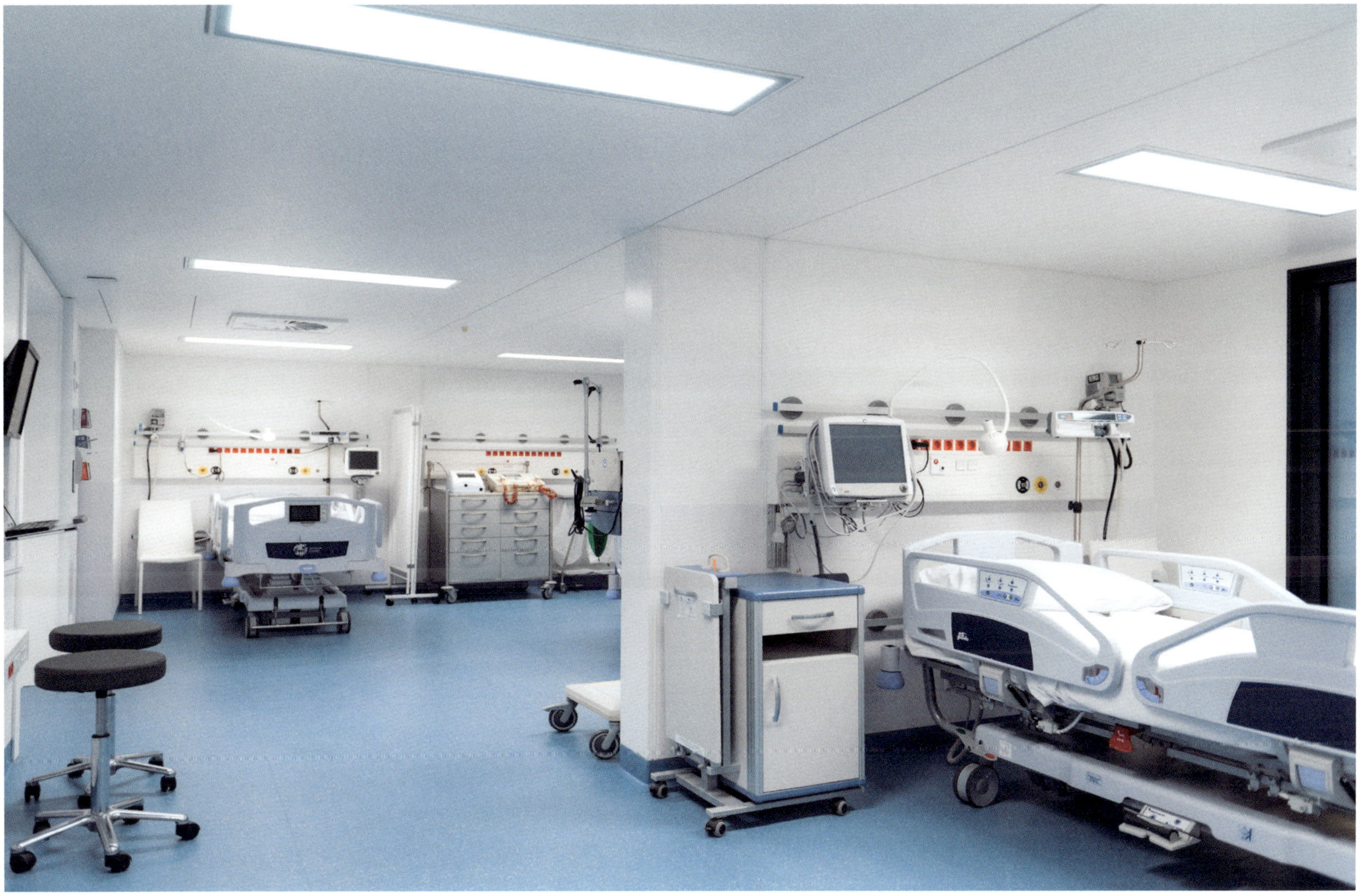

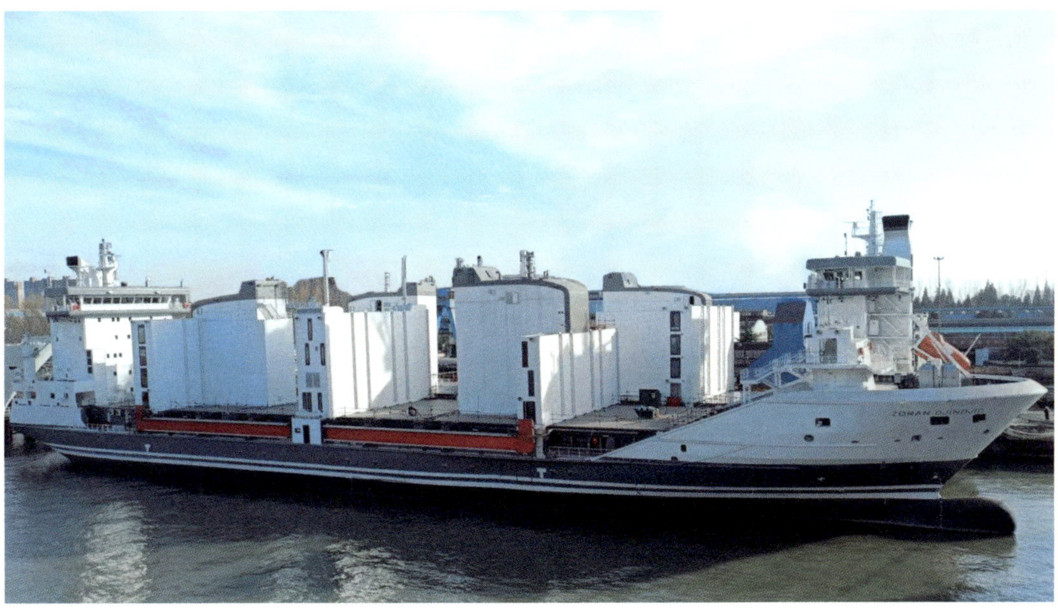

The 11 inpatients beds include 12 ICU beds.

The 129.6 meter-long and 20.6 meter-wide ship offers 9,300 square meters of efficient clinical space across seven levels.

Level 2 floor plan.

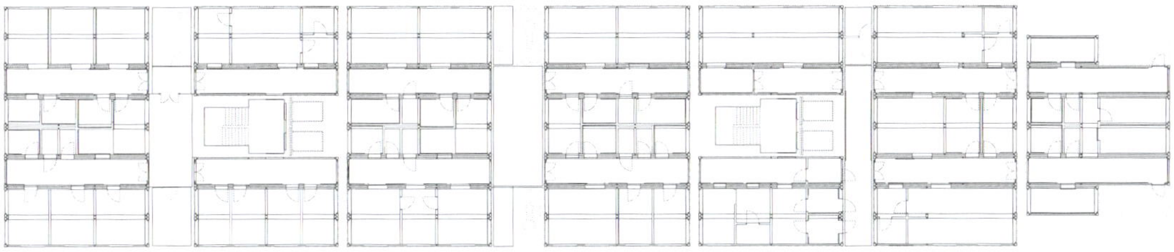

wörner traxler richter

Karlsruhe
Germany

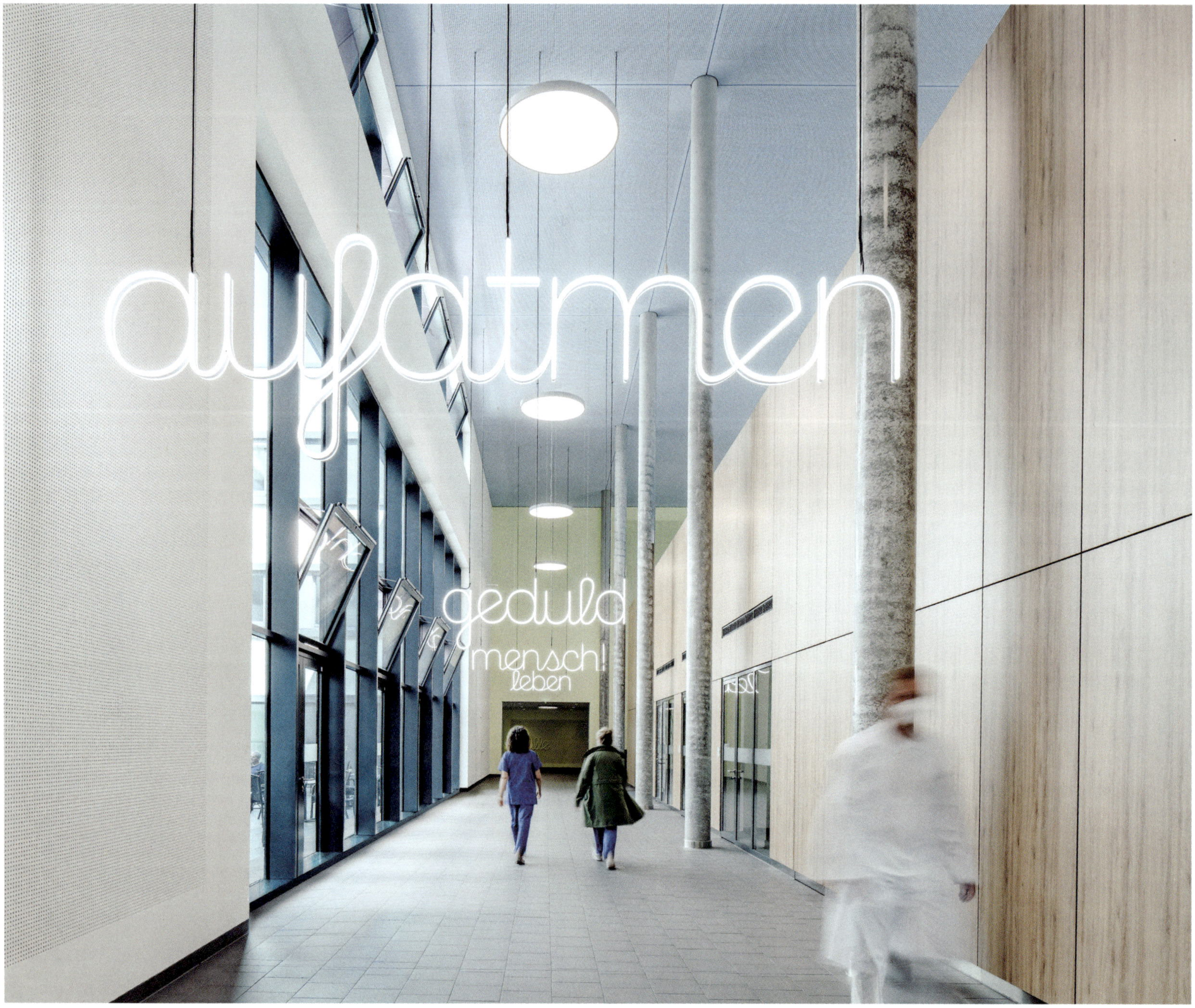

View of the entrance hall with illuminated lettering.

Operating room.

Sign indicating St. John's wort, a medicinal plant that helps with depression.

Karlsruhe Municipal Hospital – House M

The new bed and functional building's urban development axes were guided by the existing Karlsruhe Municipal Hospital complex, parts of which are listed as historic monuments. It was build by Wilhelm Strieder at the end of the 19th. century. The urban character was preserved in its openness: varying heights, proportions, and materials were harmonized, and the reddish hue of the sandstone from the historic hospital buildings was incorporated into the façade of the new structure. The hospital's new center gained a central focal point in its entrance hall. All who arrive here are welcomed with luminous words: terms related to work and the hospital stay evoke emotions and seek to acknowledge fears and concerns. The graphics, color scheme, and signage were developed in collaboration with communication designer Andreas Uebele, artist Harald F. Müller, and philosopher Hannes Böhringer.

Address: Moltkestraße 90, 76133 Karlsruhe, Germany | **Client:** Städtisches Klinikum Karlsruhe | **Completion:** 2021 | **Size:** 48,000 m² | **Original building:** Wilhelm Strieder, 19th century | **Sector:** public | **Signage:** büro uebele visuelle kommunikation

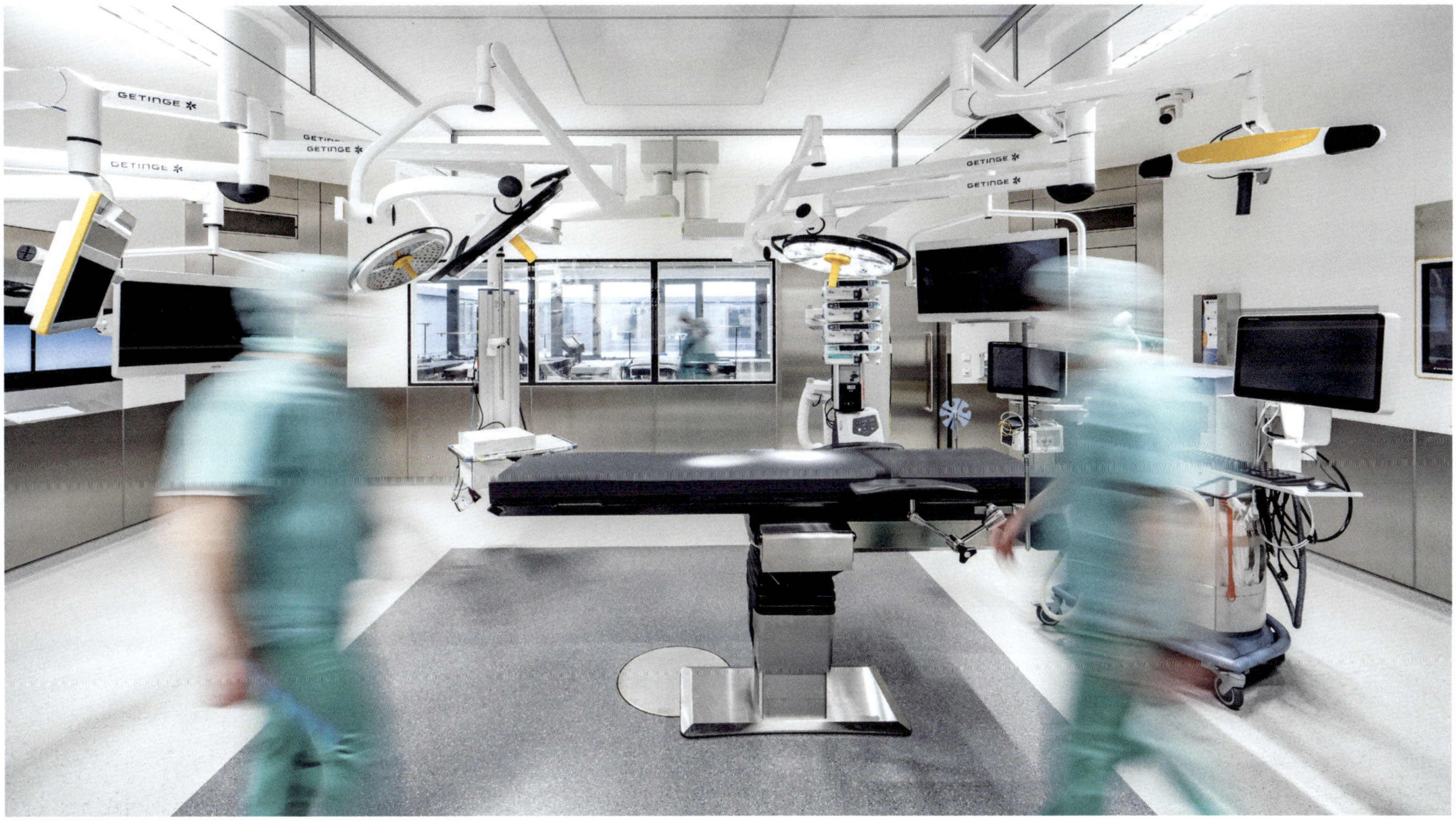

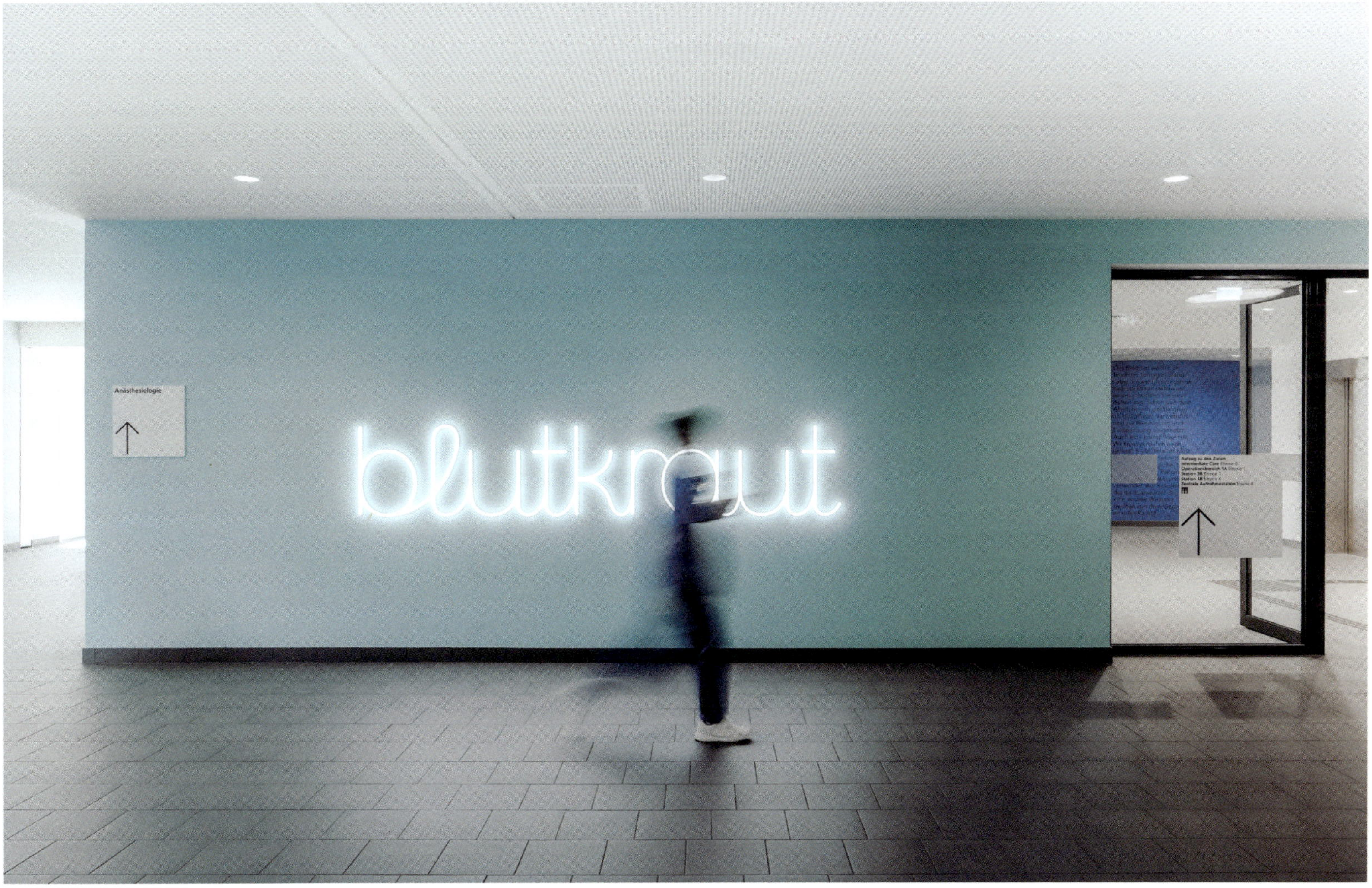

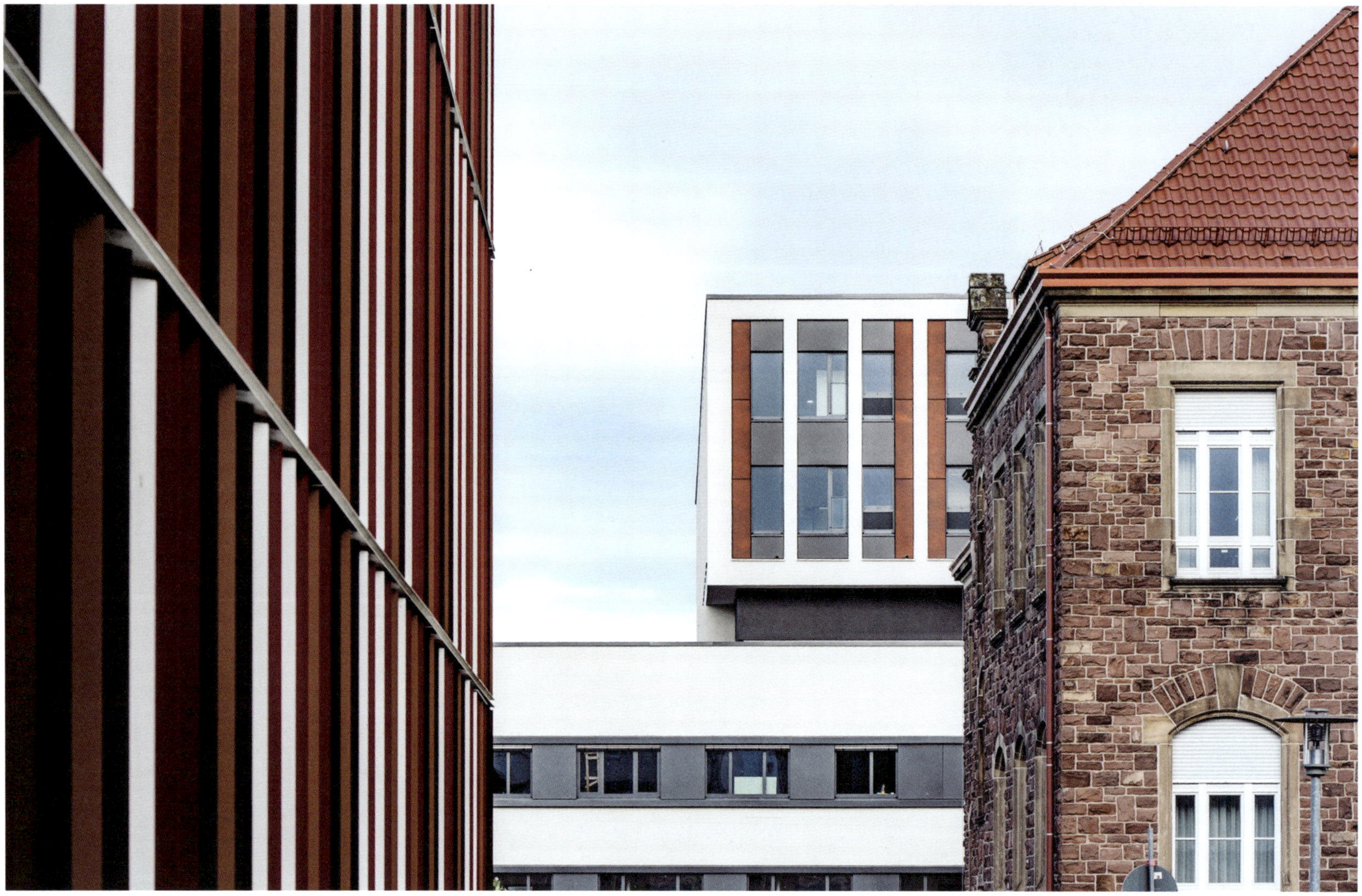

Exterior view in the context of the surrounding buildings.

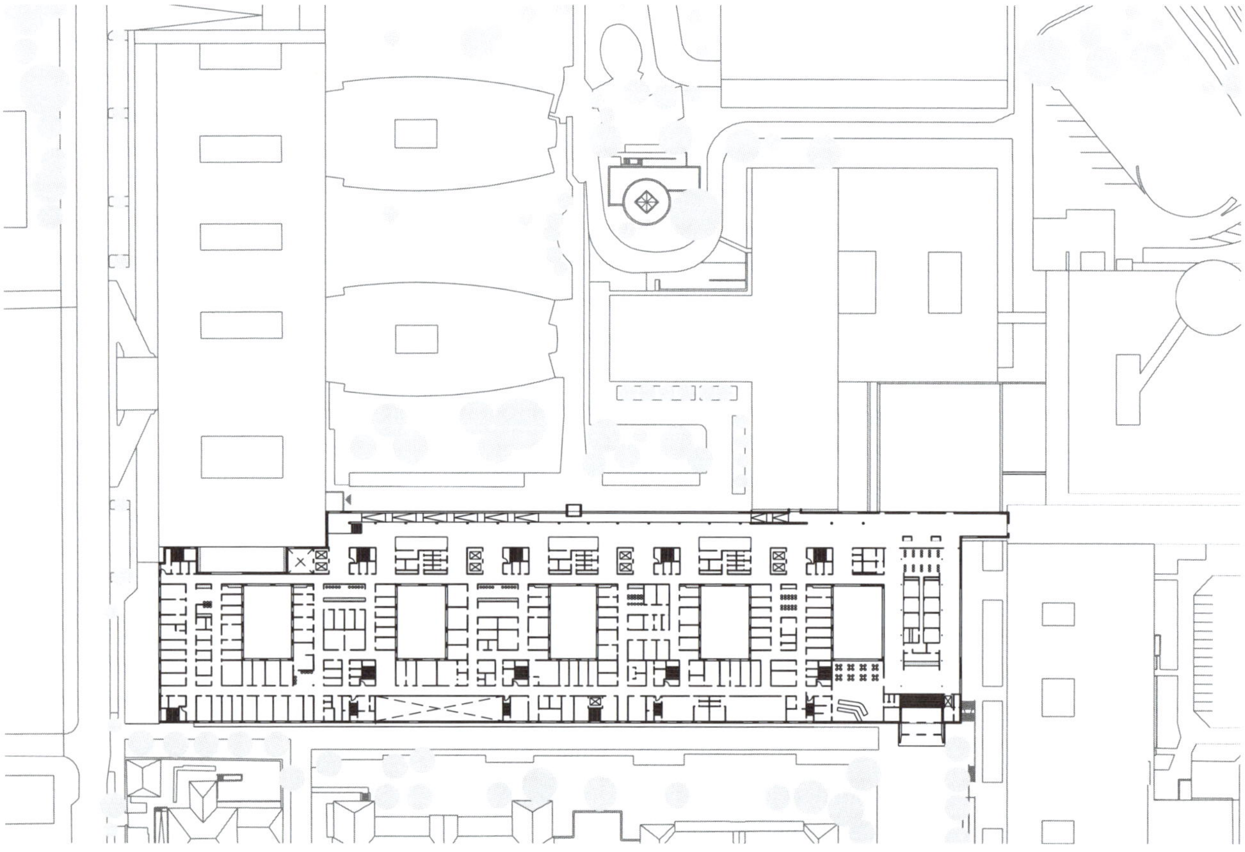

Site plan.

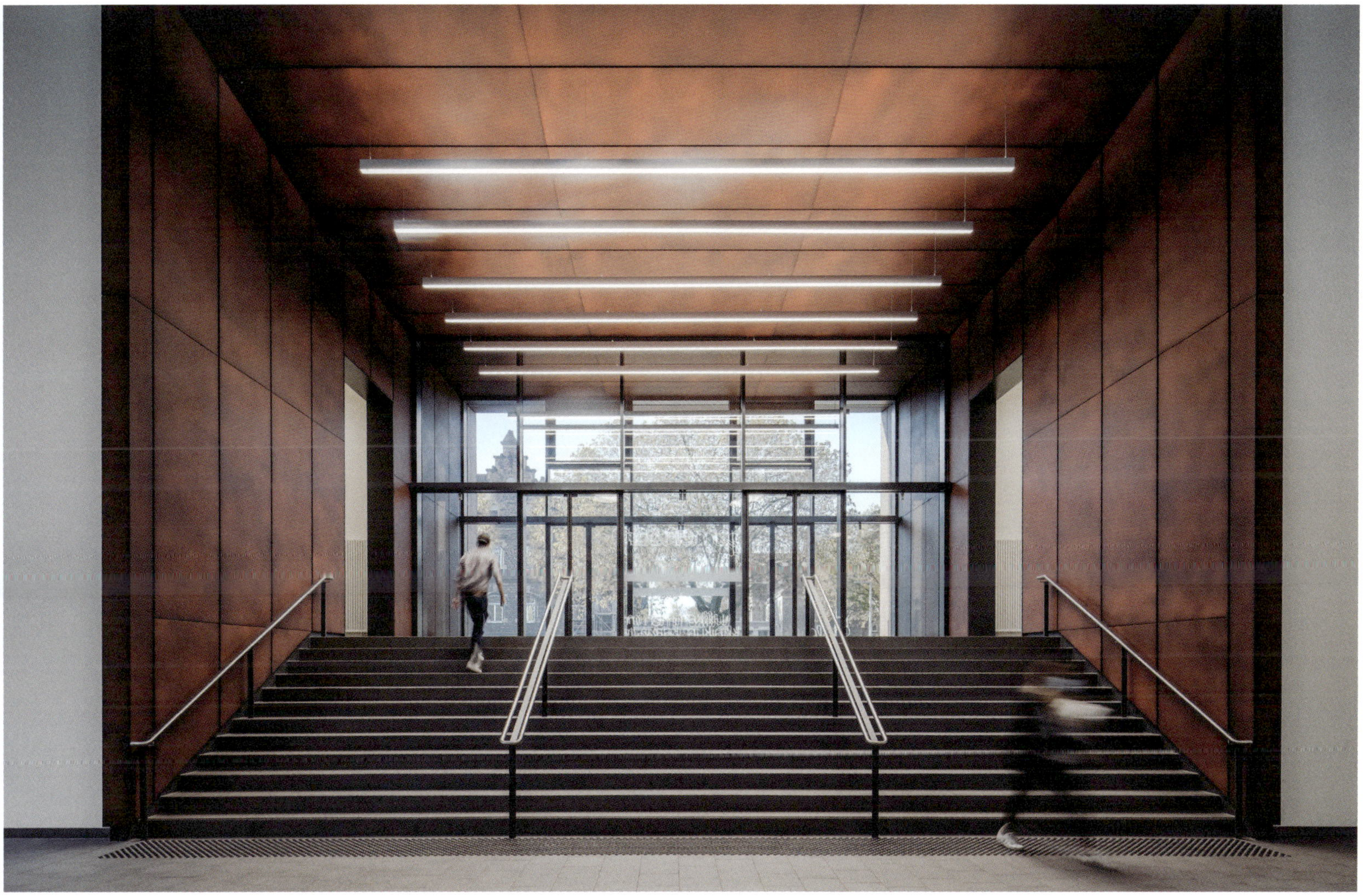

Entrance portal.

Floor plan of the nursing wards based on the floating principle.

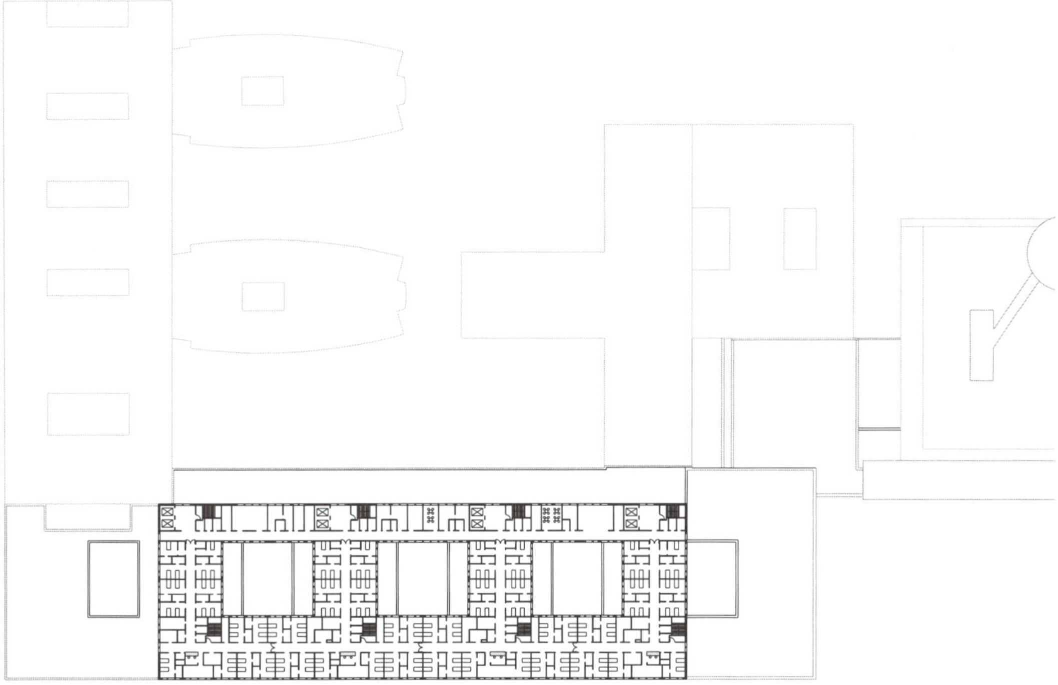

Renzo Piano Building Workshop
Studio TAMassociati

Entebbe
Uganda

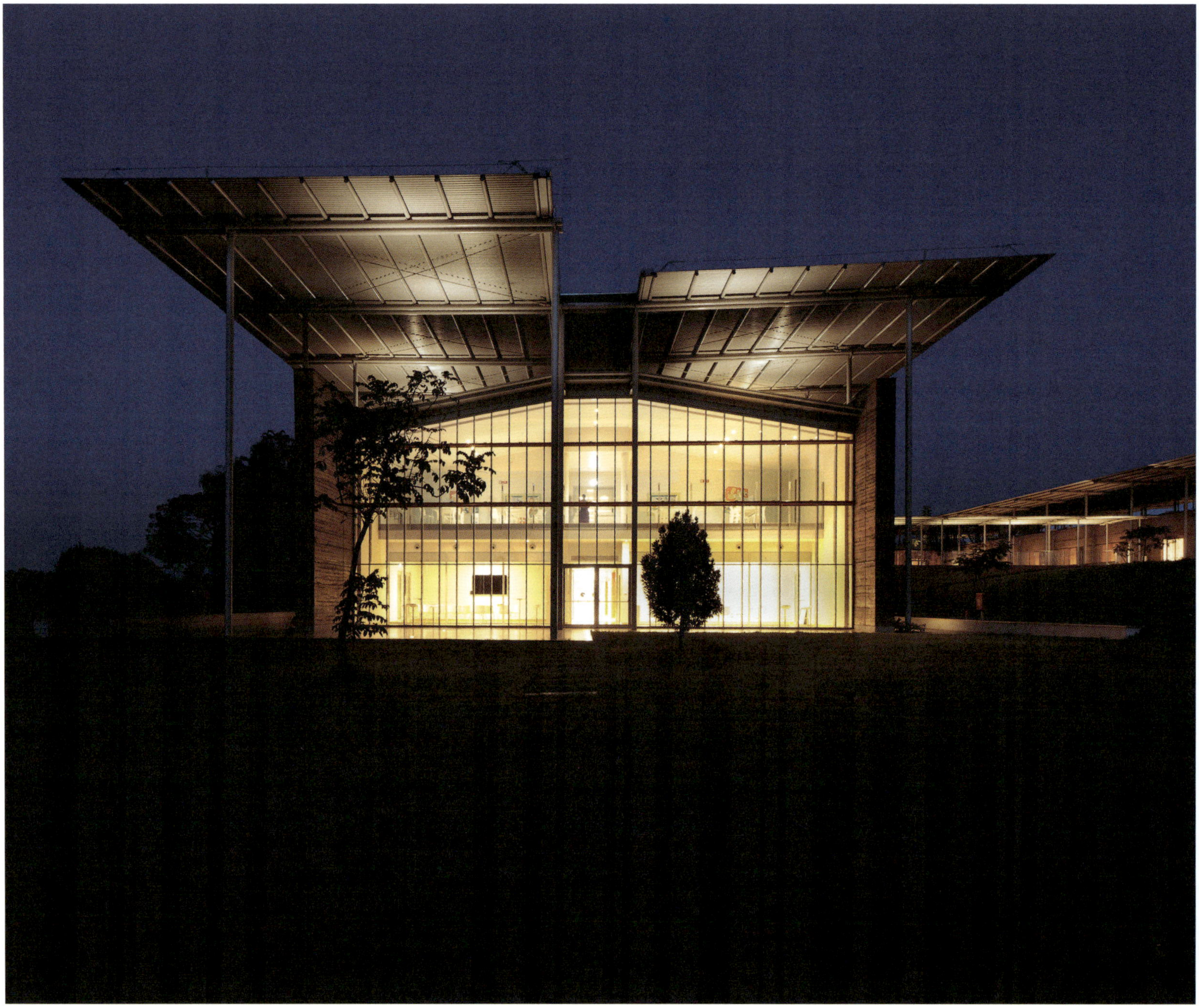

Glazed front view at night.

Façade made of natural materials.

Emergency Children's Surgical Hospital

The hospital combines the practical requirements of a pediatric surgery hospital in Africa with the desire to create a model piece of architecture. The first architectural work in Africa designed by RPBW is a sign of extreme symbolic importance for the promotion of health care in Uganda. By following the course of the land, the building creates a terraced, spatial continuum between interior and exterior, above and below. Raw earth was used as a cheap and simple construction method, which should be given back its original dignity instead of being perceived as a material for the poor. The roof is made from a suspended canopy structure supporting 3,600 square meters of photovoltaic panels. This system will ensure that the hospital has an autonomous electricity supply during the day. The photovoltaic roof floating above the building will also guarantee shade for the hospital and all the uncovered walkways.

Address: Nsubuga Road, 120-122 Bishop Dunstan, Entebbe, Uganda | **Client:** Emergency NGO Onlus | **Completion:** 2021 | **Size:** 9,695 m² | **Sector:** other | **Specialization:** children surgery | **Number of treatment rooms:** 3 | **Number of patient rooms:** 66

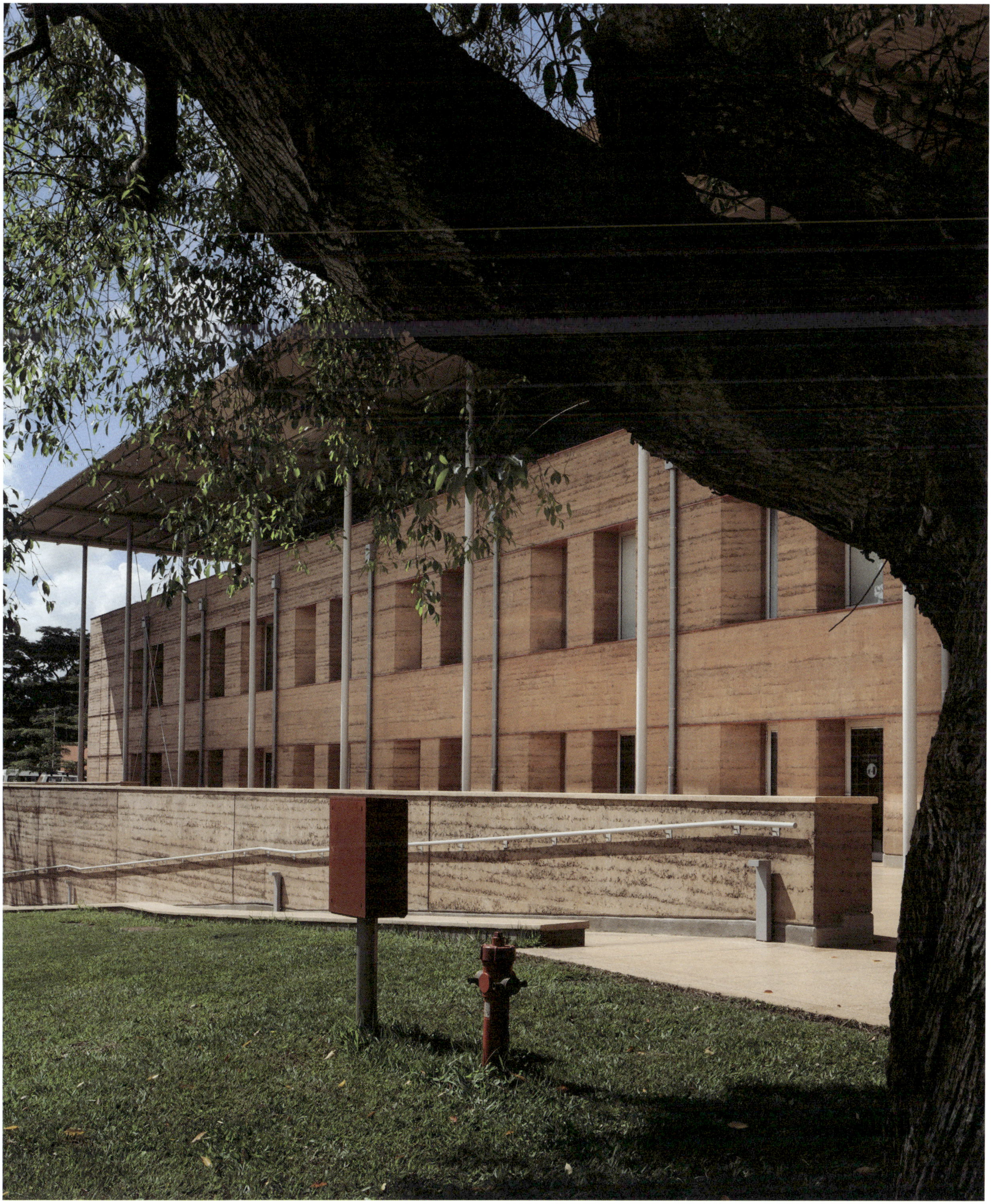

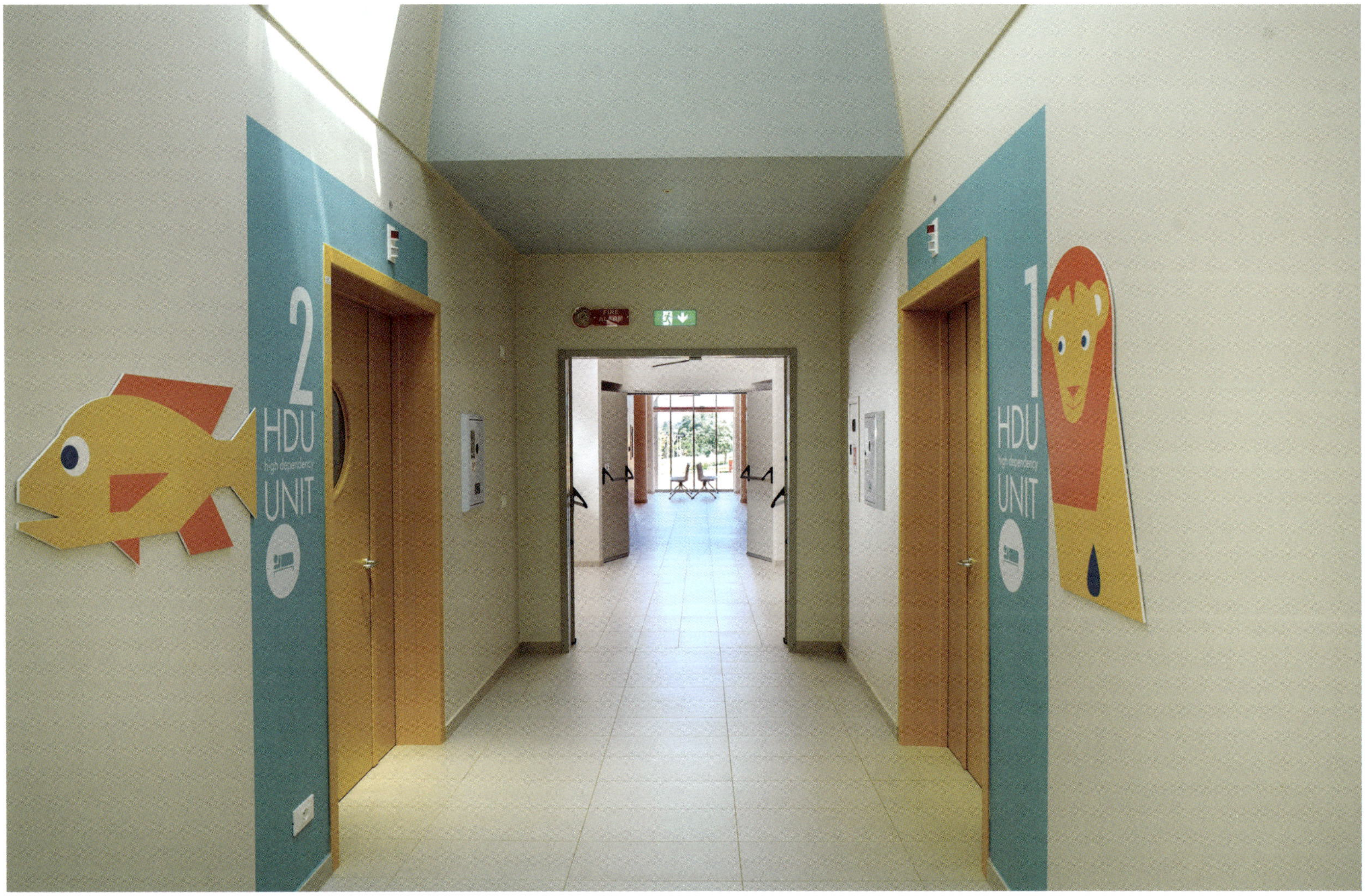

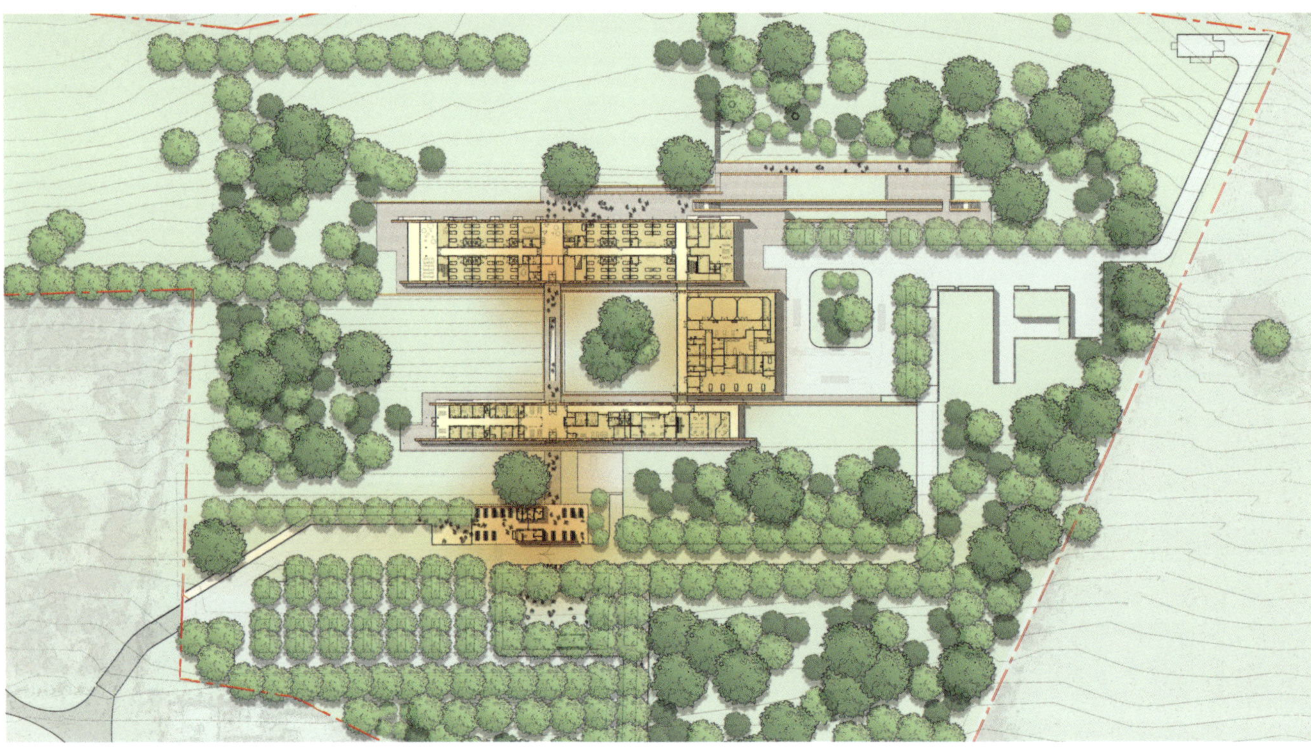

Child-friendly interior design.

Site plan.

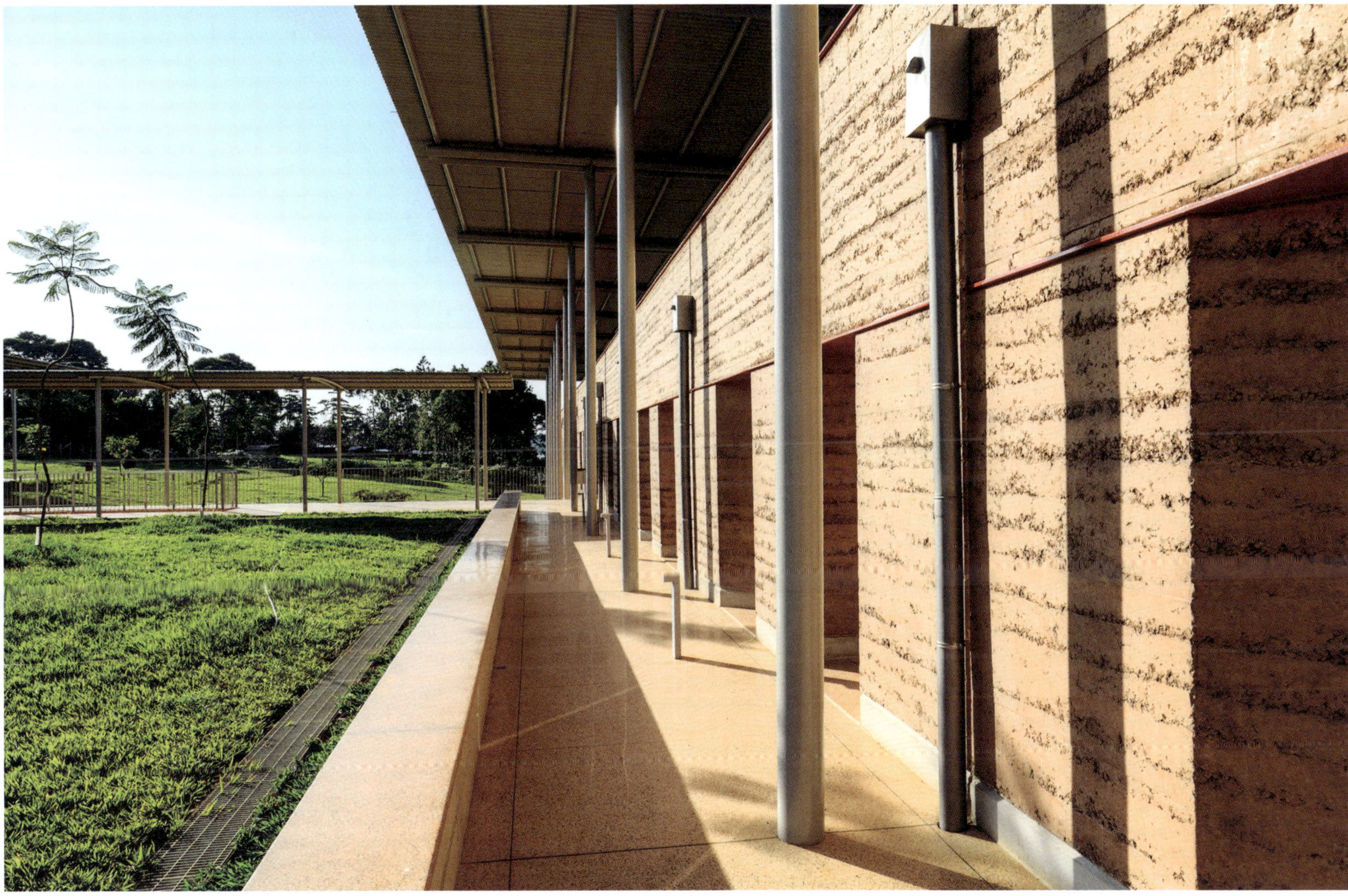

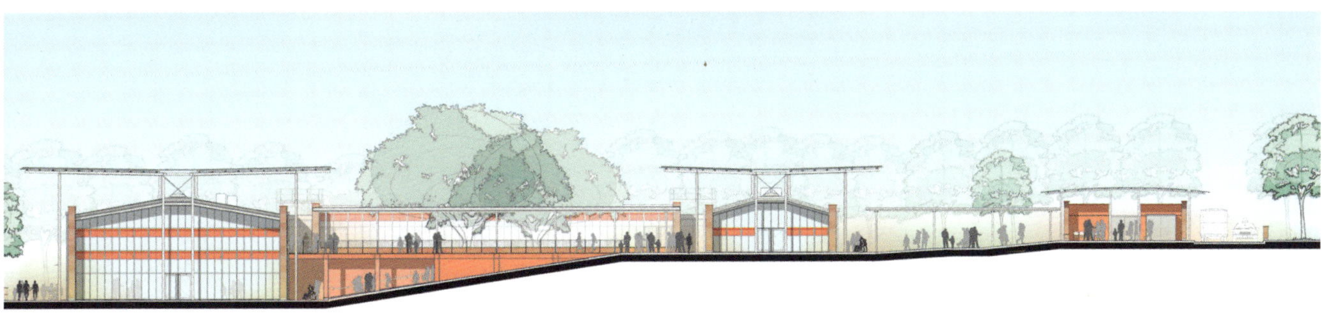

Load-bearing walls made of rammed earth.

Section.

Sketch.

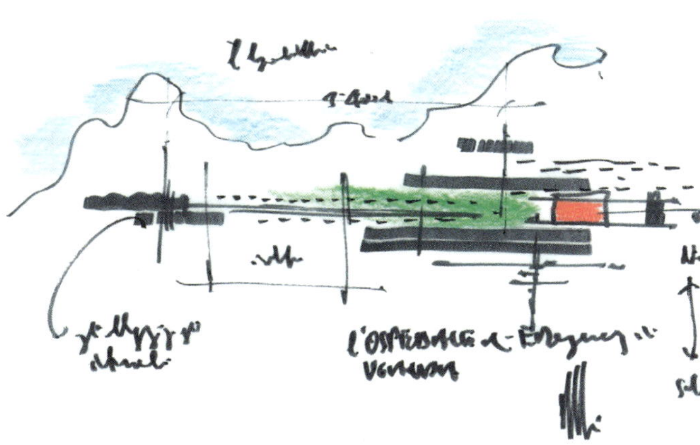

Carlos Martinez Architekten

Zihlschlacht
Switzerland

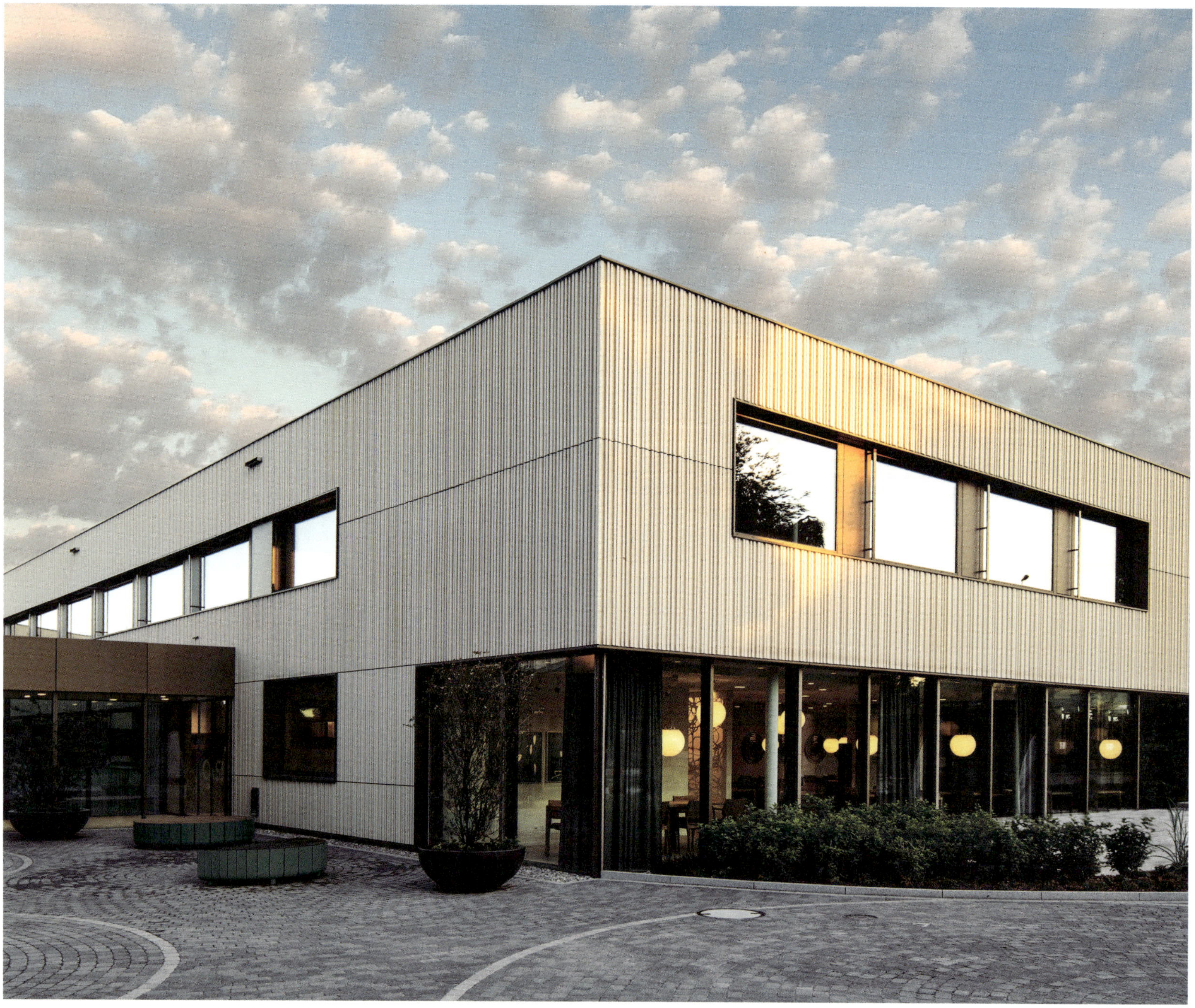

The angled cubature with its white ceramic façade.

The new building of the neurological rehabilitation center.

Patient rooms in the south open up to the Alpstein.

Zihlschlacht Rehabilitation Clinic New Building 2

Conceived as an extension of a neurological rehabilitation center, the clinic combines medical precision with the atmosphere of a high-end hotel. Positioned along the building line, its angled form and white ceramic façade respond to the topography while defining the edge of the hospital complex. The three-story structure connects seamlessly to the existing buildings and is accessed via a passerelle leading to a bright, welcoming lobby. Organized in a ring around a central core, the layout ensures clarity and efficiency. Treatment, administration, and service areas are located to the north, while the south-facing patient rooms open towards the Alpstein mountains. Flexible room layouts allow adjacent units to merge into spacious suites. Artistic interventions inspired by neural networks subtly extend the medical narrative into the architectural language, creating an environment of care, comfort, and identity.

Address: Hauptstrasse 2–4, 8588 Zihlschlacht, Switzerland | **Client:** Helsana Insurance AG | **Completion:** 2022 | **Size:** 3,500 m² | **Sector:** private | **Specialization:** neurological rehabilitation | **Number of treatment rooms:** 9 | **Number of patient rooms:** 28 | **Landscape design:** Plankton Media

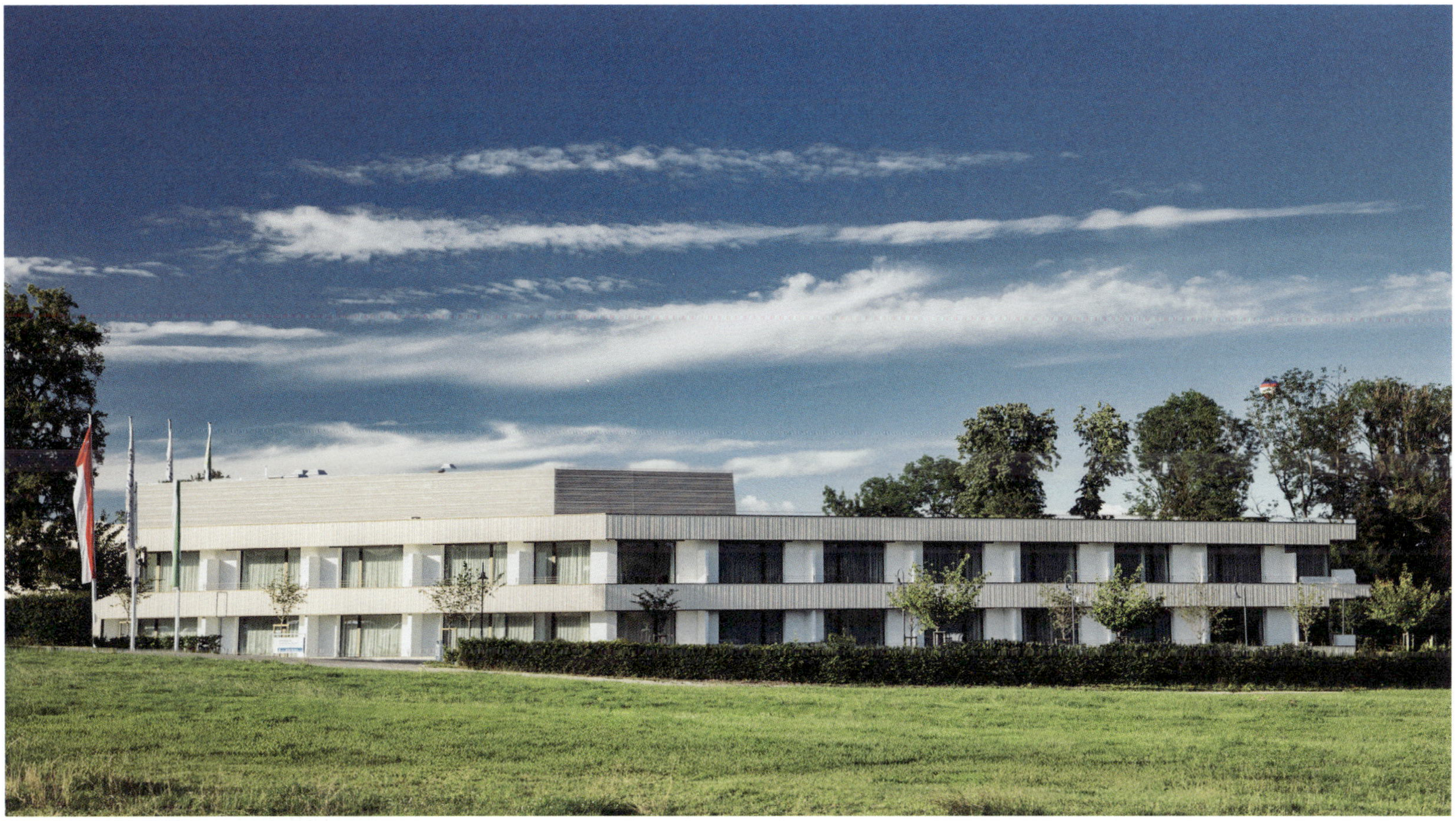

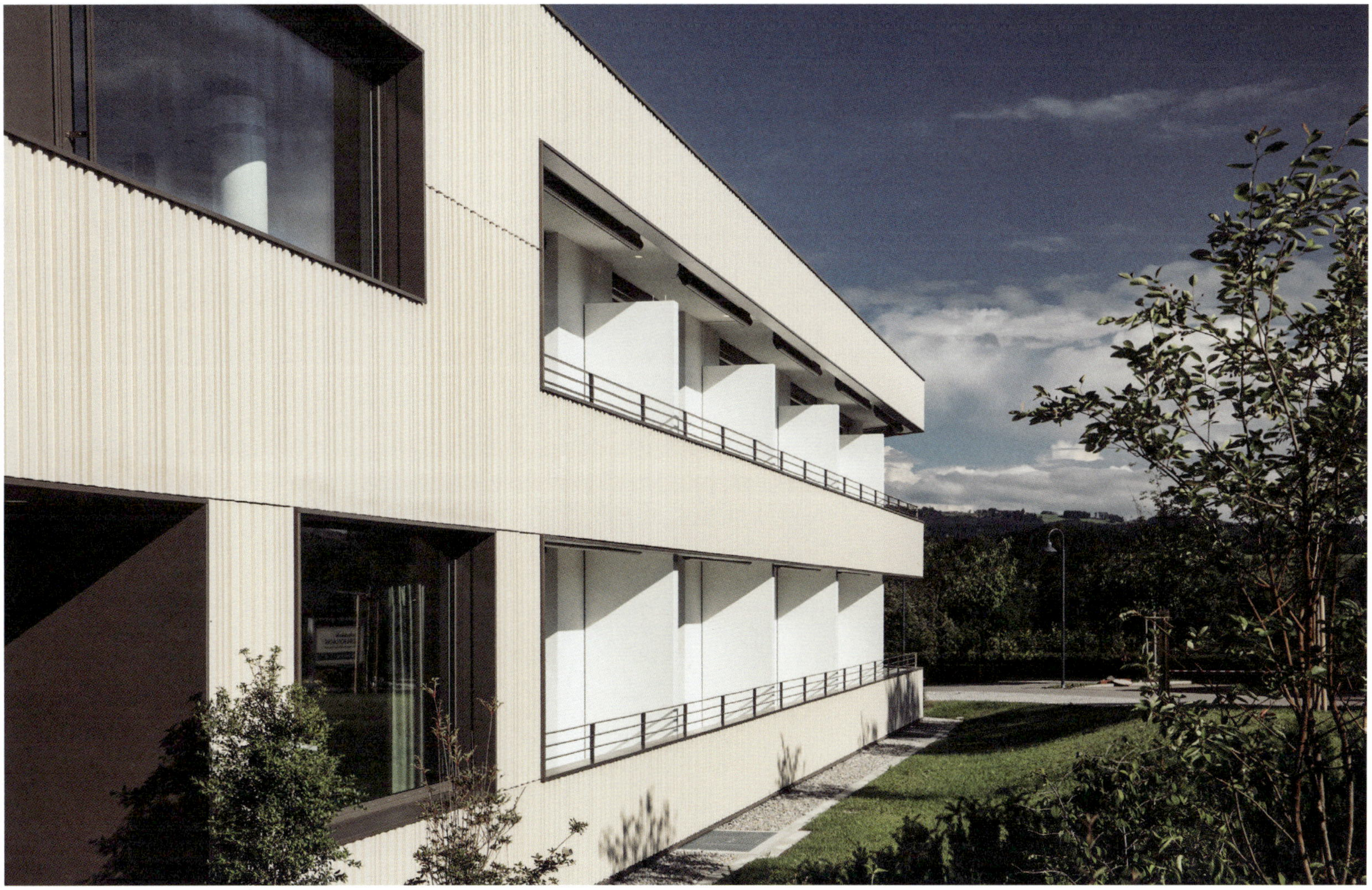

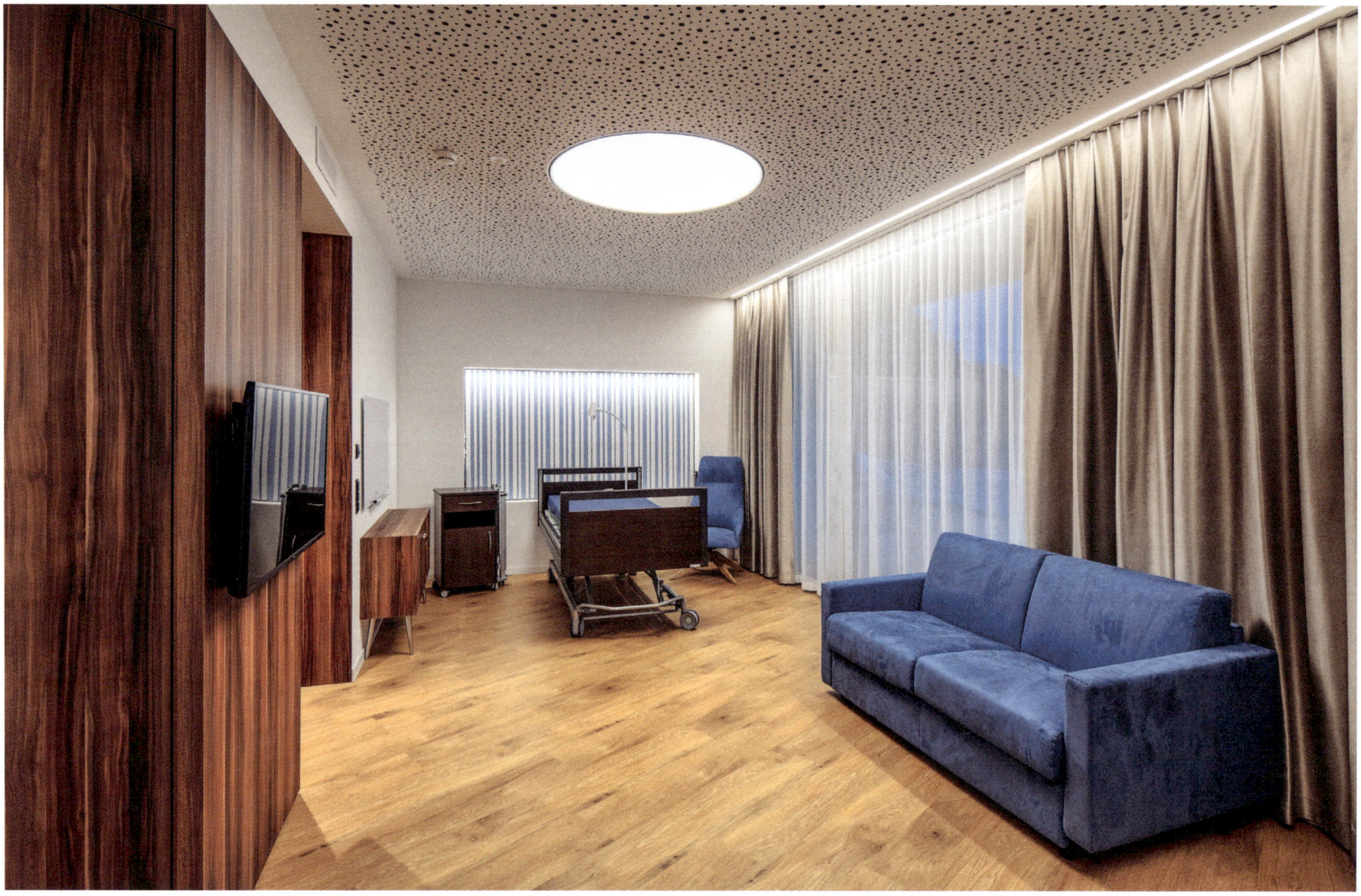

Tastefully designed patient's room.

Floor plan.

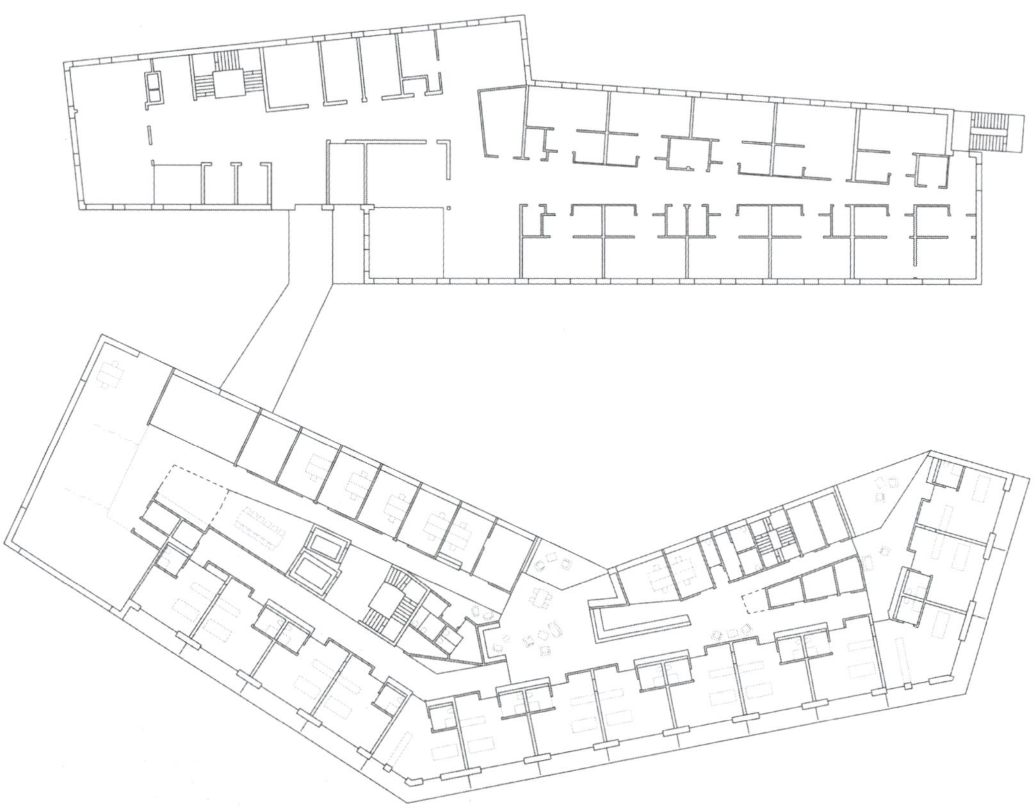

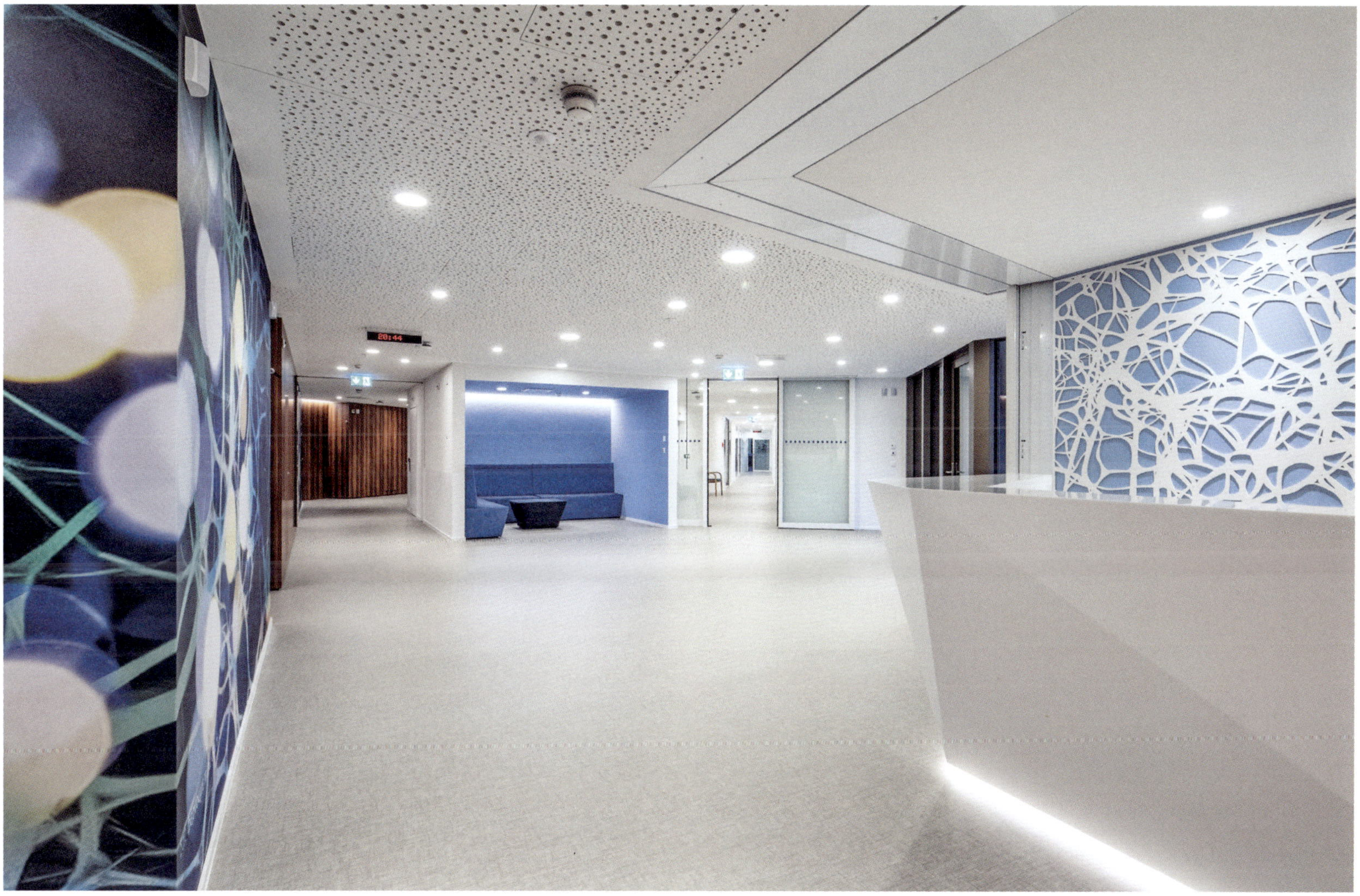

Lobby and reception area.

Site plan.

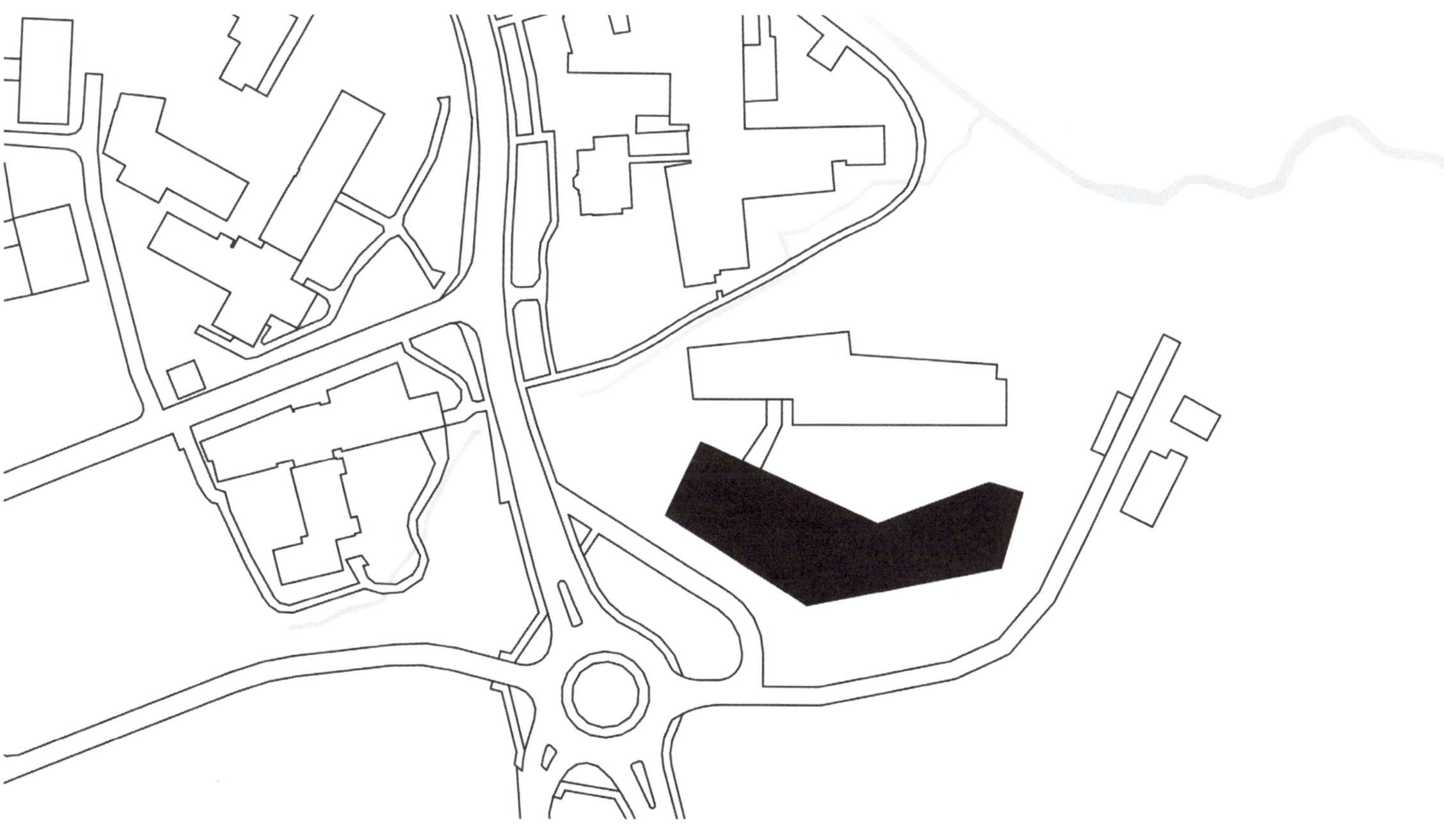

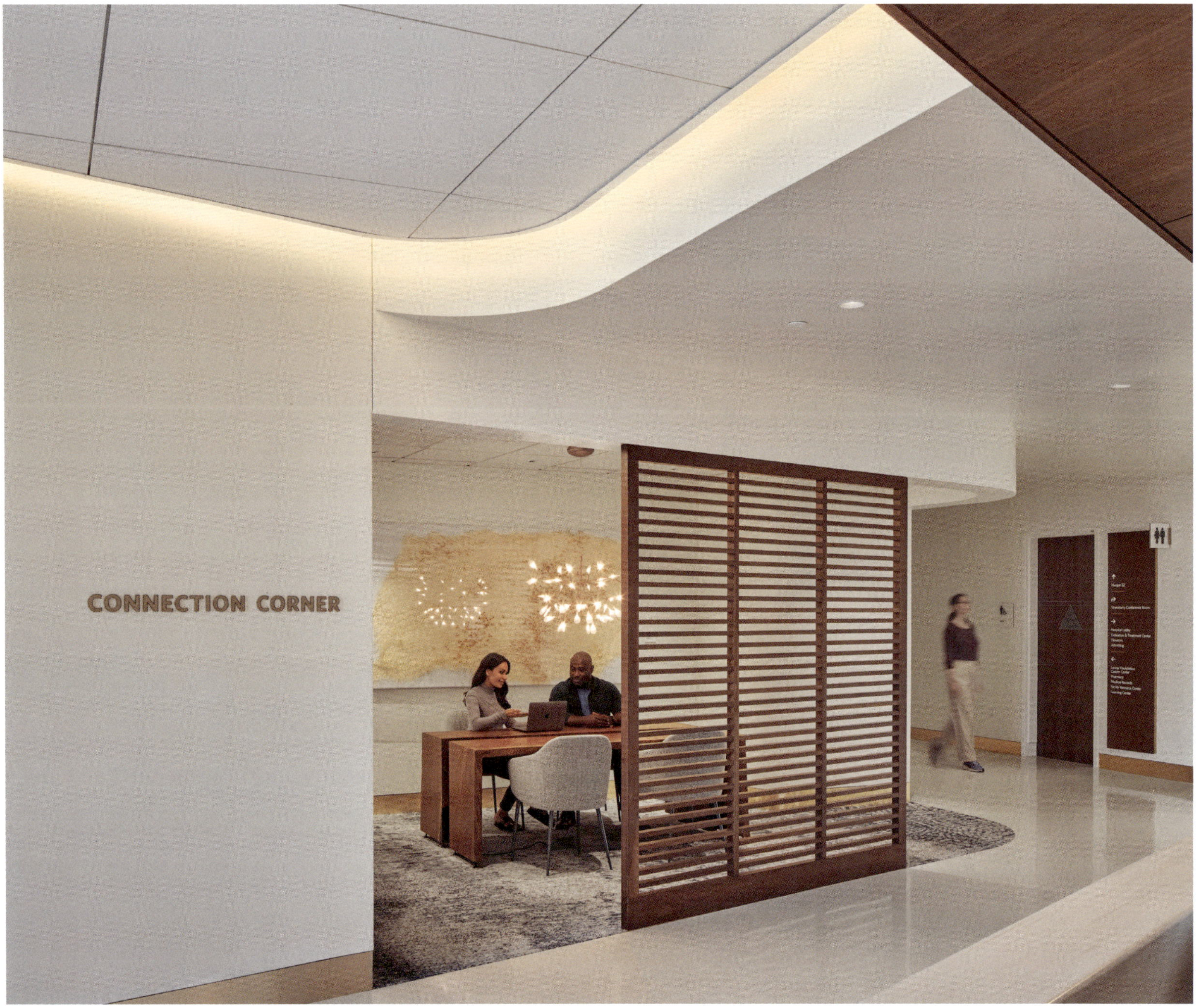

A semi-private workspace supports patients and visitors during extended stays.

The double-height lobby lounge is filled with natural light.

City of Hope Orange County Cancer Specialty Hospital

HOK designed the City of Hope Orange County Cancer Specialty Hospital – the only facility of its kind in the region – on the nearly 30-hectare City of Hope campus in Irvine. The six-story, 73-bed facility connects directly to the adjacent Lennar Foundation Cancer Center, providing a comprehensive range of inpatient and outpatient cancer services on a single campus. Each patient room is private with an en-suite bathroom and a calming color scheme. The hospital's human-centred approach manifests in its use of Feng Shui principles, daylight access in virtually every clinical space, and outdoor terraces at every level. A multi-faith spiritual care center, hospitality lounges on each floor, and a specialized Evaluation and Treatment Center complete a patient experience designed for extended stays. LEED Gold certification is anticipated.

Address: 1000A Fivepoint, Irvine, CA 92618, USA | **Client:** City of Hope | **Completion:** 2025 | **Size:** 16,165 m² | **Sector:** private | **Specialization:** oncology | **Number of treatment rooms:** 6 | **Number of patient rooms:** 73 | **Contractor:** Hensel Phelps | **Medical planning:** HOK's Los Angeles Studio | **Architecture:** HOK's Los Angeles and Chicago Studios | **Interior design:** HOK's San Fransisco and Seattle Studios

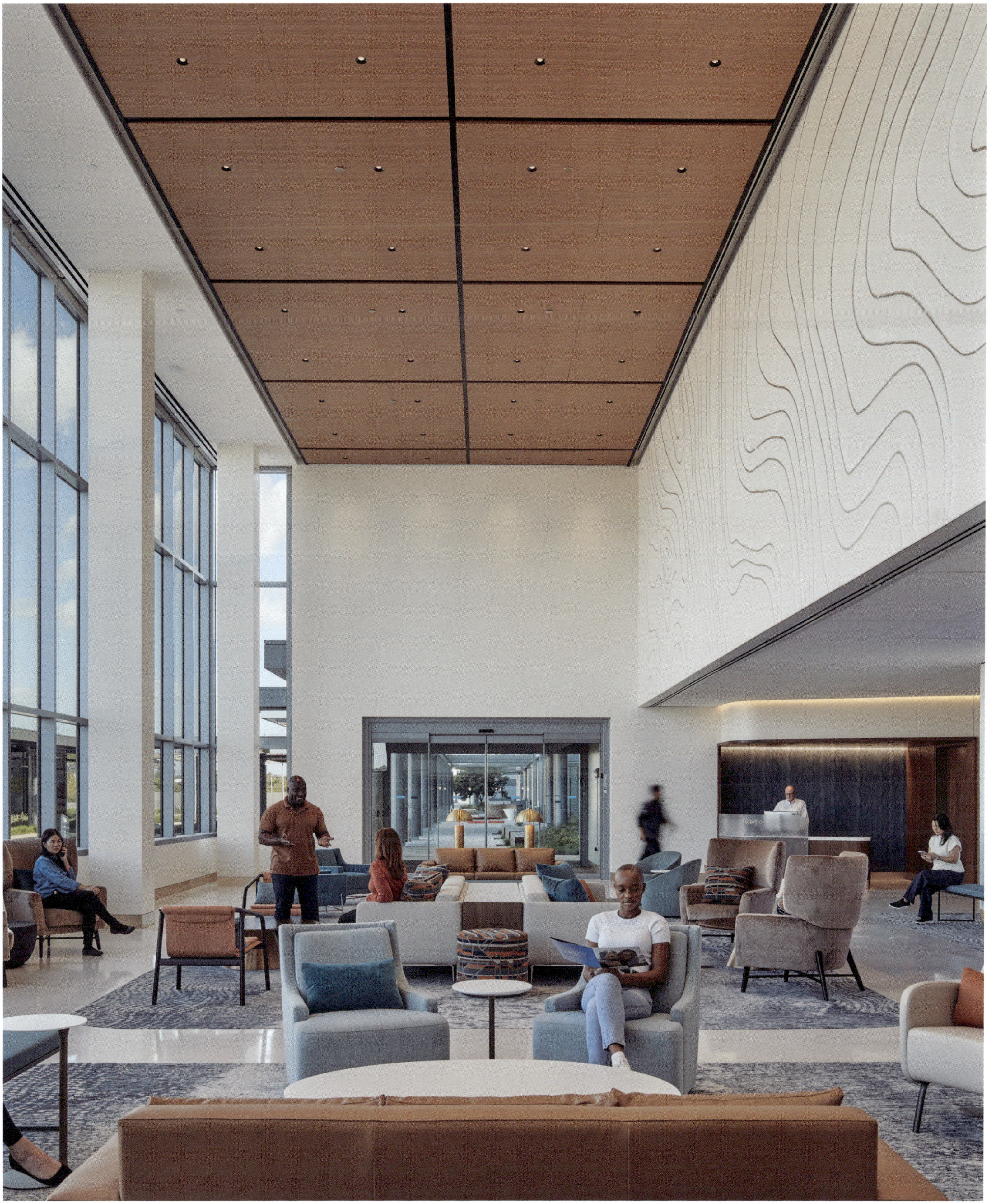

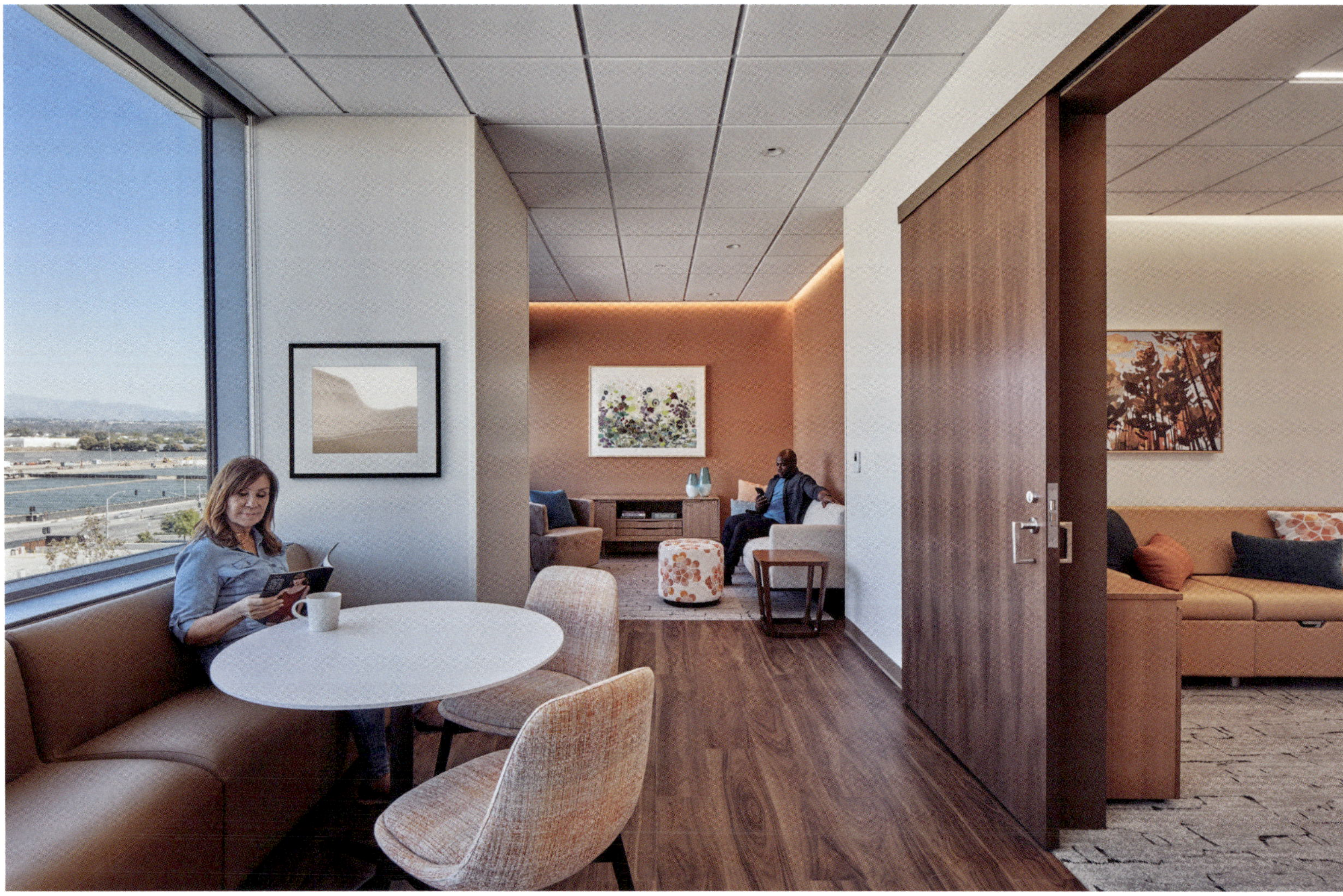

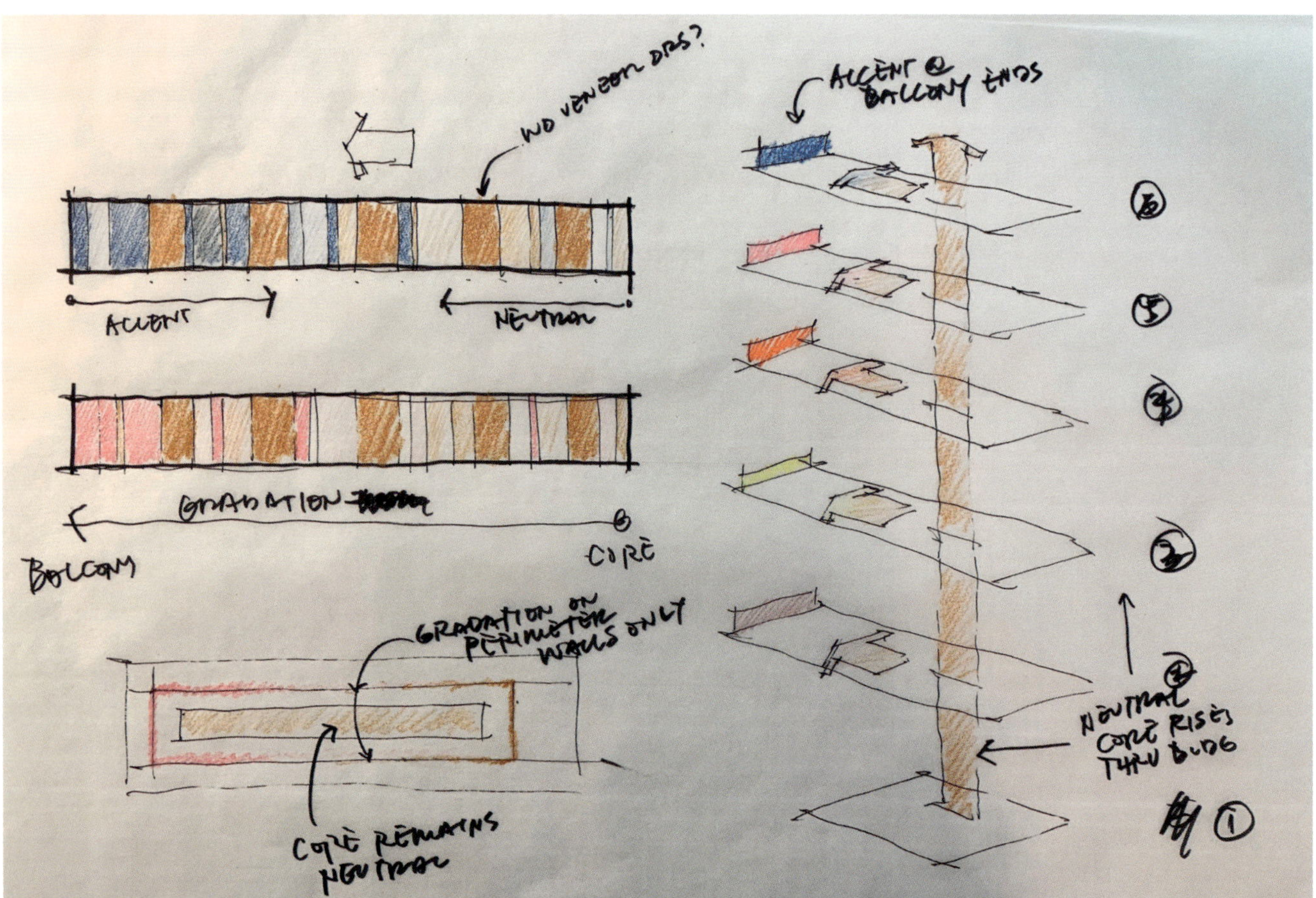

Hospitality suites on each floor serve as gathering spaces with mountain views.

Color application sketch.

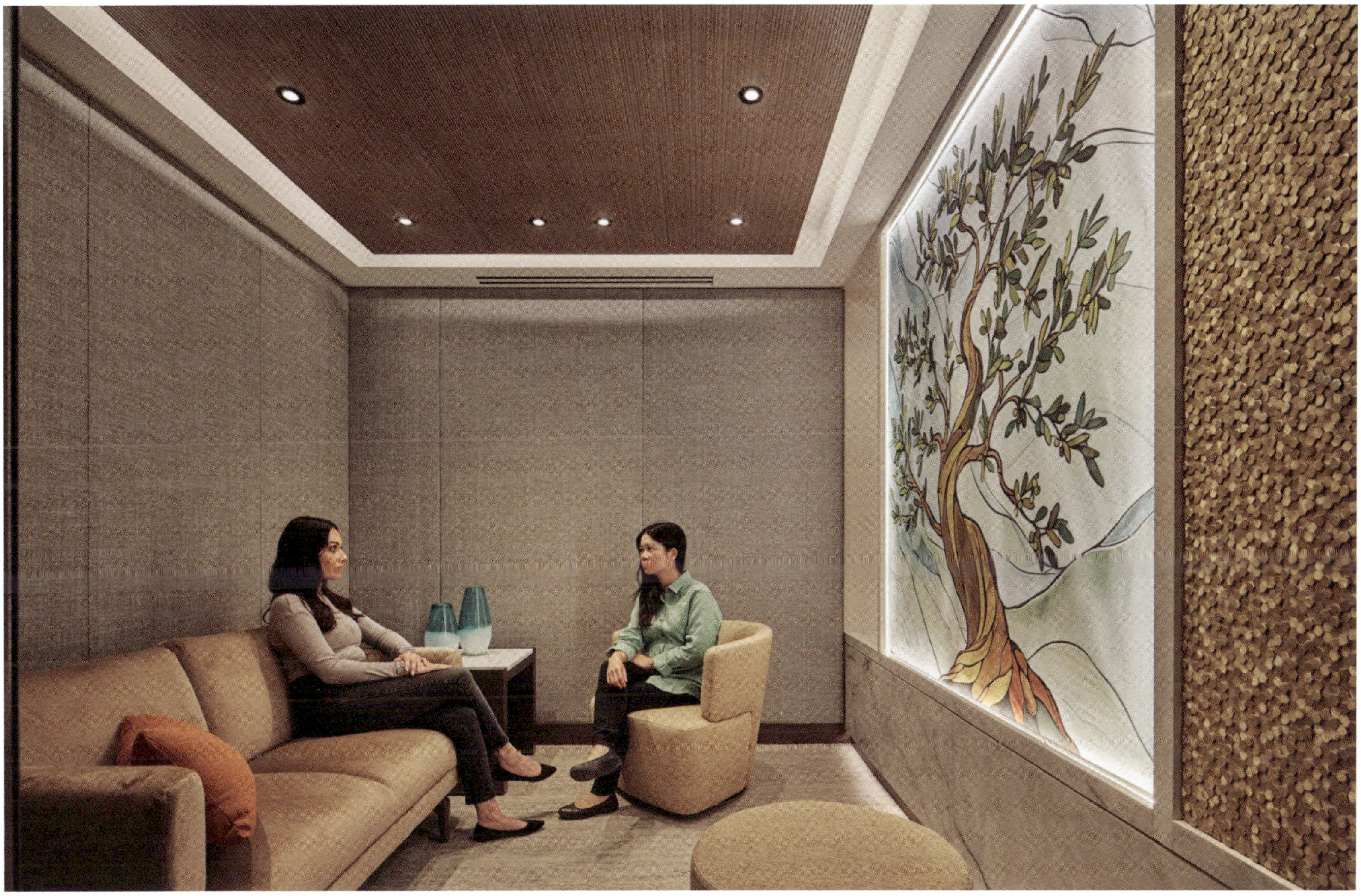

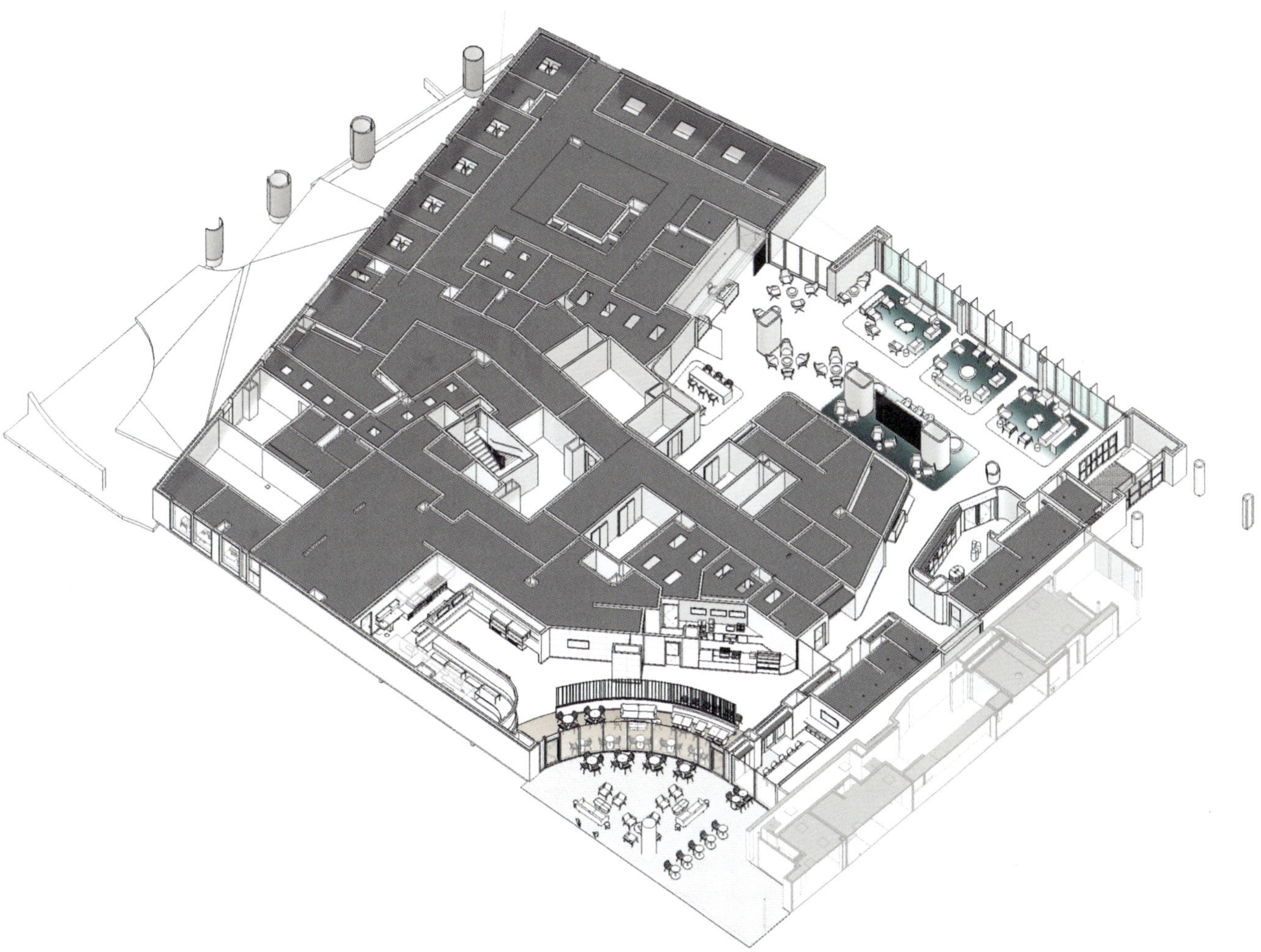

The multifaith spiritual care center provides an intimate, contemplative space.

Level 1 floor plan.

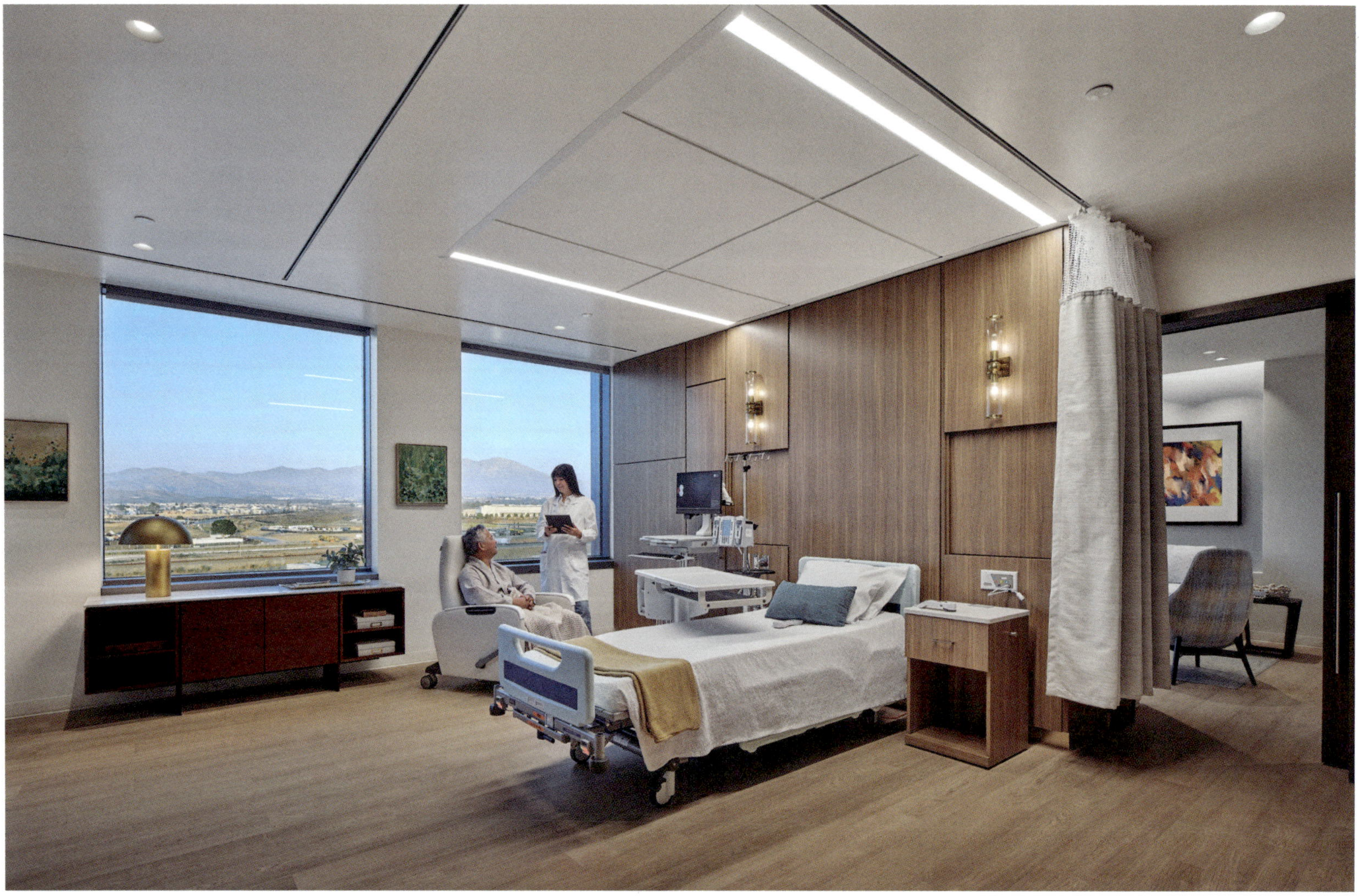

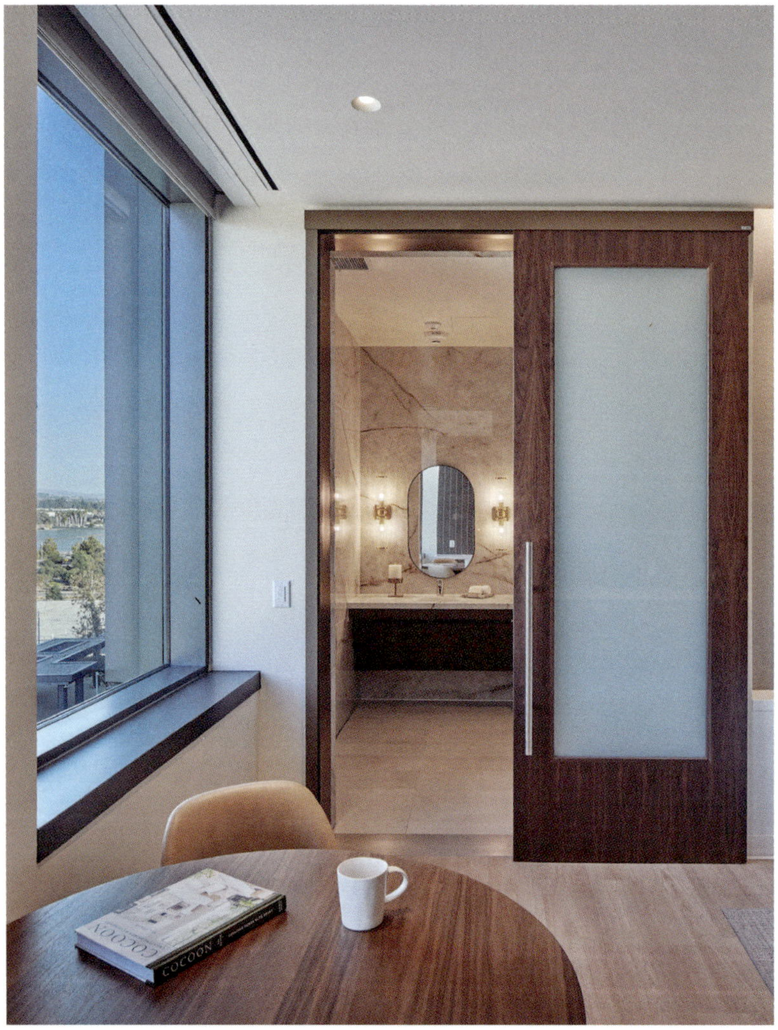

Concealed clinical utilities in family suites promote a sense of calm.

En-suite bathrooms improve comfort and privacy.

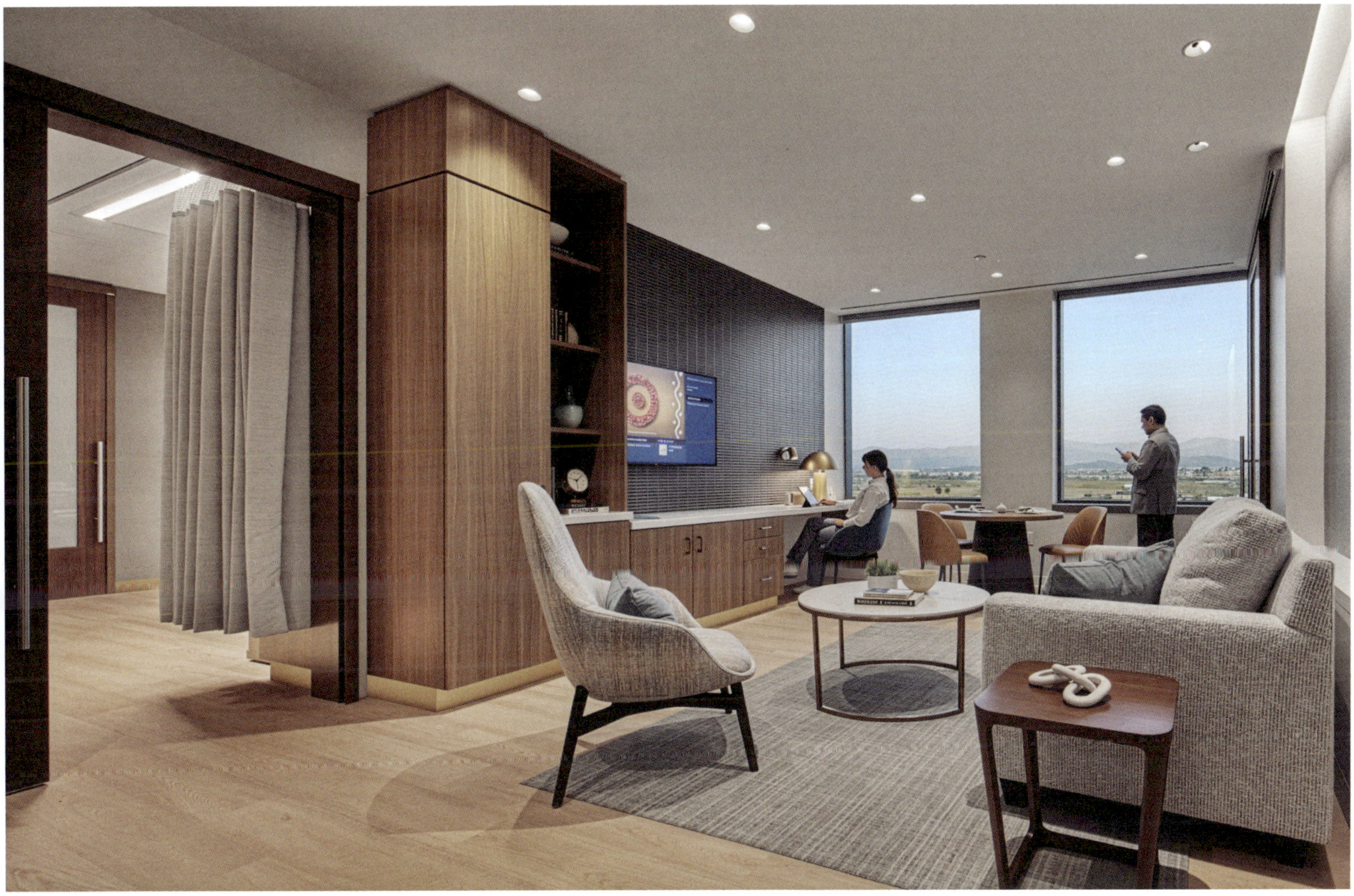

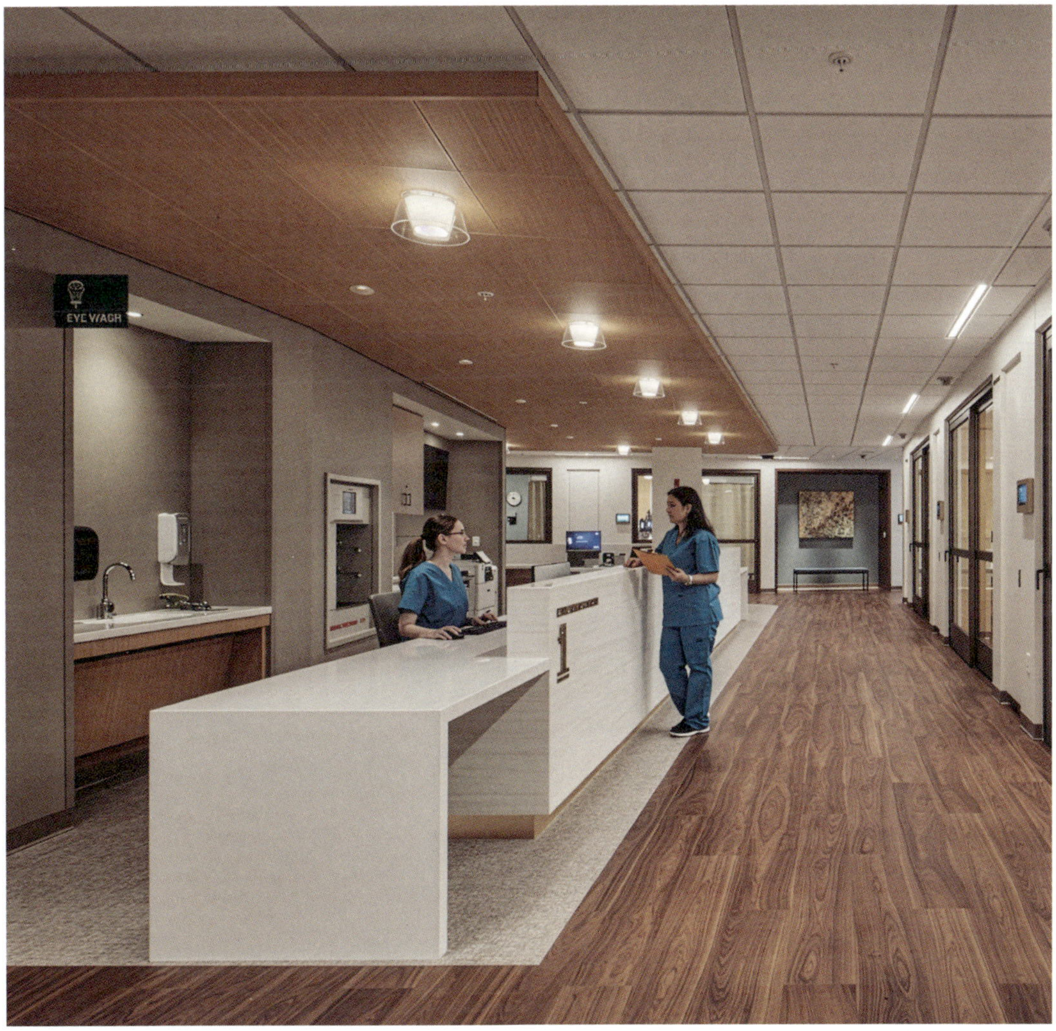

Family suites offer flexible seating for spending time with loved ones.

The Evaluation and Treatment Center provides prompt assessment and care.

FTA |
Filippo Taidelli Architetto

Misterbianco
Italy

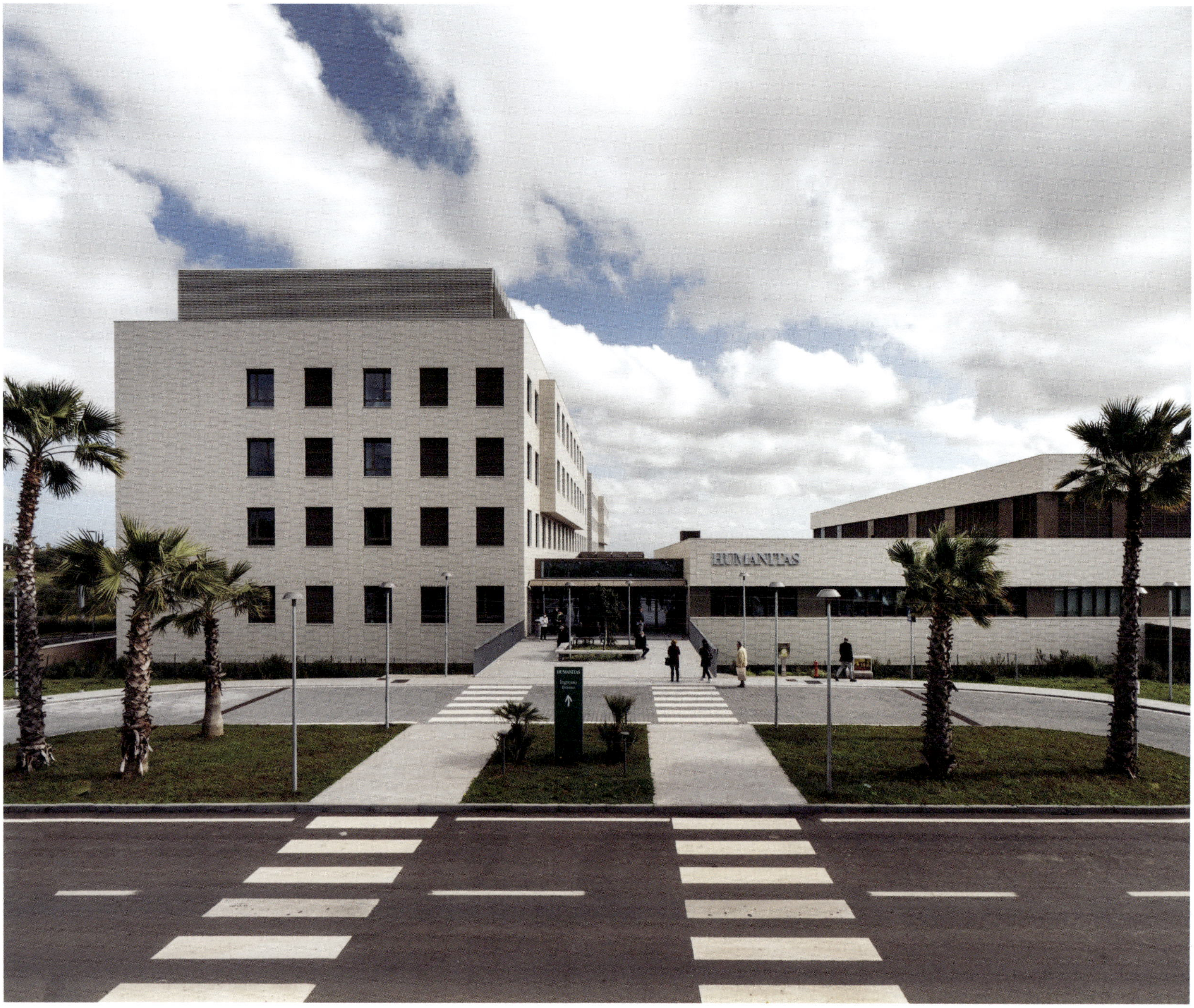

Front view with entrance.

Landscaped courtyard as one of the major design elements.

Catanese Clinical Institute

Serving as a regional reference center for oncological, neurosurgical, and orthopedic care, as well as a center of excellence for postgraduate specialist medical training, this hospital facility is situated in the calm Catalan landscape. The building comprises two regular volumes arranged side by side and a lower block. The two guiding design principles were a focus on the humanization of healthcare environments and the pursuit of a strong continuity between interior and exterior. In this interest the green surrounding extends into the building in the form of a boulevard with courtyards for recreation. The overall site layout thus merges with the surrounding landscape, extending even onto part of the roof of the lower block. In all areas, natural light is employed as a key design element, both to ensure a high level of comfort for patients and staff and to achieve significant energy savings.

Address: Contrada Cubba Marletta, 11, 95045 Misterbianco CT, Italy | **Client:** Humanitas Istituto Clinico Catanese | **Completion:** 2020 | **Size:** 25,000 m² | **Sector:** private and public | **Number of treatment rooms:** 60 | **Number of patient rooms:** 80

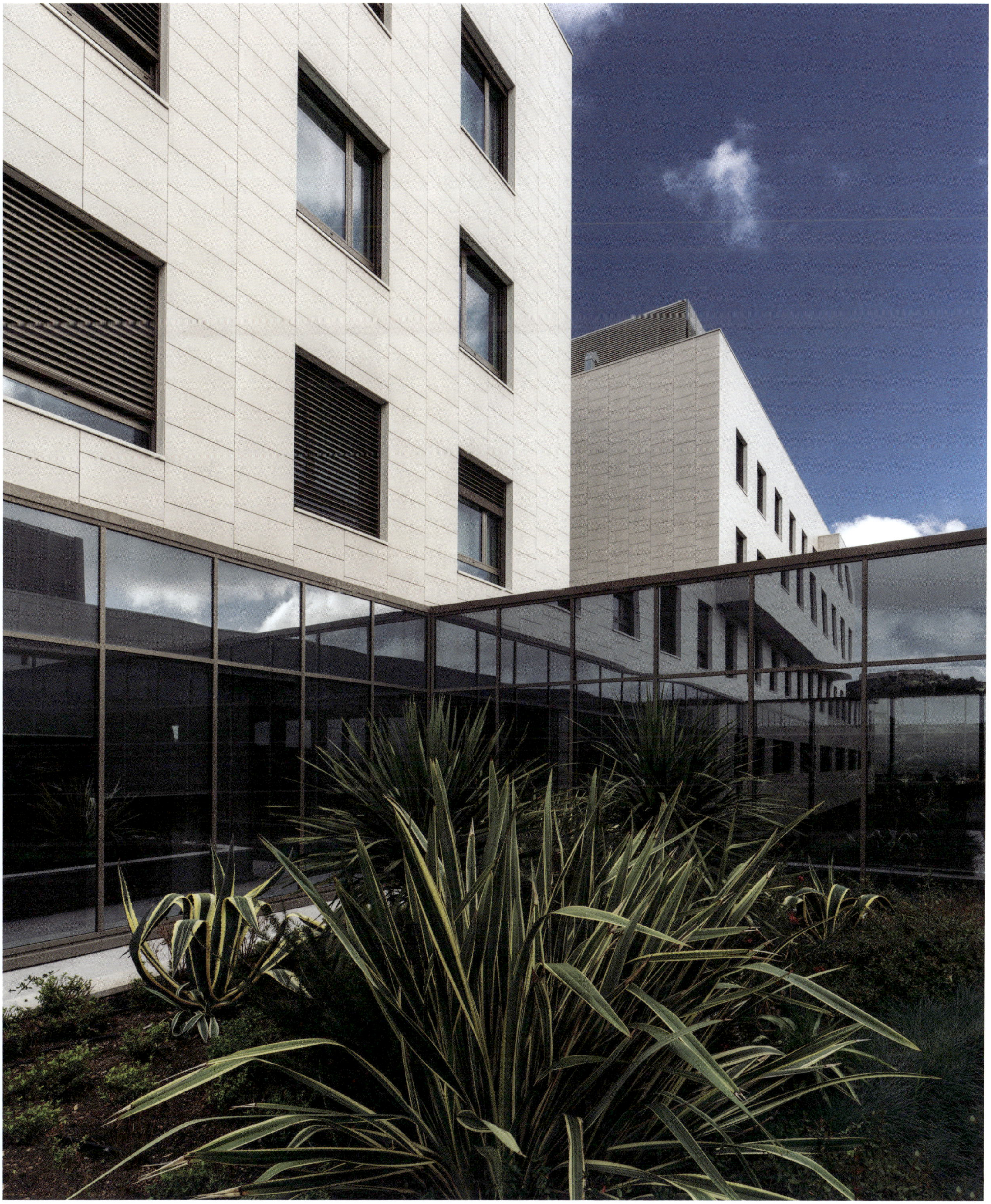

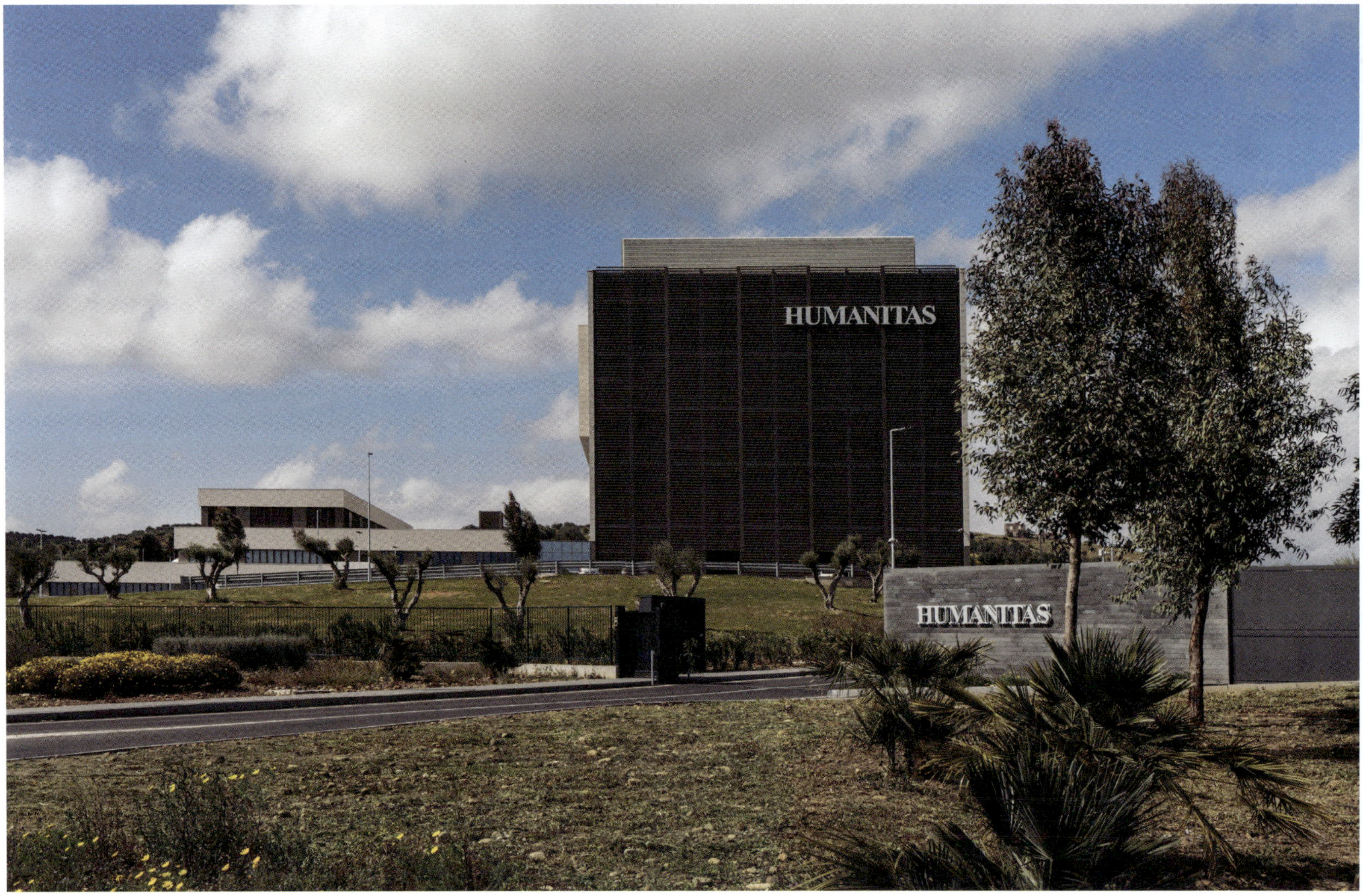

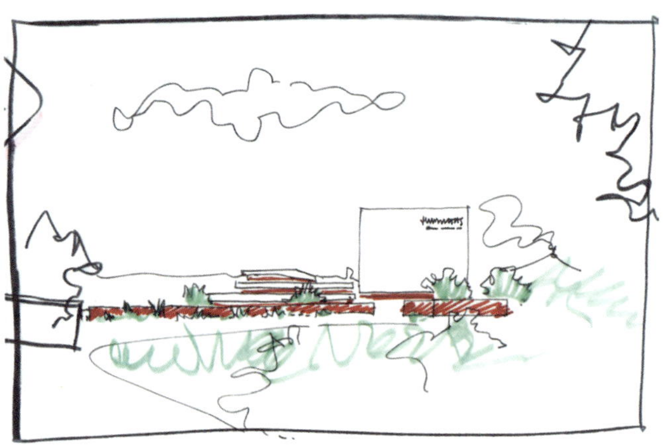

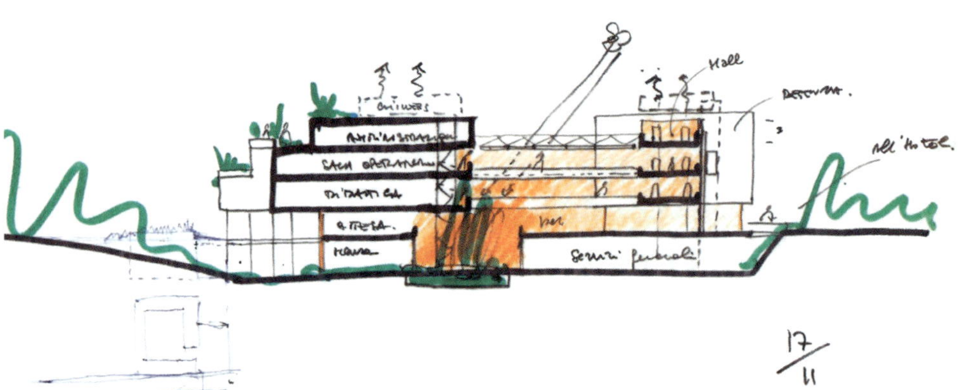

The hospital's setting in the landscape, surrounded by olive trees.

Original sketch.

Sketch underlining the original idea of merging the building with its surrounding.

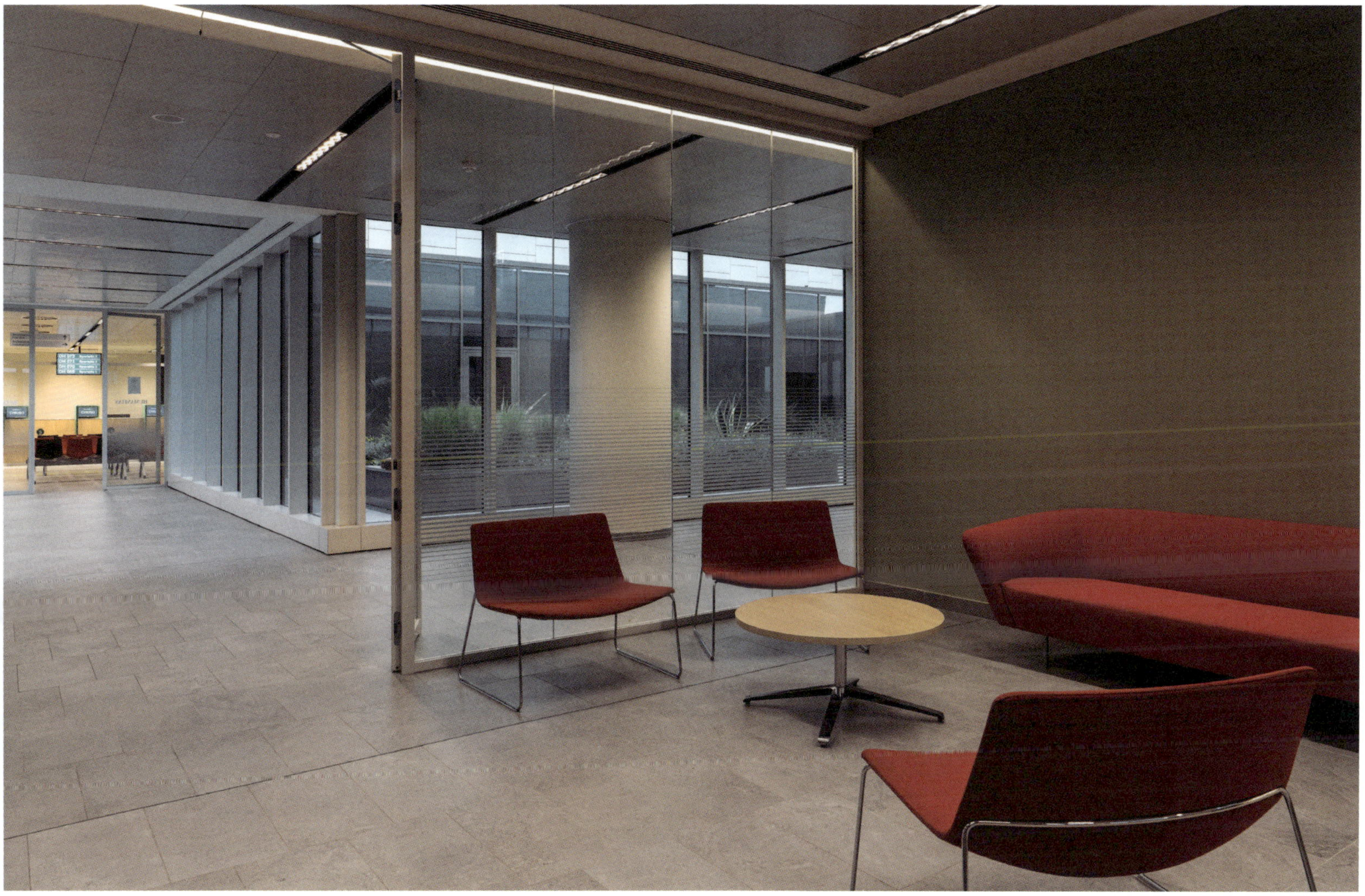

Waiting area with adjacent courtyard.

Section.

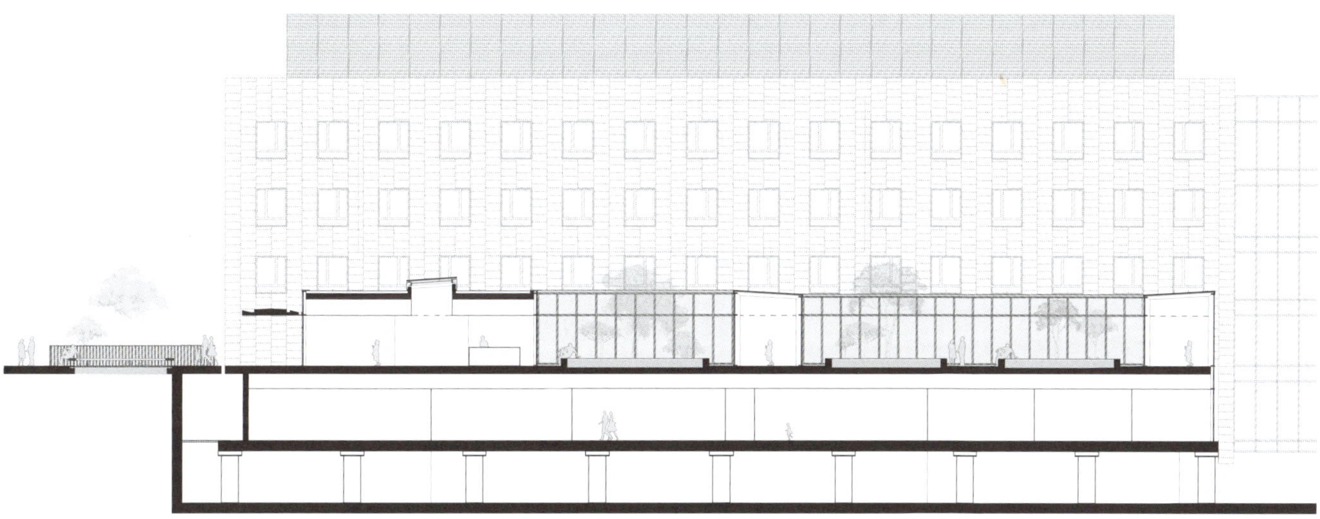

M.R Architekten
Thomas Rinne
Karsten Gottwald
Partnerschaftsgesellschaft

Berlin
Germany

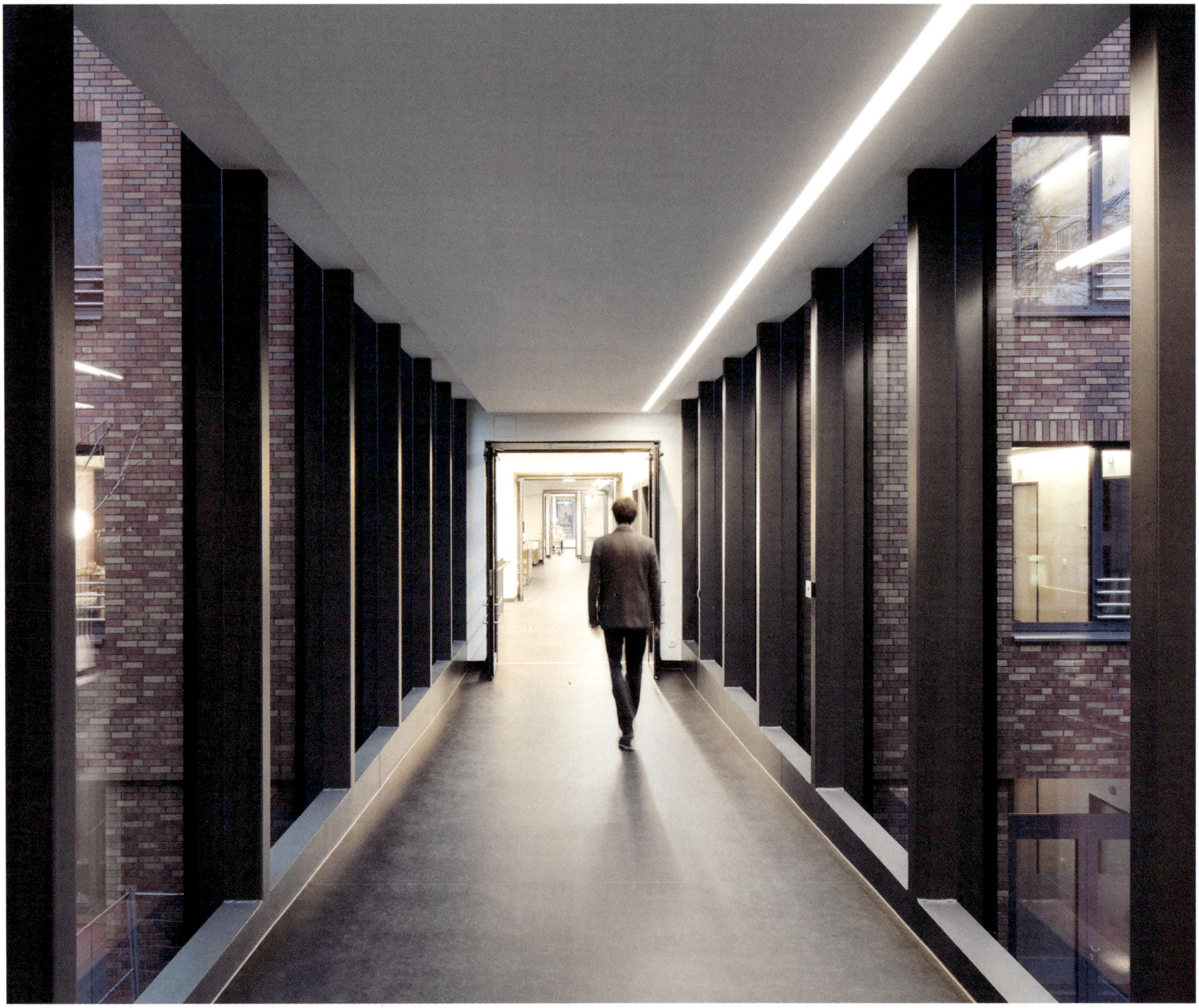

Tunnel and a glass bridge connect the new building to the existing structures.

Hospital's northwest view.

New Building 100 – Queen Elisabeth Herzberge Evangelical Hospital

The New Building 100 designed by Thomas Rinne and Karsten Gottwald of M.R Architekten complements the historic campus of the Queen Elisabeth Herzberge Evangelical Hospital in Berlin-Lichtenberg. The hospital dates back to Hermann Blankenstein's design from 1893 and is part of the Herzberge Landscape Park. The four-story new building provides functional spaces for neurology, diabetology, a comfort ward, and a medical care center. Positioned at the western edge of the site, it blends into the park's historic network of paths and sightlines, and its materials harmonize with the existing, historically protected buildings. Two courtyards provide natural light and ventilation, as well as clear orientation and a high quality of stay for patients and nursing staff. A tunnel and a glass bridge connect the new building to the existing structures.

Address: Herzbergstraße 79, 10365 Berlin, Germany | **Client:** Queen Elisabeth Herzberge Evangelical Hospital (KEH) – New Building 100 | **Completion:** 2020 | **Size:** 6,640 m² | **Original building:** Hermann Blankenstein, 1893 | **Sector:** other | **Specialization:** neurology, diabetology | **Number of treatment rooms:** 27 | **Number of patient rooms:** 37

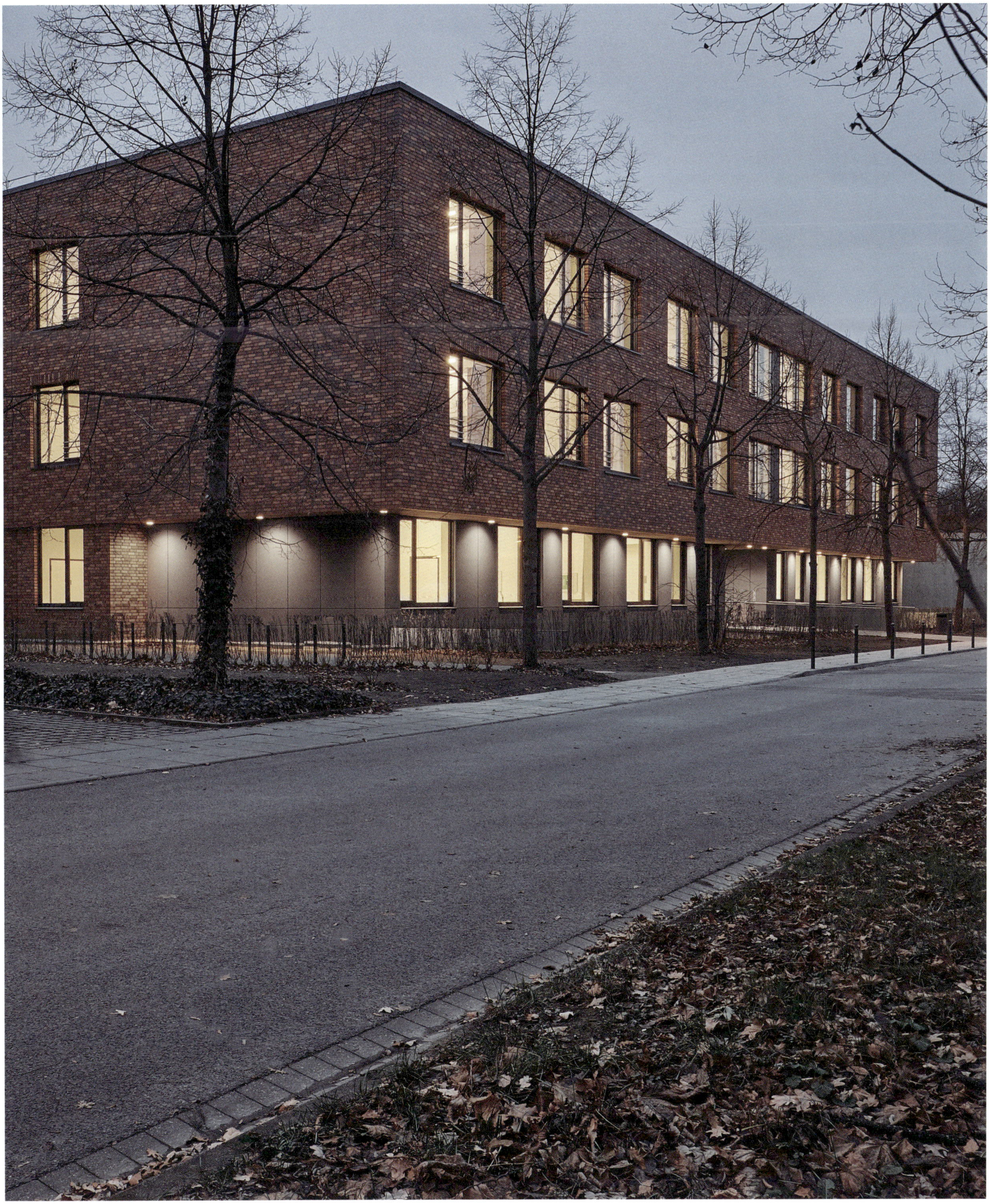

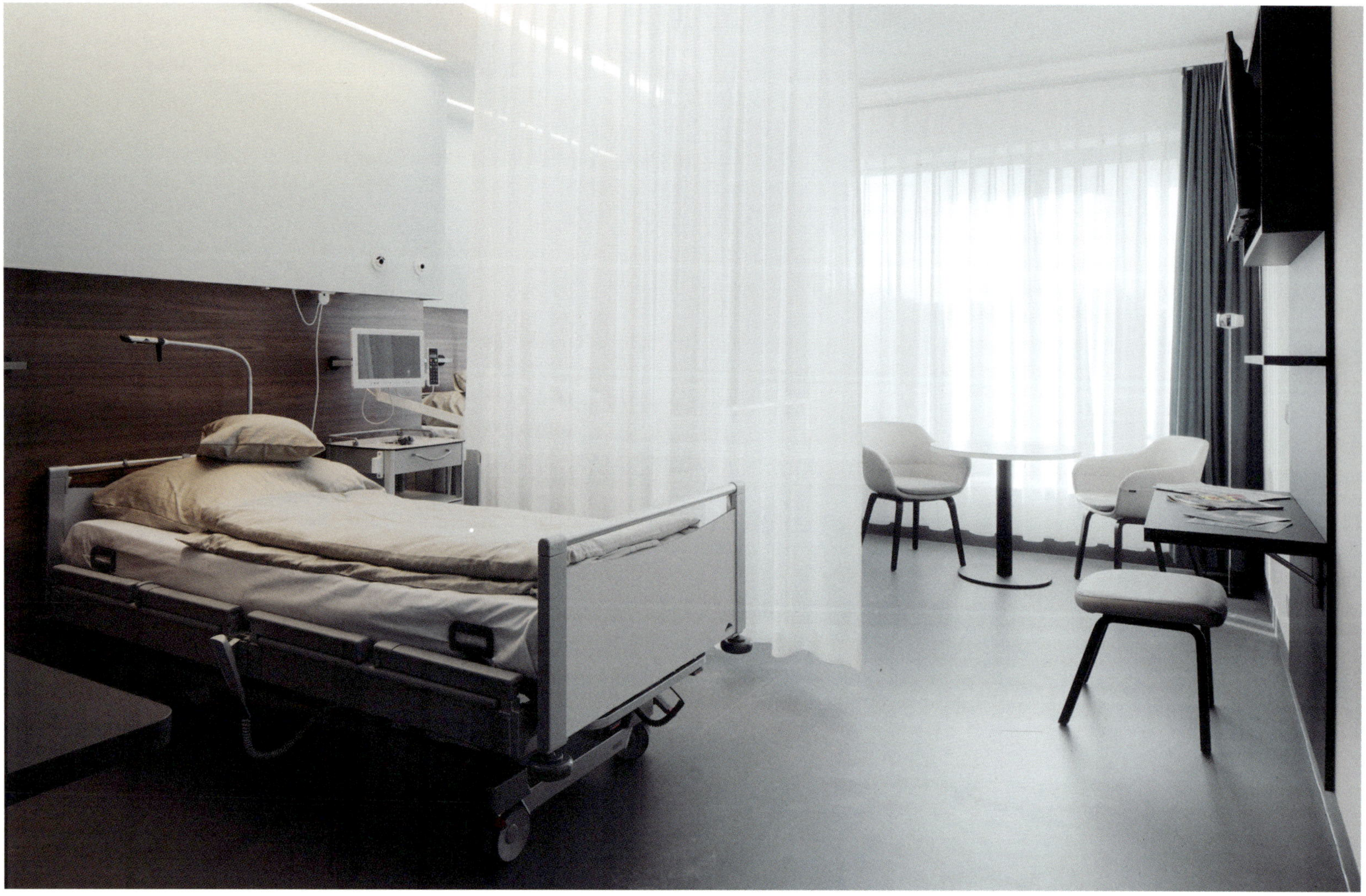

Well designed and spacious patient's room.

First floor plan with nursing ward.

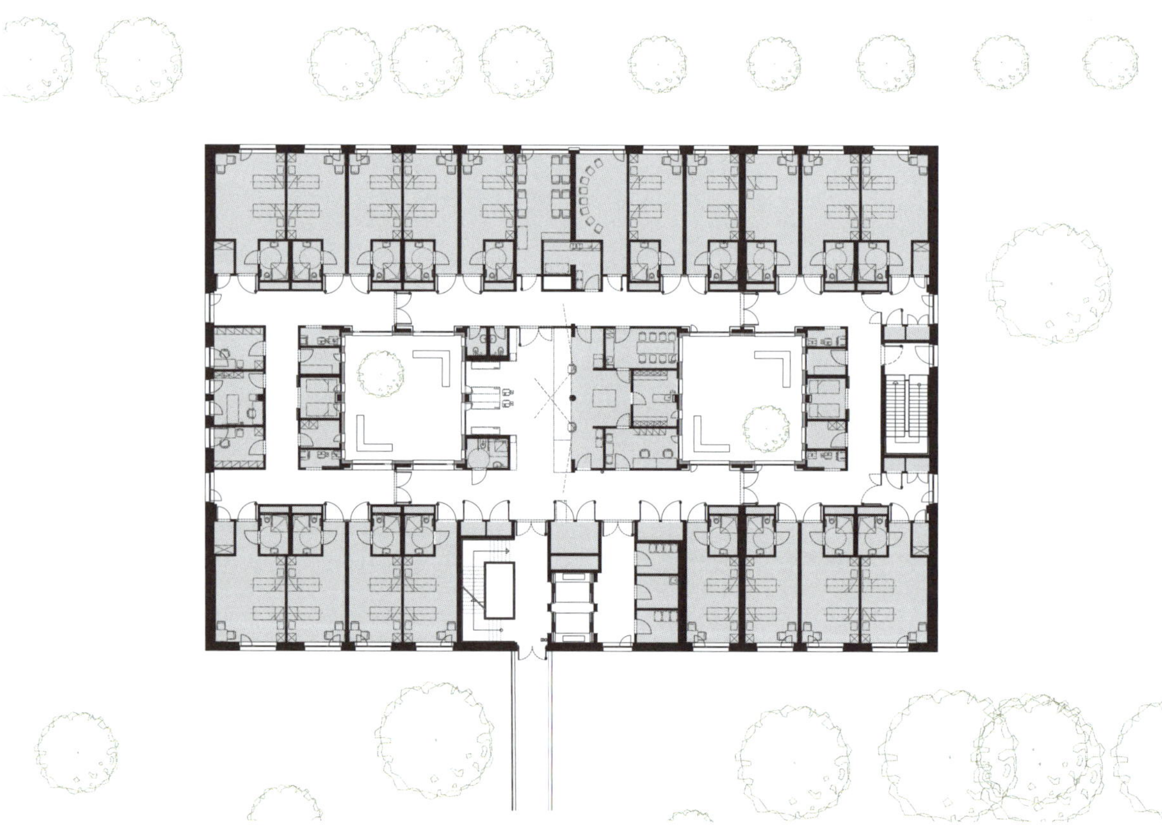

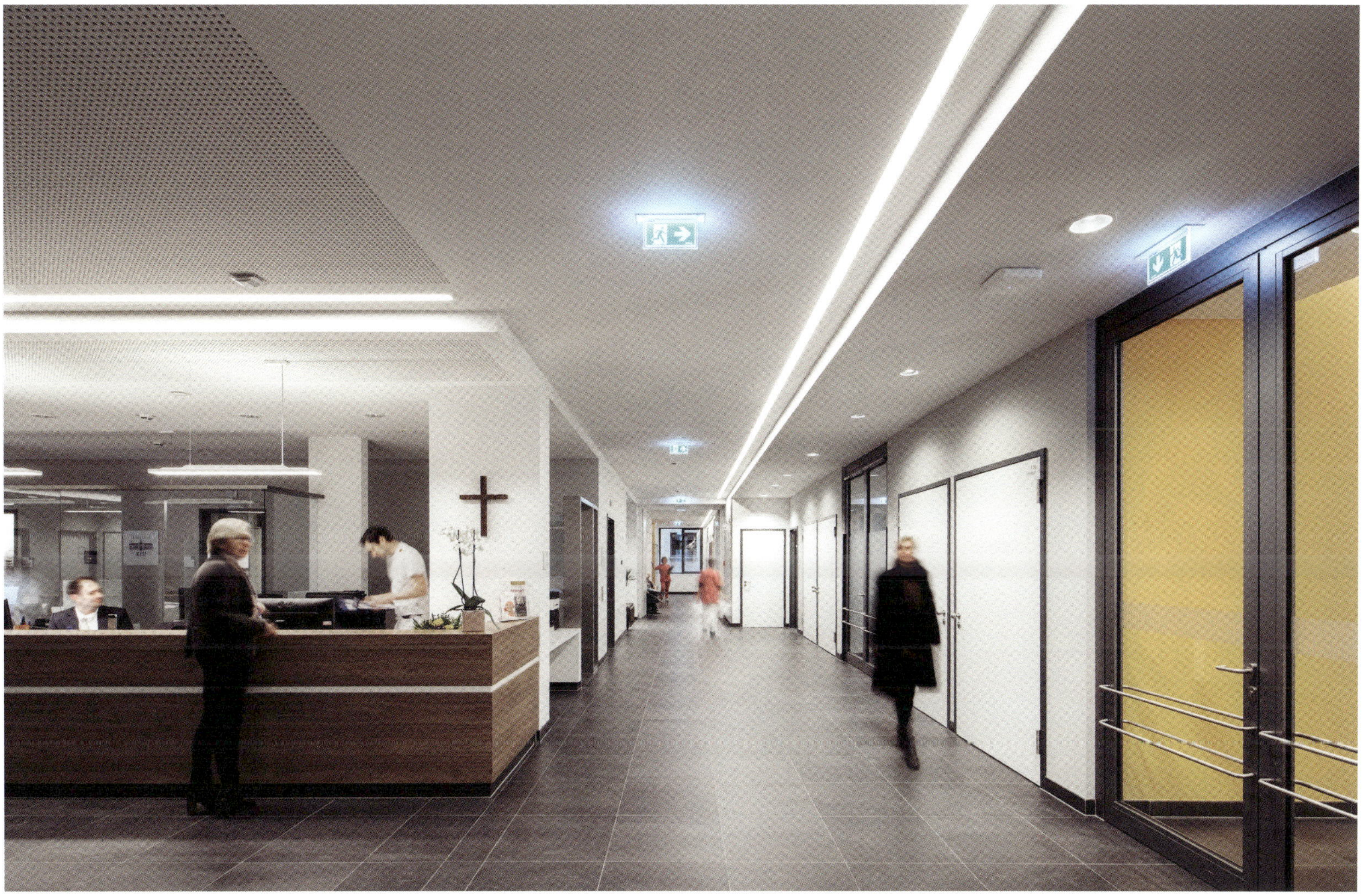

Clearly structured reception desk.

Section.

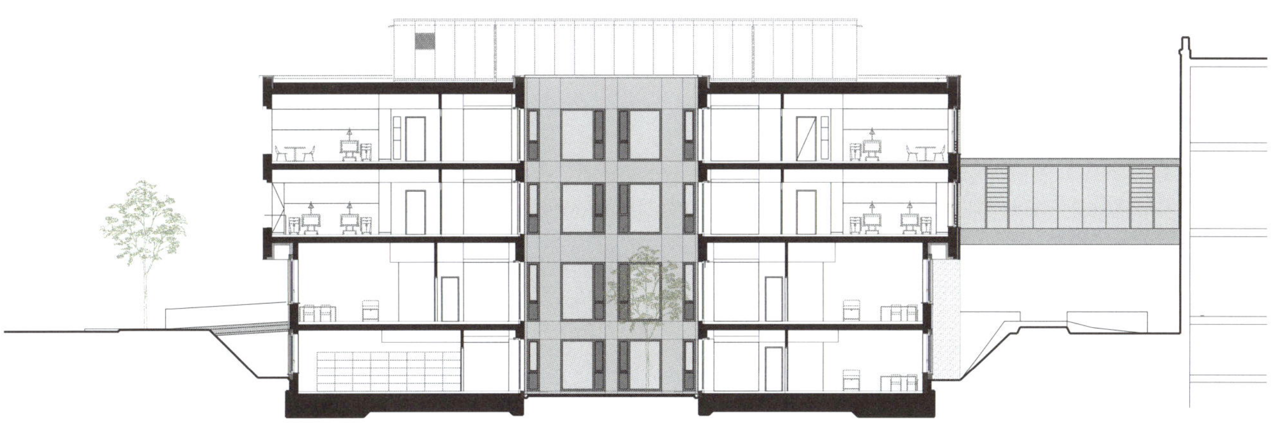

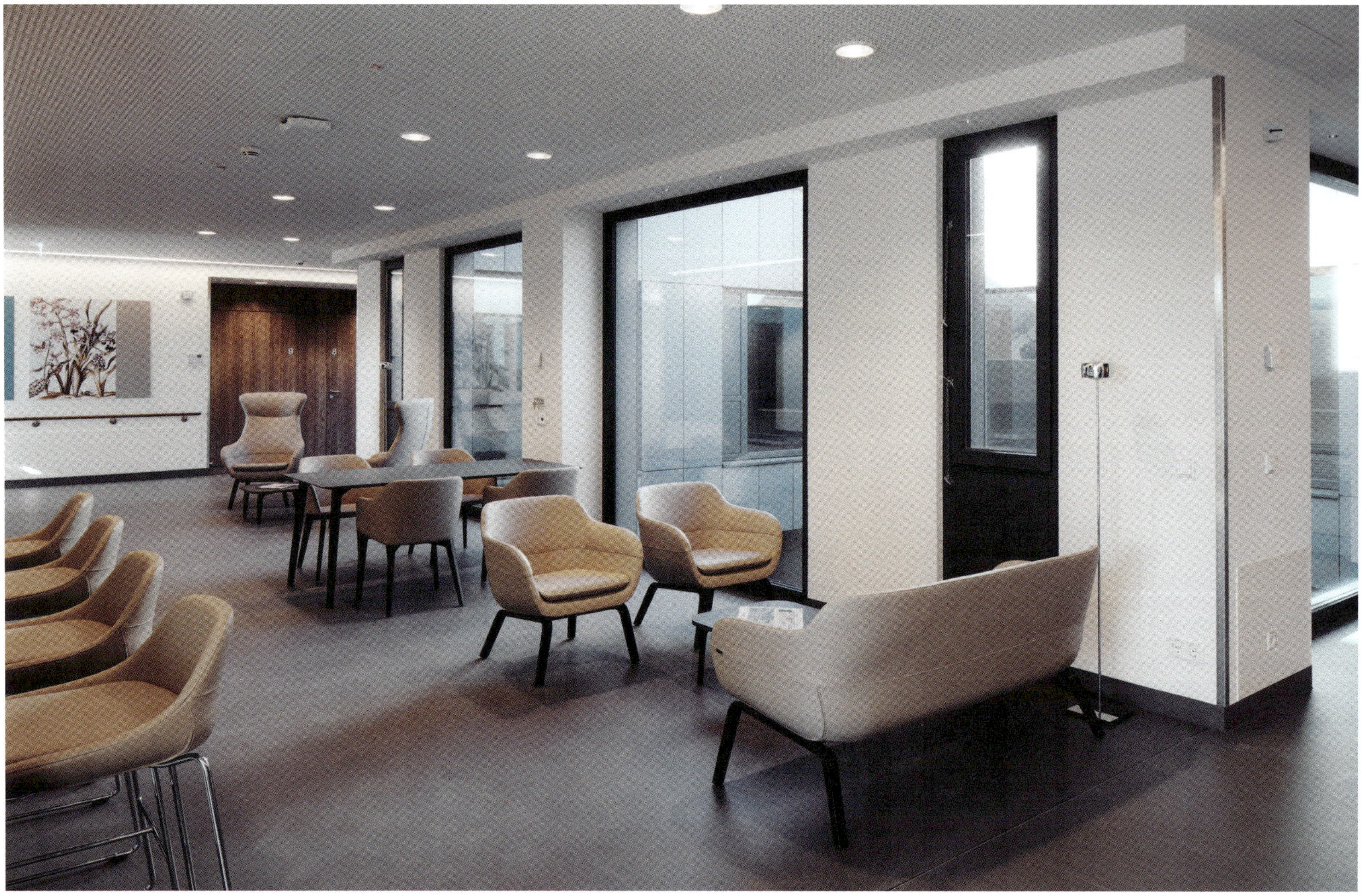

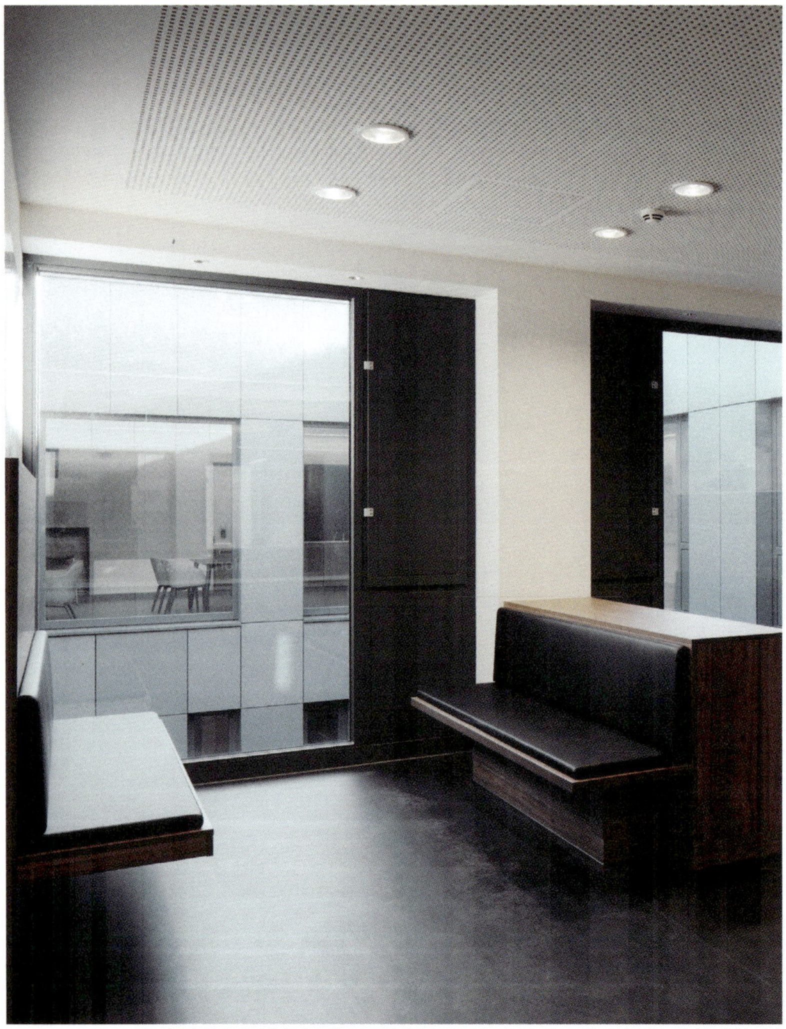

Waiting area looking out into the courtyard.

Private patient area with large windows to the court-yard.

Figure-ground plan.

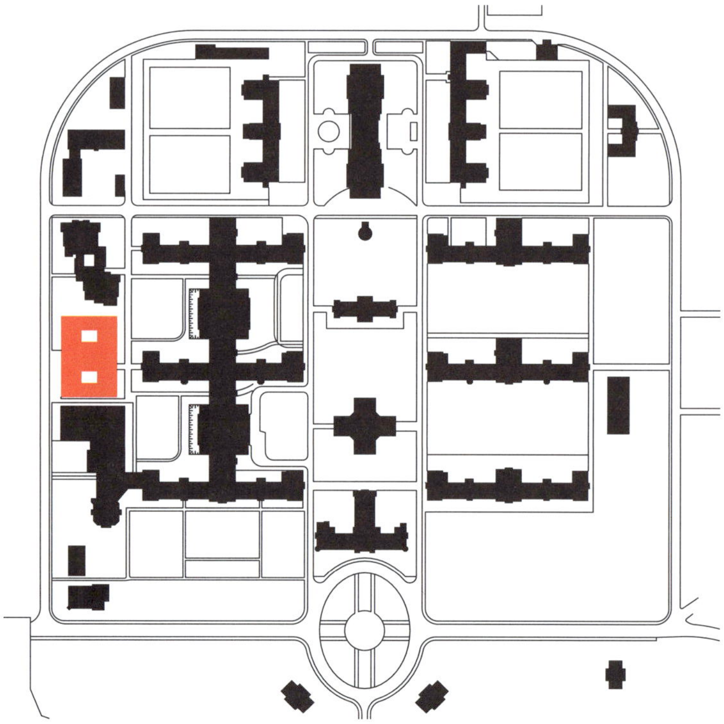

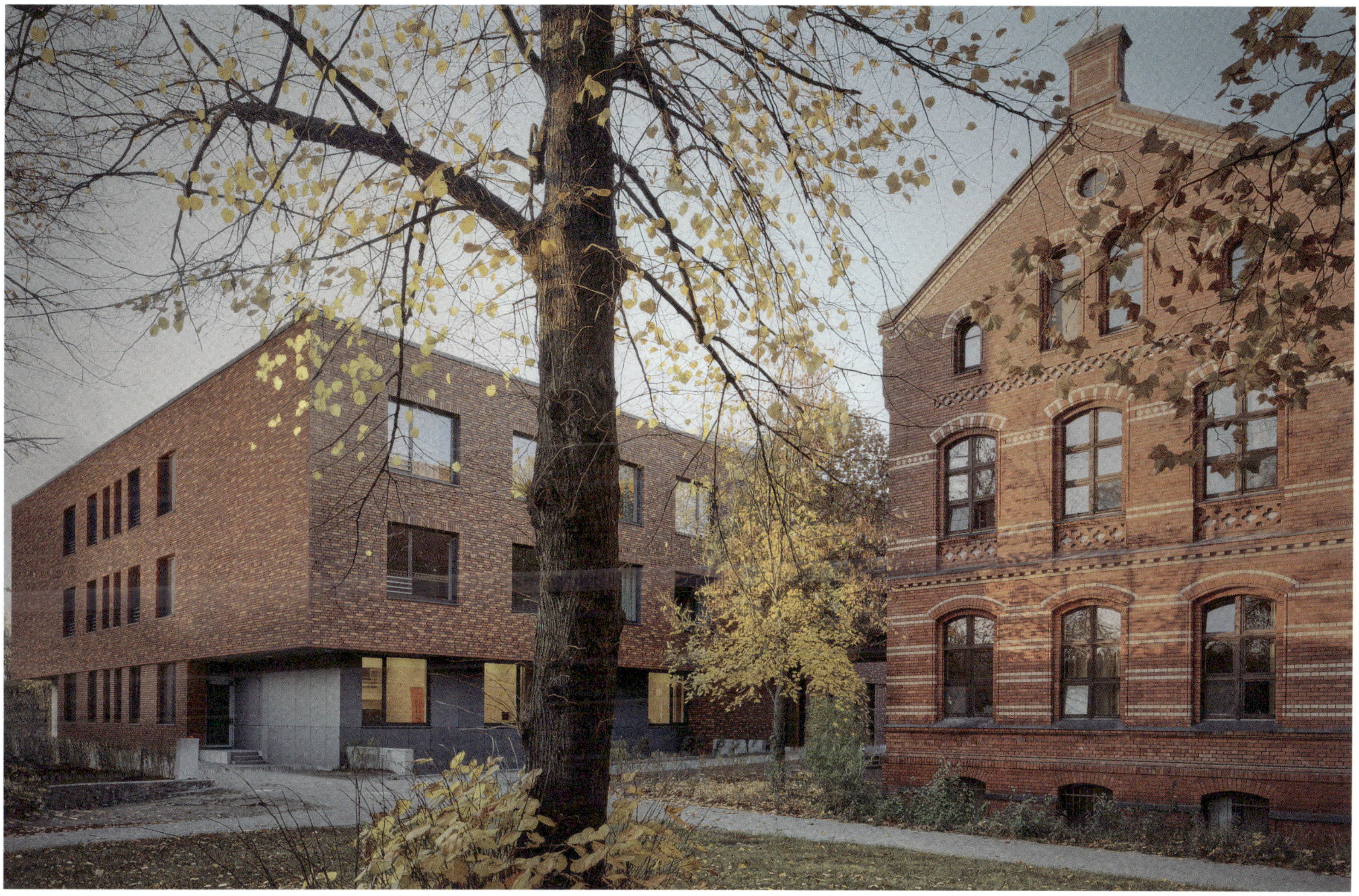

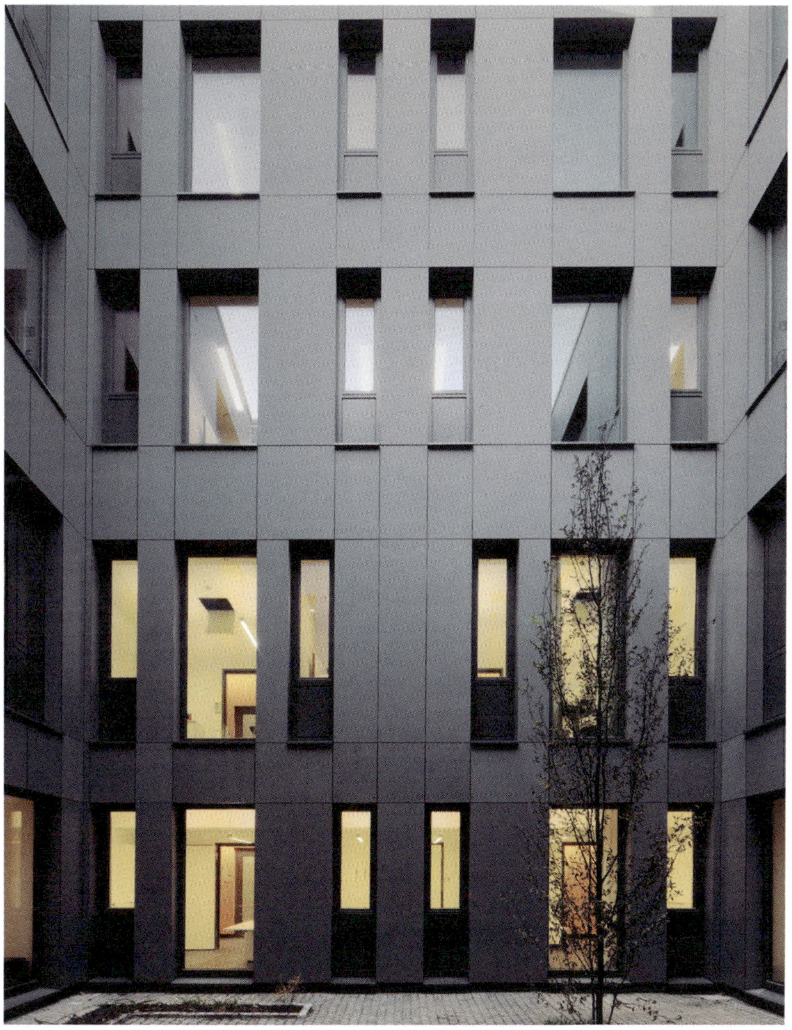

Hermann Blankensteins building from 1893 and the brick-faced extension.

The courtyard uses the same material as the street façade of the ground floor.

3XN
LINK Arkitektur

Copenhagen
Denmark

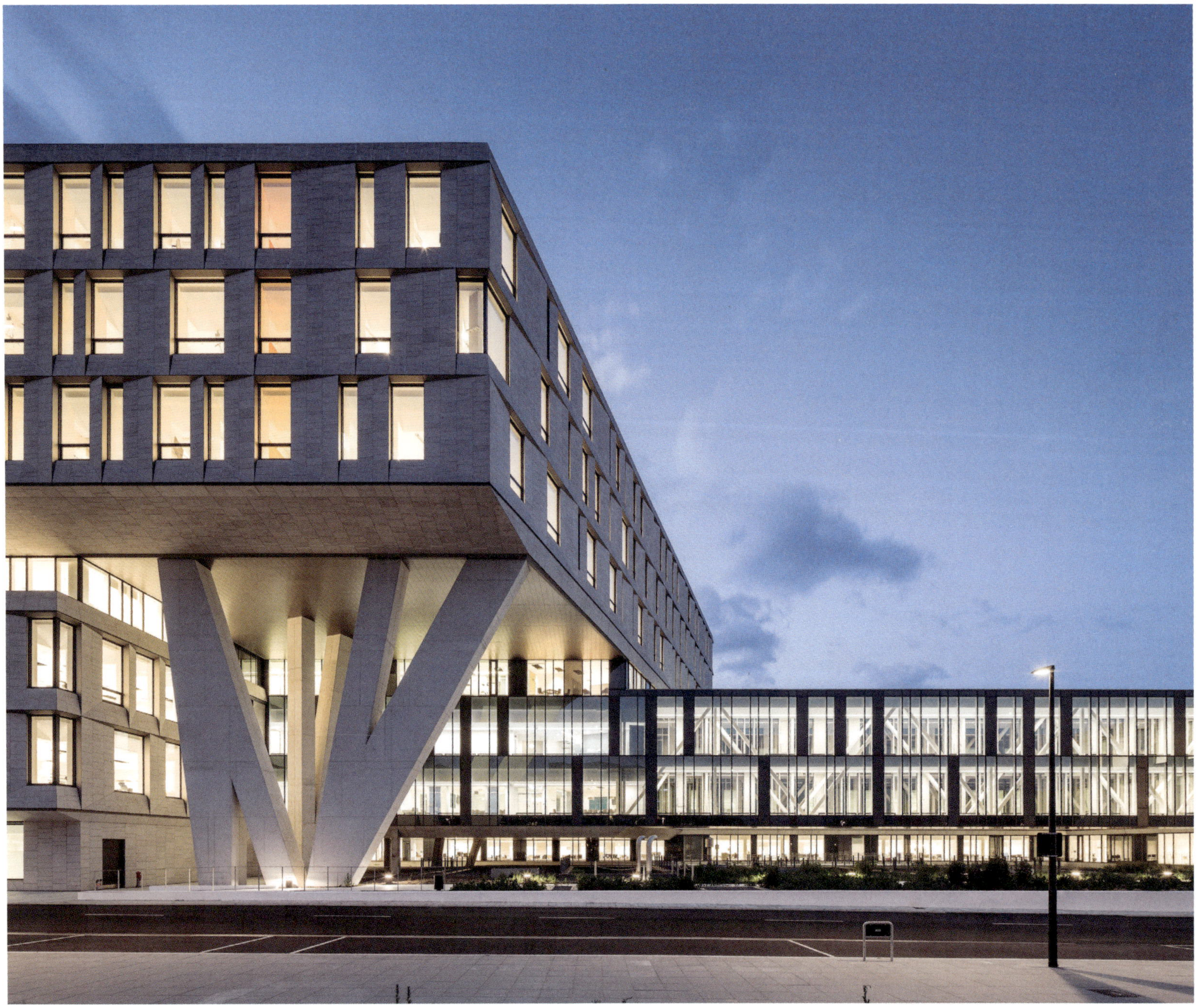

A natural light stone was chosen for the façade to give it a bright and welcoming appearance.

The staircases are located in the open atria, where daylight flows into the building from the glass ceiling.

Nordfløjen Rigshospitalet – The North Wing

Advances in medical treatment and digital healthcare technologies are reshaping hospital design, with the North Wing of Rigshospitalet Copenhagen University Hospital – designed in close collaboration between 3XN and LINK Arkitektur – increasingly emphasizes flexibility and long-term adaptability to meet evolving clinical needs. Carefully integrated into its surroundings, the building unfolds through five central zones that support orientation and create restorative environments. From the combination of a healing-oriented approach and sustainable strategies results a calm, green healthcare setting. Two spiral staircases and four elevator cores structure intuitive vertical circulation, guiding movement through light-filled interiors with glazed ceilings and façades. While floor-specific color schemes support wayfinding, artworks by Olafur Eliasson, Malene Landgreen, and Erik A. Frandsen soften the clinical atmosphere and define key points.

Address: Blegdamsvej 9, 2100 Copenhagen, Denmark | **Client:** The Capital Region of Denmark | **Completion:** 2020 | **Size:** 65,200 m² | **Sector:** public | **Number of treatment rooms:** 43 | **Number of patient rooms:** 209 | **Landscape design:** Kristine Jensens Tegnestue

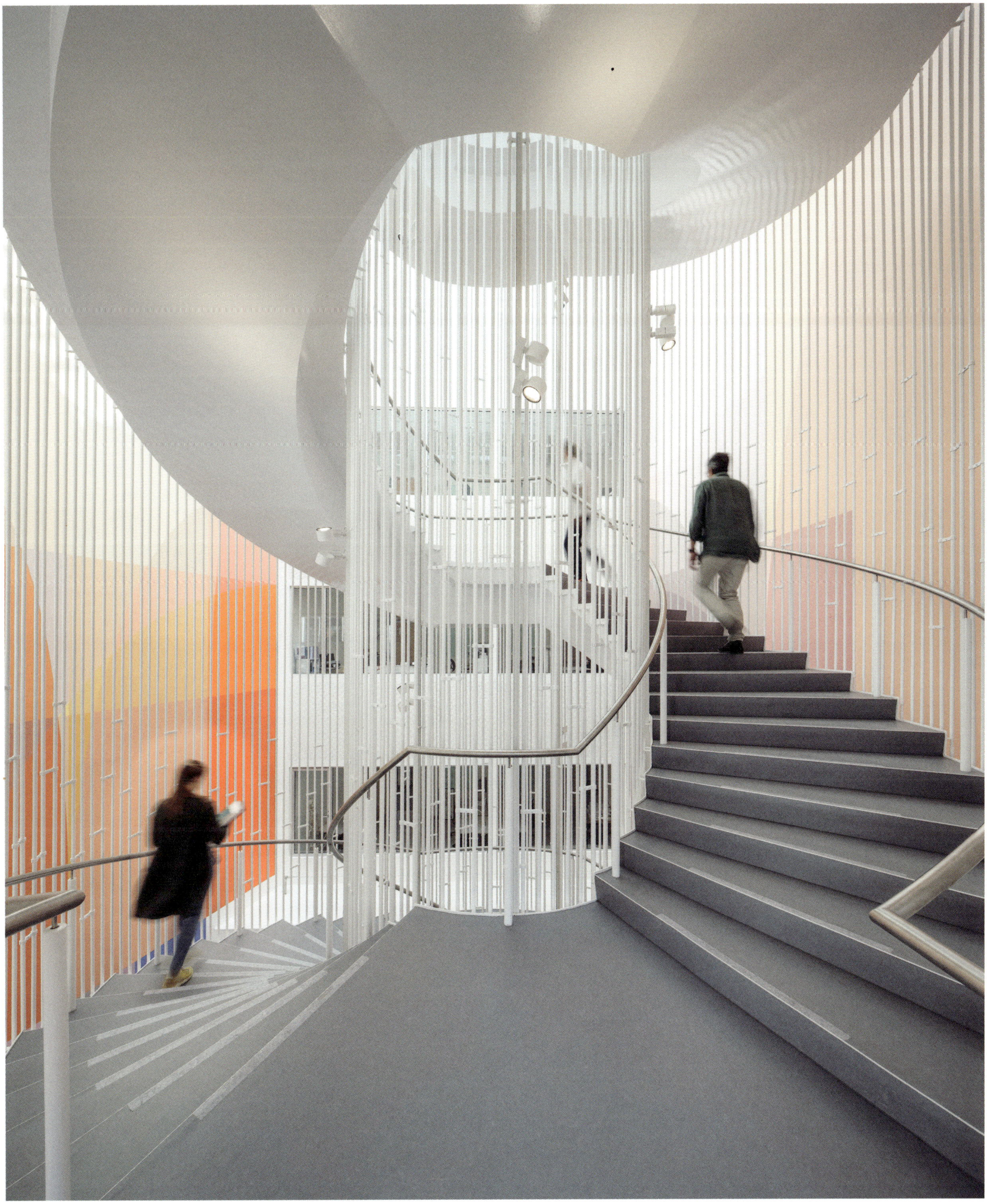

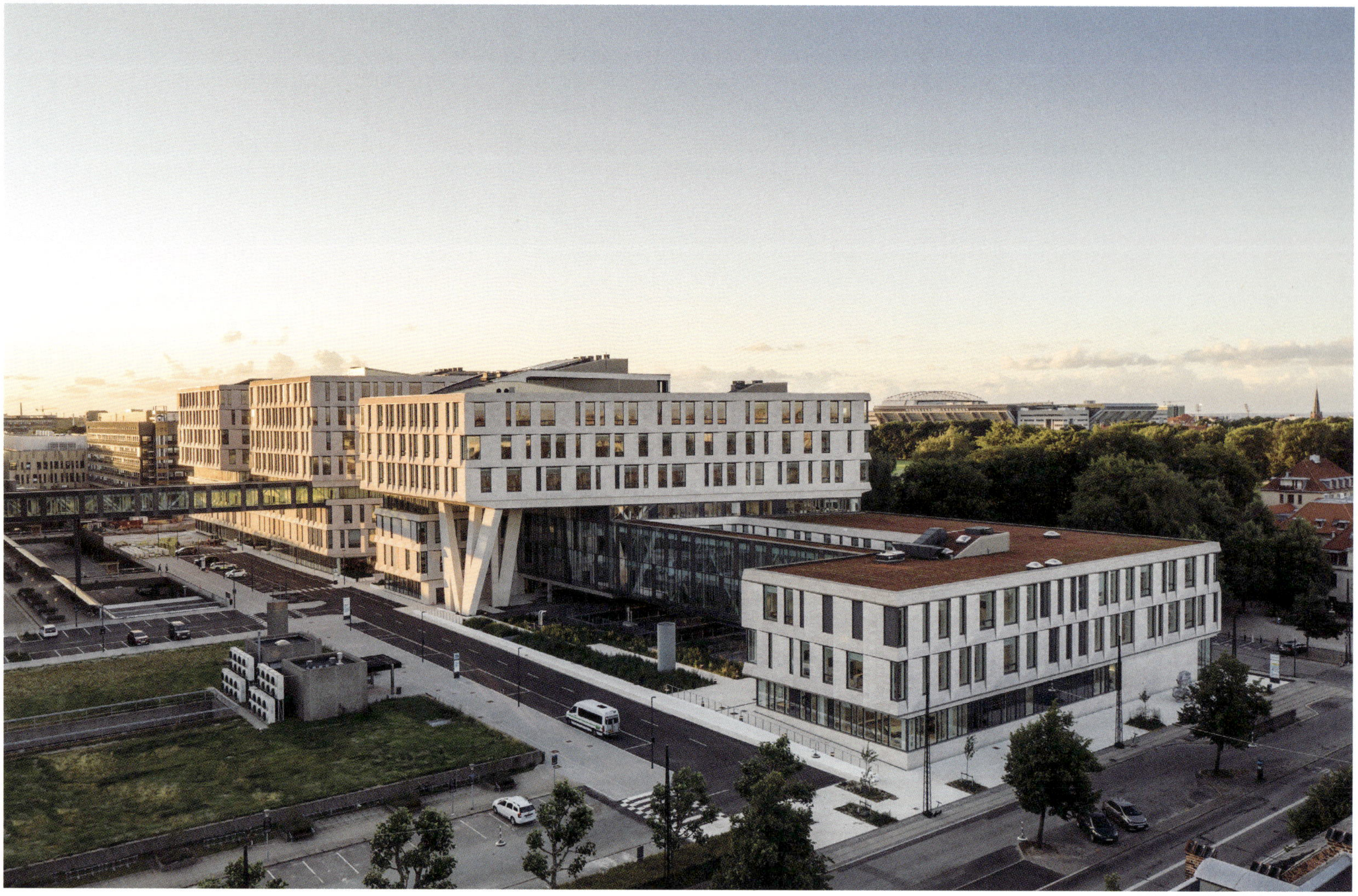

The hospital combines sustainable solutions with natural elements inside and outside to create a greener environment.

Ground floor plan.

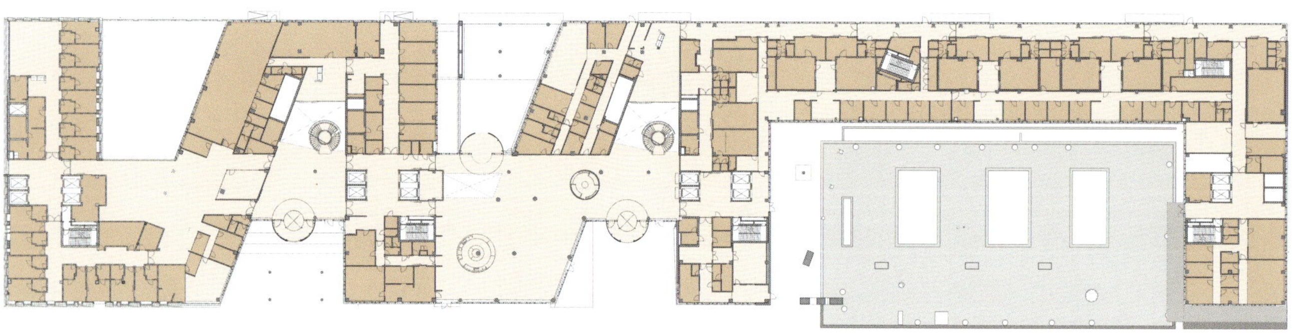

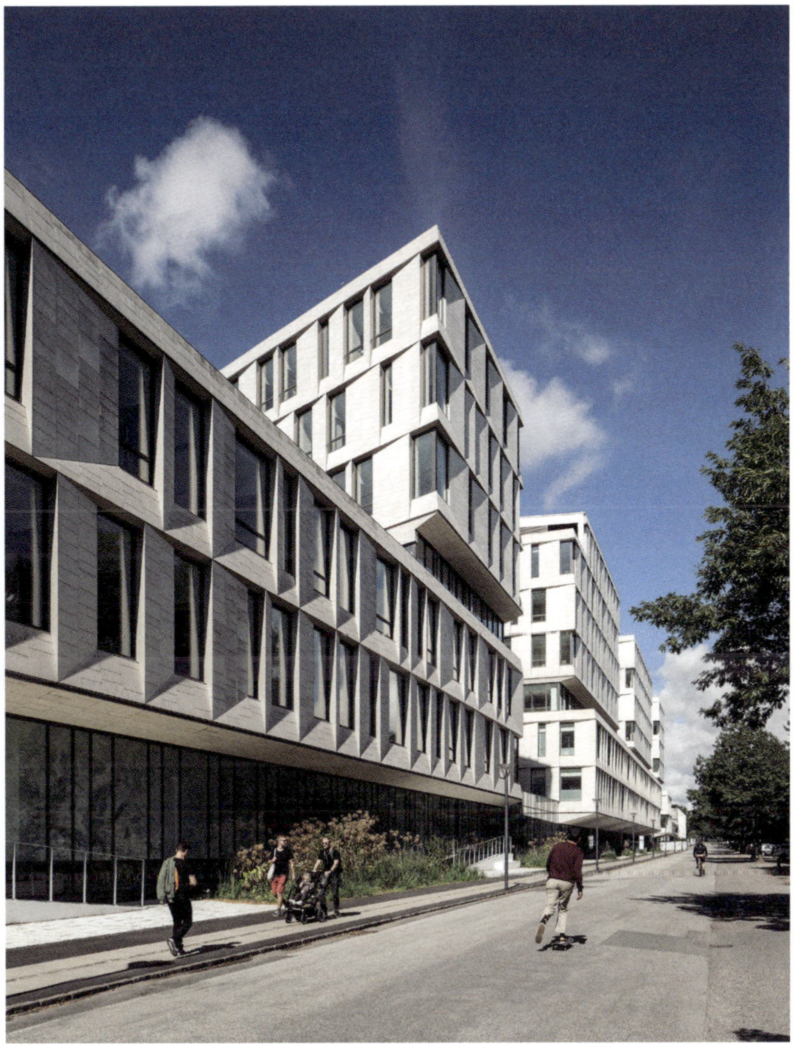

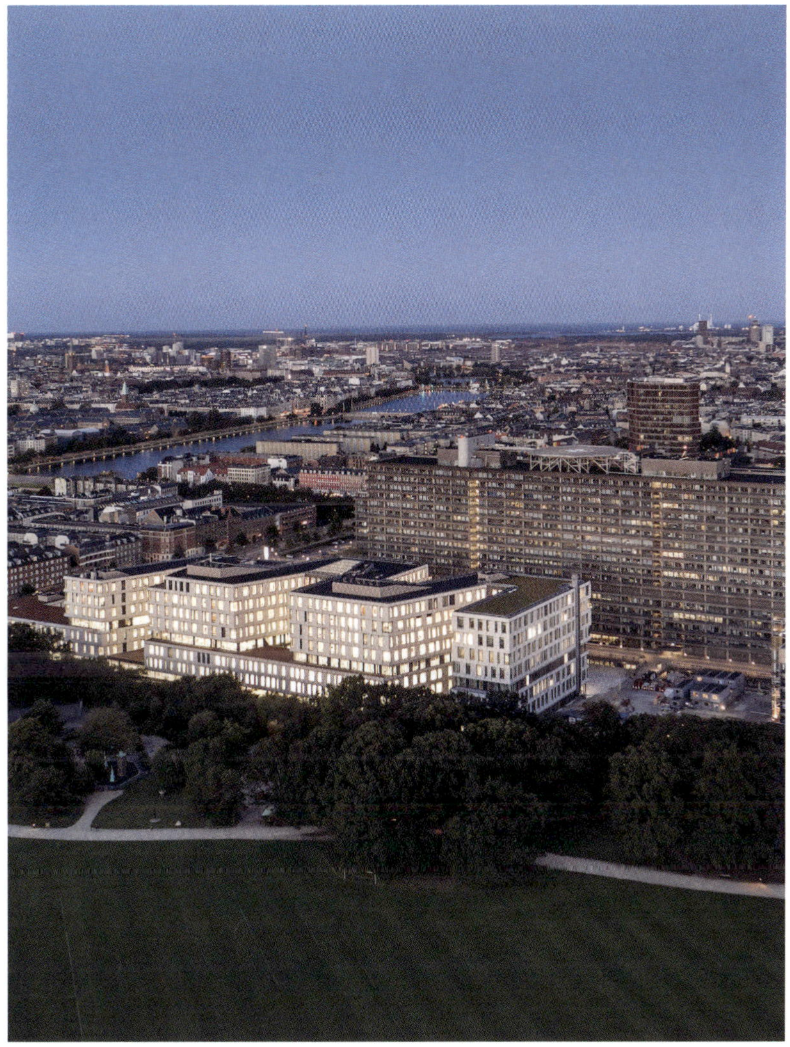

A natural light stone was chosen for the façade to give it a bright and welcoming appearance.

The building is located near the park and residential areas.

Second and first floor plan with folded V-structures.

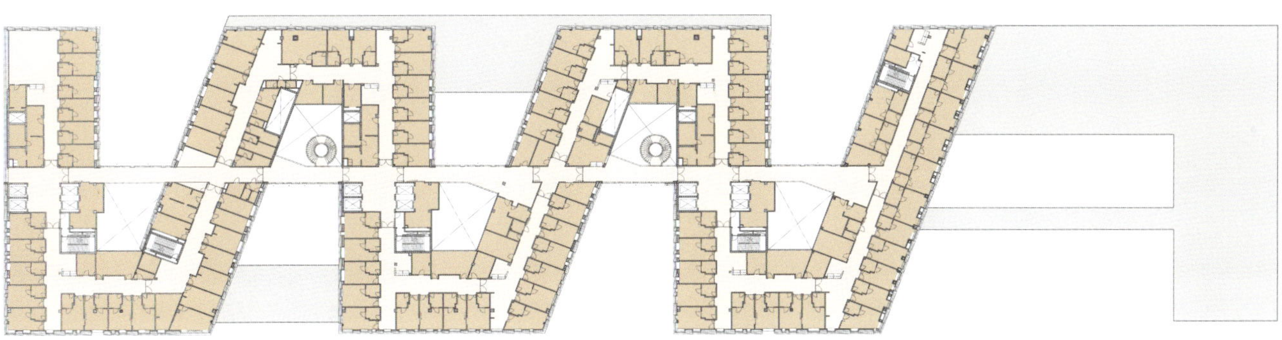

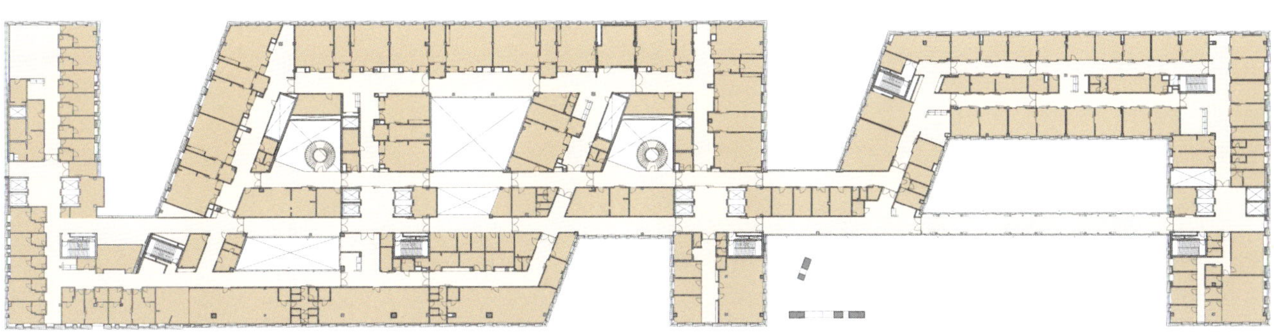

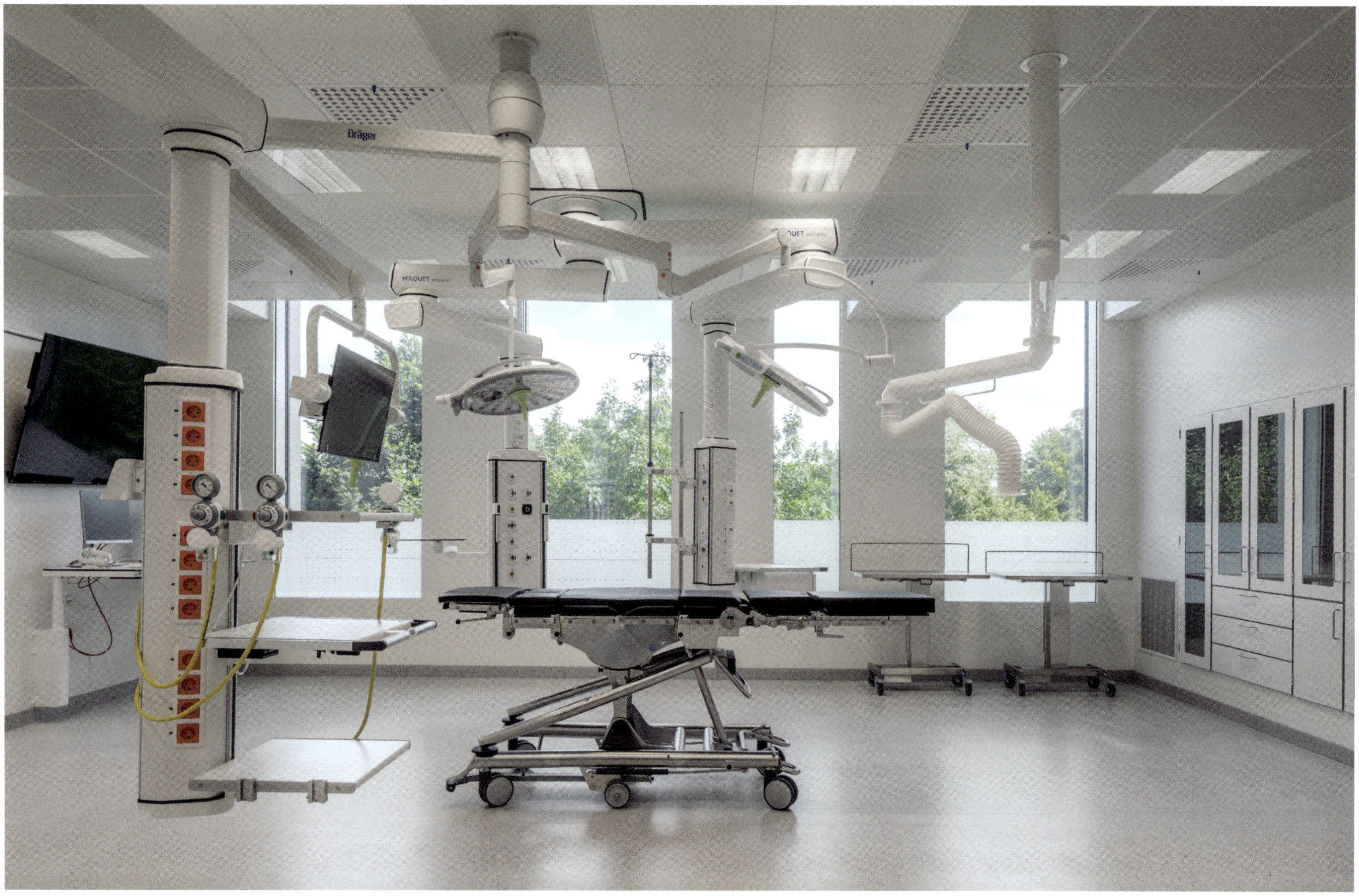

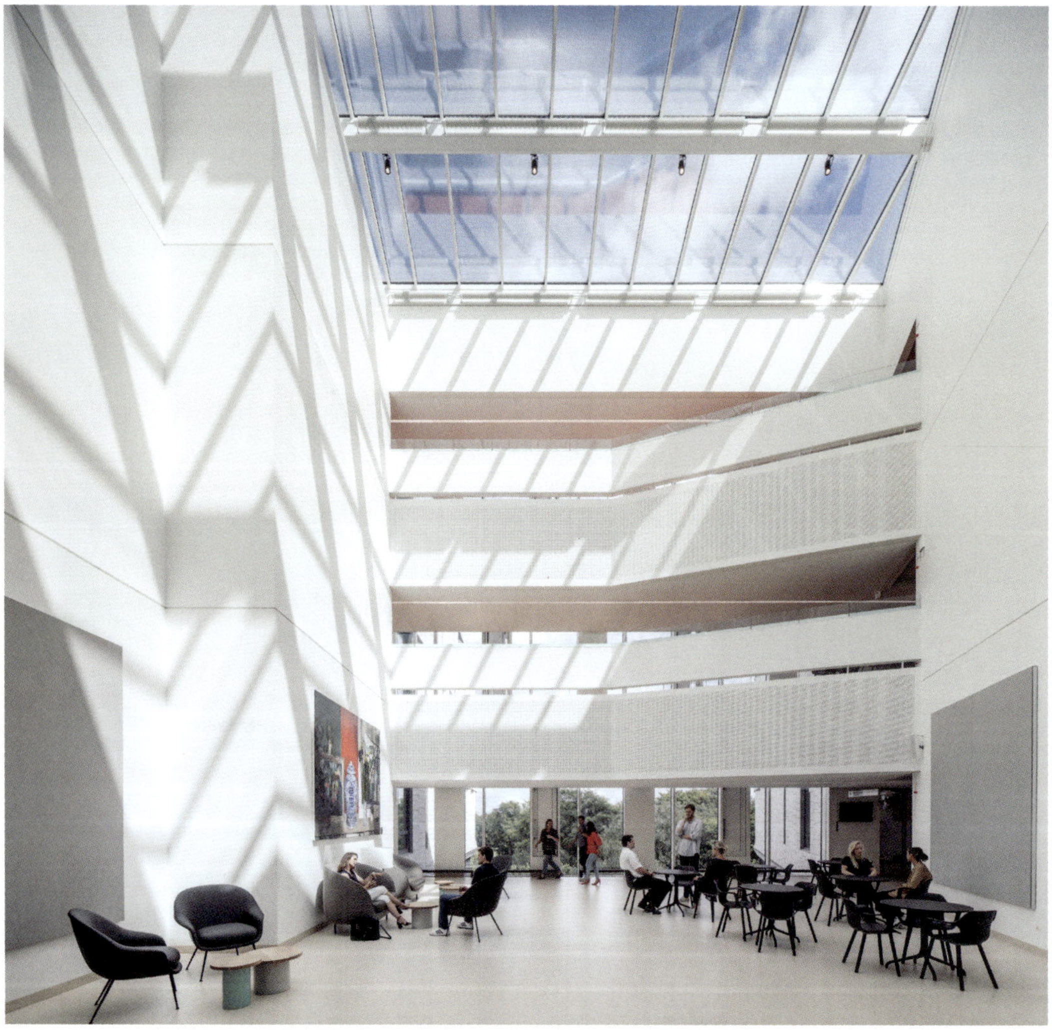

The design is based on simple principles that ensure flexibility and allow adaptation to future needs.

Roof glazing brings natural daylight into the waiting areas.

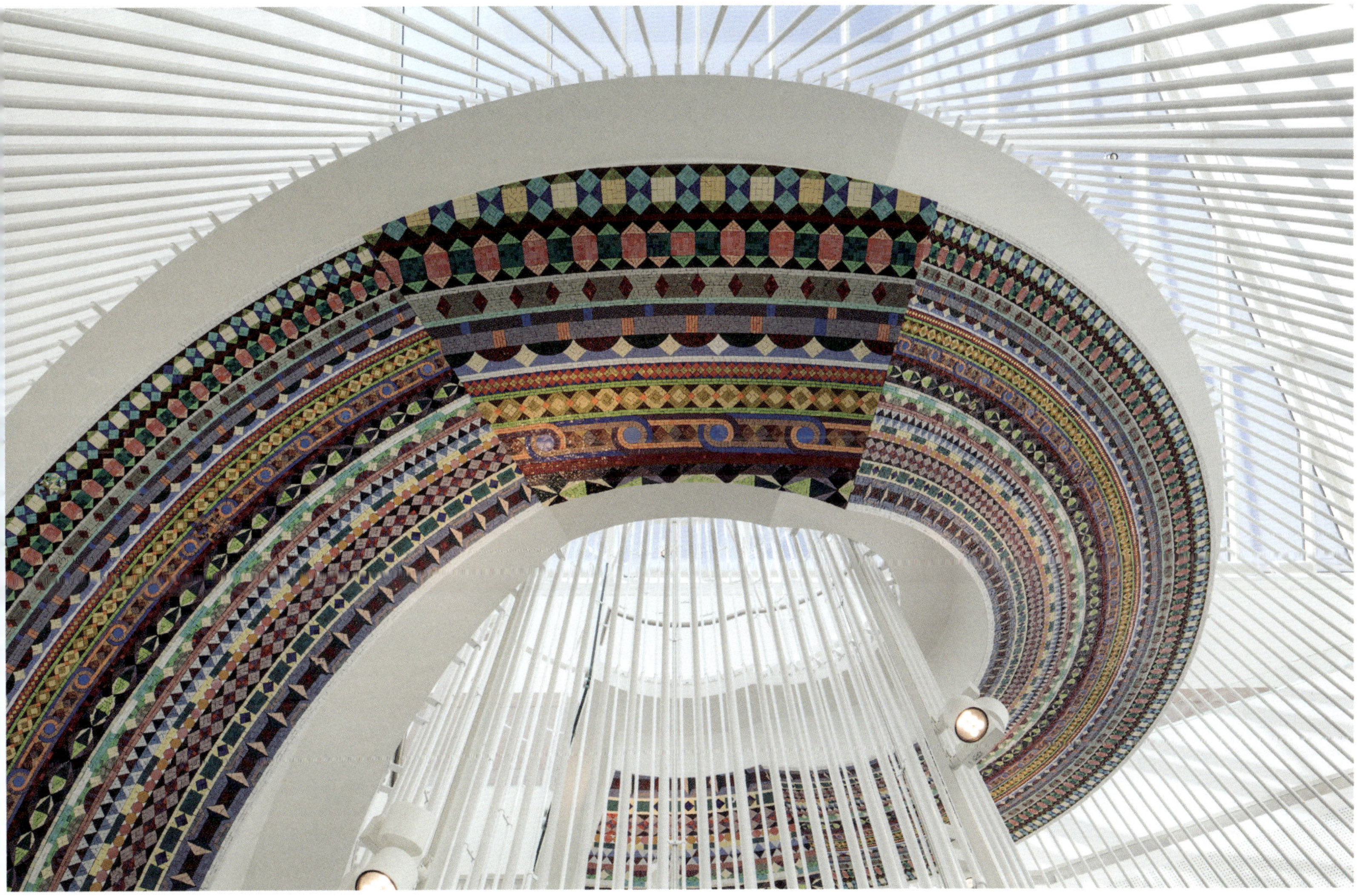

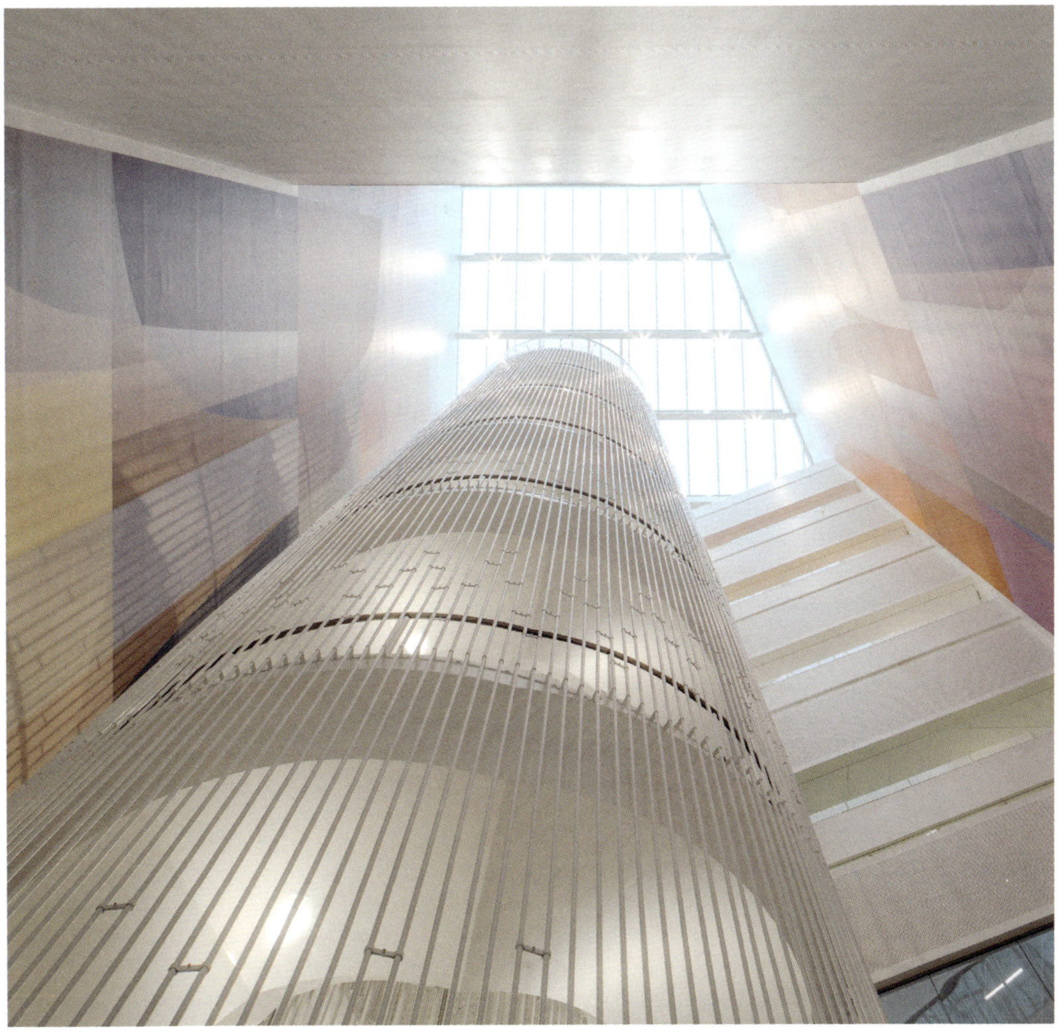

Erik A. Frandsen's mosaic decoration is located around the spiral staircase.

Malene Landgreen's 40-meter-high wall paintings add color to the building's design.

alsh sander.hofrichter architekten
H2M Architekten

Kulmbach
Germany

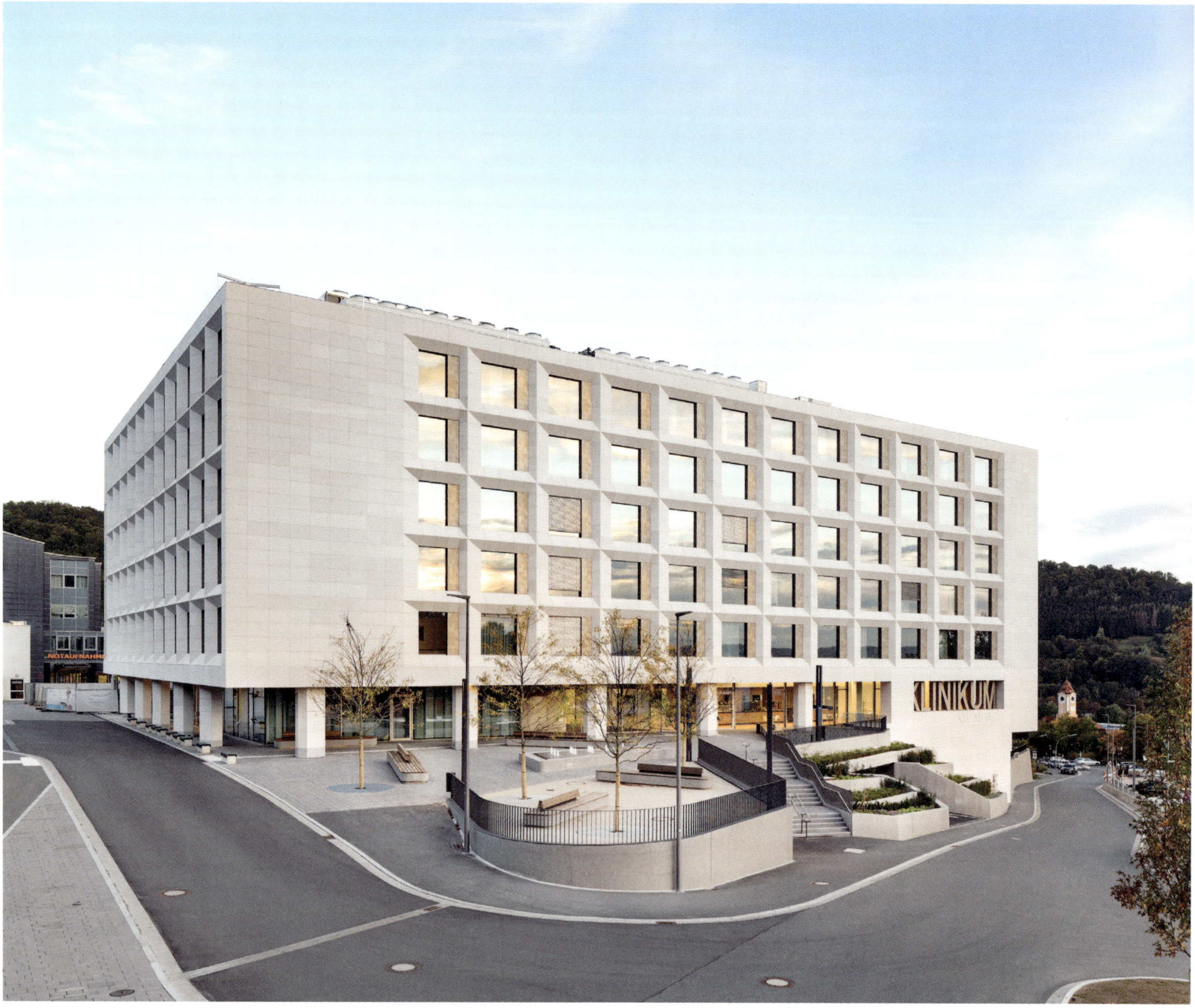

Hospital's bright, sculptural natural stone façade.

Inner courtyard with a deck.

Kulmbach Hospital

The hospital was developed as a double-ring structure through two strategically placed new wings, transforming the existing 1970s building into a modern hospital with short pathways. The new buildings, in conjunction with the existing structure, create modern care facilities: large, interconnected wards with single and double rooms allow for a high degree of flexibility in occupancy. Due to the steep slope, new diagnostic and therapy were created in the well-lit basements of the South New Building; the ring-shaped arrangement around the inner courtyard ensures optimal lighting. The existing ribbon façade is contrasted by a modern structural façade, which gives the building a light, striking appearance. Both inside and out, the use of natural materials – from wood surfaces to the natural stone façade – creates a cohesive, serene overall appearance that harmonizes with the surrounding landscape.

Address: Albert-Schweitzer-Straße 10, 95326 Kulmbach, Germany | **Client:** Zweckverband Klinikum Kulmbach | **Completion:** 2024 | **Size:** 36,700 m² | **Original building:** began operations in 1972 | **Sector:** other – City and District of Kulmbach | **Specialization:** municipal level II hospital | **Number of treatment rooms:** 61 | **Number of patient rooms:** 235

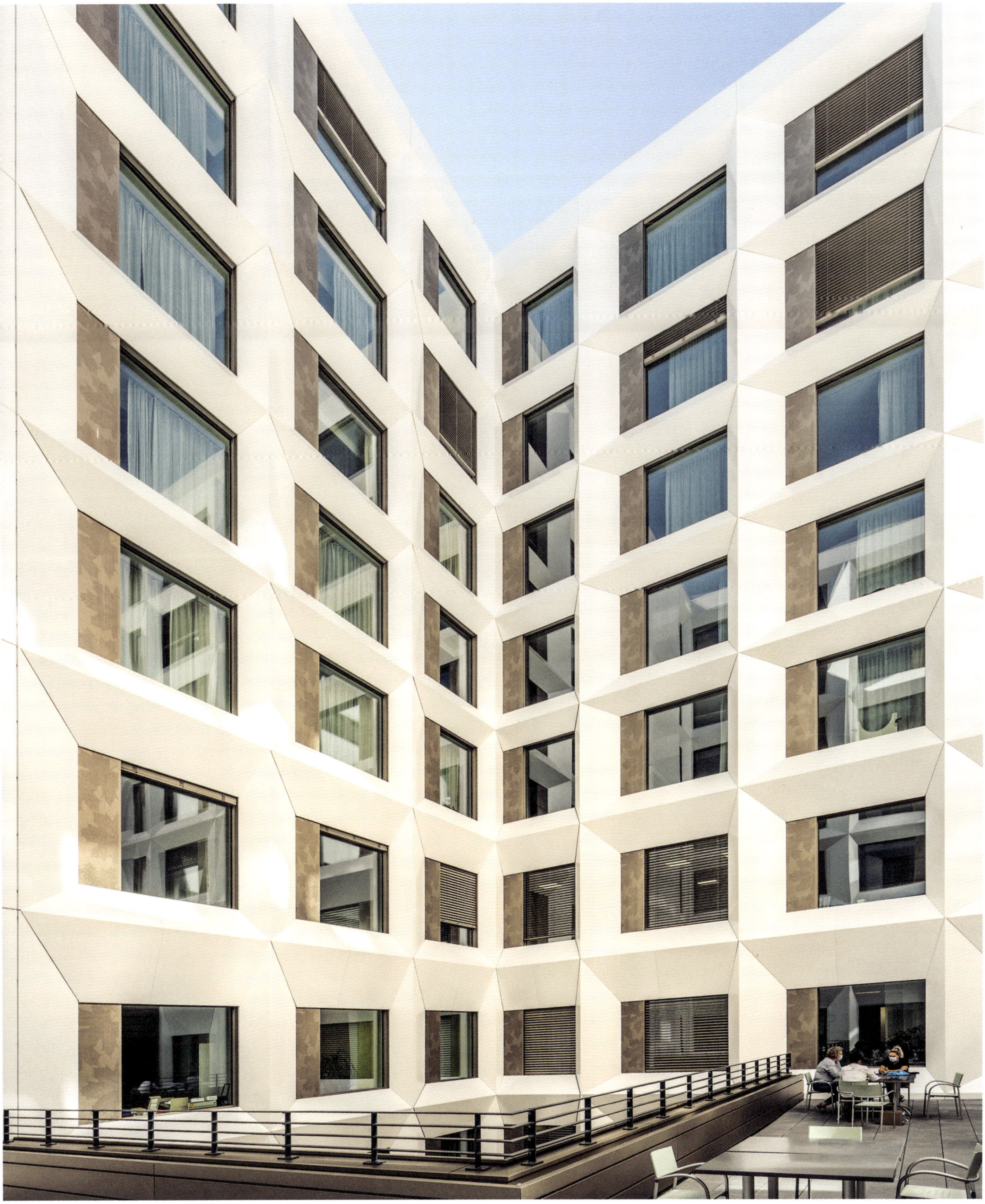

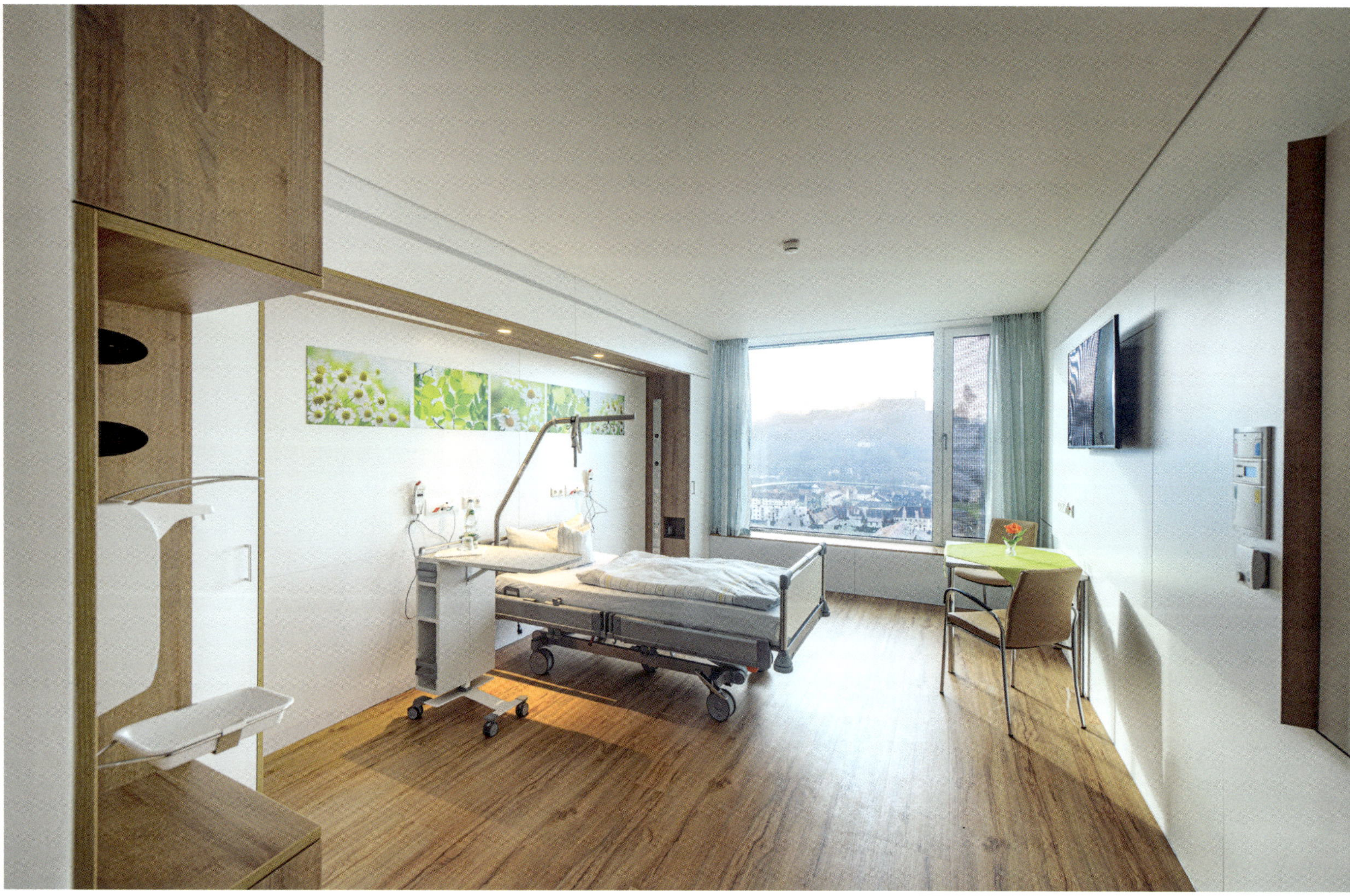

Patient's room with large, finely detailed panoramic window.

Ground floor plan.

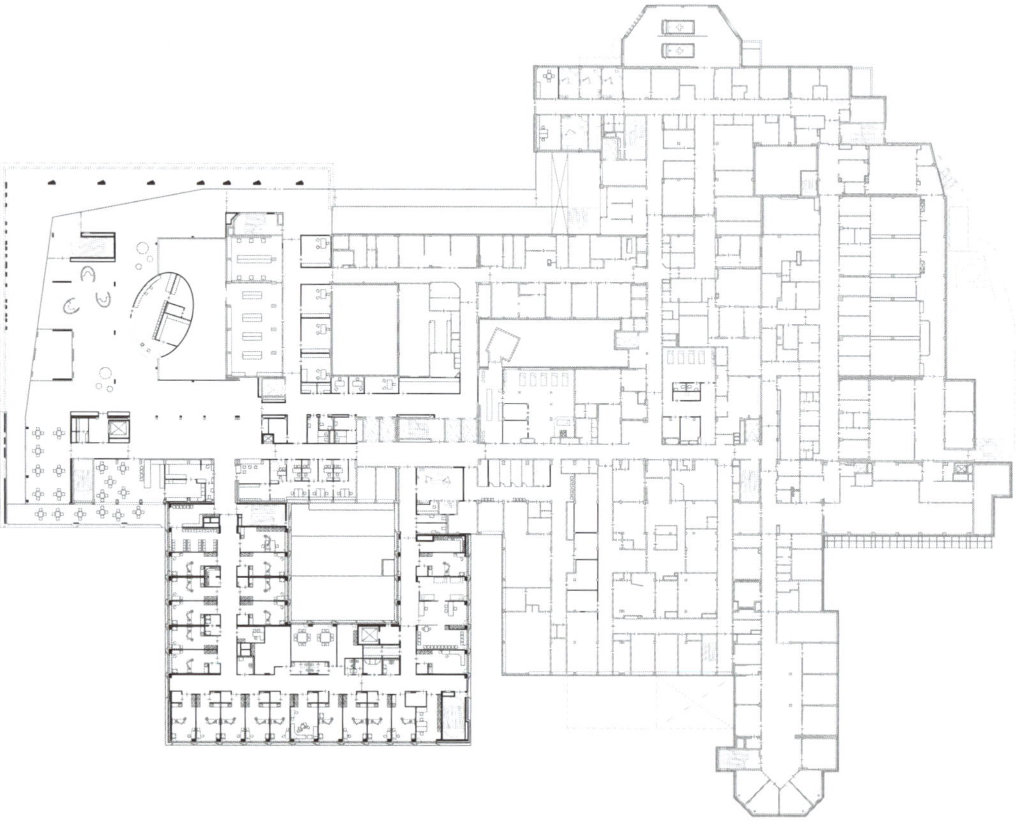

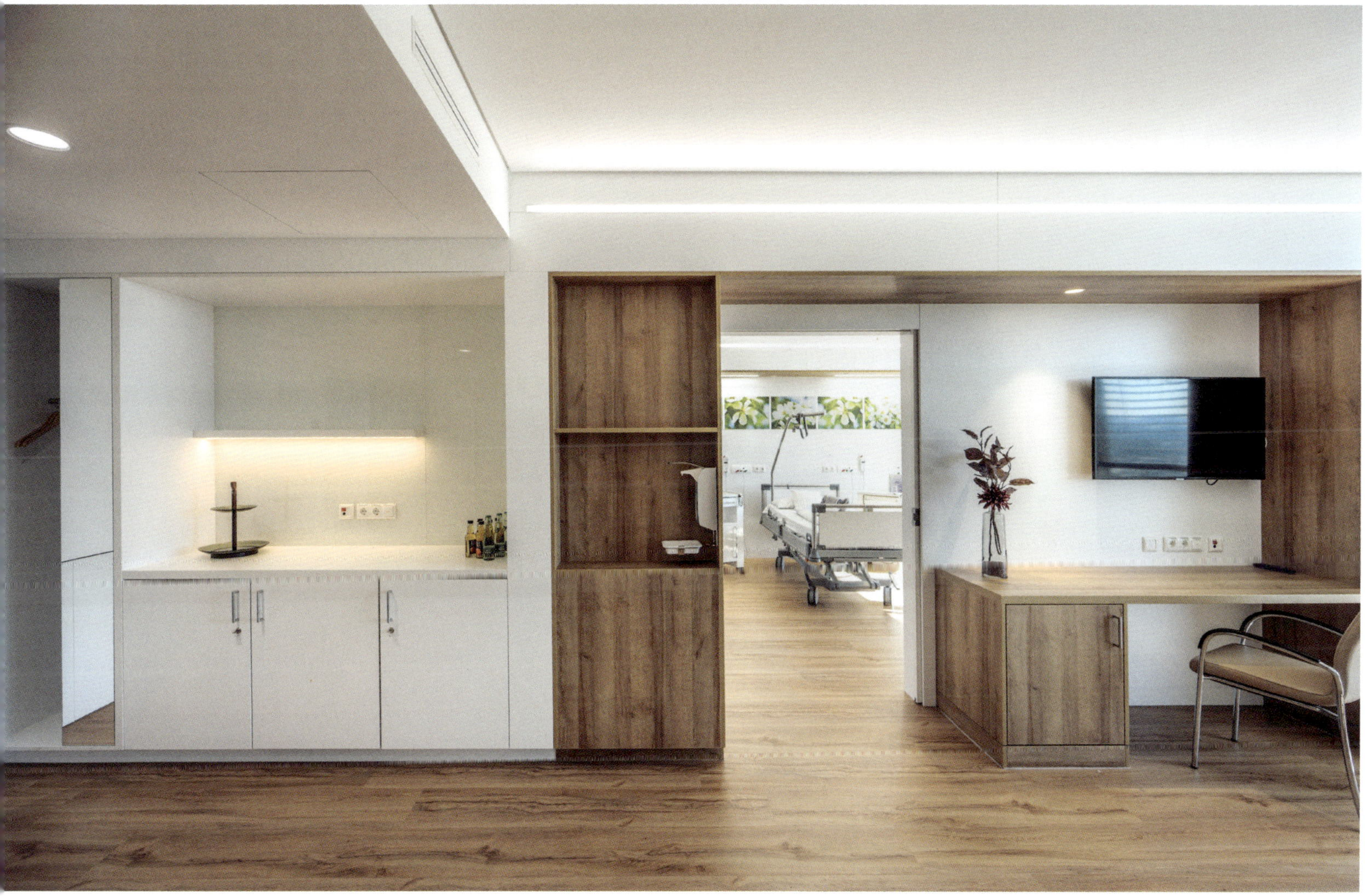

A feel-good atmosphere created by natural materials.

First floor plan.

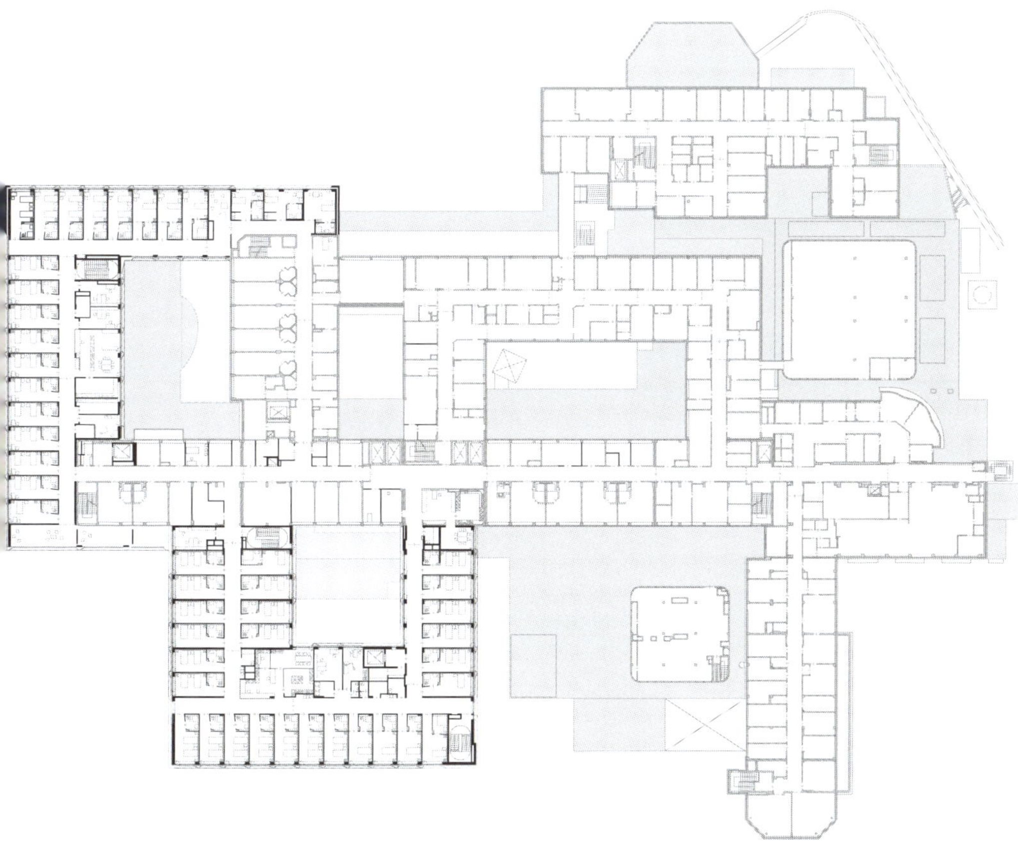

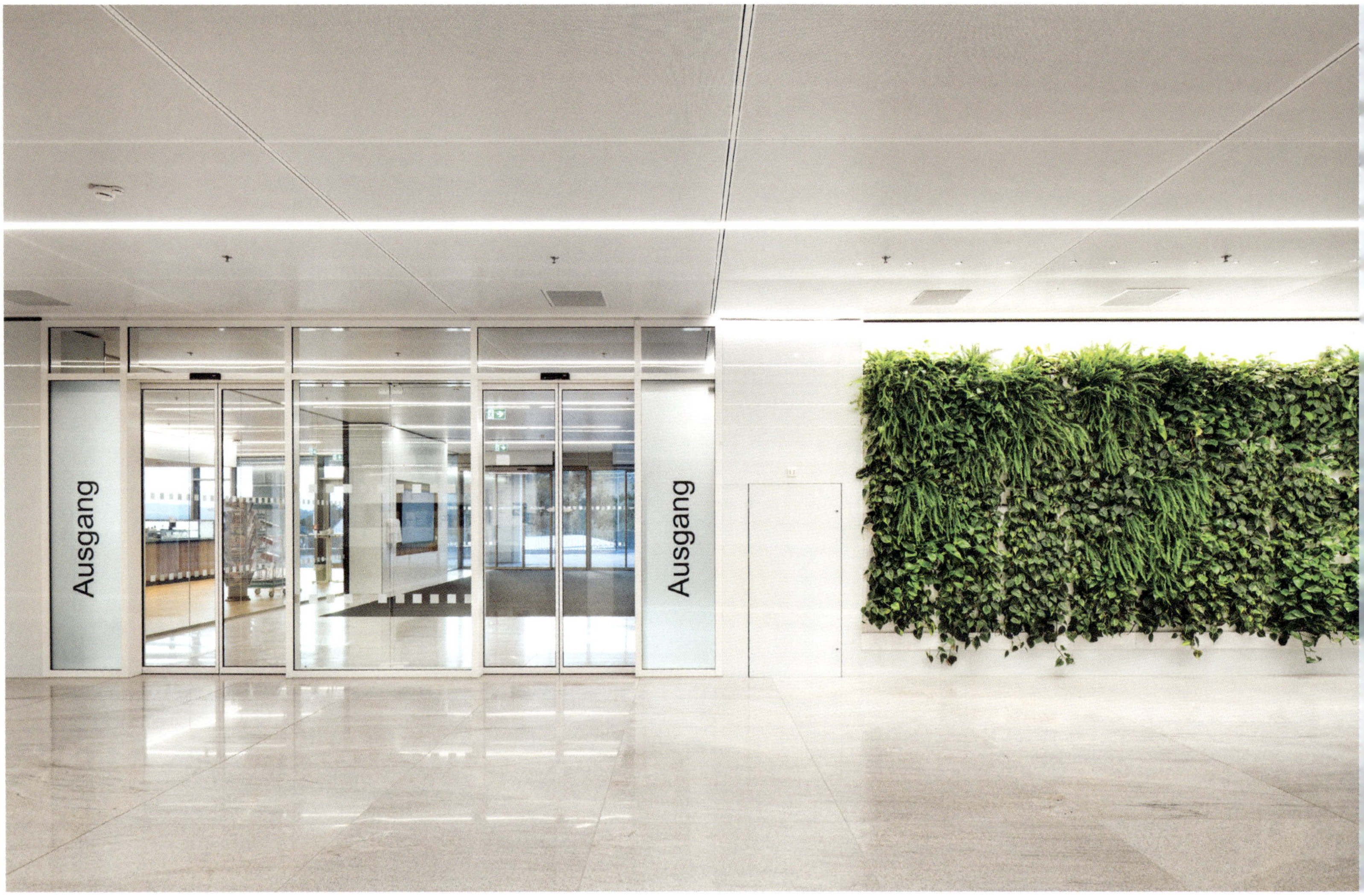

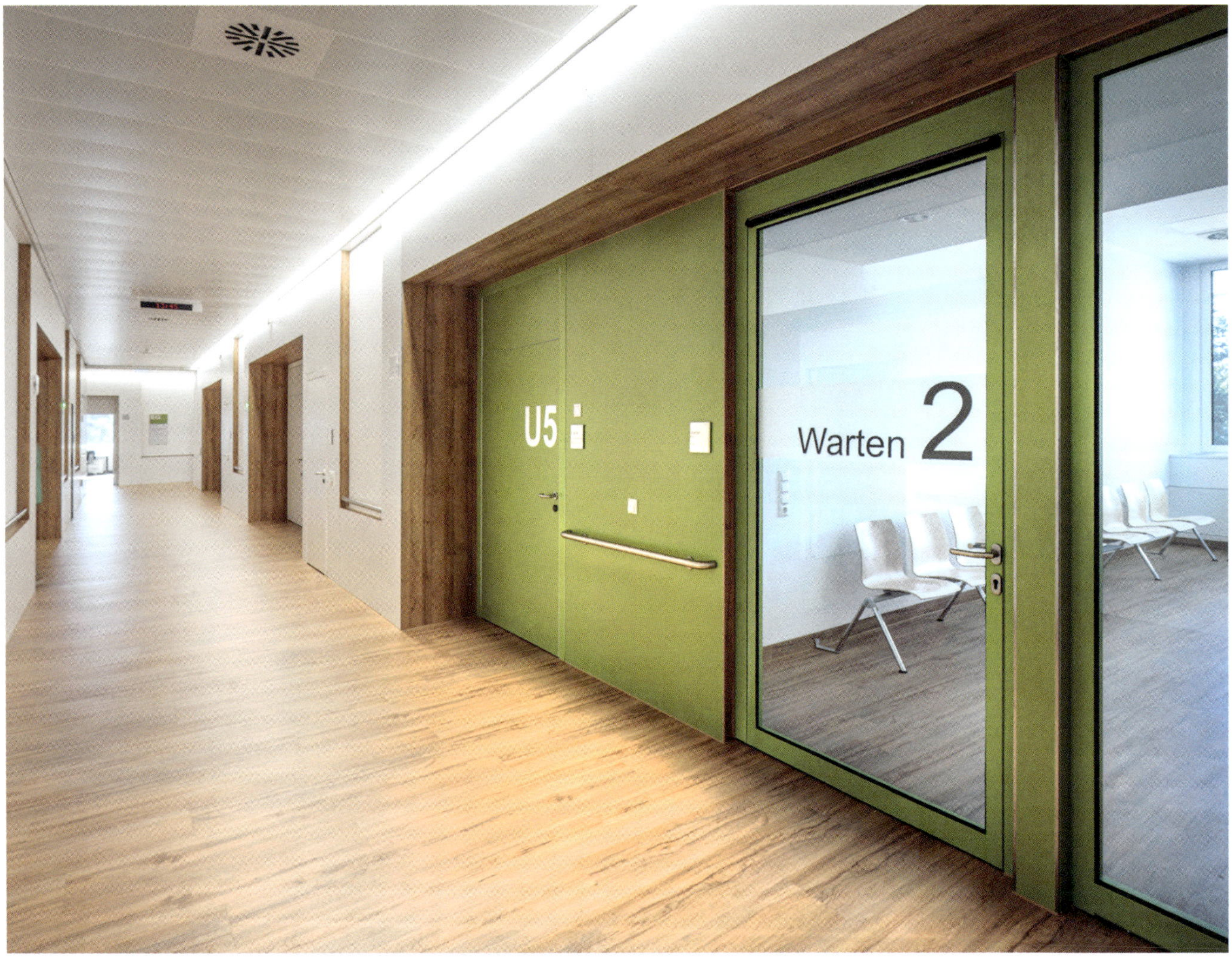

The bright and attractive new entrance area.

Spacious inner corridor with waiting room.

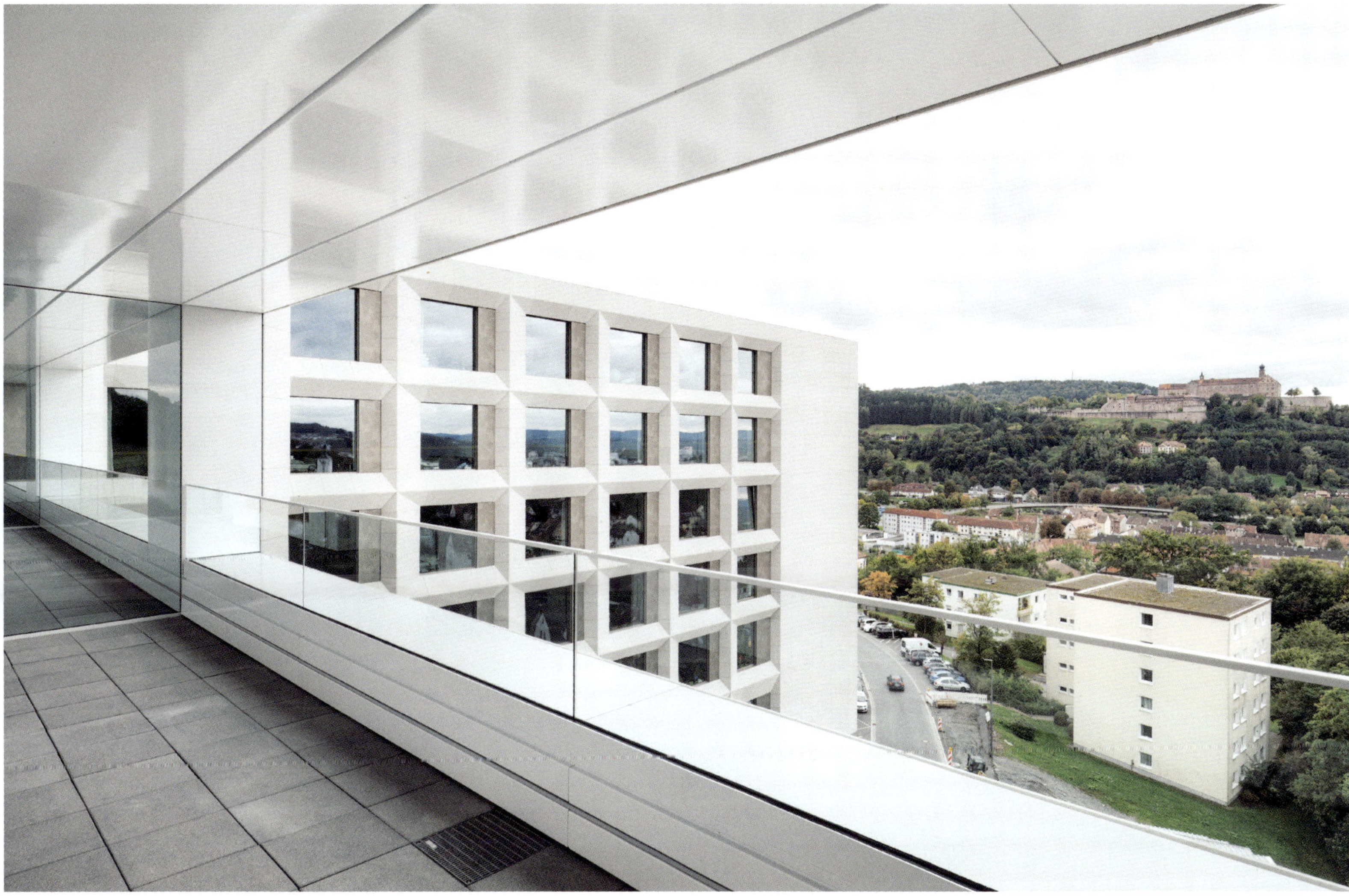

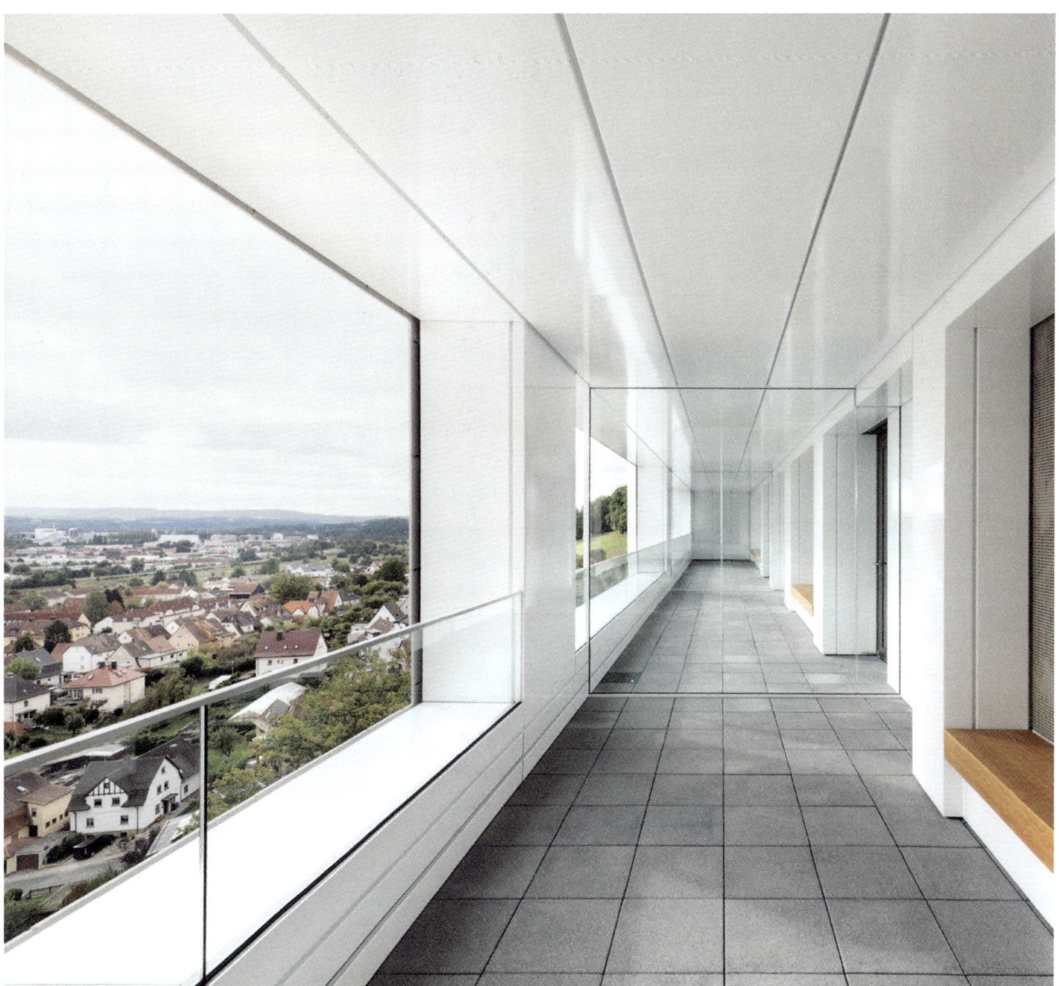

Beautiful view of Kulmbach's Plassenburg.

Serene views of the city and surrounding from the exterior hospital passages.

Nickl & Partner Architectural Design Consulting (Beijing) Ltd.

Shenzhen China

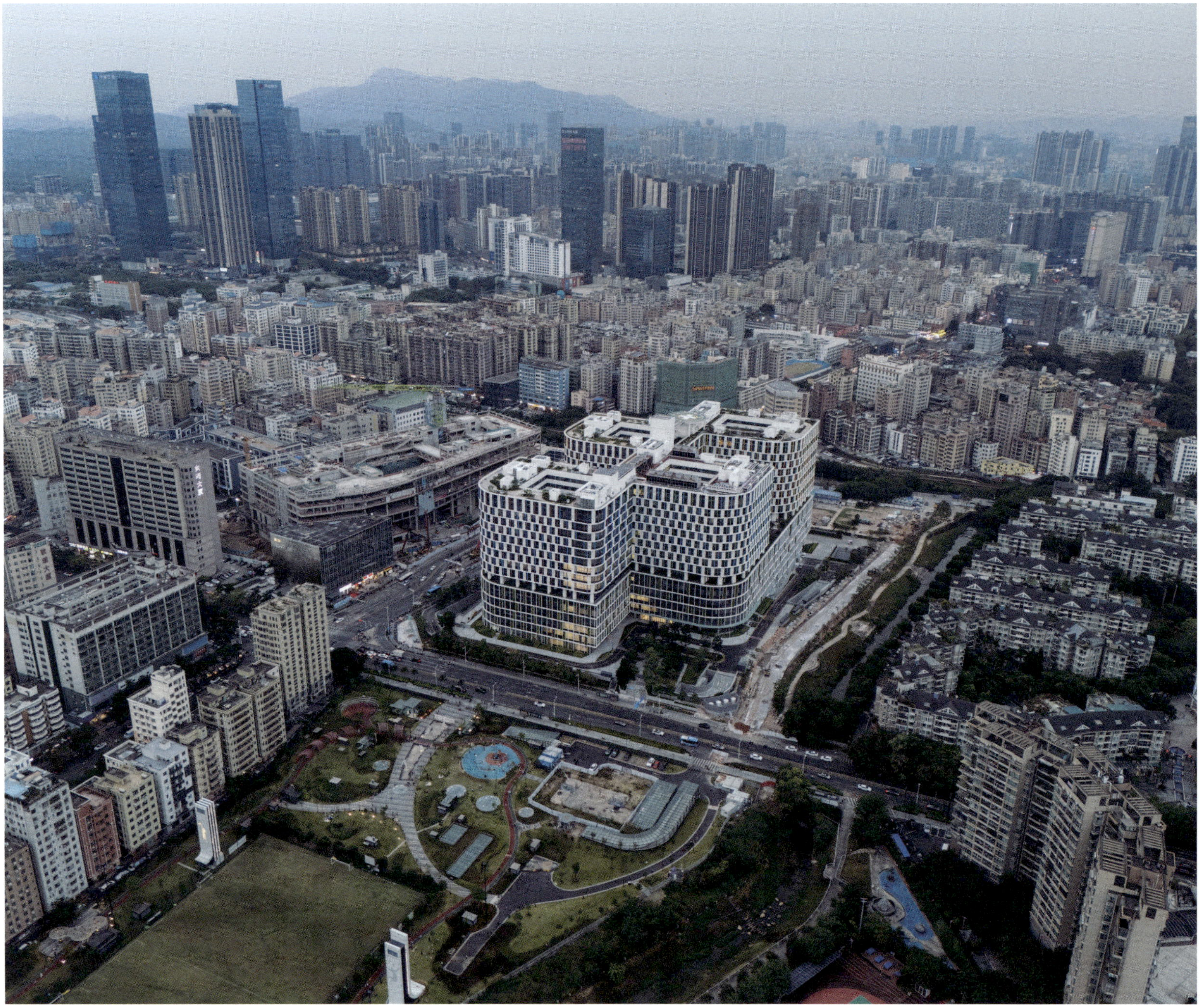

Shenzhen Children's Hospital Longhua Campus

Hospital as a healing mega structure within the city.

The design is reinforced by a coordinated façade and a strong structural grid.

Healing playground for children on intermediate level.

The Shenzhen Children's Hospital Longhua Campus is a milestone for healthcare in the vibrant metropolis of Shenzhen. With a capacity of 1,500 beds, it sets new standards in pediatric care, emphasizing the integration of health and innovation at the highest level. The hospital's size, double that of the previous Futian campus, and its seamless connection to the urban infrastructure through the Minzhi subway station, highlights the close relationship between architecture and urban life. The 360,000-square-meter facility integrates state-of-the-art functions for medicine, science, research, and education. With a daily outpatient volume of up to 10,000 patients, the hospital responds to the growing demand and significantly reduces waiting times – an authentic model for the future of medical efficiency.

Address: No. 7019 Yitian Road, Lianhua Subdistrict, Futian District, Shenzhen, Guangdong Province, China | **Client:** Shenzhen Municipal Bureau of Construction and Public Works | **Completion:** 2025 | **Size:** 360,000 m^2 | **Sector:** public | **Specialization:** pediatric care | **Number of treatment rooms:** 150 | **Number of patient rooms:** 1,500

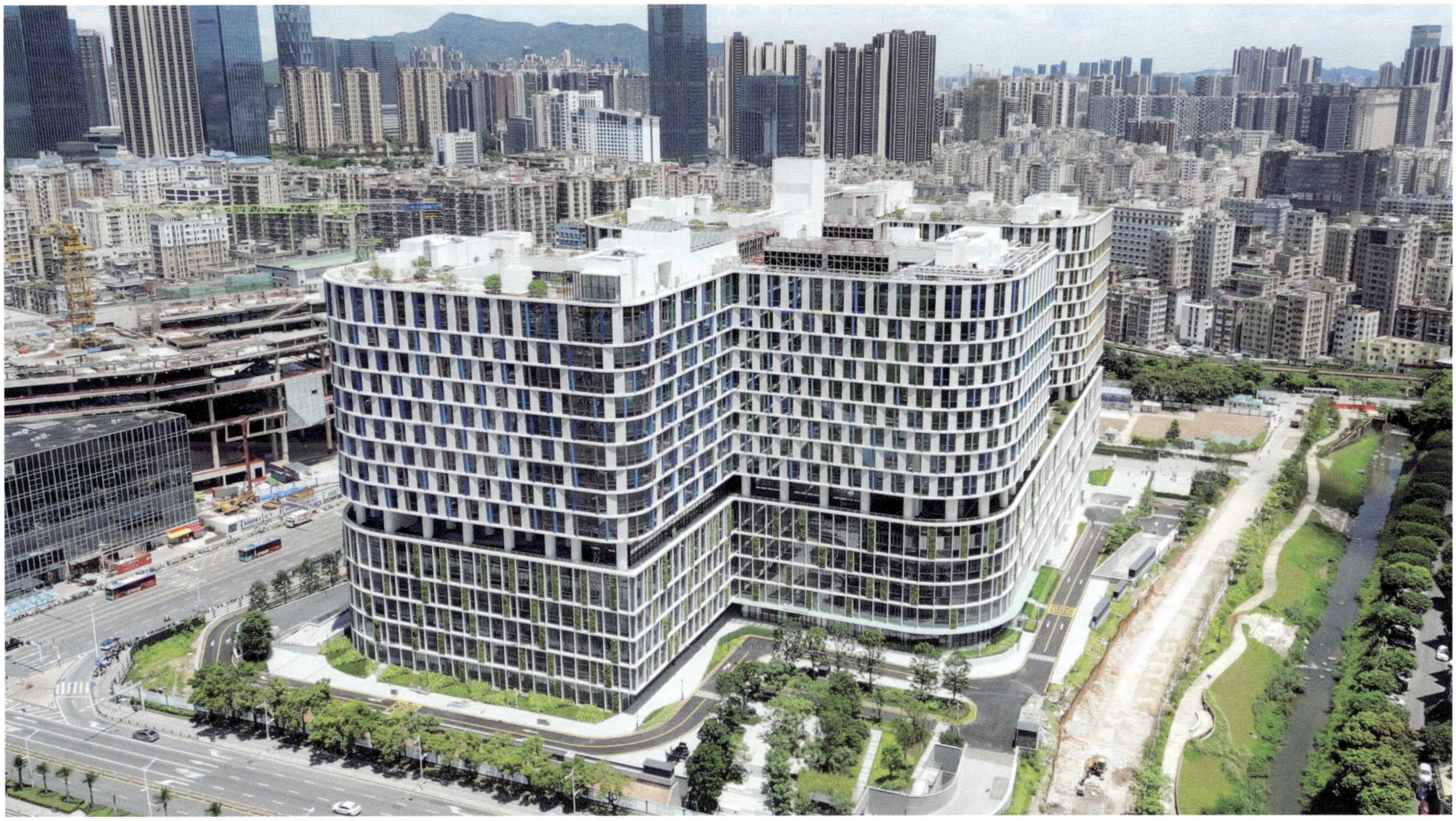

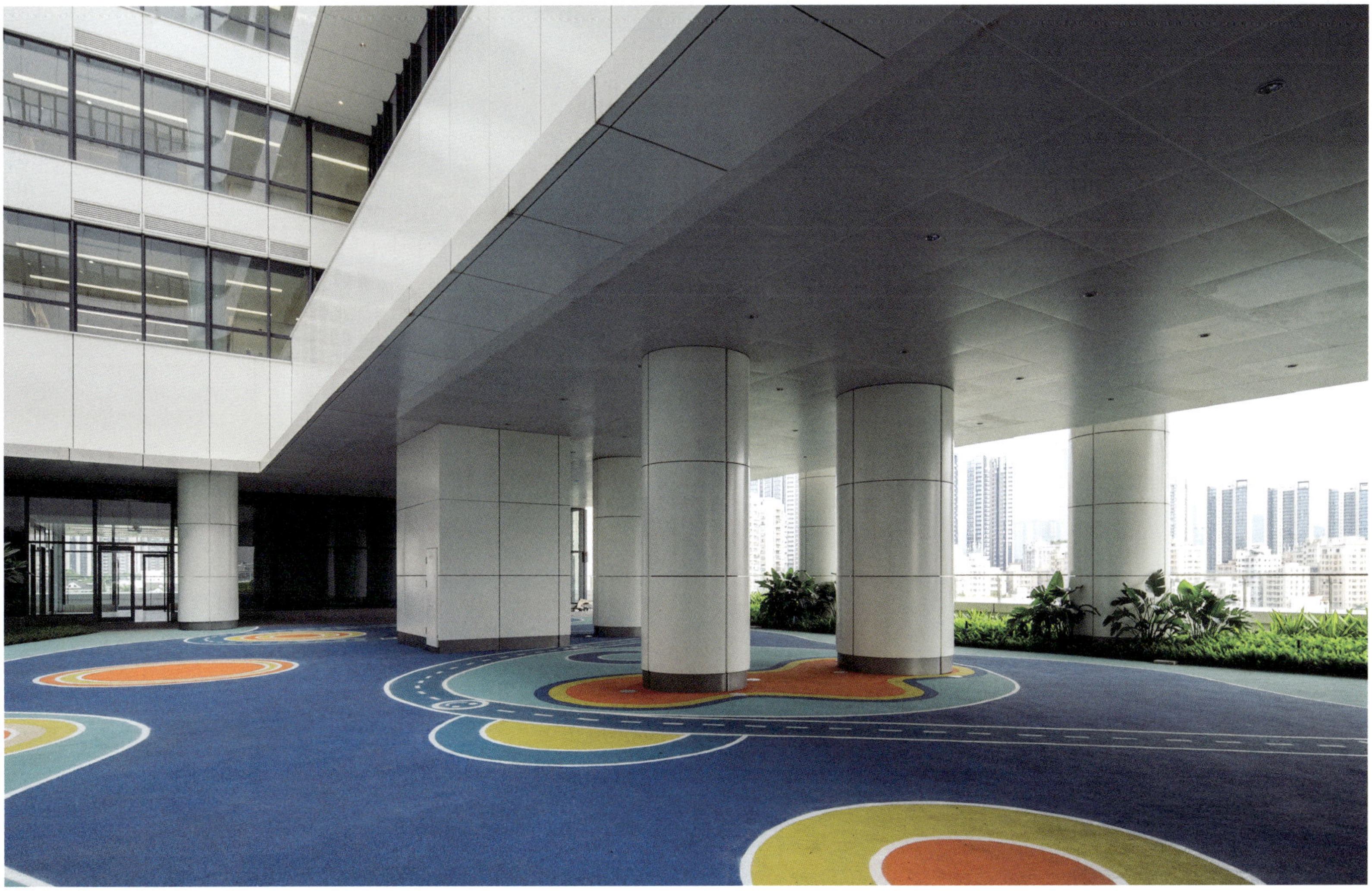

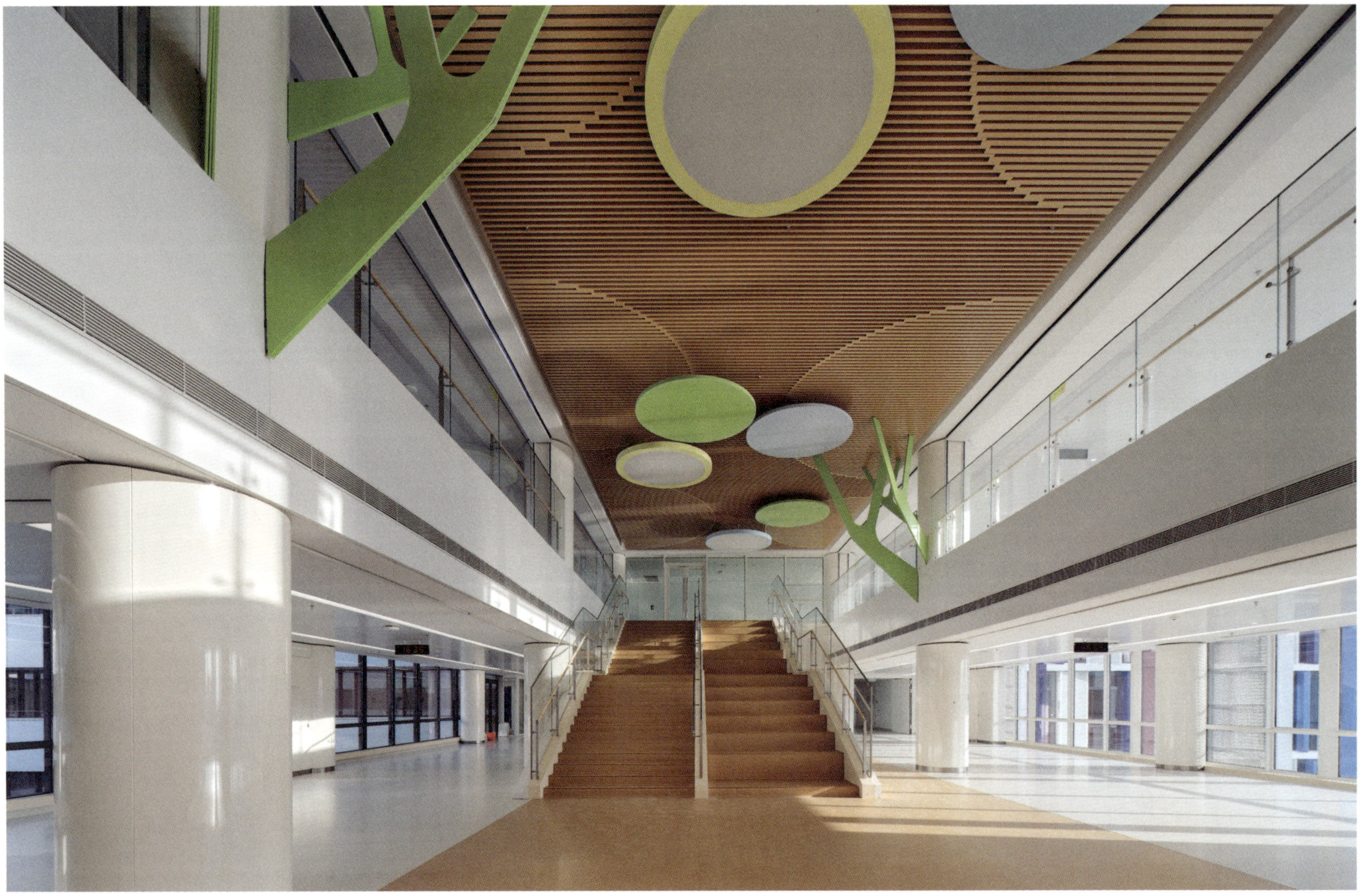

Interior spaces are designed at a child-friendly scale, with abundant daylight, warm colors, and intuitive orientation.

Ground floor plan.

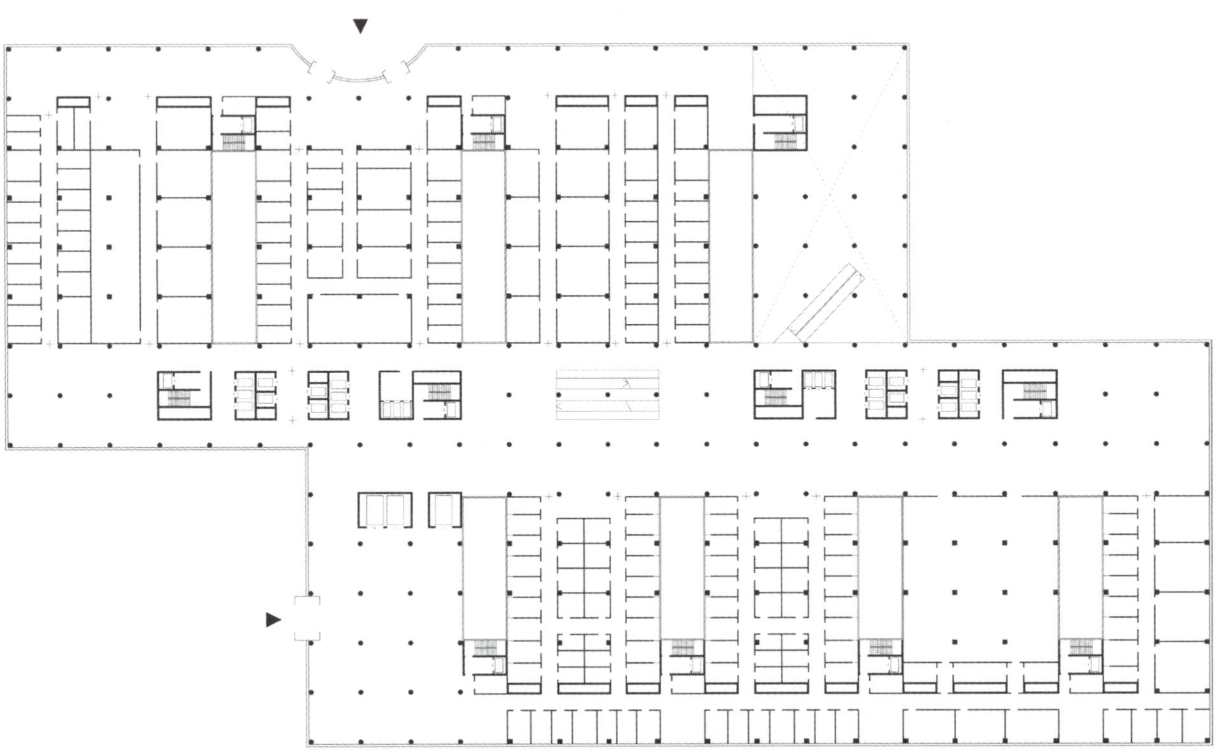

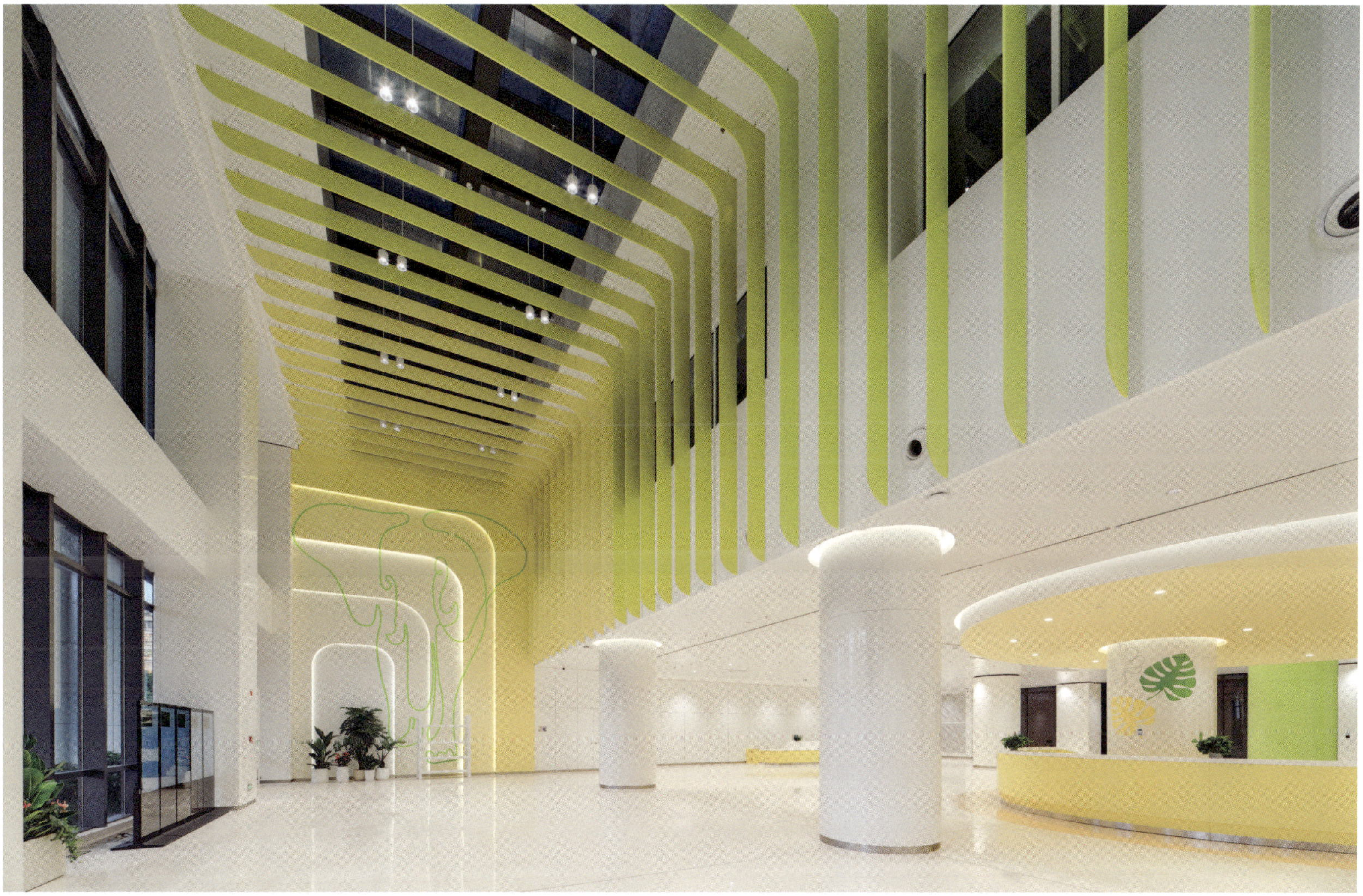

Structural and spatial frameworks enable reconfiguration and expansion without disrupting ongoing hospital operations.

Explosion.

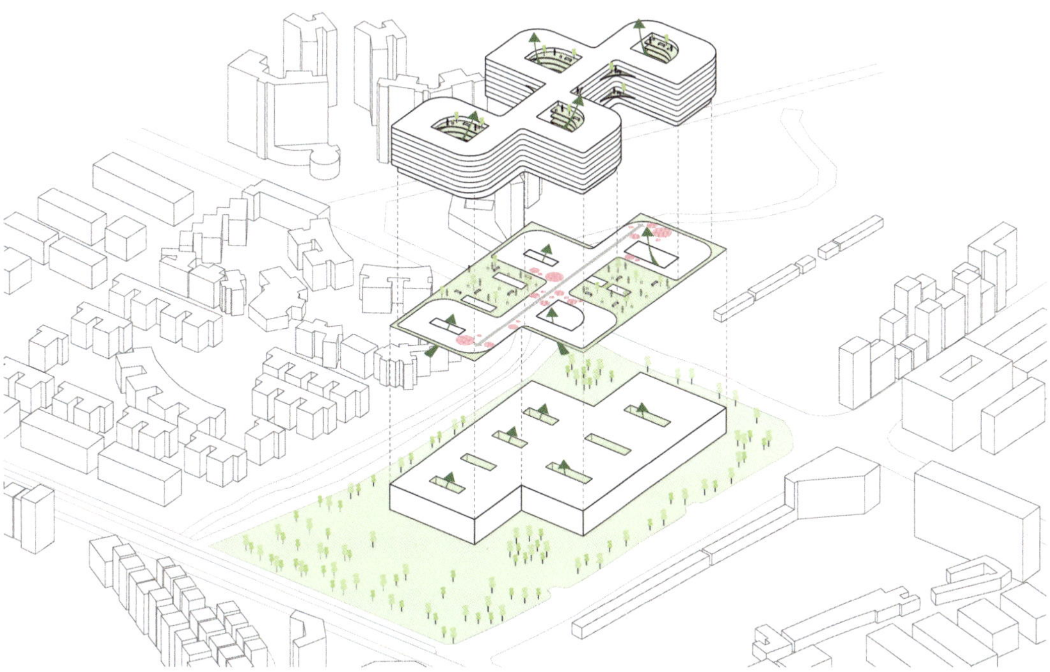

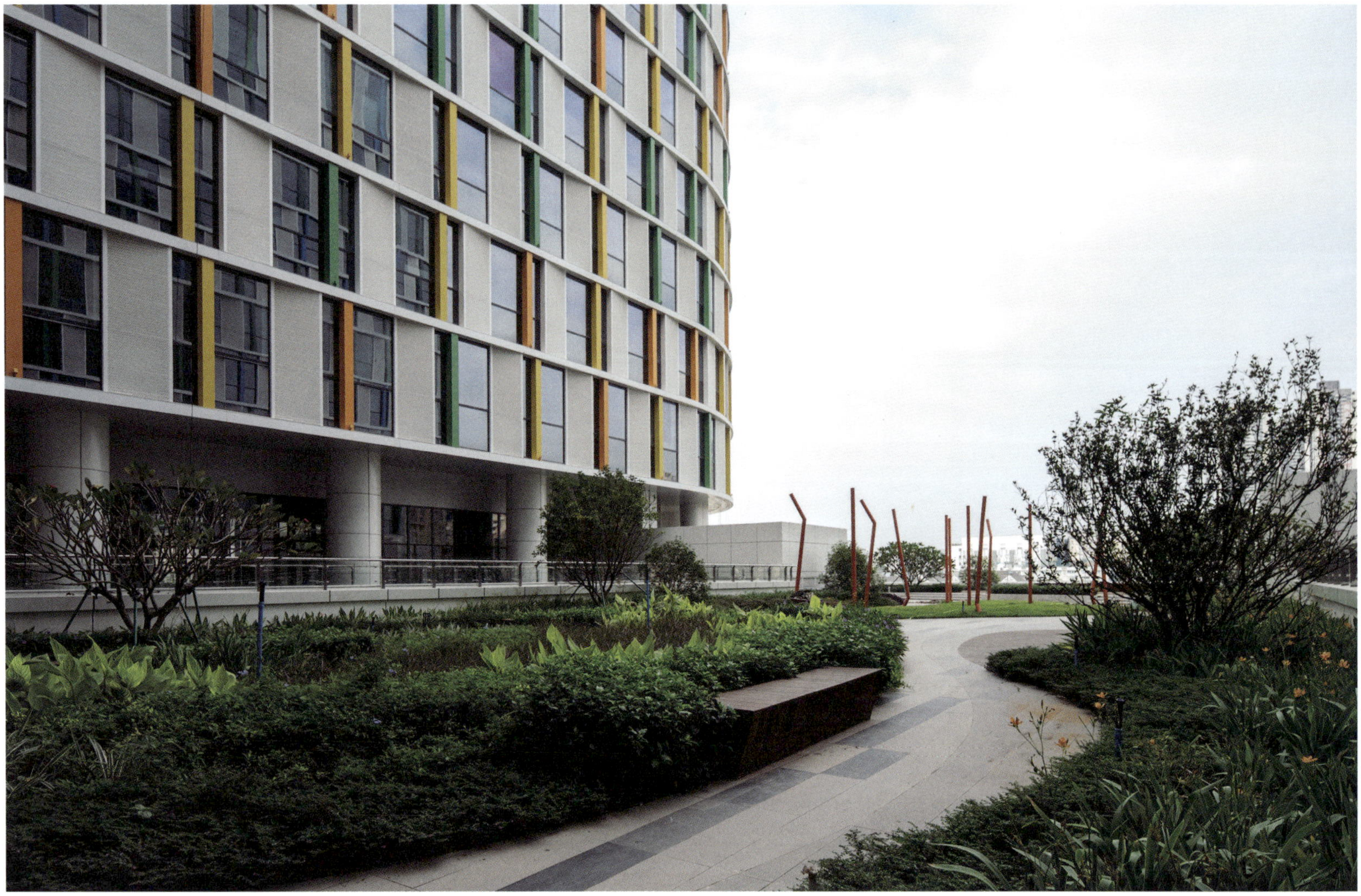

Courtyards, atria, and views to greenery support emotional wellbeing for patients, families, and staff.

Solar cycle.

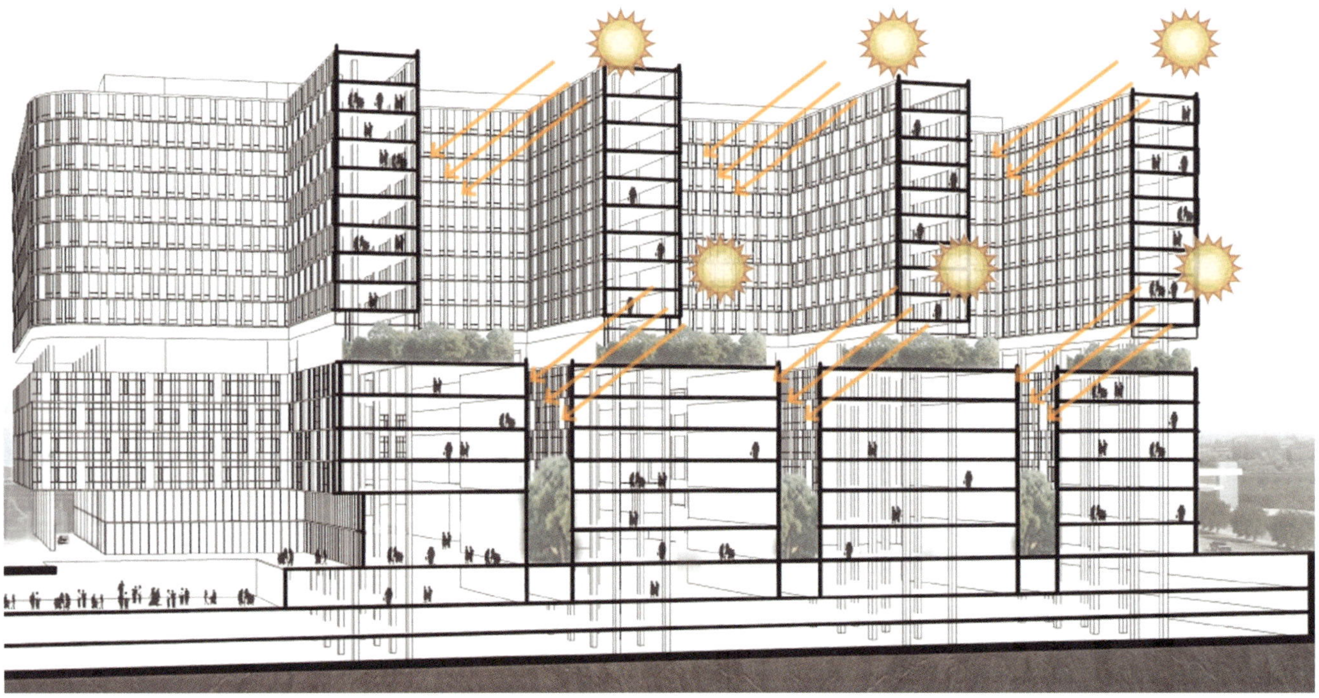

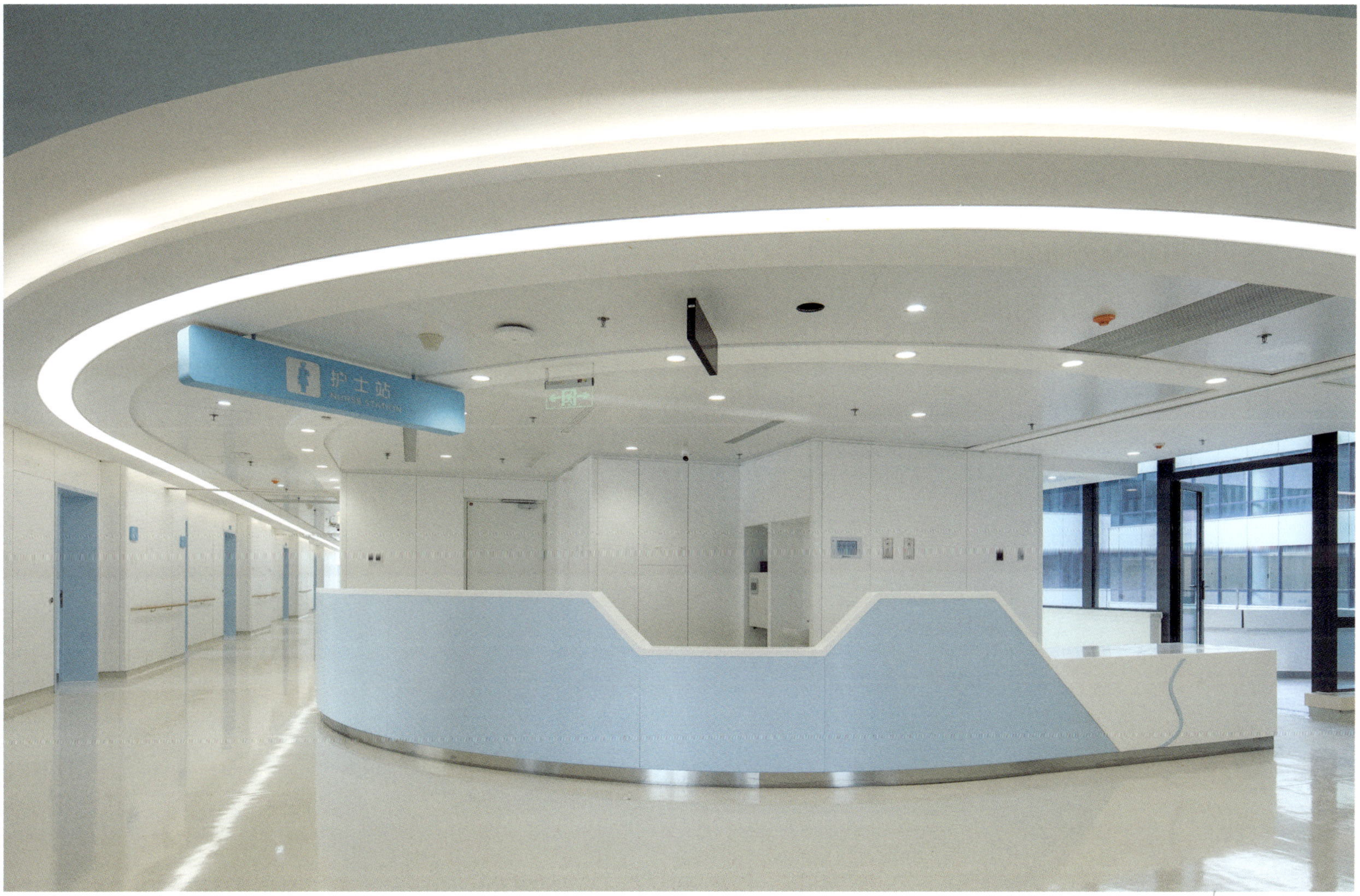

Operational performance is enhanced through the clear separation of public, clinical, and service zones, ensuring privacy, dignity, and infection control.

Section.

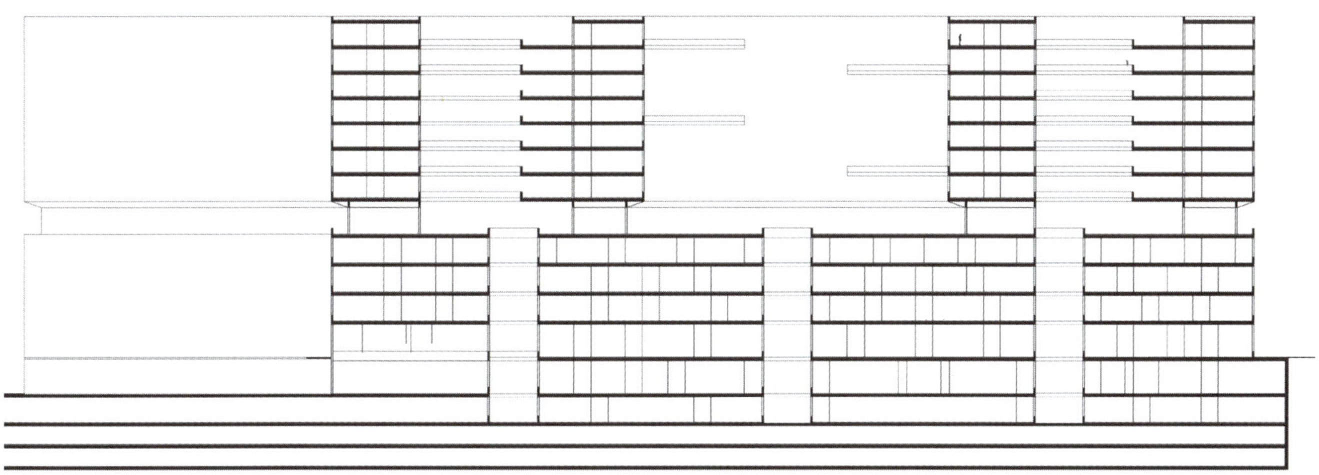

Krampe Schmidt Architekten

Gelsenkirchen Germany

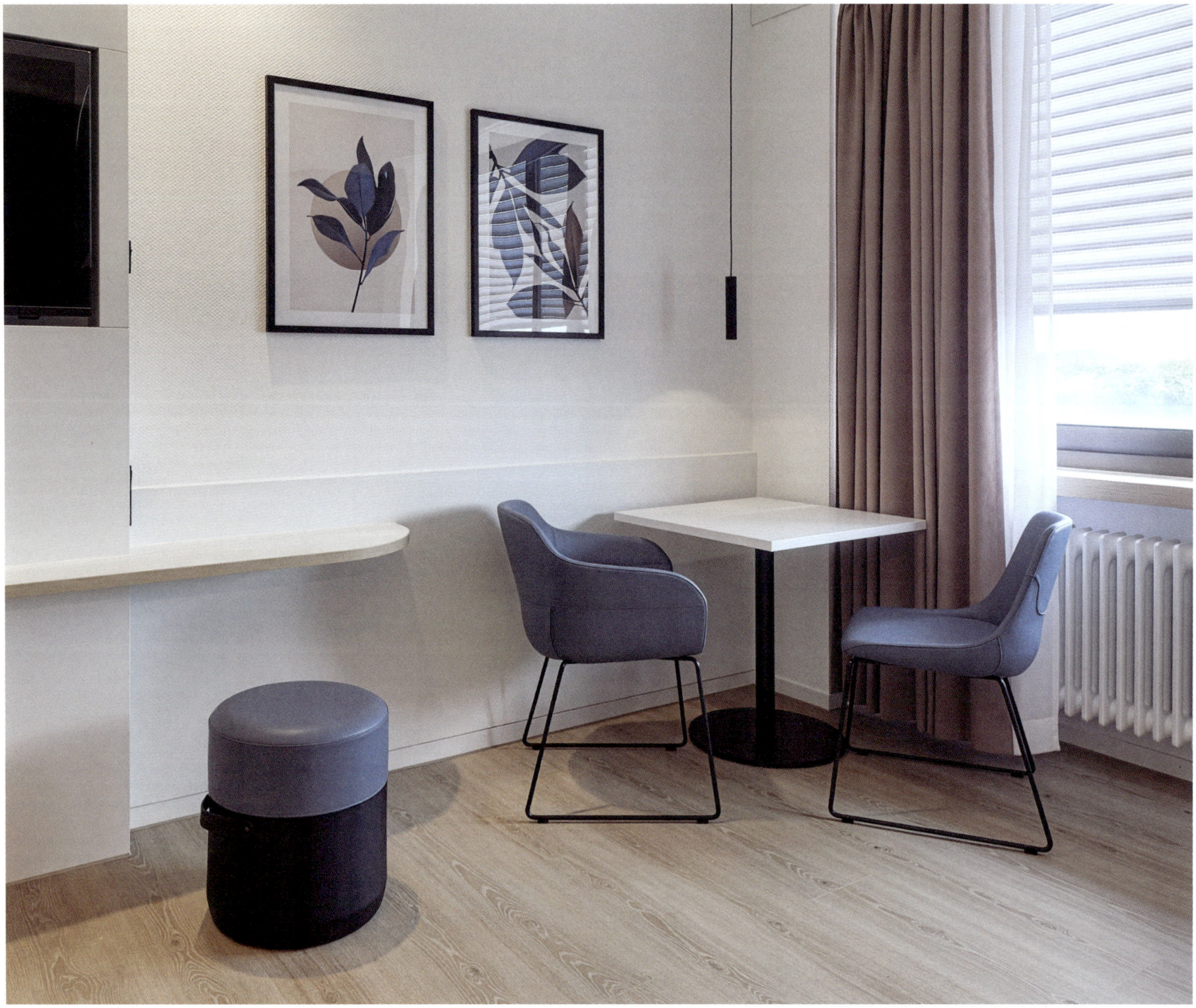

Patient rooms' sitting areas offer views of greenery and plenty of natural light.

The nursing supply cabinet provides quick and efficient access to medical items.

Private Patient Unit Marienhospital Gelsenkirchen

Krampe Schmidt Architekten converted the top patient floor of the 1970s-era Marienhospital Gelsenkirchen into a private patient unit – featuring a contemporary, clearly structured spatial and design concept. A striking color scheme, inspired by the original blue of the exterior façade, defines the identity of the space and aids in wayfinding. Light-colored materials, wood finishes, and warm lighting create a calm, hotel-like atmosphere. Open areas such as the patient lobby and nursing station promote communication and enhance the quality of the patient experience. The rooms combine functionality with home-like comfort and each of them features separate bathroom and toilet areas. To achieve this, the old prefabricated wet rooms were preserved in an environmentally conscious manner and adapted to today's comfort standards. The blue theme has been carried through in the custom-designed bathroom fixtures.

Address: Virchowstraße 122, 45886 Gelsenkirchen, Germany | **Client:** KERN – Katholische Einrichtungen Ruhrgebiet Nord GmbH | **Completion:** 2024 | **Size:** 2,000 m² | **Original building:** Nikolaus Rosiny, 1978 | **Sector:** ecclesiastical | **Specialization:** acute care and trauma | **Number of patient rooms:** 32

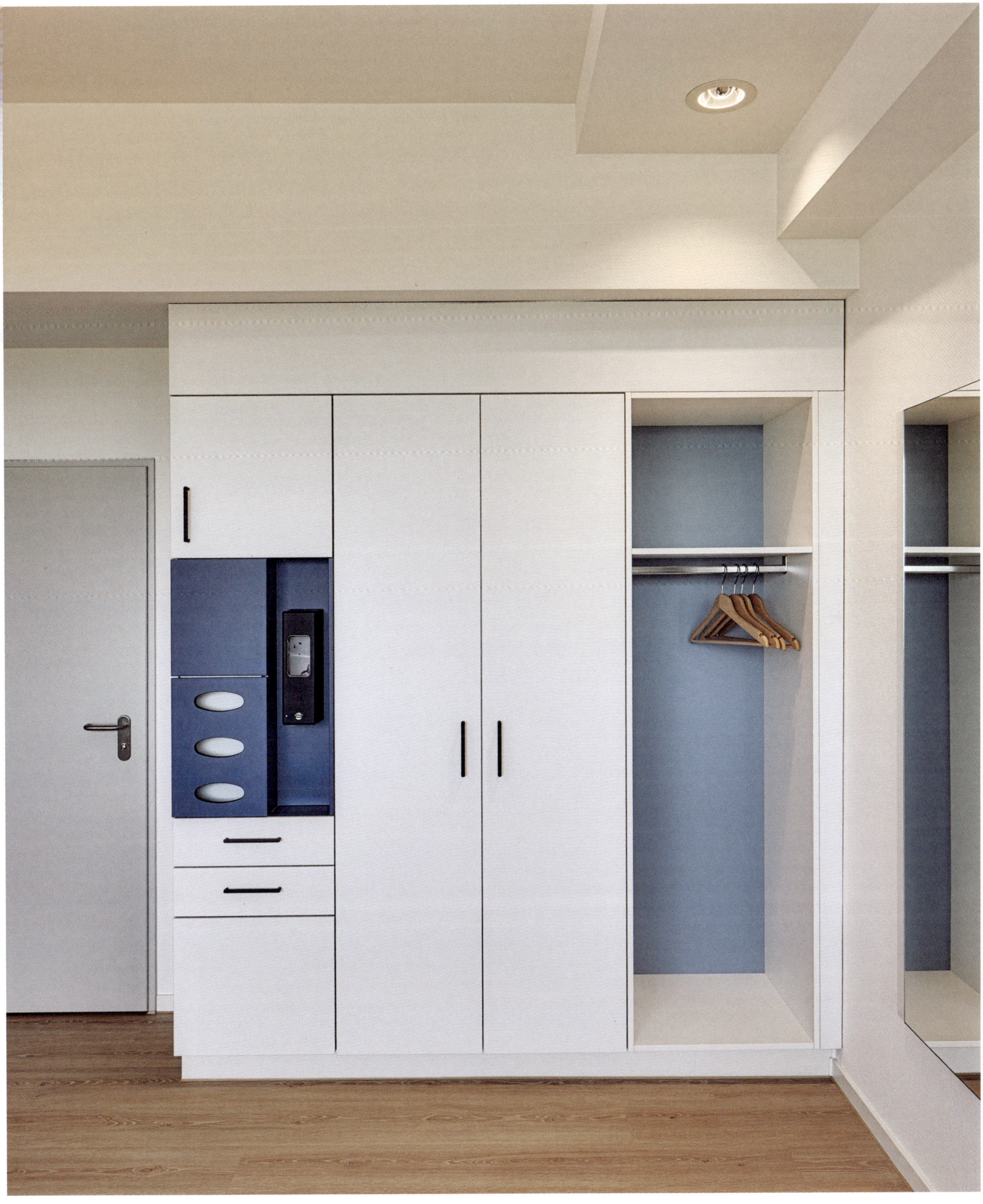

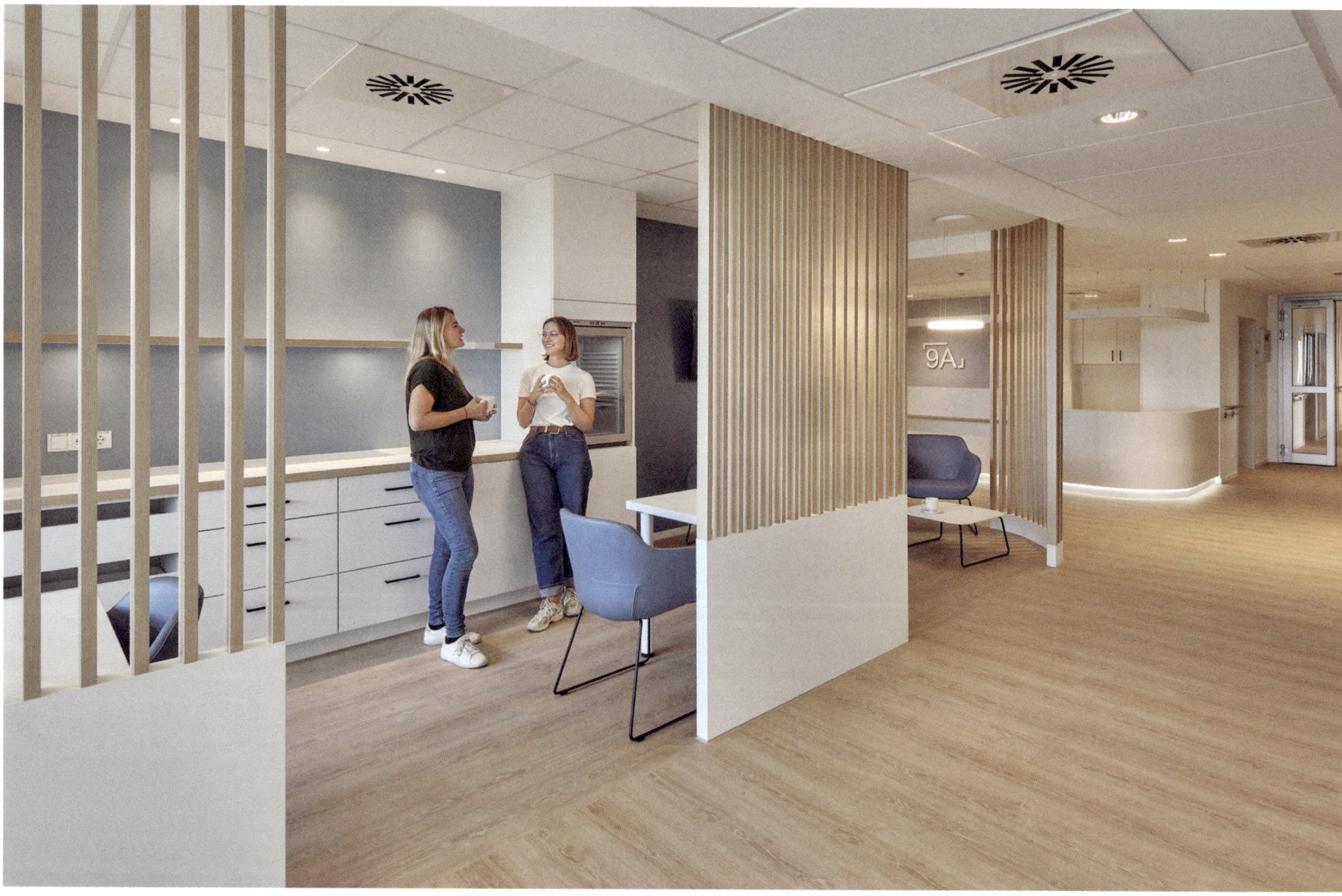

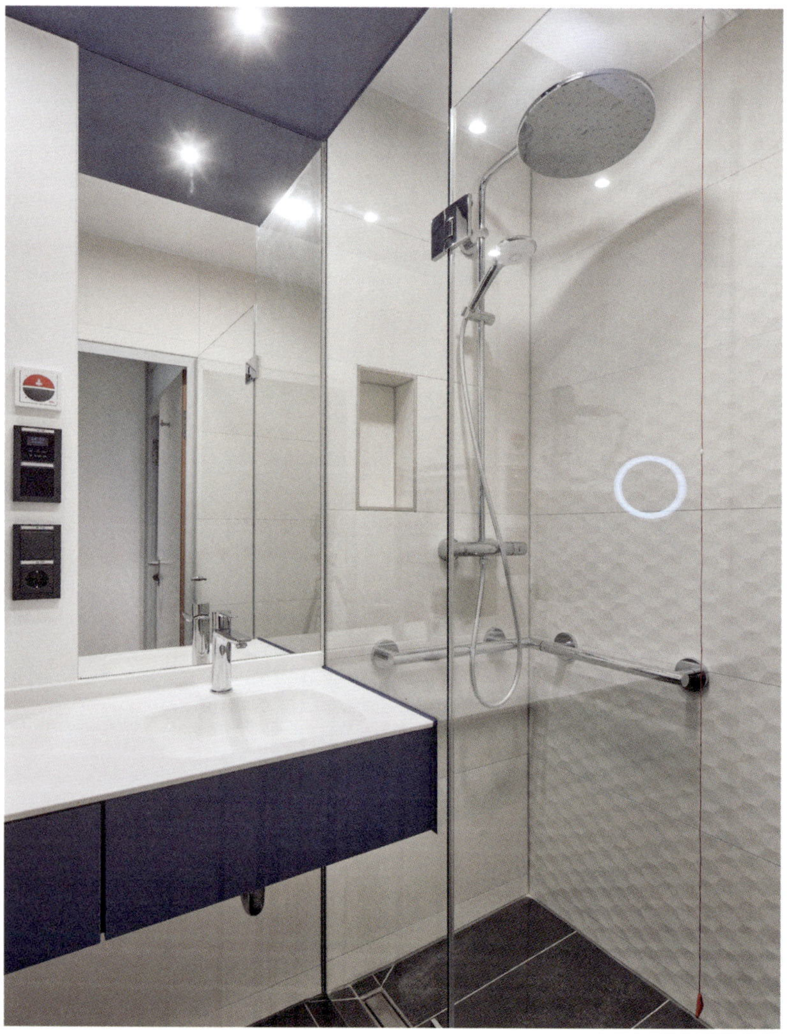

Open-concept patient lobby with coffee service in welcoming atmosphere.

The old wet rooms were preserved but equipped with modern features.

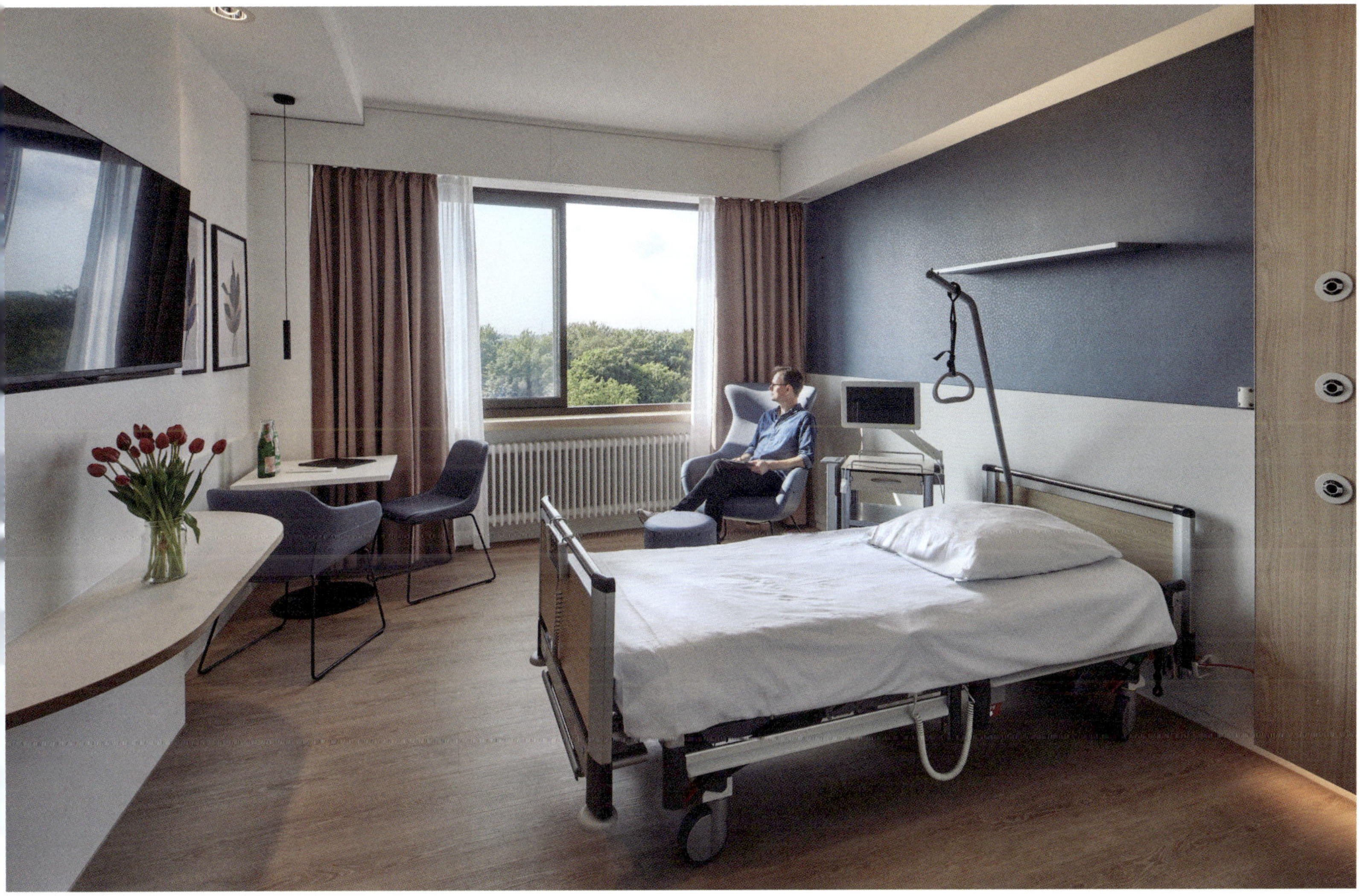

Light colors and wood finishes create a soothing atmosphere.

Floor plan.

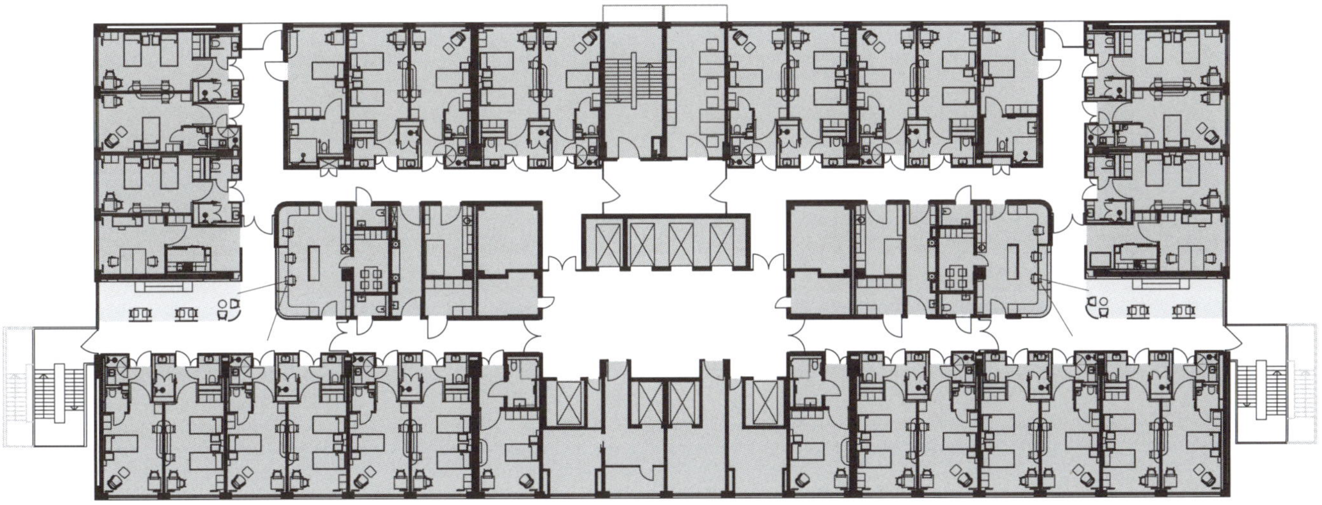

La – Hoz Arquitectura
Construcciones
Planificadas

Bogotá
Colombia

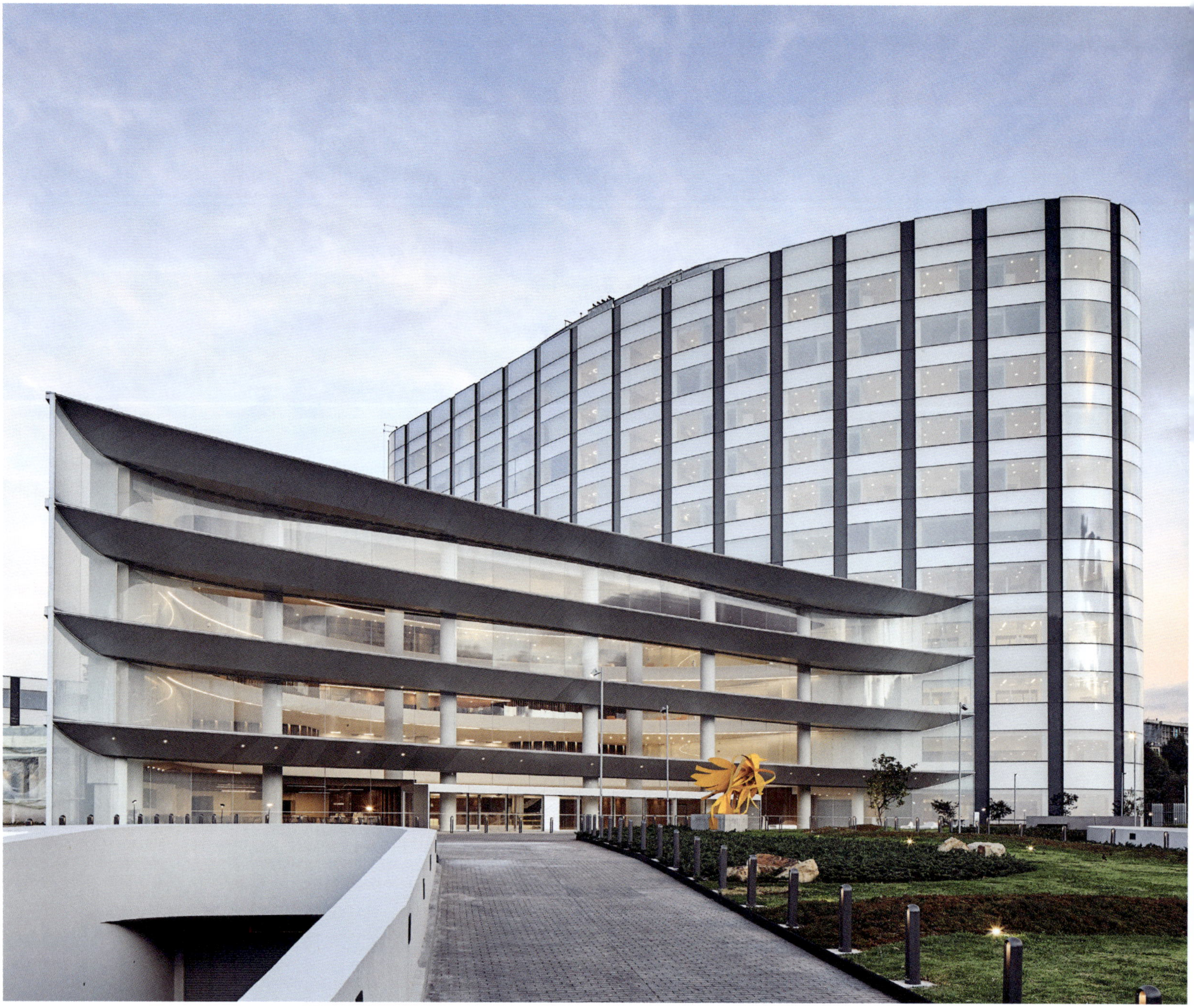

CTIC Luis Carlos Sarmiento Angulo Cancer Treatment and Research

The Luis Carlos Sarmiento Angulo Cancer Treatment and Research Center (CTIC) redefines healthcare through an architecture shaped by light, landscape, and human dignity. Conceived as a comprehensive oncology campus, the project combines treatment, research, and education within a cohesive environment. Curved volumes and an east–west orientation maximize daylight, while extensive glazing frames views of Bogotá's Eastern Hills. A landscaped podium frees the ground plane for gardens and contemplative outdoor spaces, transforming the campus into a place of encounter rather than a conventional hospital complex. Interior spaces prioritize openness, orientation, and comfort through warm materials and natural light. Terraces, resting areas, and a mountain-facing chapel reinforce the project's therapeutic character, integrating nature into experiences of care, recovery, and reflection.

Main façade providing access to the lobby, waiting areas, and interior terraces.

The helical staircase linking the priority care area with the grand lobby while drawing natural light into the basement.

Interior view of the circulation corridor distributing movement throughout the building.

Address: Rd. 168 N° 14-42, Bogotá, Colombia | **Client:** Fundación CTIC, Grupo AVAL | **Completion:** phase 1: 2022 | **Size:** 100.490 m² | **Sector:** public-private institution | **Number of patient rooms: 160** | **Number of treatment rooms: 170** | **Specialization:** Cancer Treatment and Research

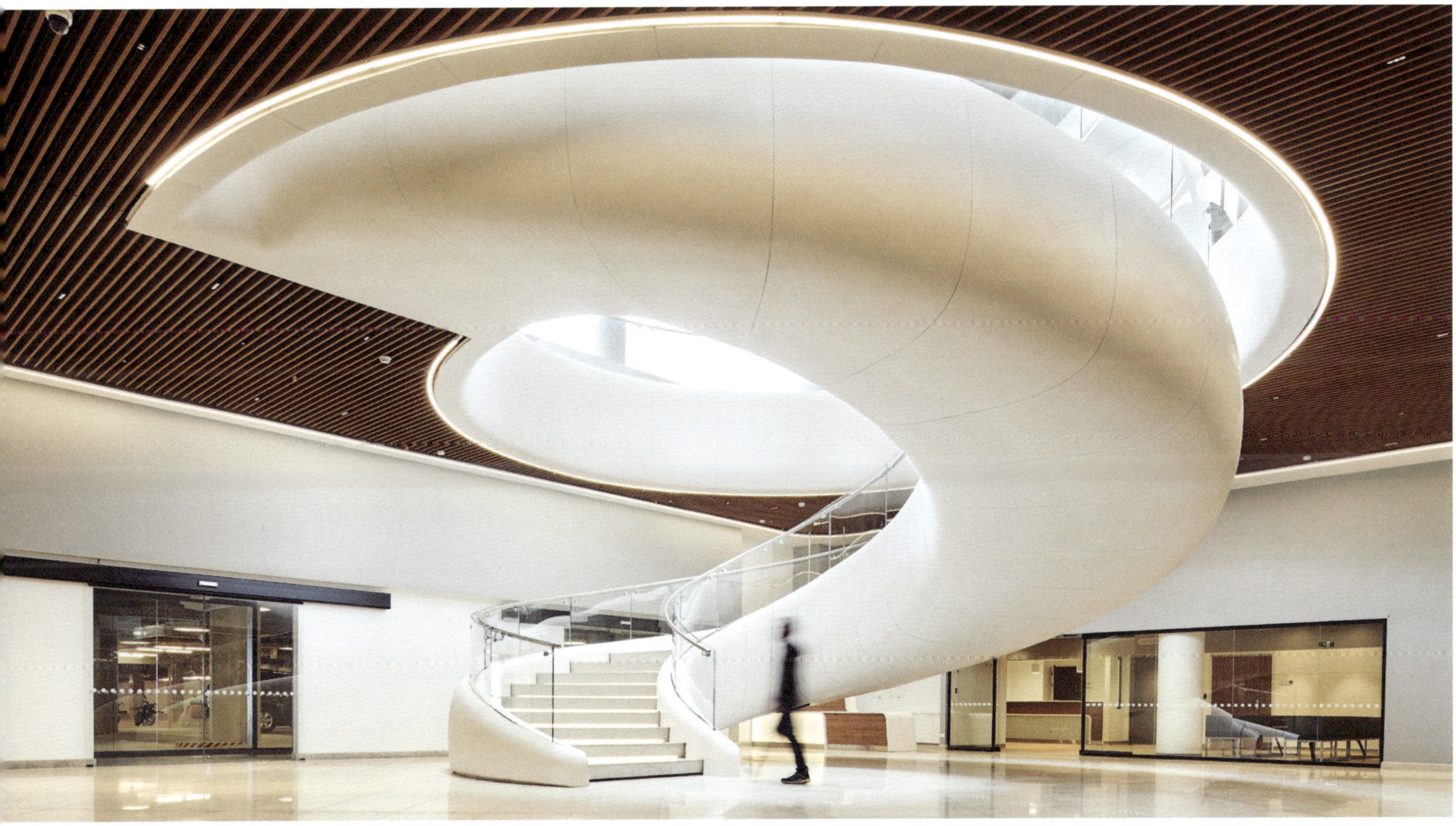

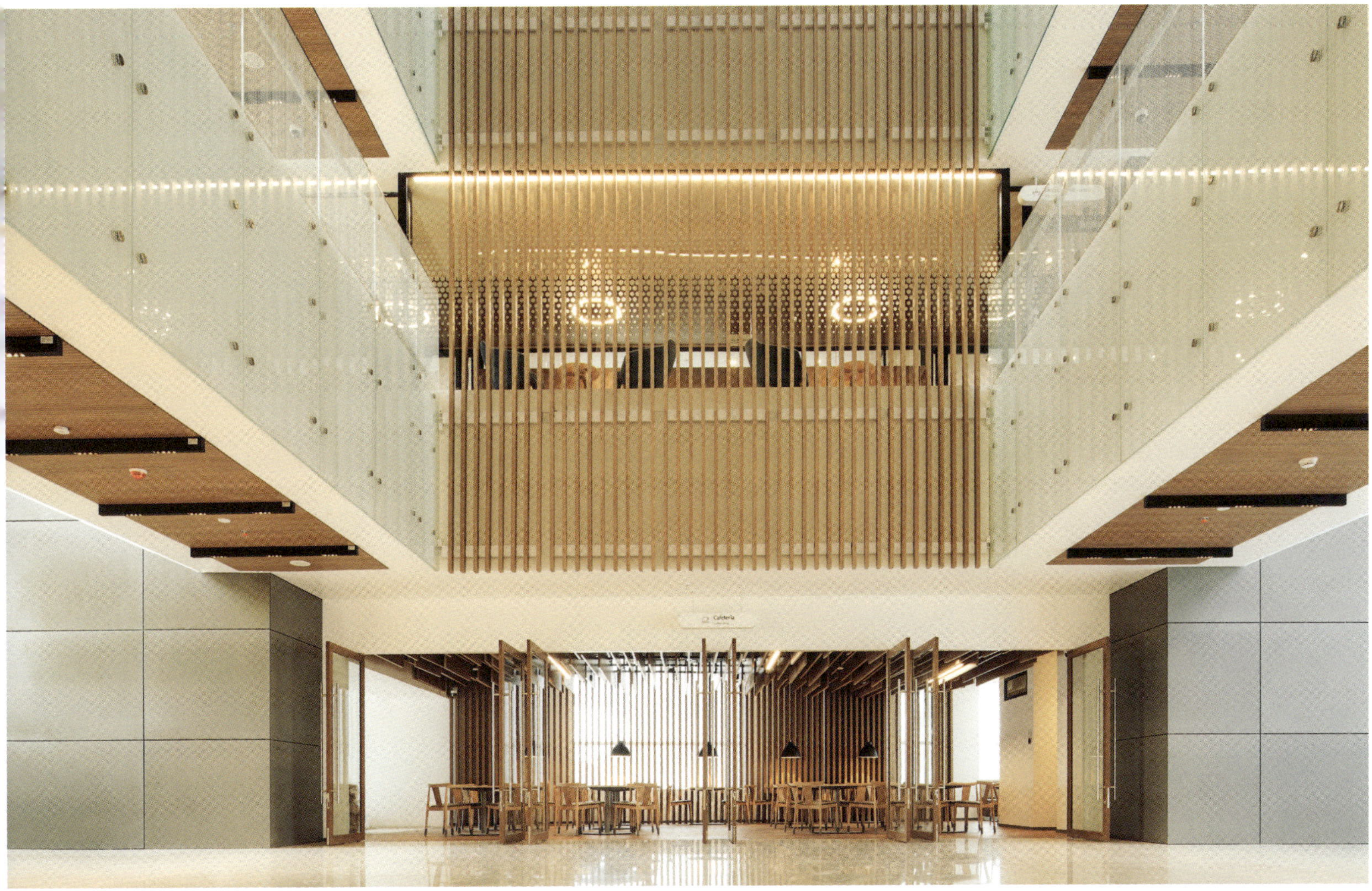

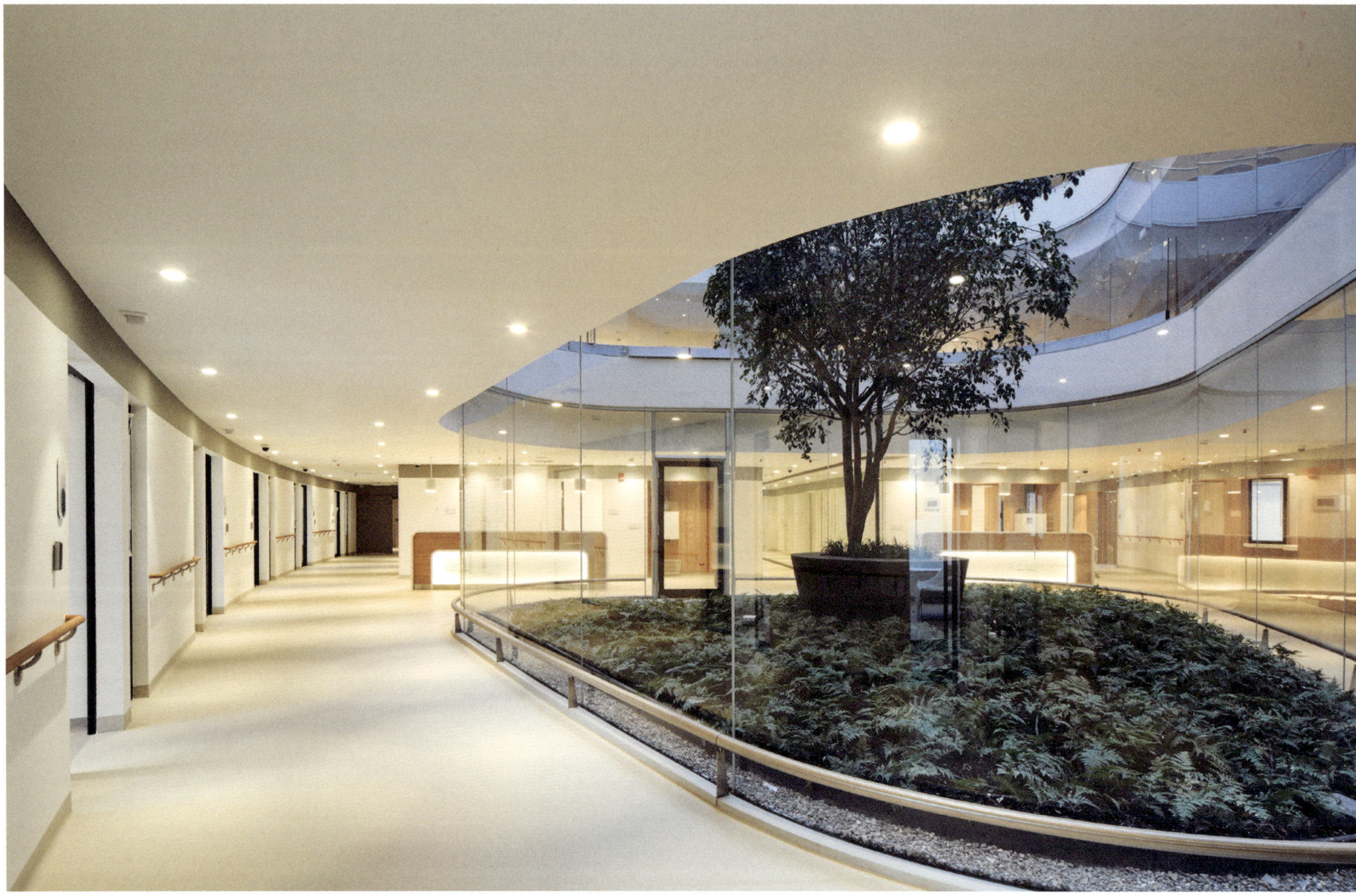

Ward central courtyard and garden serving as a source of natural light, creating generous, human-scaled spaces.

Typical floor plans of levels 3 and 8.

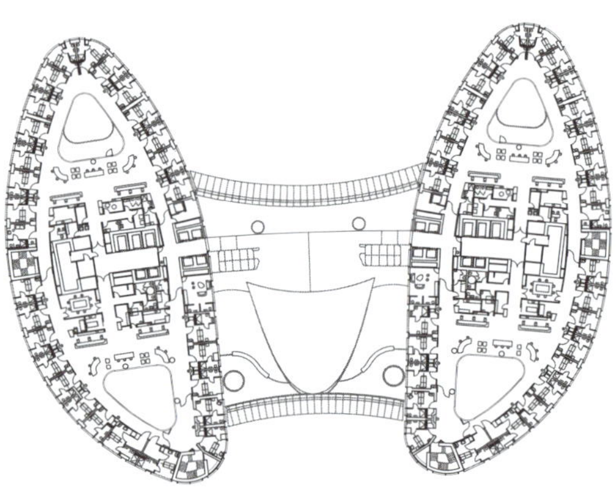

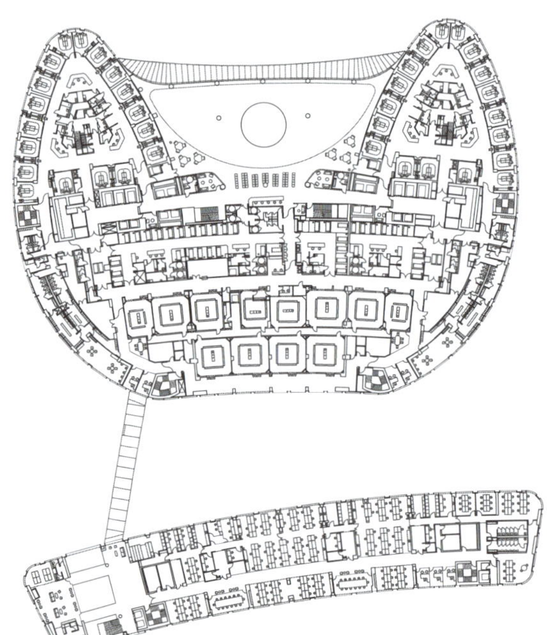

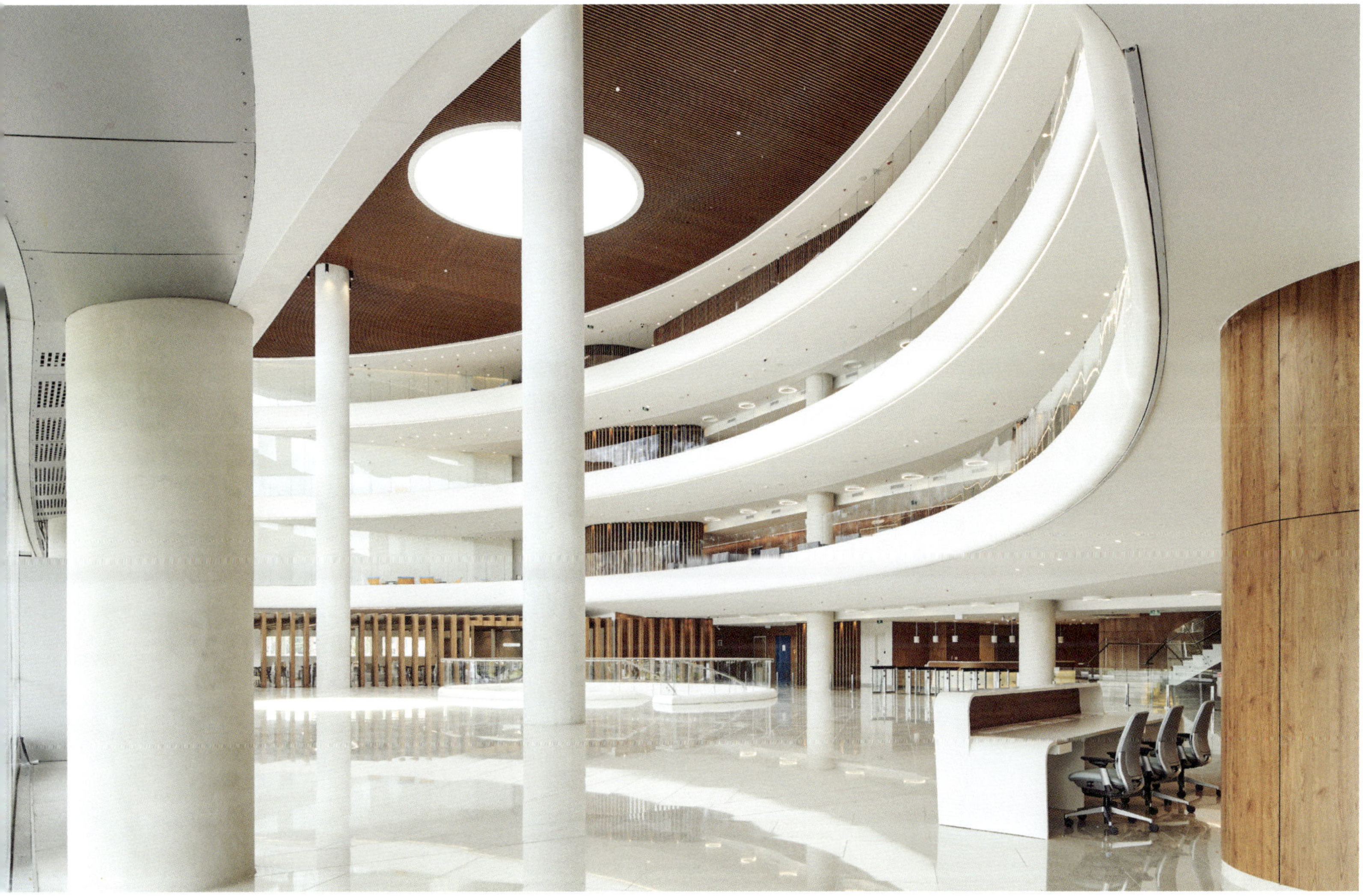

The grand lobby entrance, featuring a composition of natural light that illuminates the waiting areas across multiple levels.

3D view of a typical patient room.

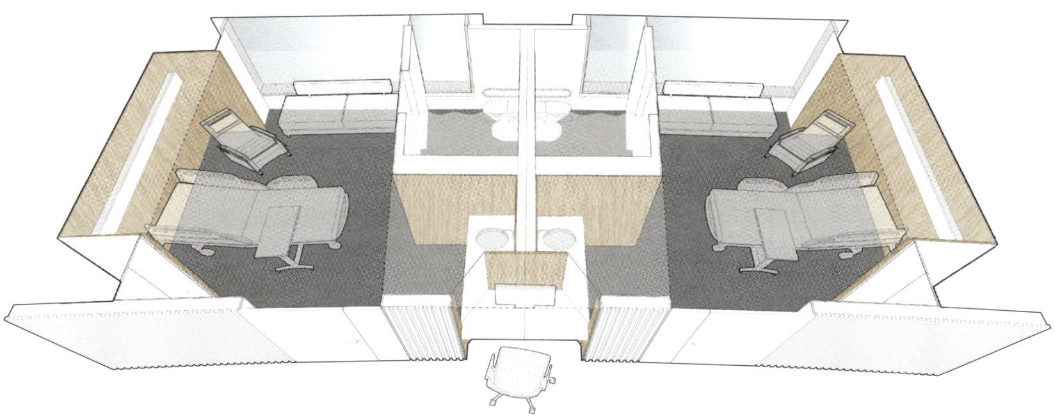

FTA |
Filippo Taidelli Architetto

Rozzano
Italy

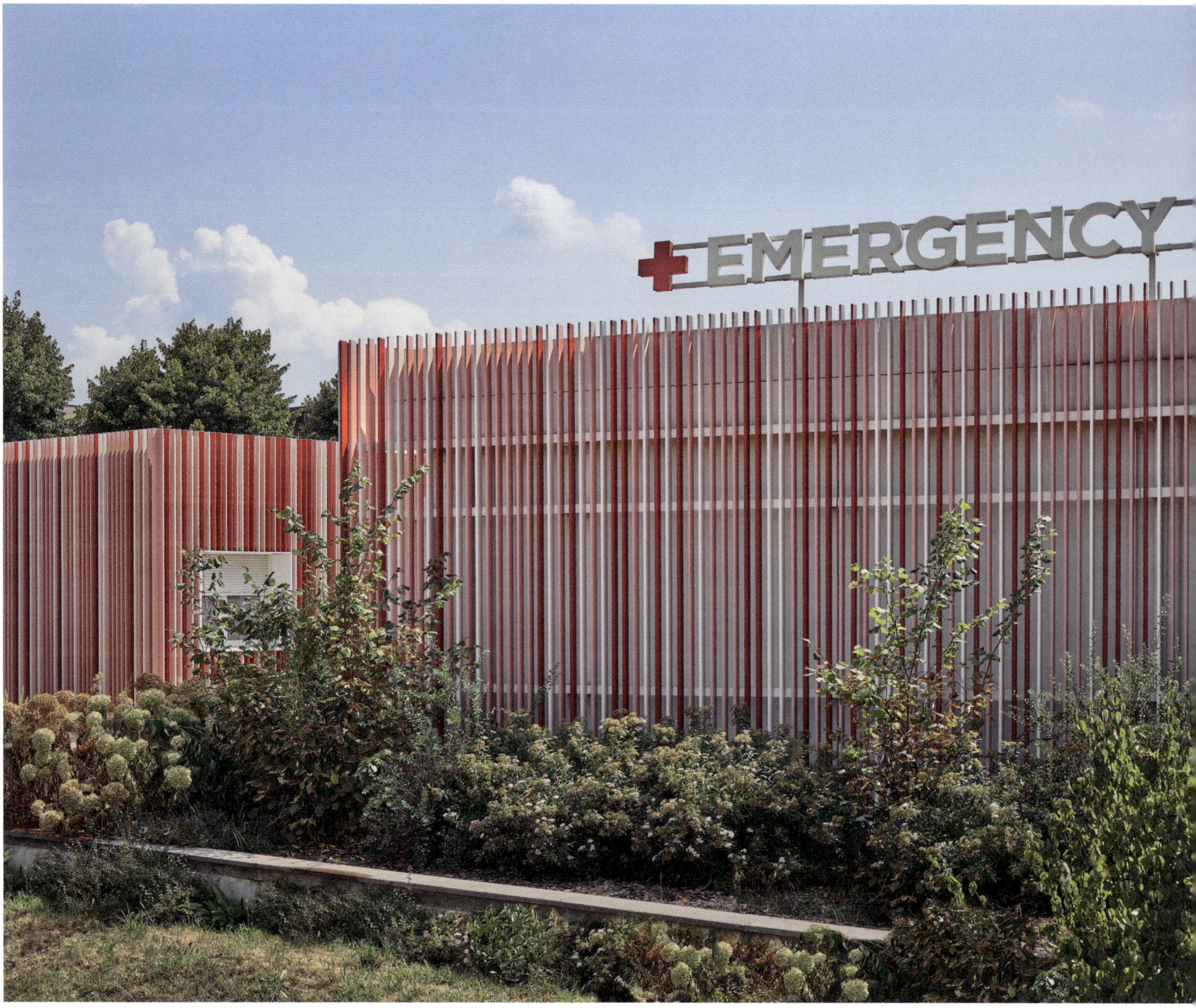

Vertical slats creating a vivid façade.

A inner green space helps creating a pleasant environment.

Emergency Hospital 19

Emergency Hospital 19 is a versatile, high-tech architecture designed for rapid response to both temporary emergencies and permanent expansions. Built in just three months using mono-blocs, it allows a rapid assembly, disassembly and an easy transport. The building is configured as a prefabricated, replicable modular system. It follows a broad sustainability approach – technical, social, energetic, and environmental. The basic module has been developed to be energetically autonomous, as well as adaptable to latitude and context. Green areas help to improve the indoor climate and serve as a therapeutic instrument for patients and healthcare workers. The external façade of Emergency Hospital 19 has an additional, modular skin, conceived as a dress, adaptable to the climatic and image conditions required by the particular geographical context.

Address: Cascina Perseghetto, 20089 Rozzano MI, Italy | **Client:** Pieve | **Completion:** 2020 | **Size:** 2,750 m^2 | **Sector:** private and public | **Number of treatment rooms:** 24 | **Number of patient rooms:** 38 | **Façade design:** Adriano Venir

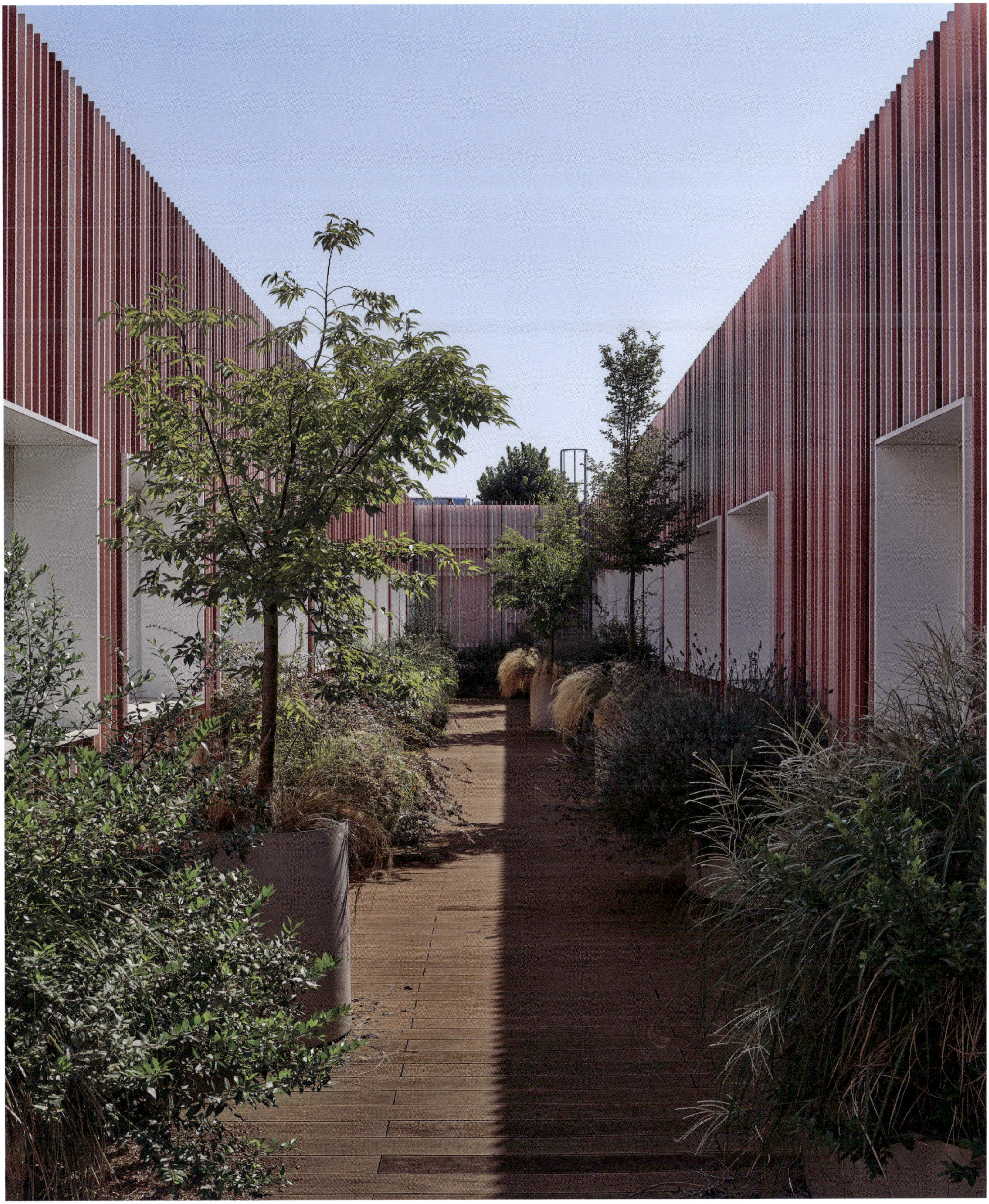

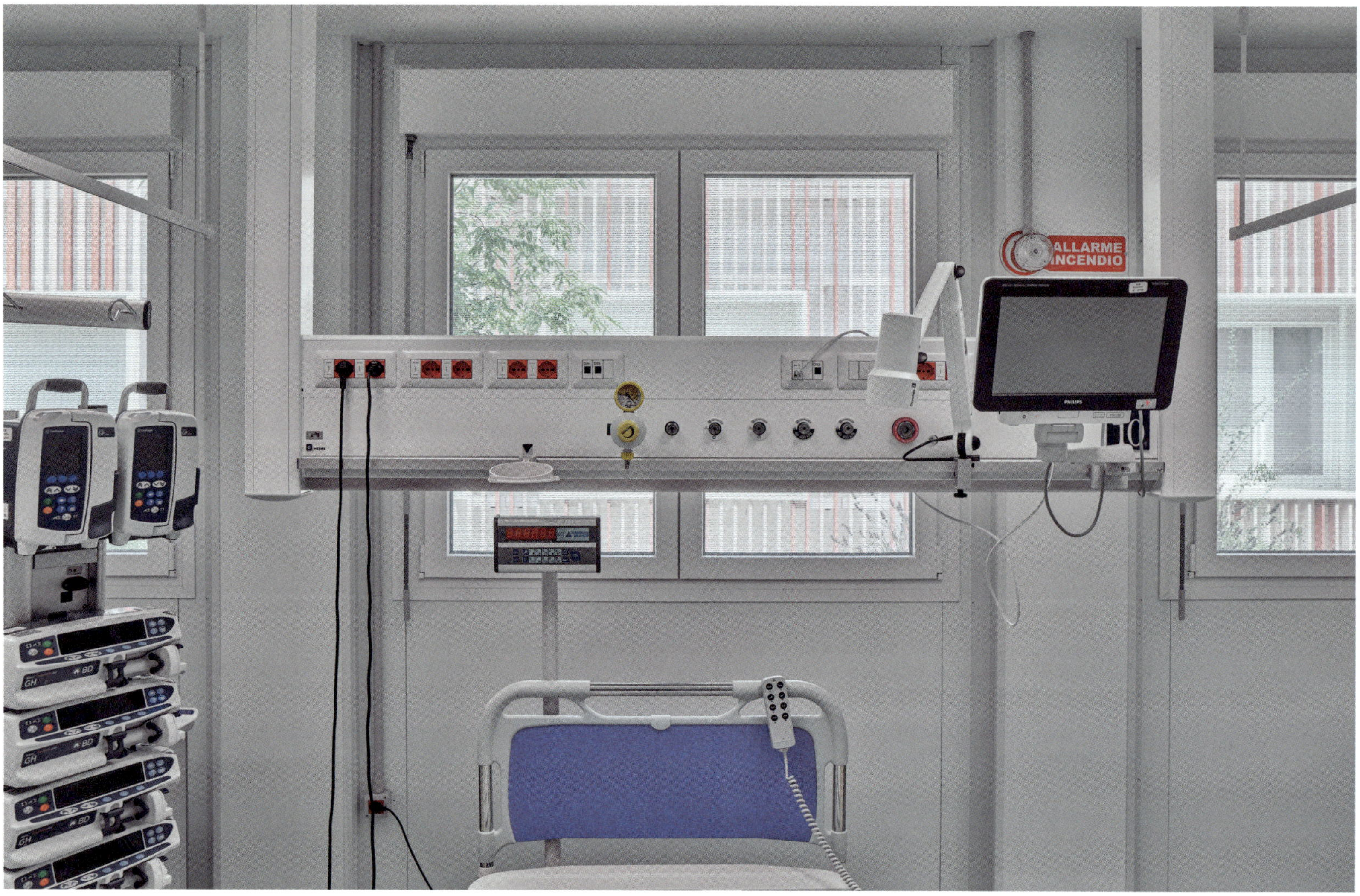

The interior is designed for functionality.

Annotated sketch showing the solar roof.

Sketch showing the different building volumes.

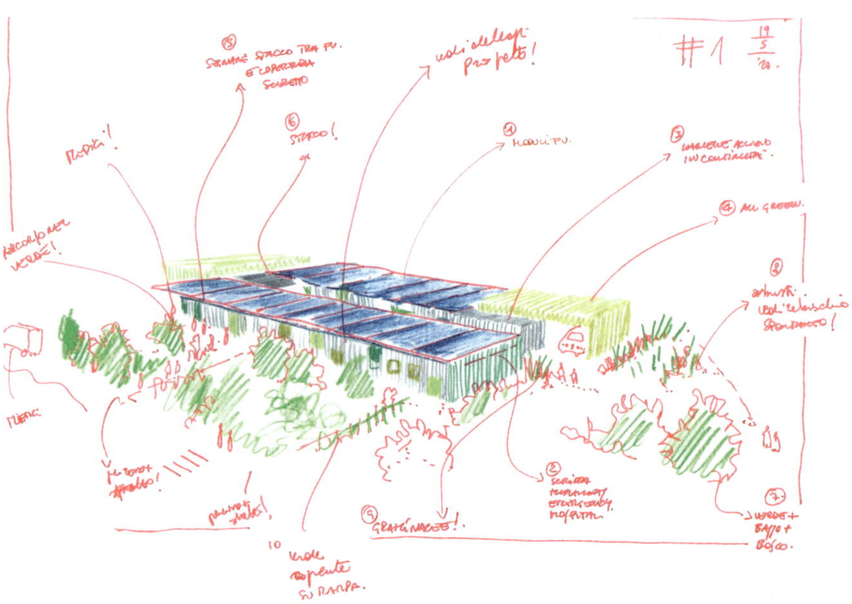

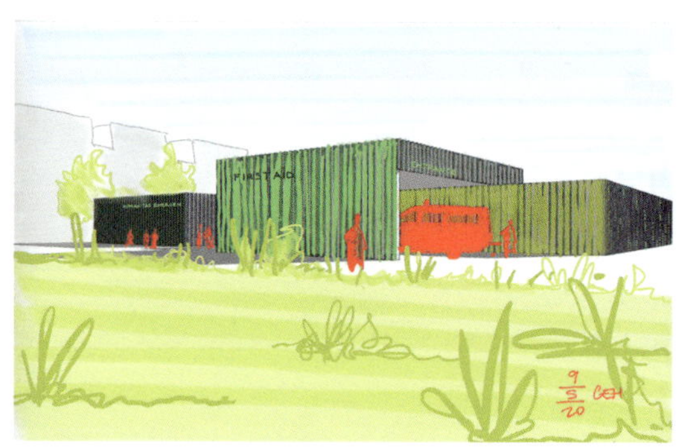

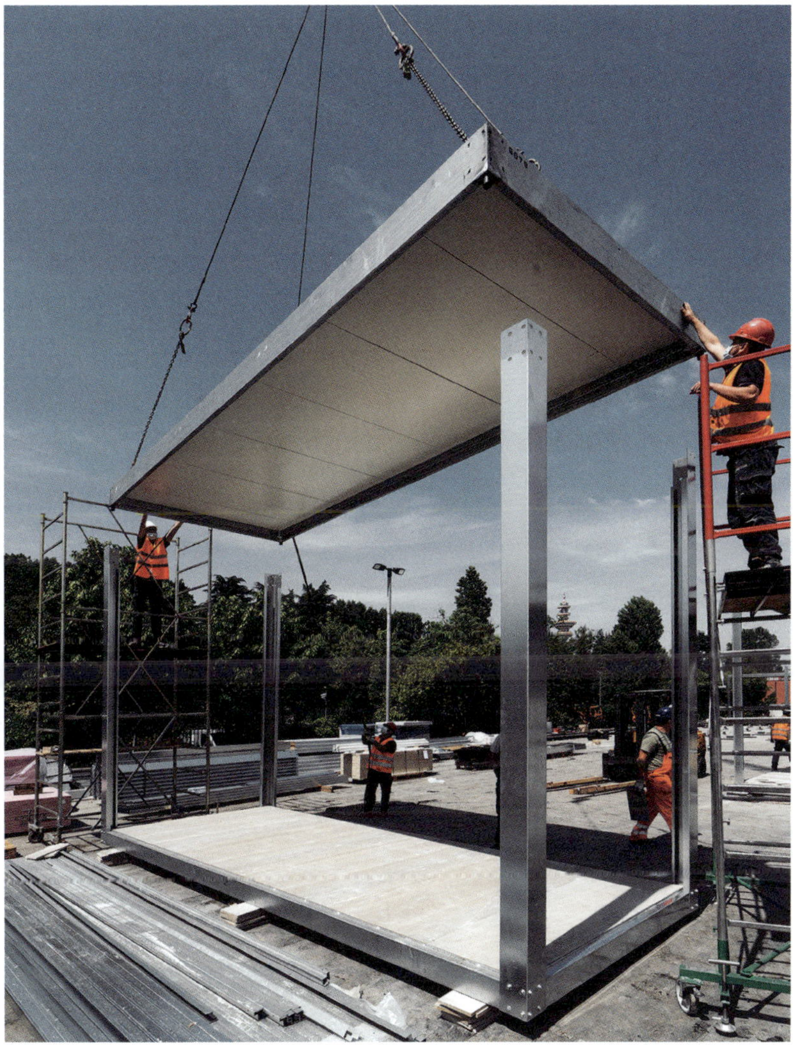

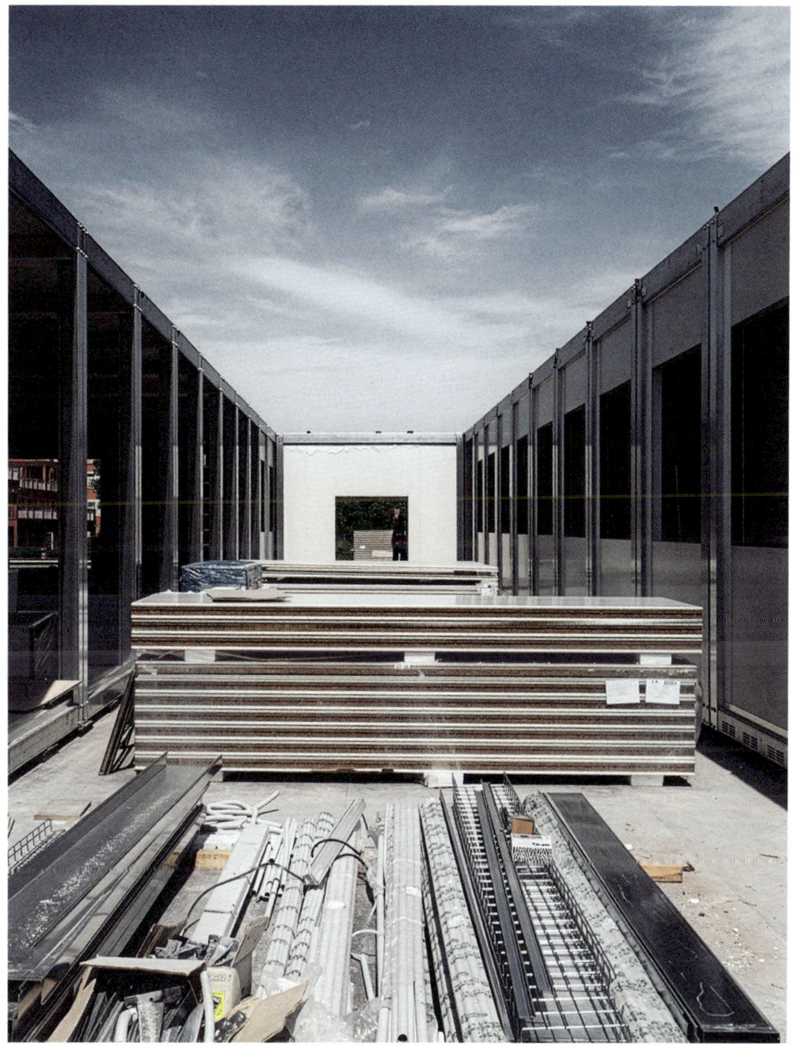

Construction site showing the assembly of a basic module.

Assembly of multiple mono-bloc modules.

Rendered cross-sectional view with layered sketching.

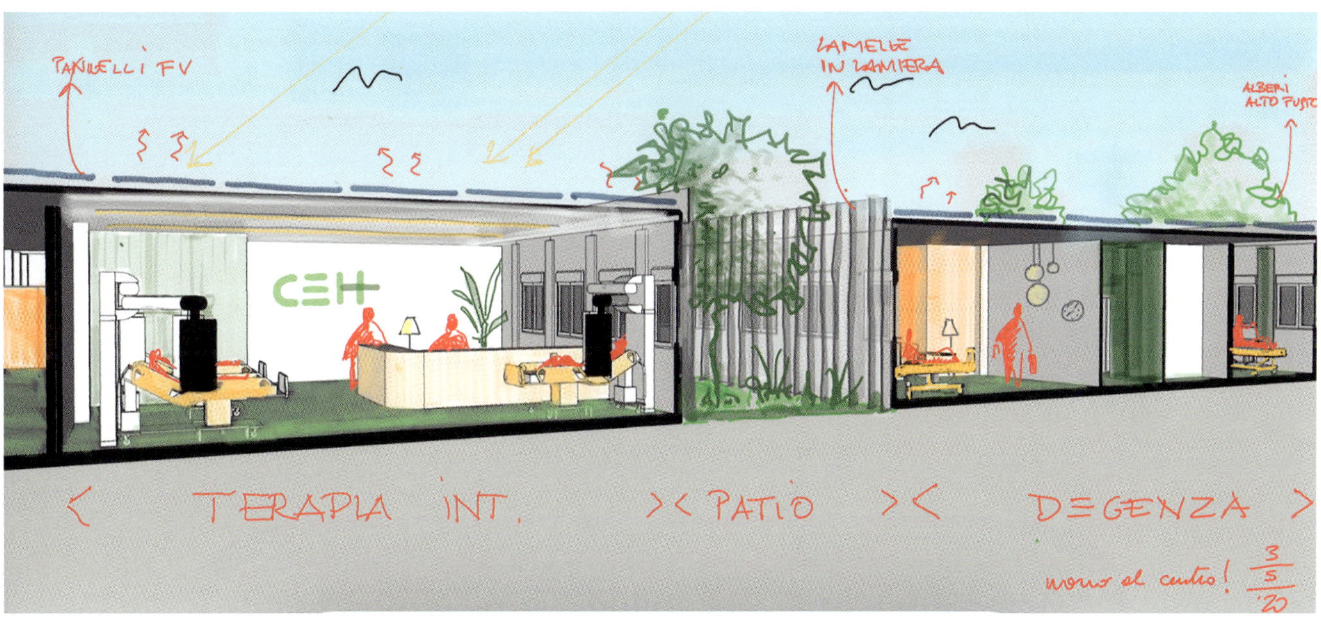

Ernst Giselbrecht + Partner

Leoben
Austria

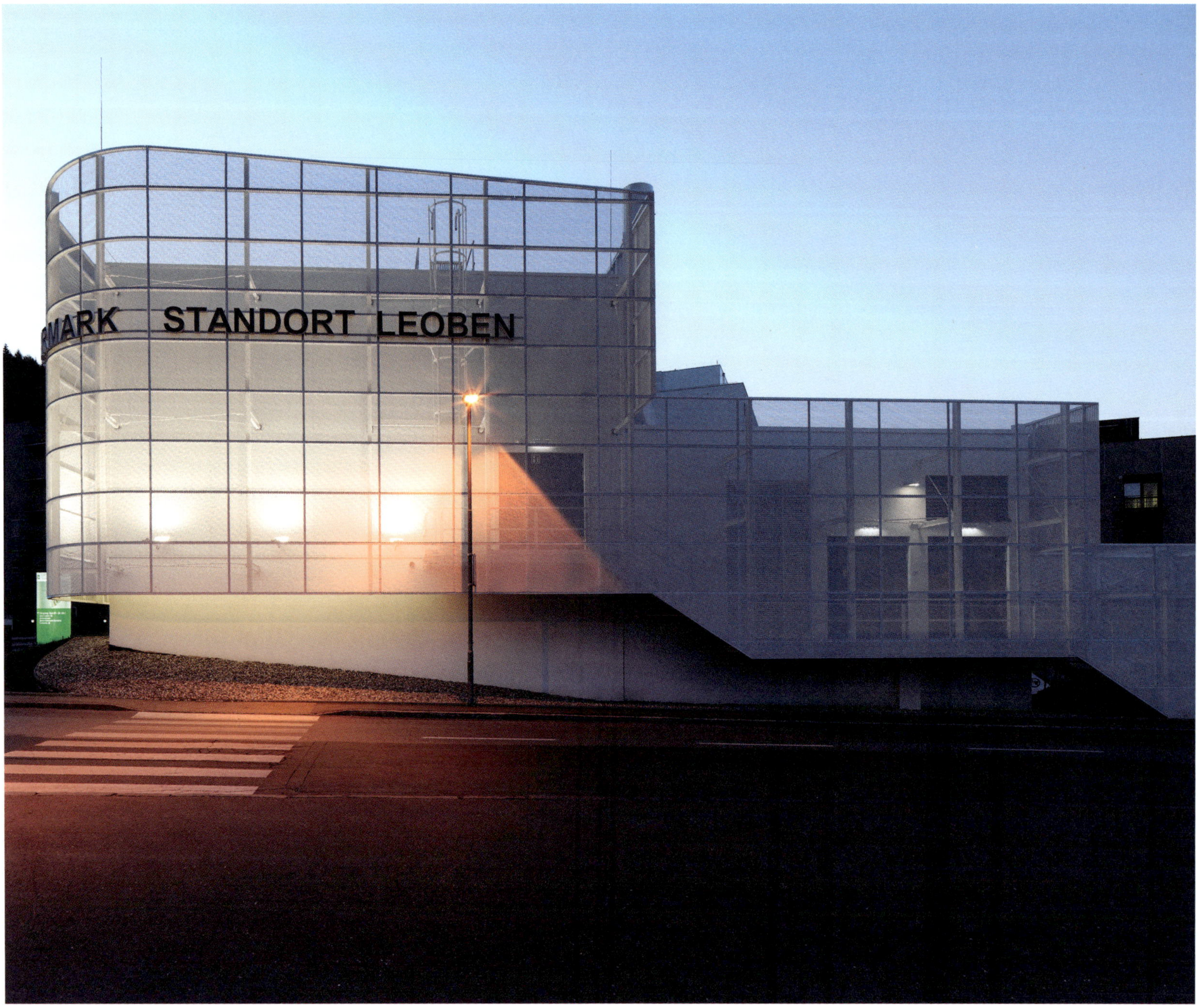

The southwest façade of the building.

Central courtyard with greenery.

LKH Leoben – Radiation Therapy

The decentralized facility for Radiation Therapy and Radiation Oncology (STZ) at LKH Leoben was constructed south of the outpatient building on the former helicopter landing pad. The sloping terrain along Vordernberger Street shapes the building's form: while the structure appears as a single-story building on the west side and extends along the street and toward the east into a two-story volume with an exposed basement. The building is directly connected to the hospital's main corridor; a central hub with a control center, waiting areas, and vertical access organizes internal processes. The ground floor houses initial intake, examination, and planning, while the basement contains the radiation treatment area with the linear accelerator. The massive construction of the radiation treatment bunker necessitates a windowless design and incorporates a strong connection to the outdoors.

Address: Vordernberger Straße, 8700 Leoben, Austria | **Client:** Steiermärkische Krankenanstalten GmbH KAGes | **Completion:** 2017 | **Size:** 2,025 m^2 | **Sector:** state | **Specialization:** radiation therapy | **Number of treatment rooms:** 6

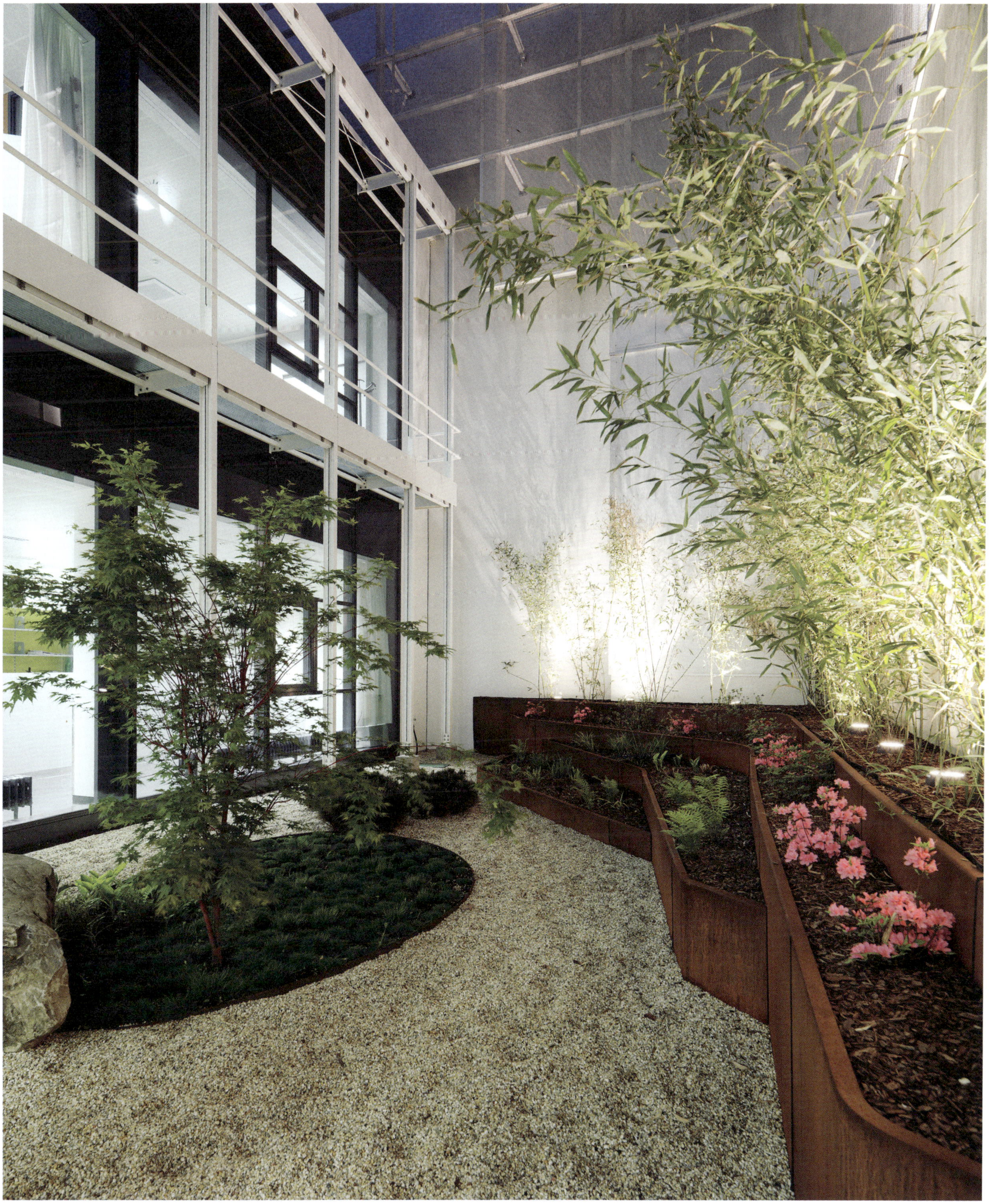

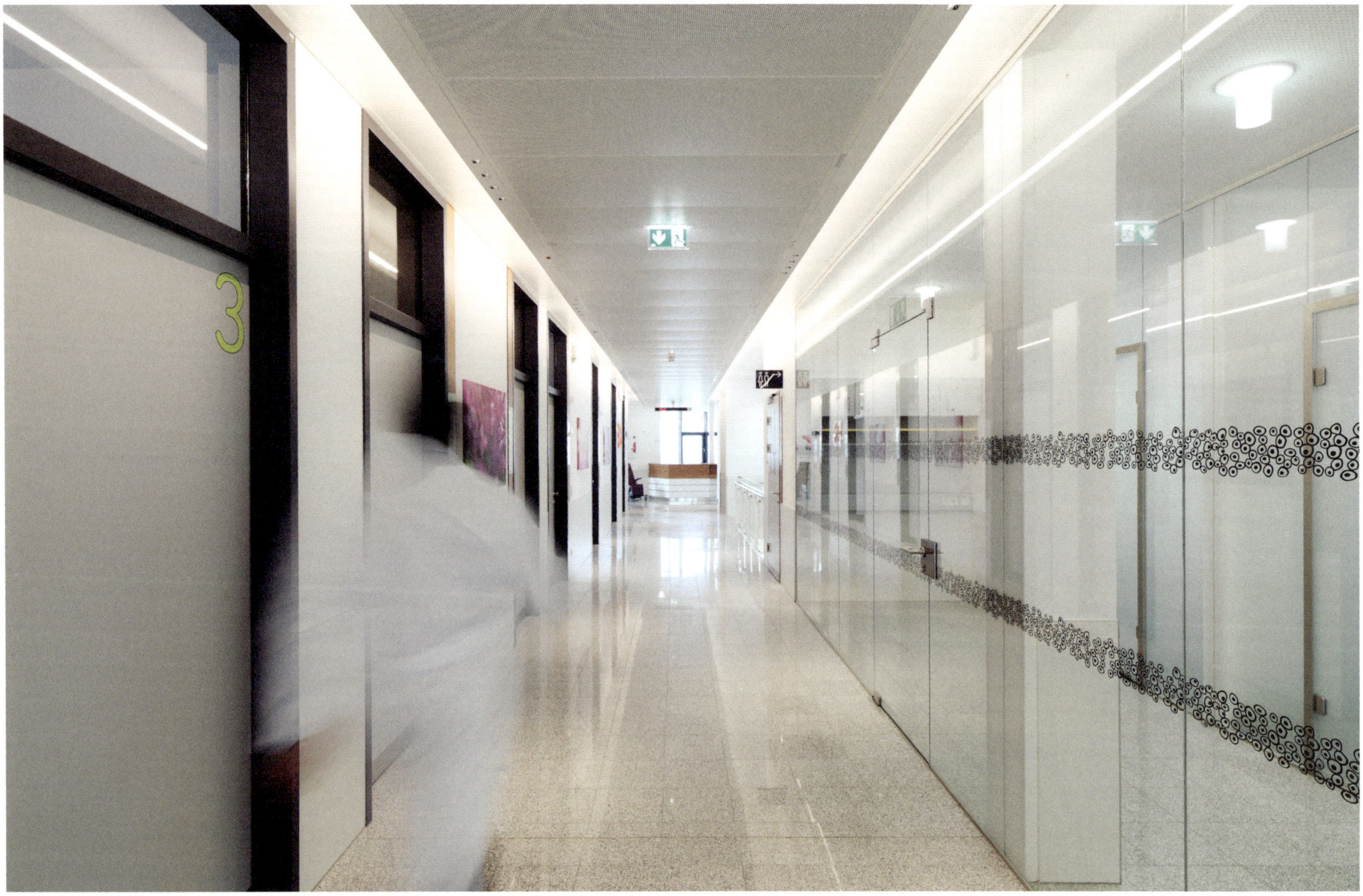

Well-lit and spacious corridor.

First floor plan.

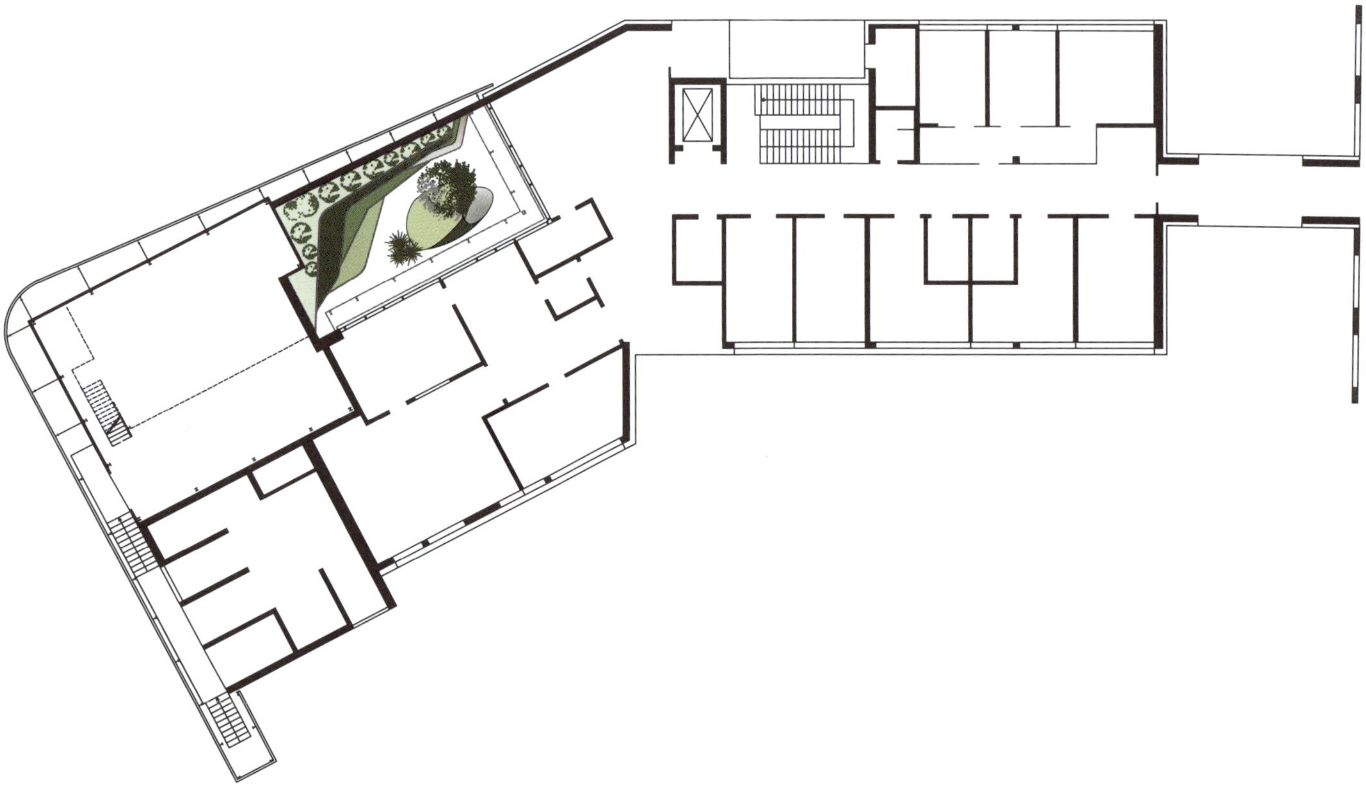

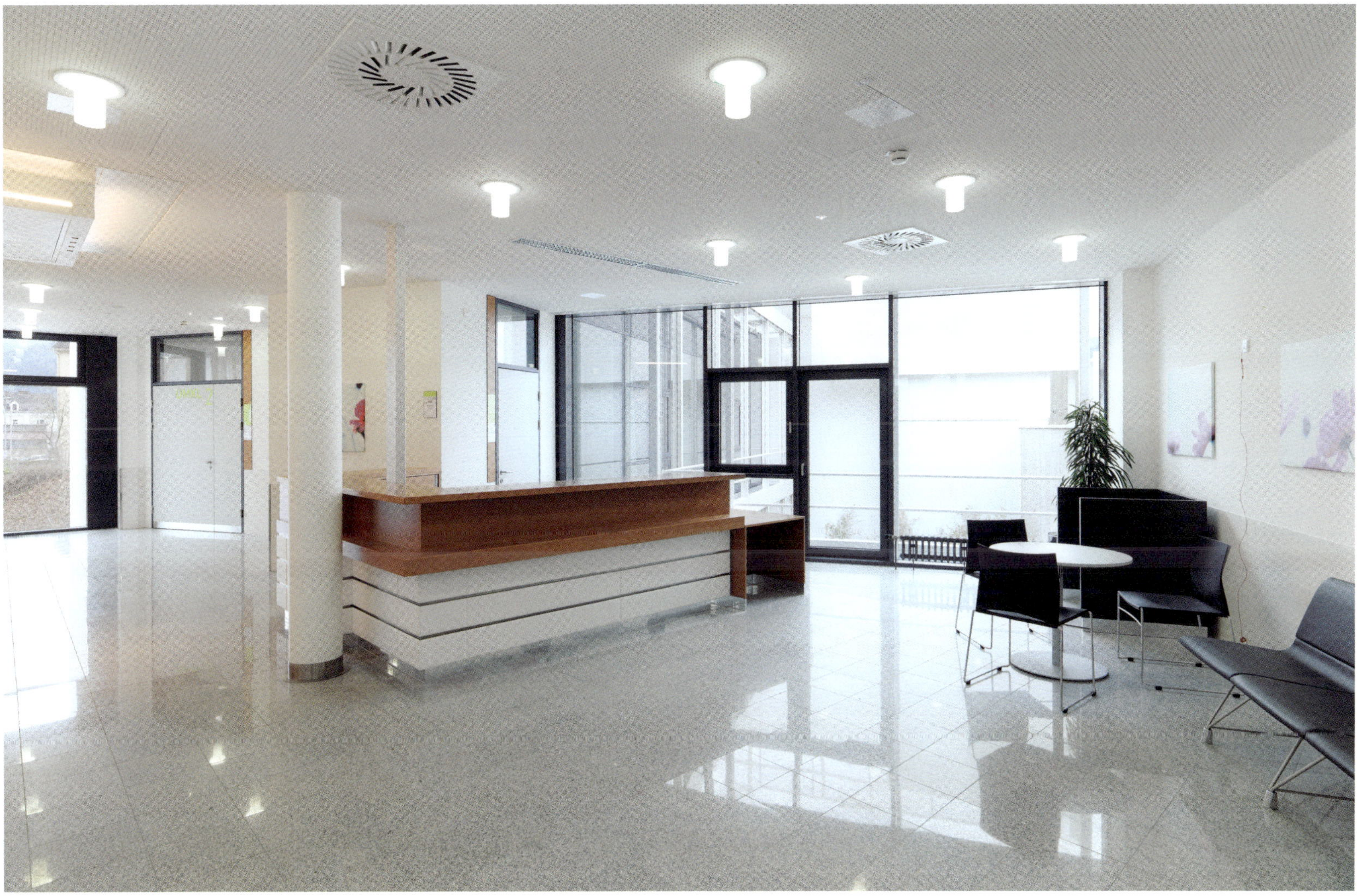

Reception and waiting area of the hospital.

Section.

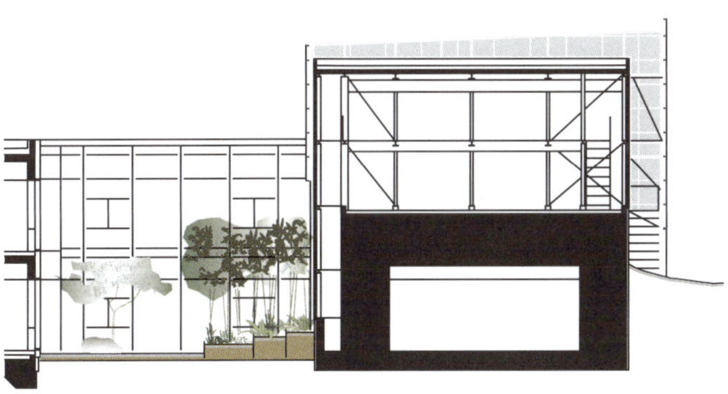

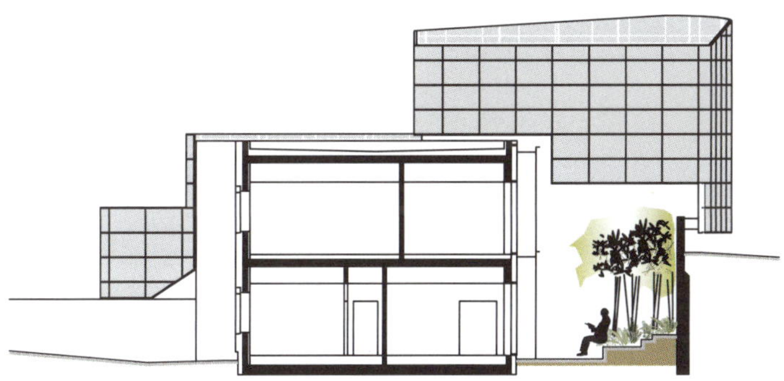

Krampe Schmidt Architekten

Herne Germany

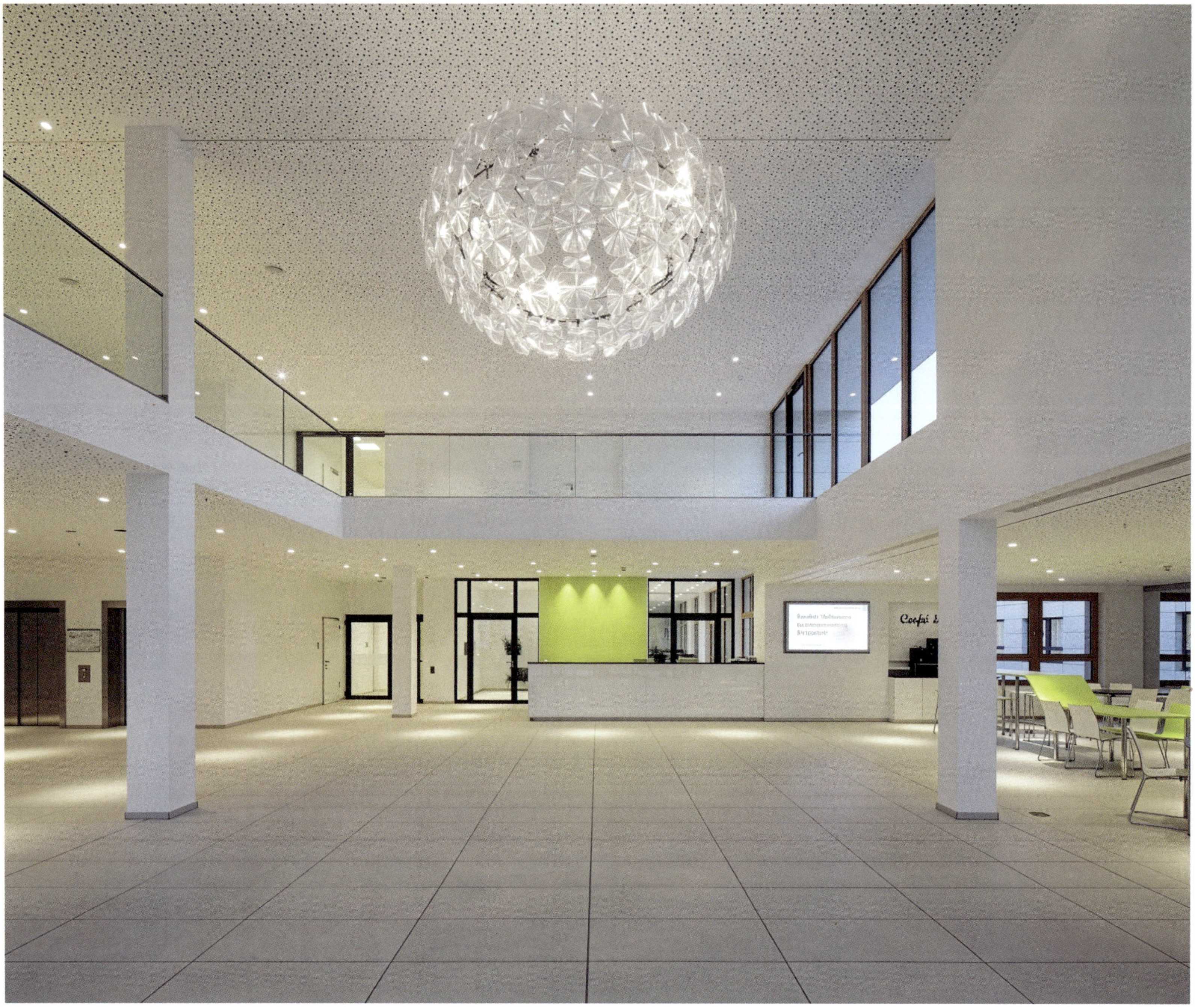

In the entrance hall, the natural stone façade is echoed in the flooring.

The new building including the addition is aligned with the residential buildings.

Balconies in front of patient rooms with floor-to-ceiling windows.

Rheumatology Center Ruhrgebiet

Nestled within a park-like, barrier-free landscape, this Rheumatology Center in the Ruhr area combines architecture and healing into a holistic space with a hotel-like character. The new building from 2014 emphasizes light, openness, and clear navigation: a spacious, two-story foyer, ring-shaped corridors, and rooms flooded with natural light throughout create a sense of clarity and tranquility. Floor-to-ceiling windows and loggias lend the light-filled patient rooms a cozy atmosphere. The 2023 addition, clad in light-colored natural stone, consistently extends this concept of health-focused architecture with a focus on well-being. It adds additional therapy and lounge areas without sealing off new spaces. The result is a place that spatially supports recovery while simultaneously fostering social interaction.

Address: Claudiusstraße 45, 44649 Herne, Germany | **Client:** St. Elisabeth Gruppe GmbH – Katholische Kliniken Rhein-Ruhr, Herne | **Completion:** 2014 / 2023 | **Size:** 17,344 m² | **Sector:** ecclesiastical | **Specialization:** rheumatology clinic | **Number of patient rooms:** 92 | **Landscape design:** SAL Landschaftsarchitektur

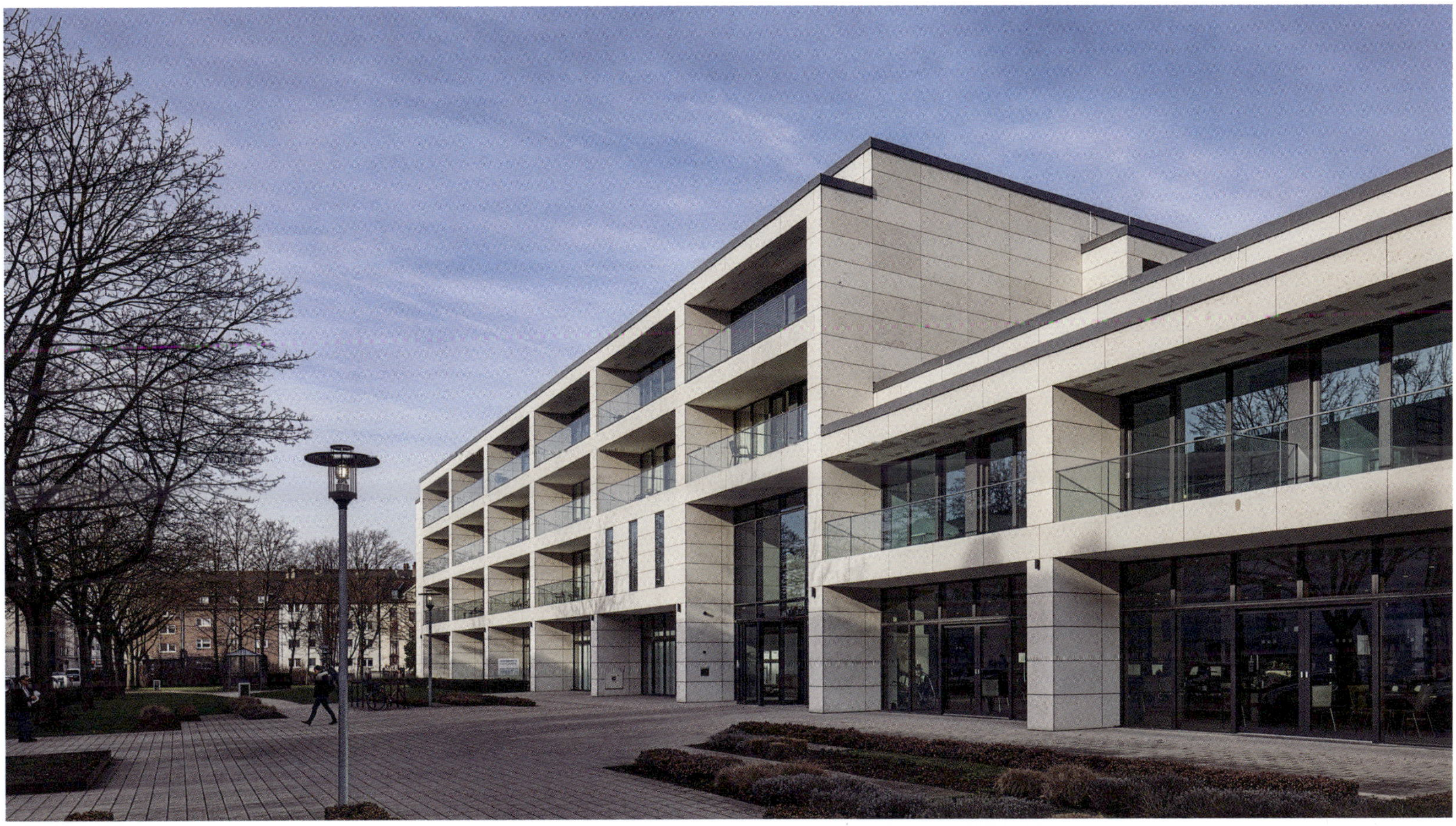

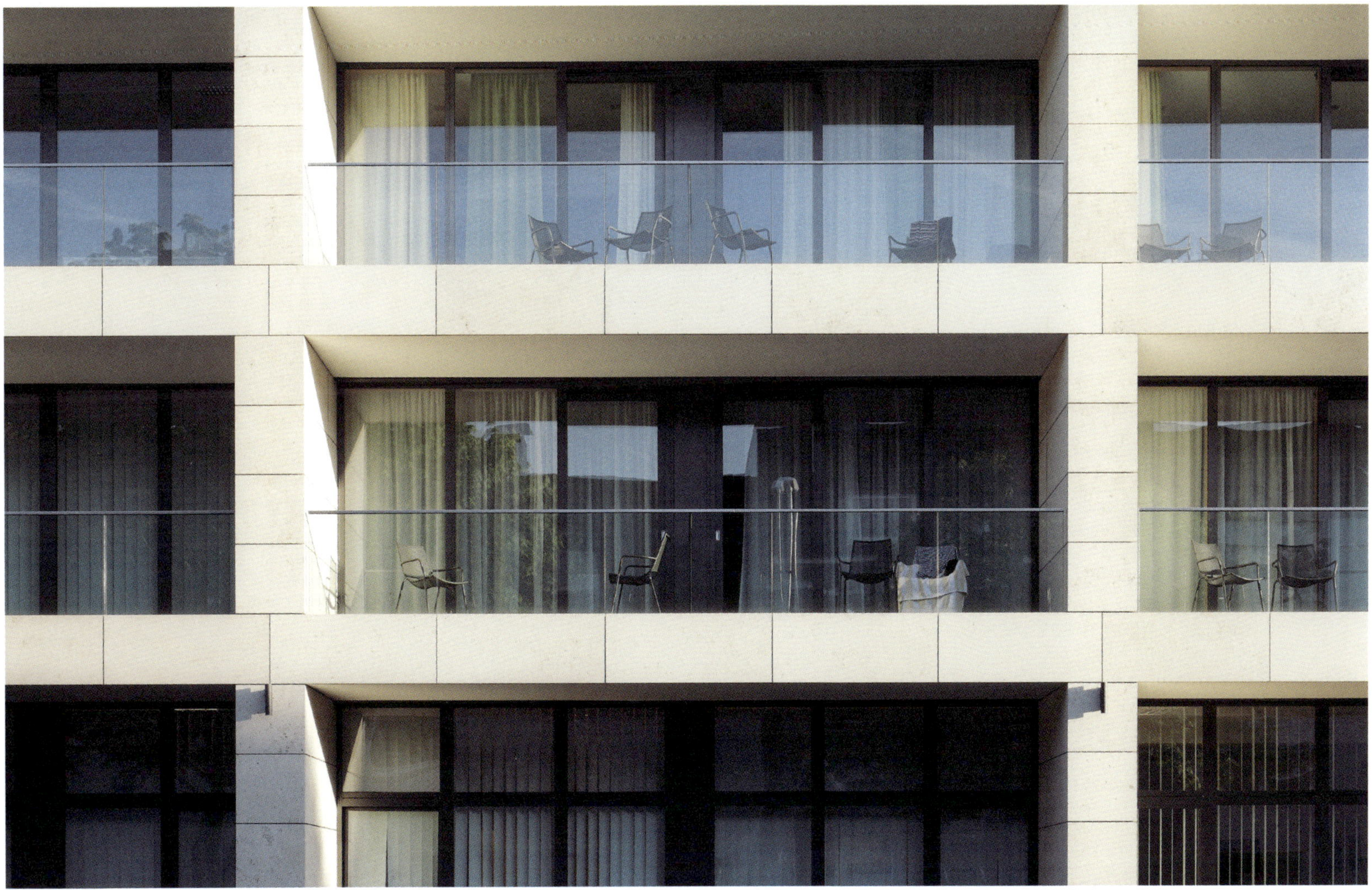

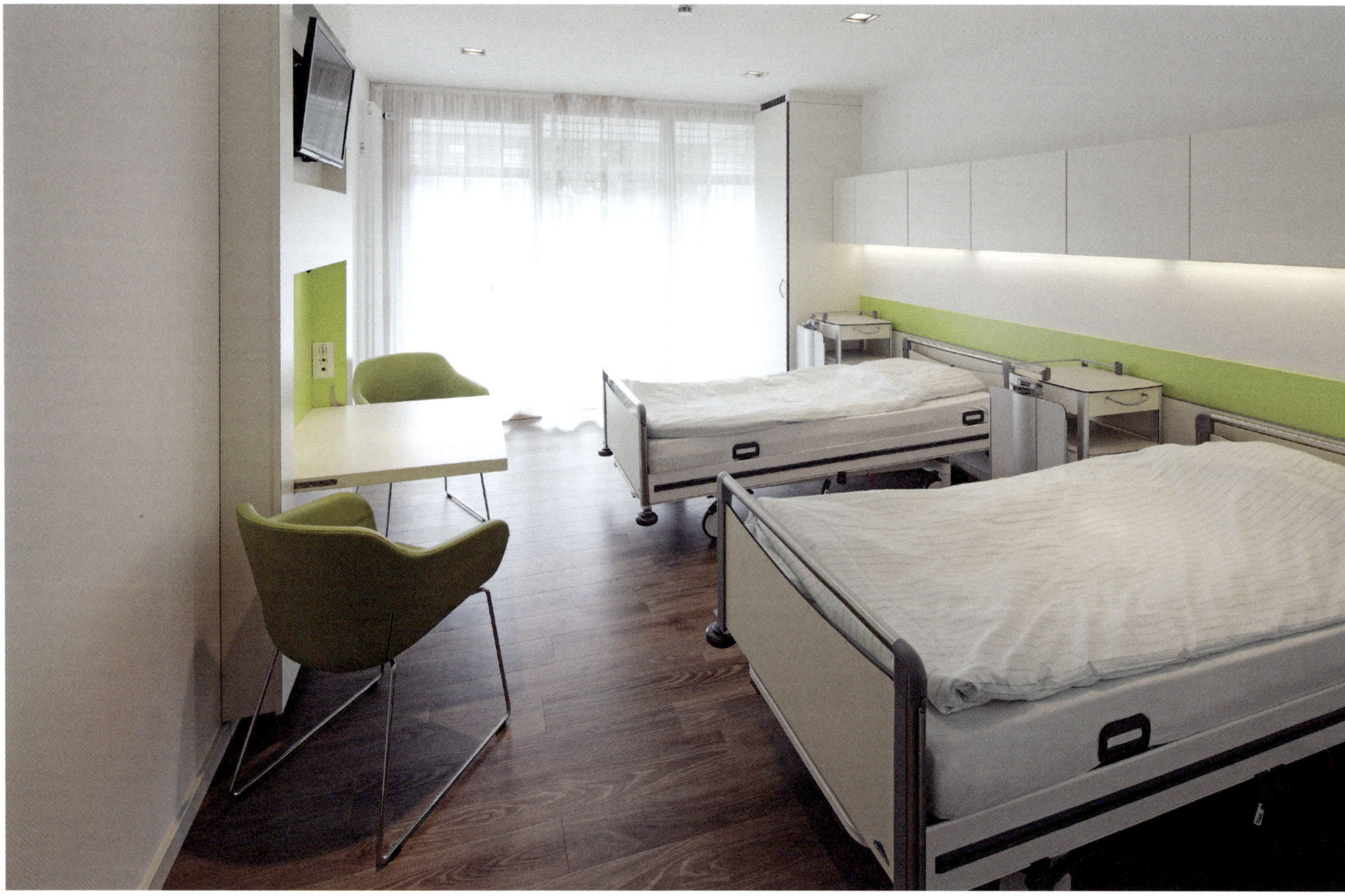

Patient room equipped with loggia, floor-to-ceiling windows, and glass railing.

Ground floor plan, 2014 original building.

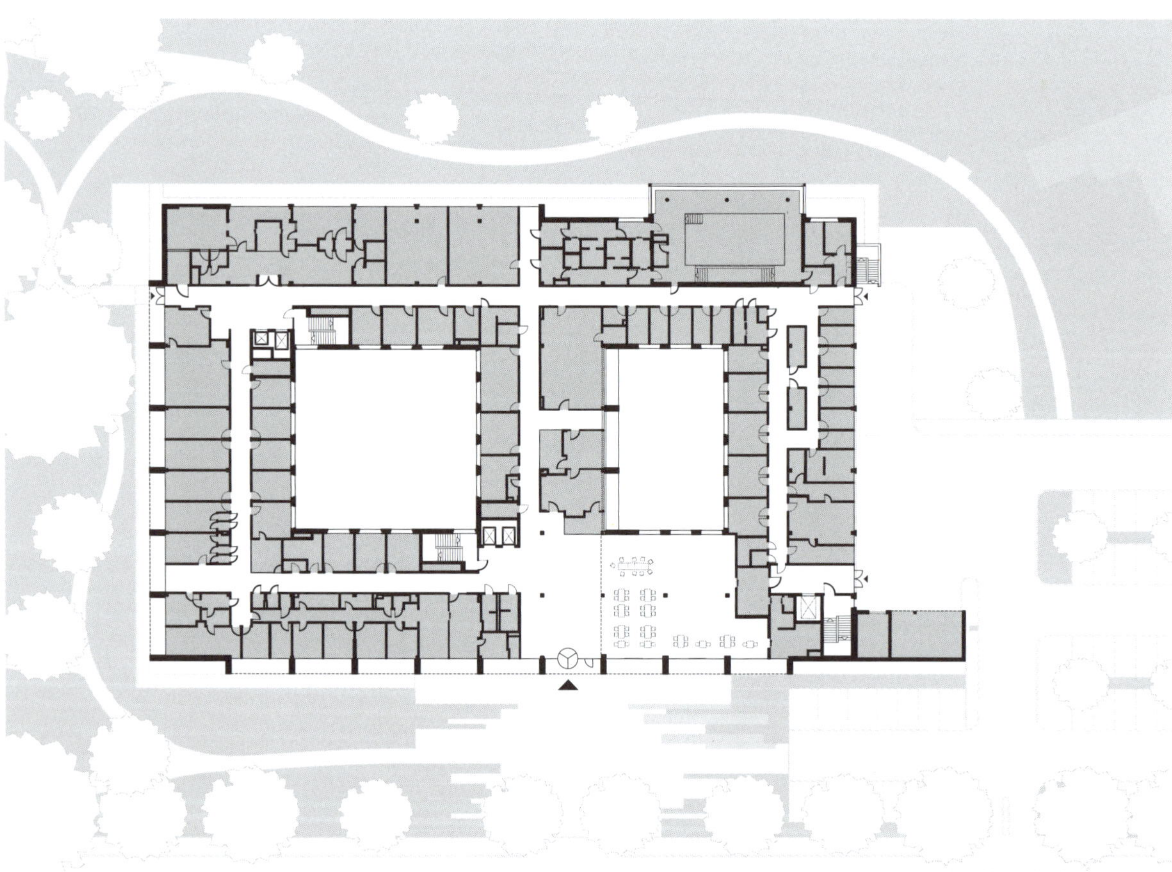

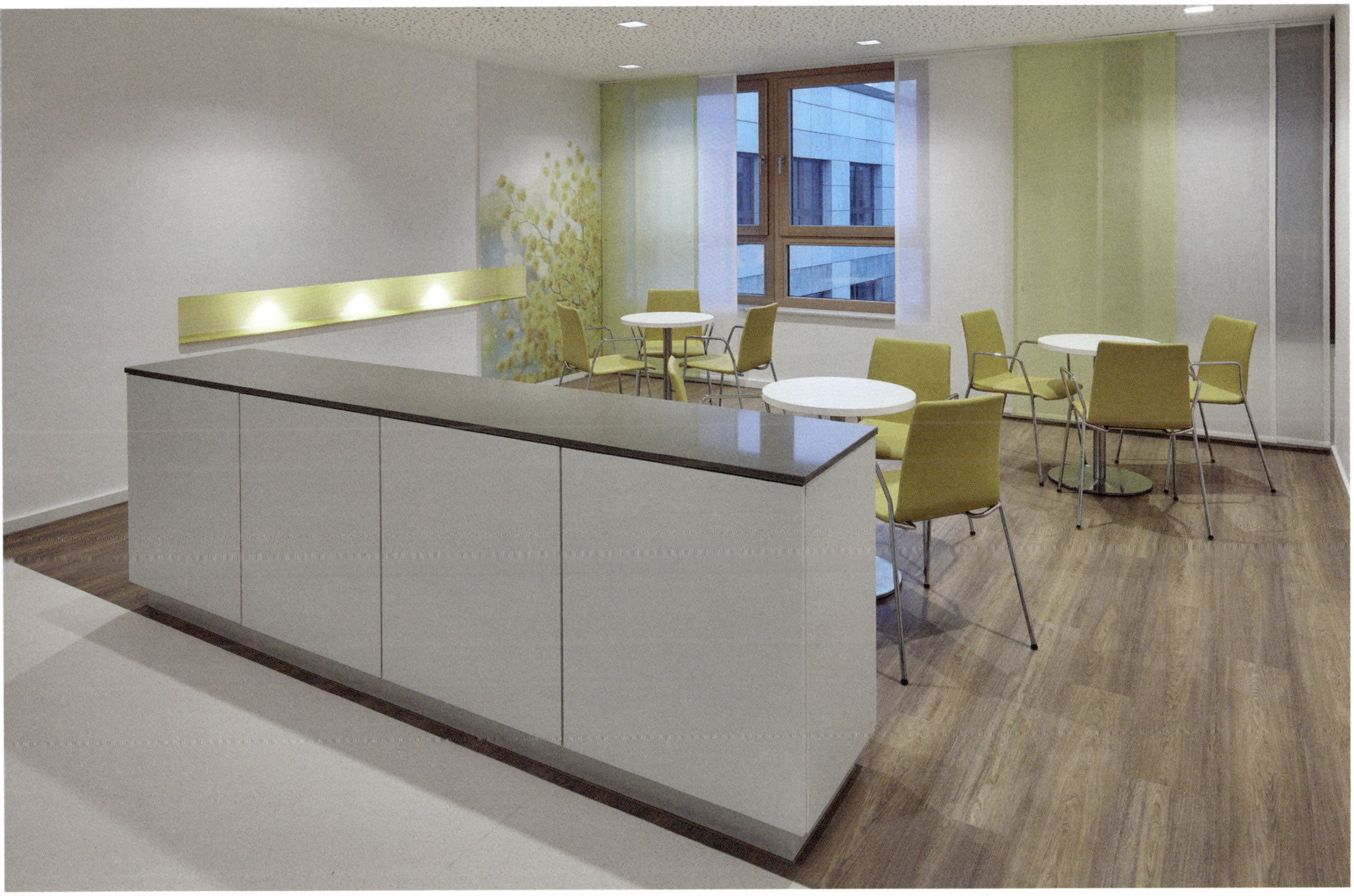

A lounge and waiting area on the newly added top floor.

Third floor plan, 2023 addition.

Perspective of the addition.

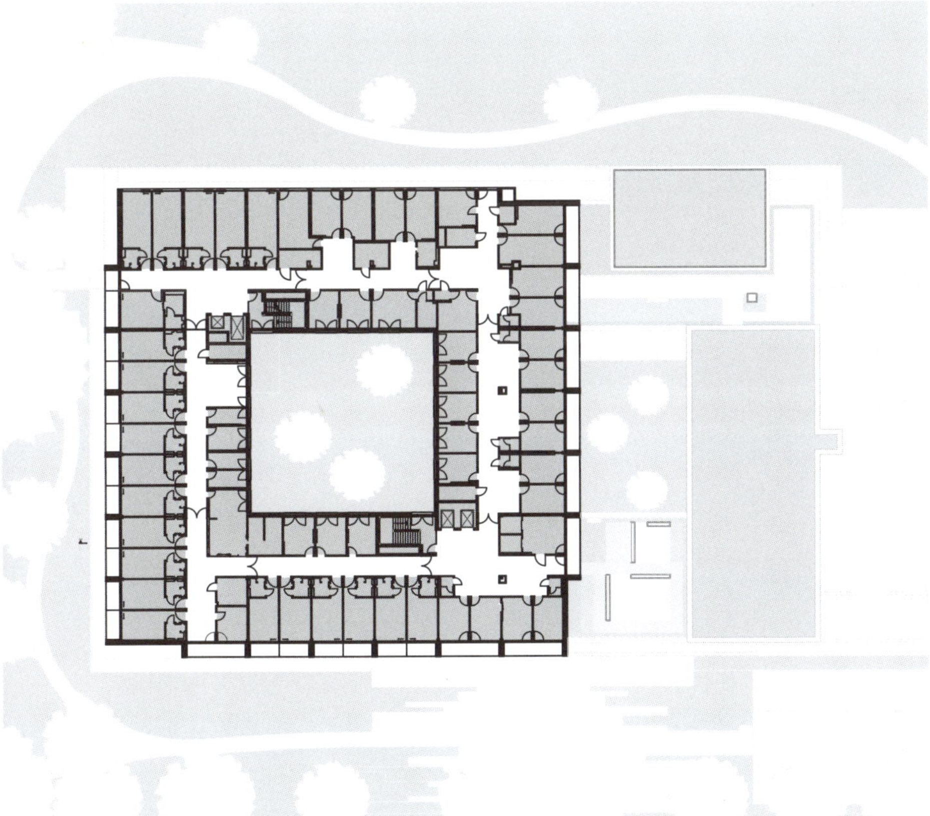

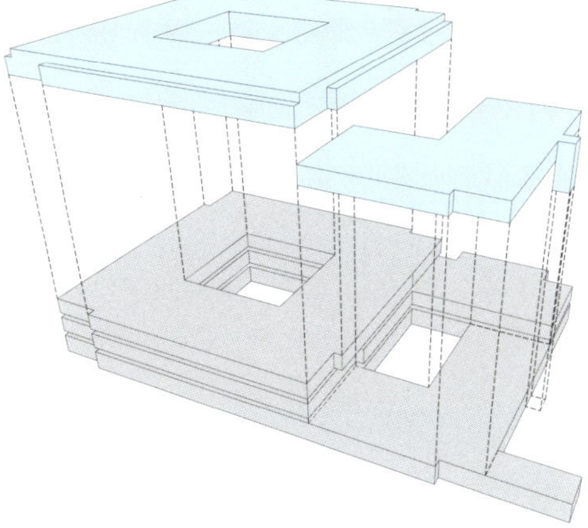

Scott Tallon Walker Architects with Medical Architecture

Dublin Ireland

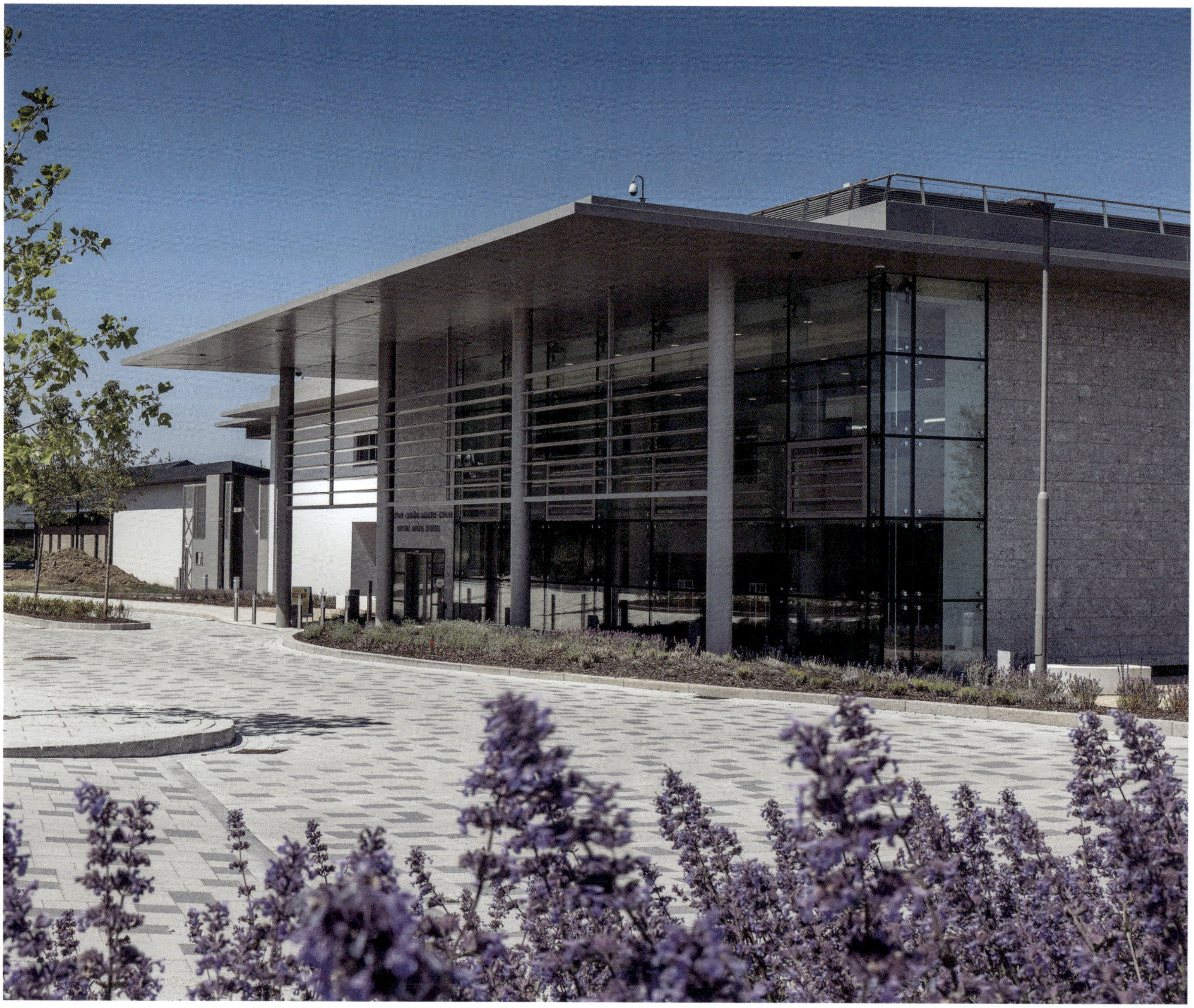

Entrance pavilion with canopy and open glazed façade, establishing a welcoming arrival space.

Community buildings around pedestrianized village green.

Patient courtyard supporting retreat and social interaction.

National Forensic Mental Health Service

Accessed through a spacious and welcoming reception pavilion, the National Forensic Mental Health Service campus is laid out as a series of buildings around a pedestrianized "village green", achieving intuitive wayfinding through a site-wide narrative of color, art, and landscaping. A "village center" provides shared recreational and therapeutic facilities including a horticultural area, while a series of courtyards and secure perimeter gardens allow patients direct access to nature from each ward. Patient bedrooms are clustered in small wards around shared indoor and outdoor spaces in which collective activities and therapies take place. Within this unifying design concept, individual buildings respond to the specific clinical requirements of distinct patient cohorts in a facility which maximizes the therapeutic value of landscape and design within the constraints of a secure setting.

Address: Portraine Demesne, Portrane, Co. Dublin, K36 FD79, Irland | **Client:** Health Service Executive Ireland | **Completion:** 2022 | **Size:** 25,000 m^2 | **Sector:** state | **Specialization:** specialist mental health hospital | **Number of patient rooms:** 170

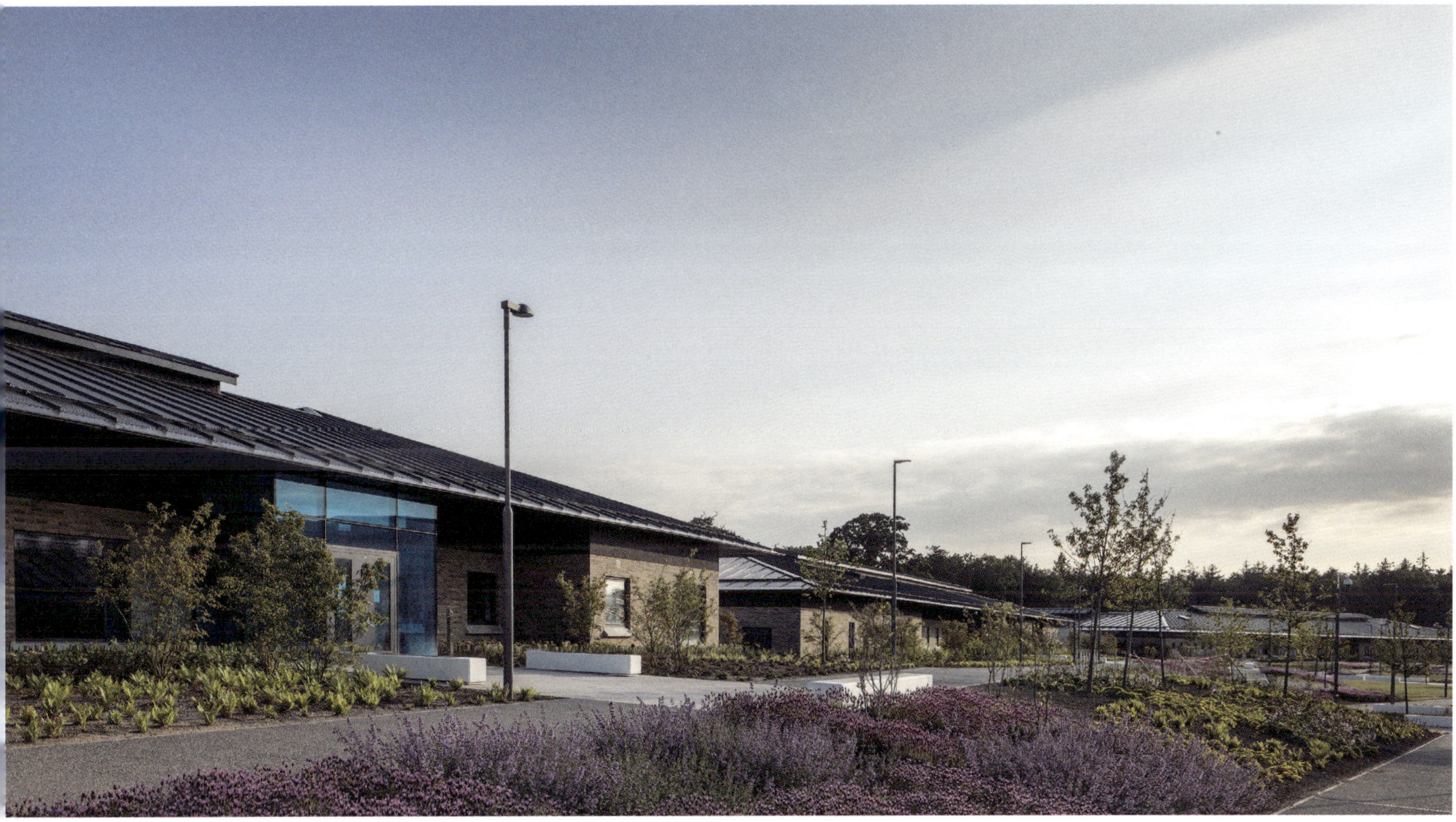

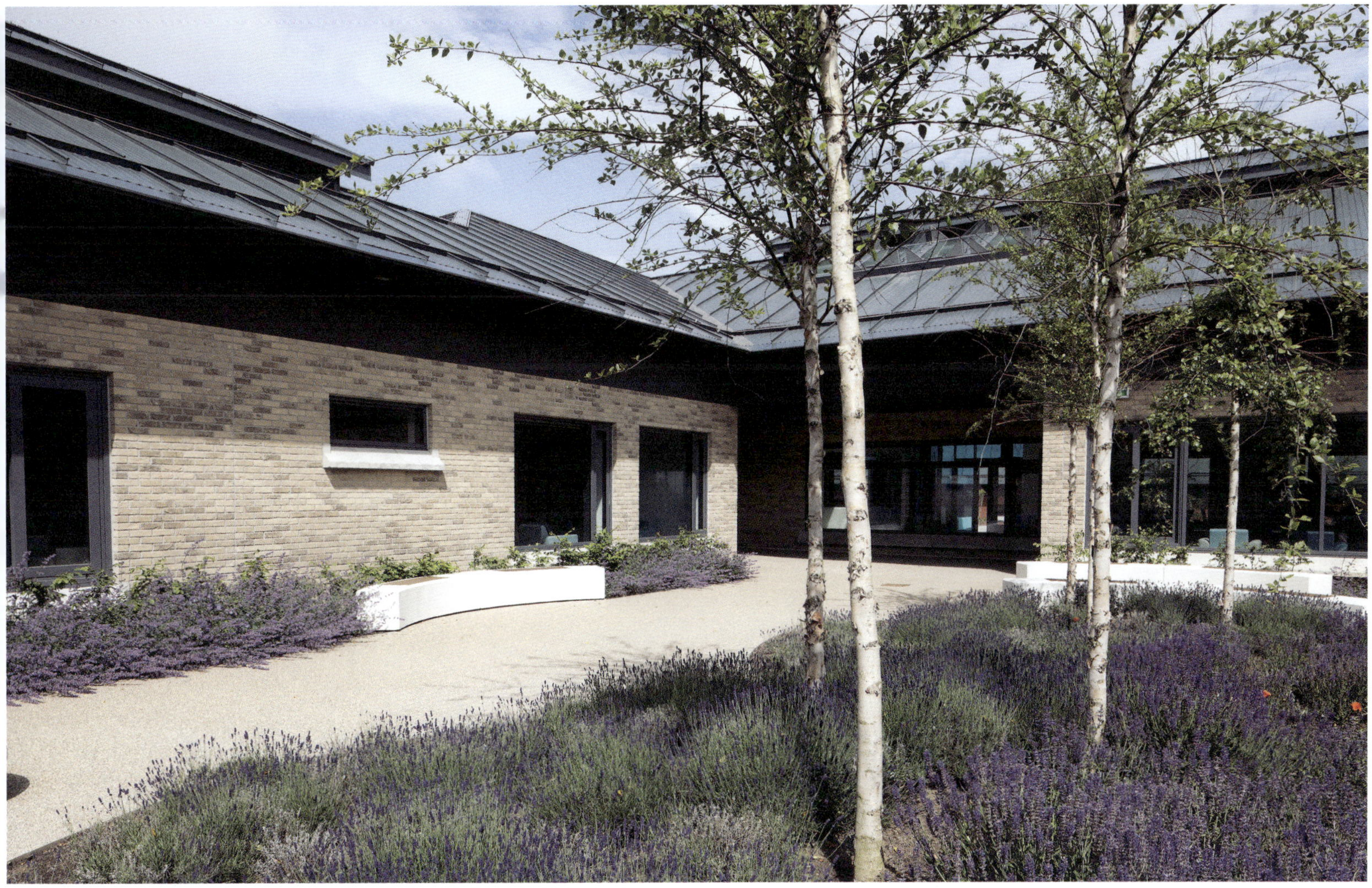

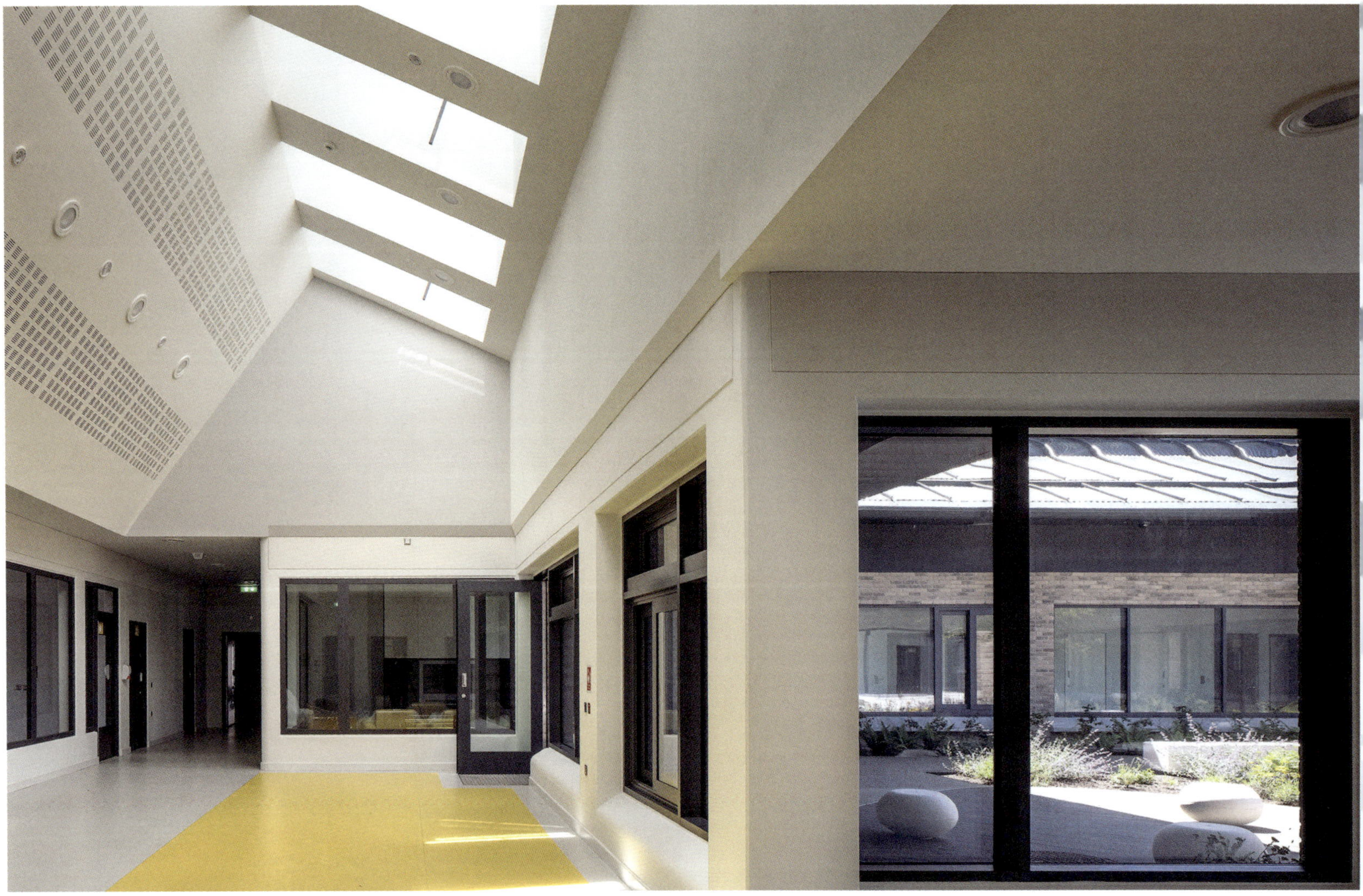

Patient milling area with warm tones, soft daylight, and open circulation zones.

Detail plan layout.

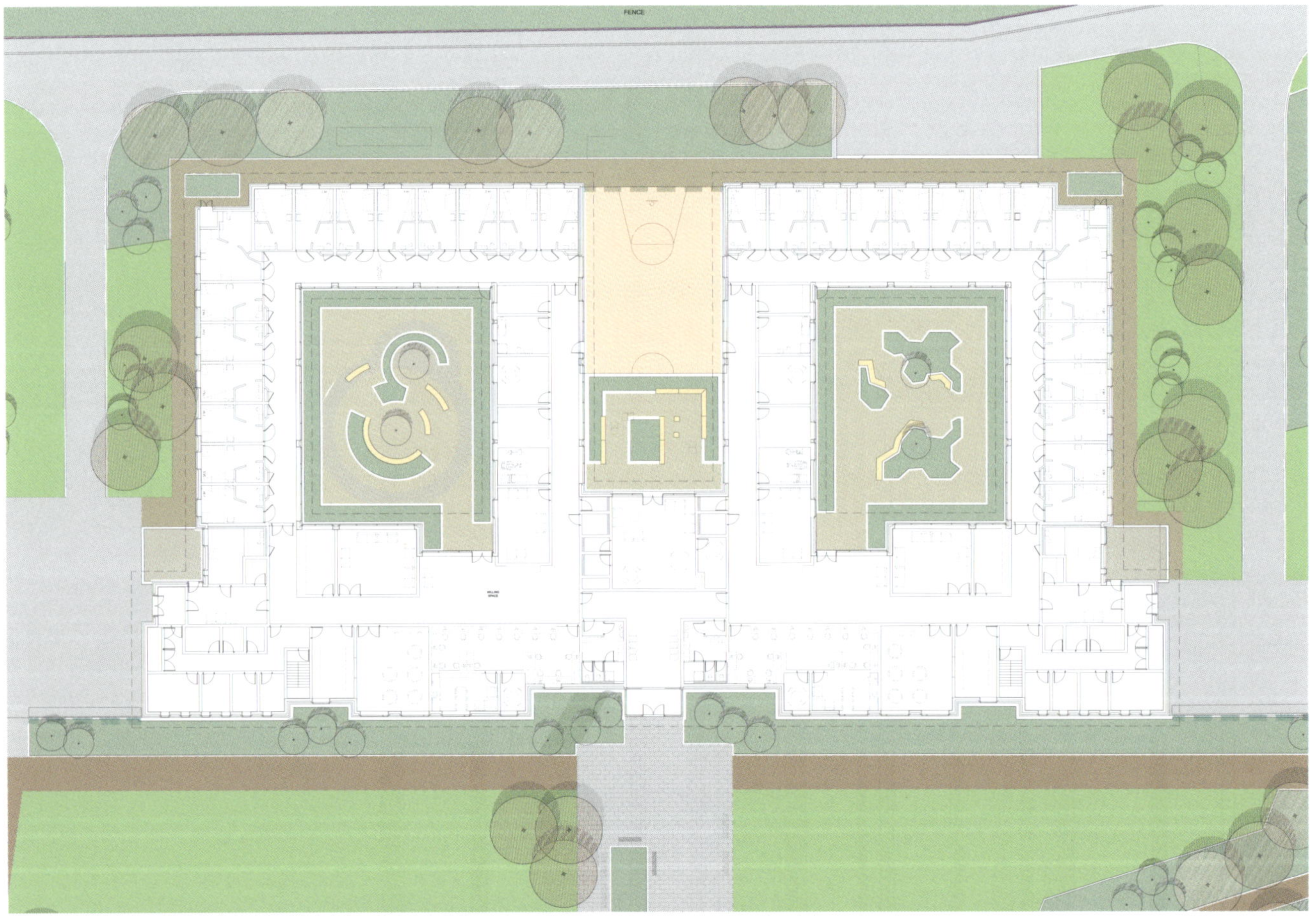

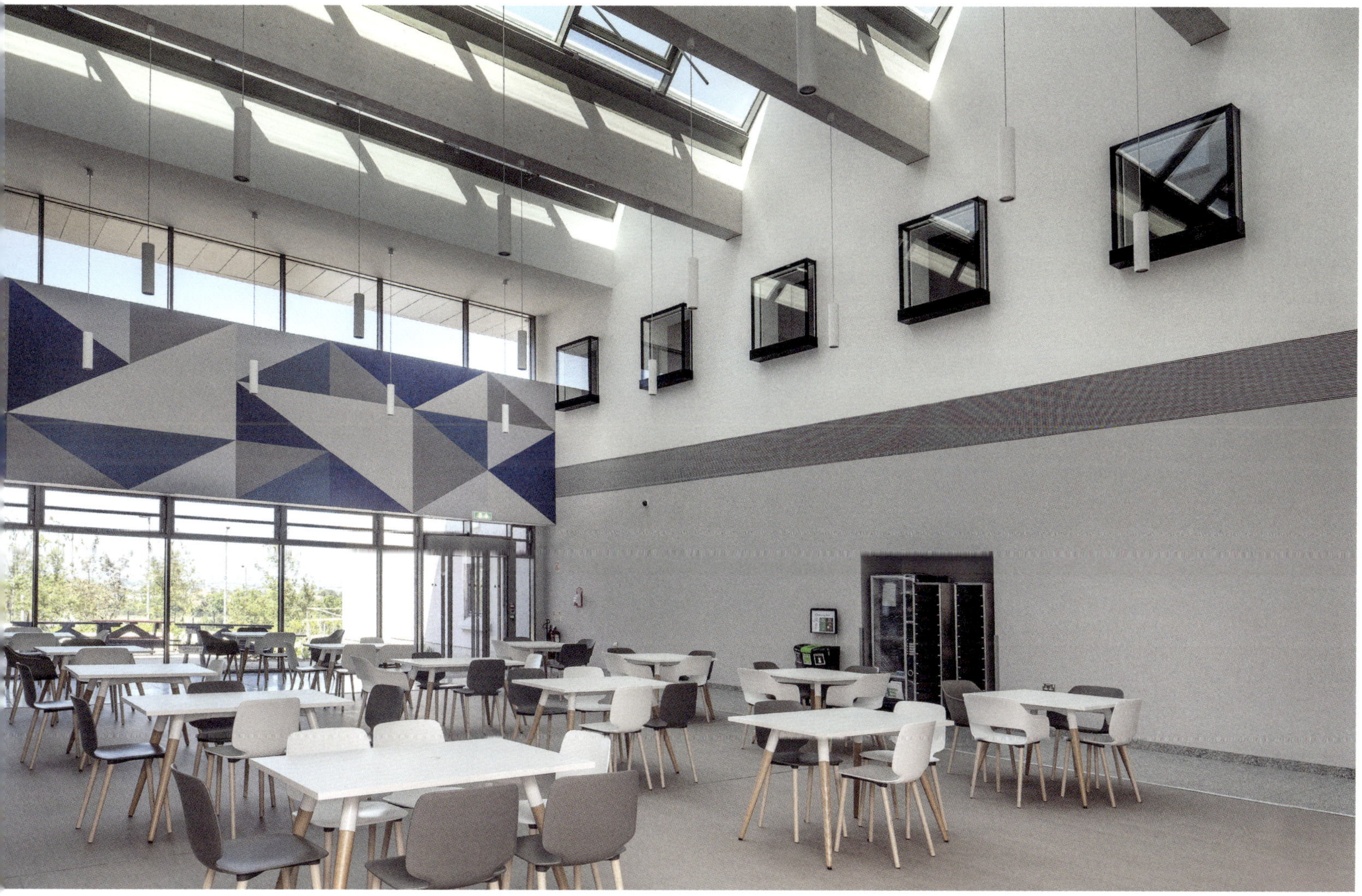

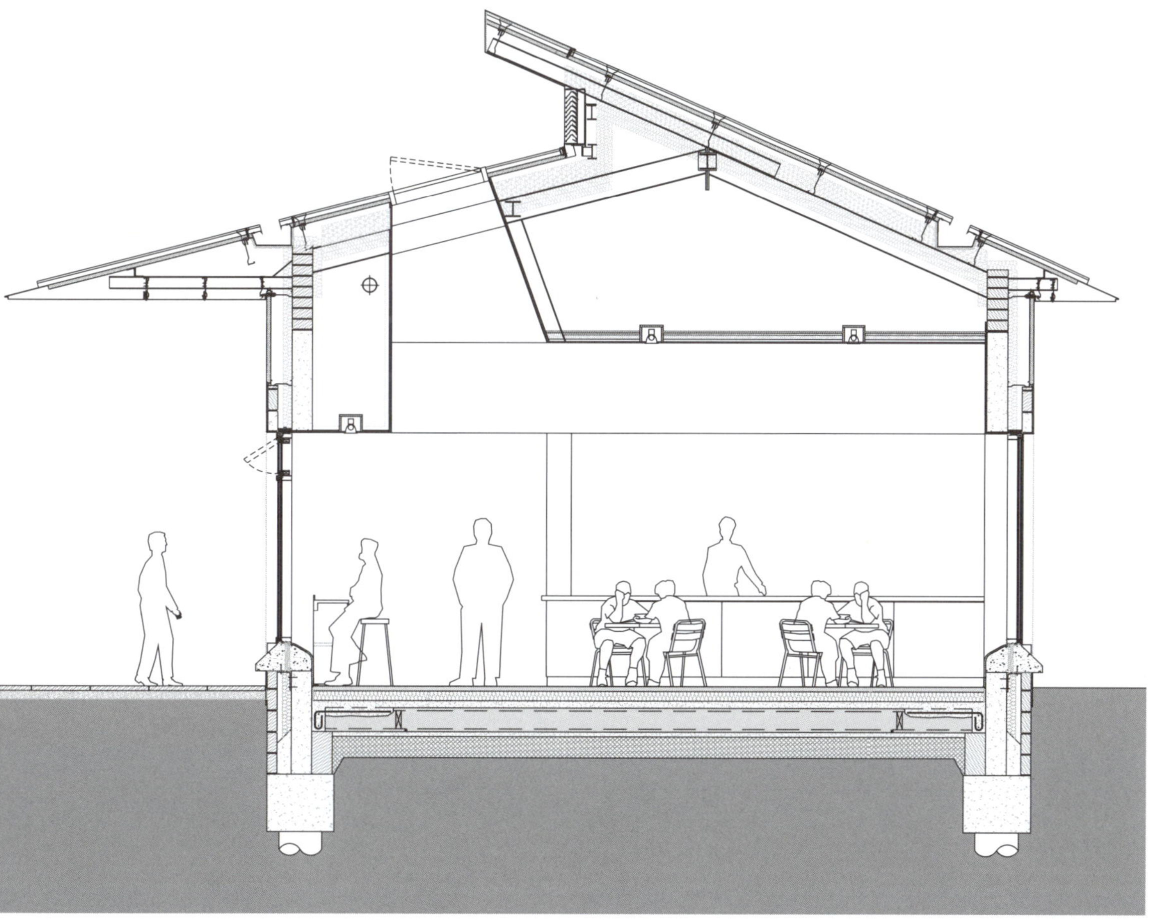

Dining area with glazed atrium and open views to greenery.

Section.

AIDAHO

Tokyo
Japan

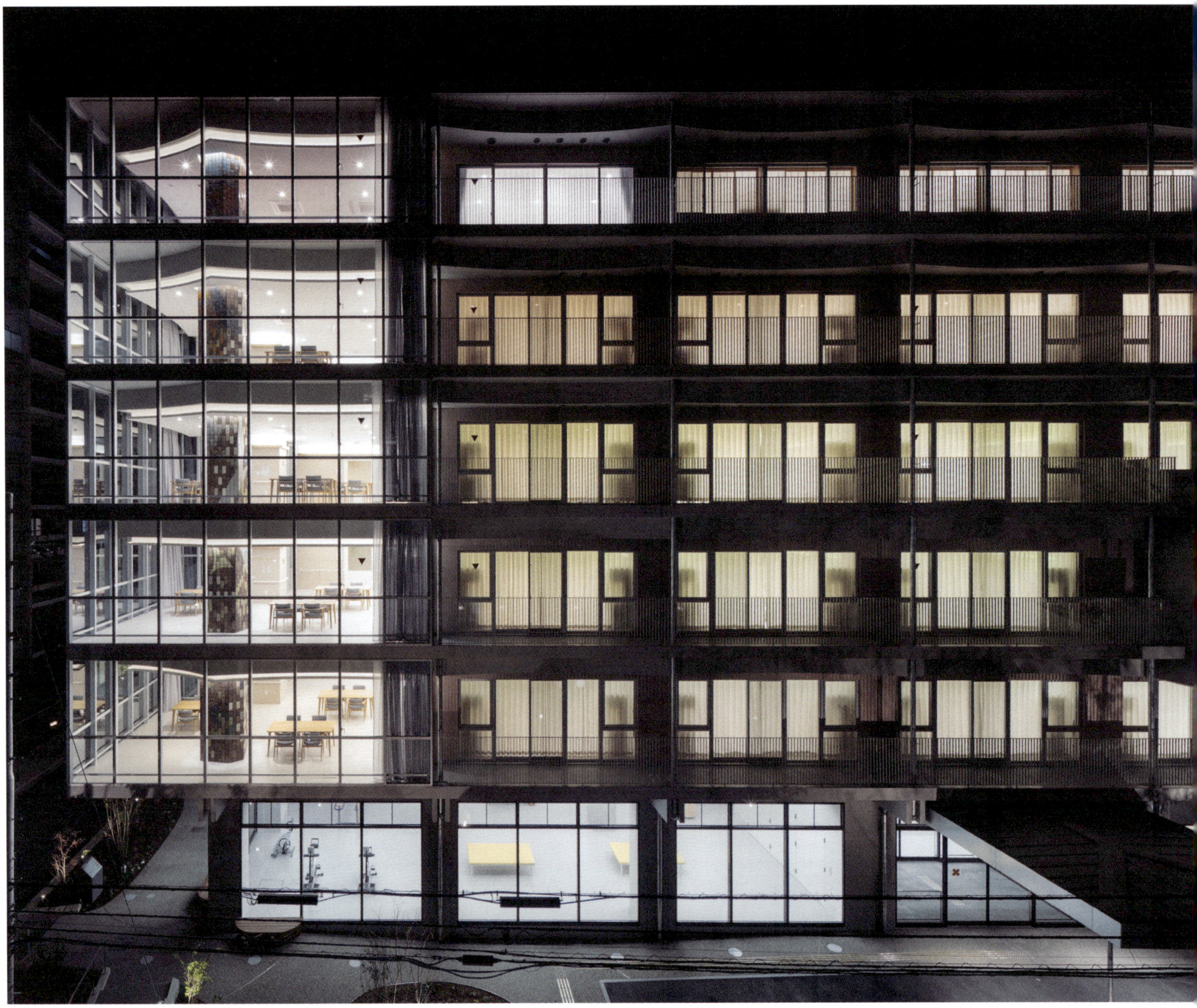

Asoka Hospital South Wing

Exterior view of the hospital's front façade, taken from the opposite building.

Daytime close-up of the distinctive curved façade at the front.

The custom art tile columns and the dining/lounge rooms on each floor.

Asoka Hospital South Wing is designed for holistic regeneration, transcending traditional medical treatment to reconnect patients with everyday life. The ground floor features a rehabilitation room opening onto a Therapy Path – a community garden with natural terrains for real-world walking practice. The rehabilitation wards are inspired by Kintsugi, the Japanese art of repairing broken pottery, symbolizing human resilience and the beauty of recovery. Conversely, the palliative care ward uses natural materials like wood and shoji screens to recreate the peaceful warmth of a home. Visible inside and out, a symbolic giant tree column pierces through each floor's lounge, clad in custom tiles collaboratively crafted by a tile manufacturer in Tokoname – a city renowned for its ceramics – and a local welfare facility.

Address: 1-18-1 Sumiyoshi, Koto-ku, Tokyo 135-0002, Japan | **Client:** Social Welfare Corporation Asokakai | **Completion:** 2024 | **Size:** 4,903 m^2 | **Sector:** private | **Number of treatment rooms:** 4 | **Number of patient rooms:** 61 | **Sign design:** Hokkyok/Hokuto Fujii | **Planting design:** Suniha Uniha/Miho Yoshida | **Artwork tiles:** Koji Takahashi Design office, Mizuno Seitoen Lab

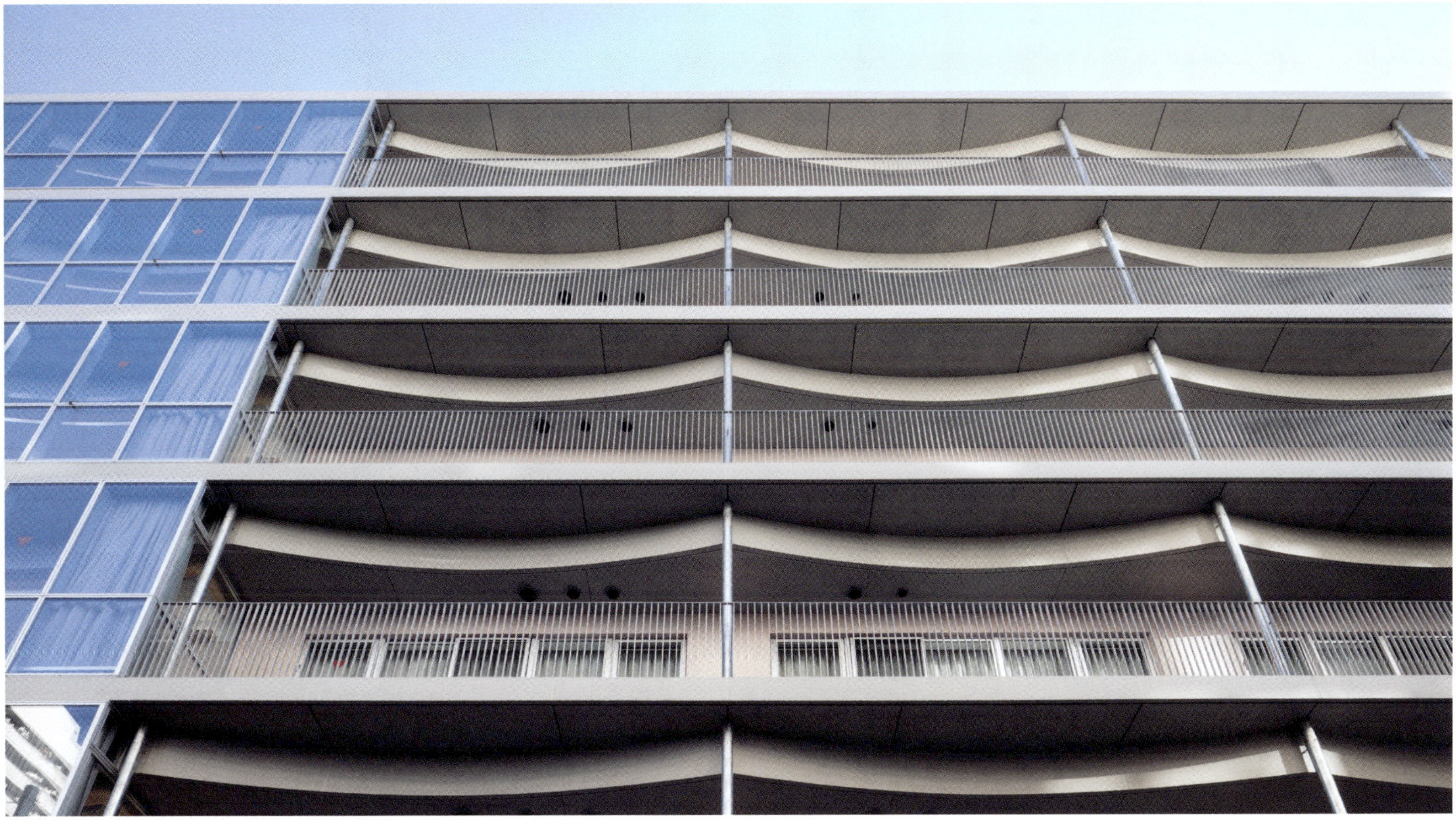

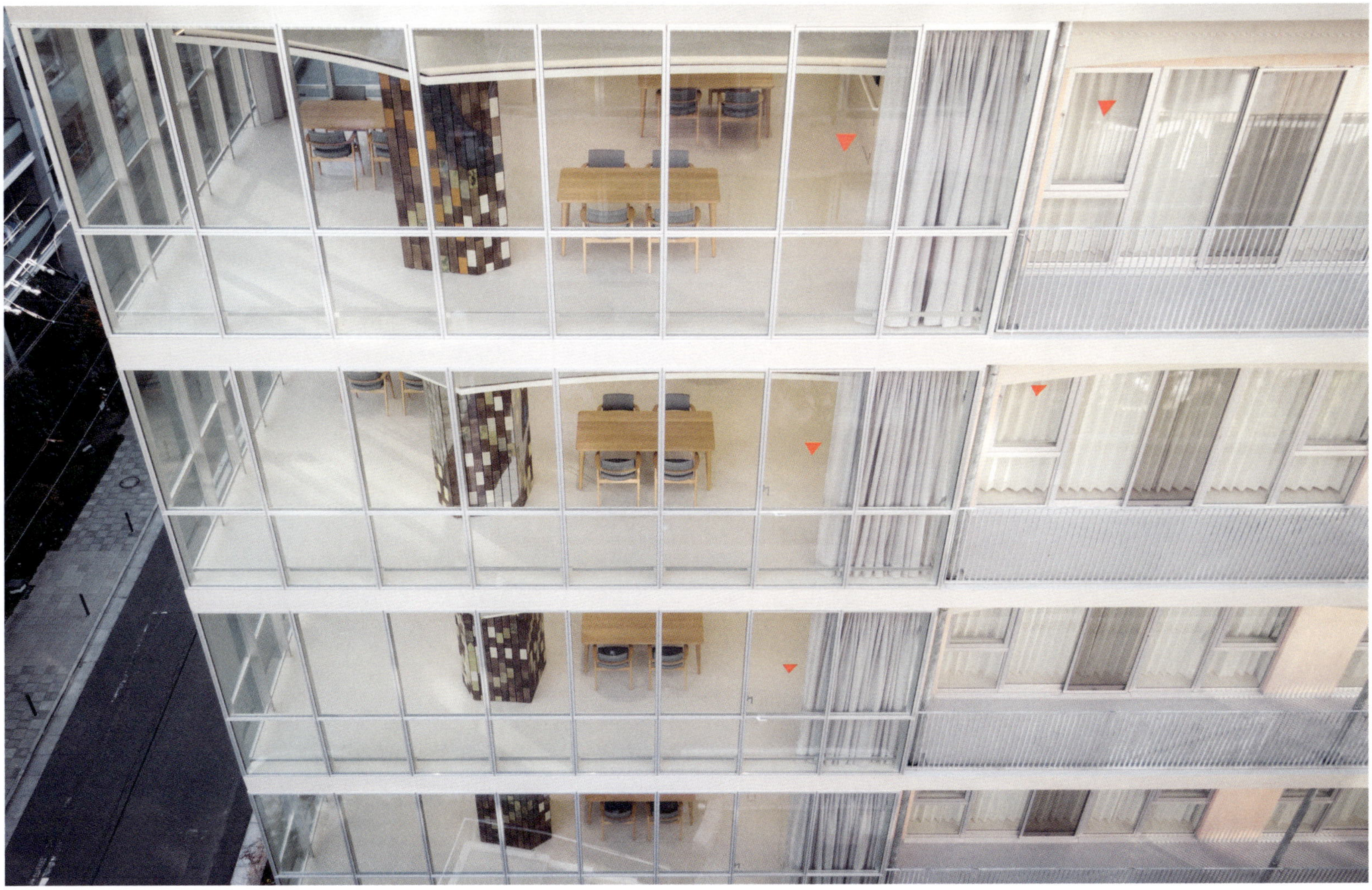

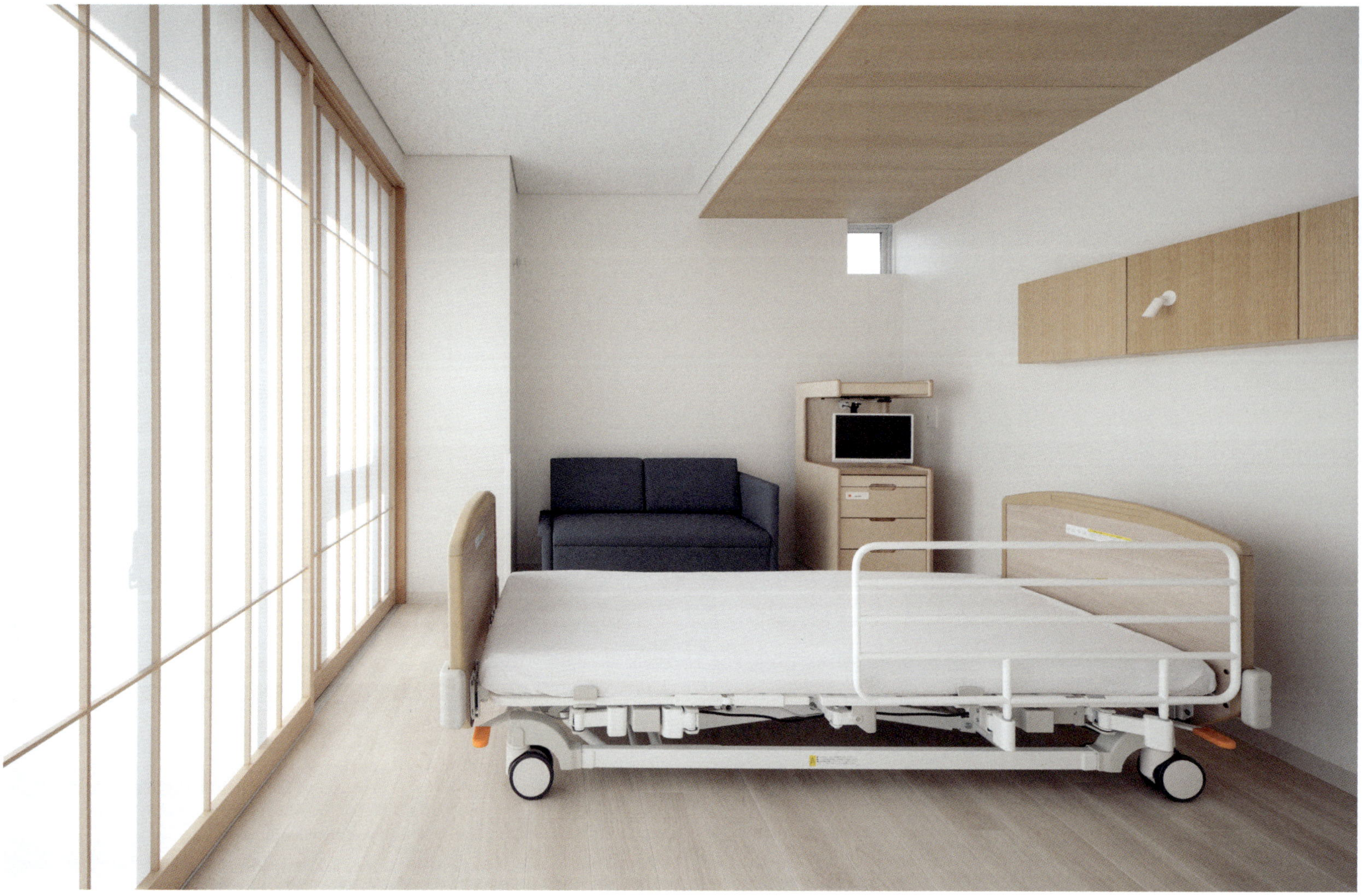

A private patient room in the palliative care ward.

East, north, and west elevation. Ground floor plan.

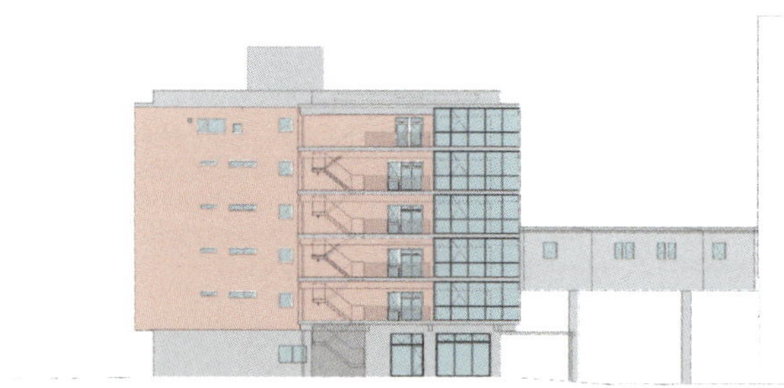

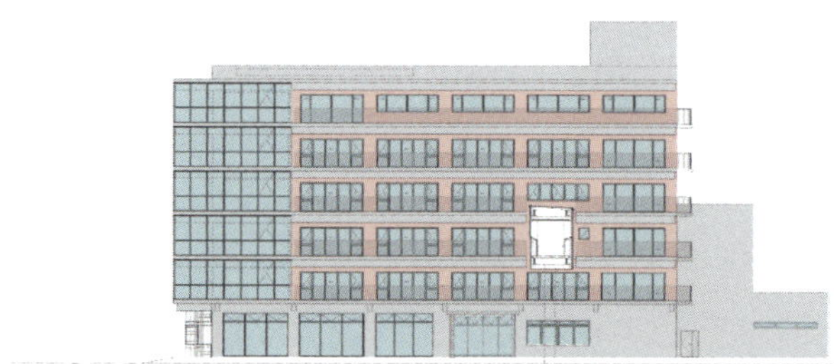

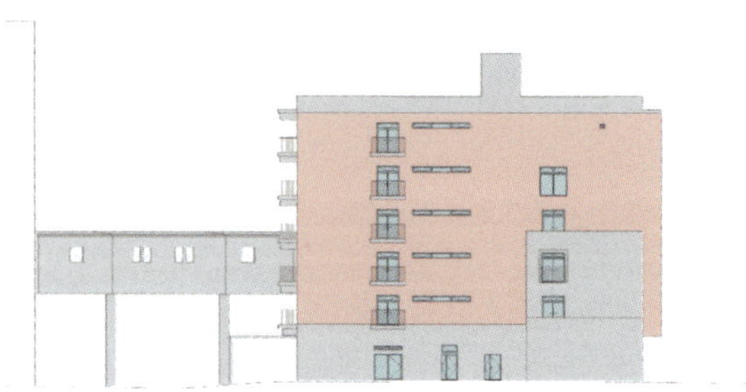

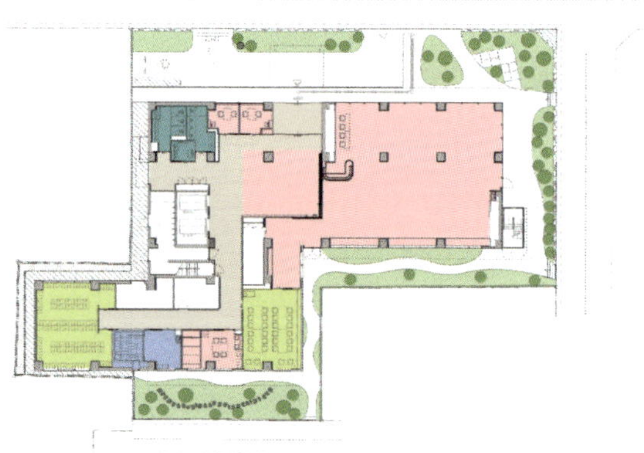

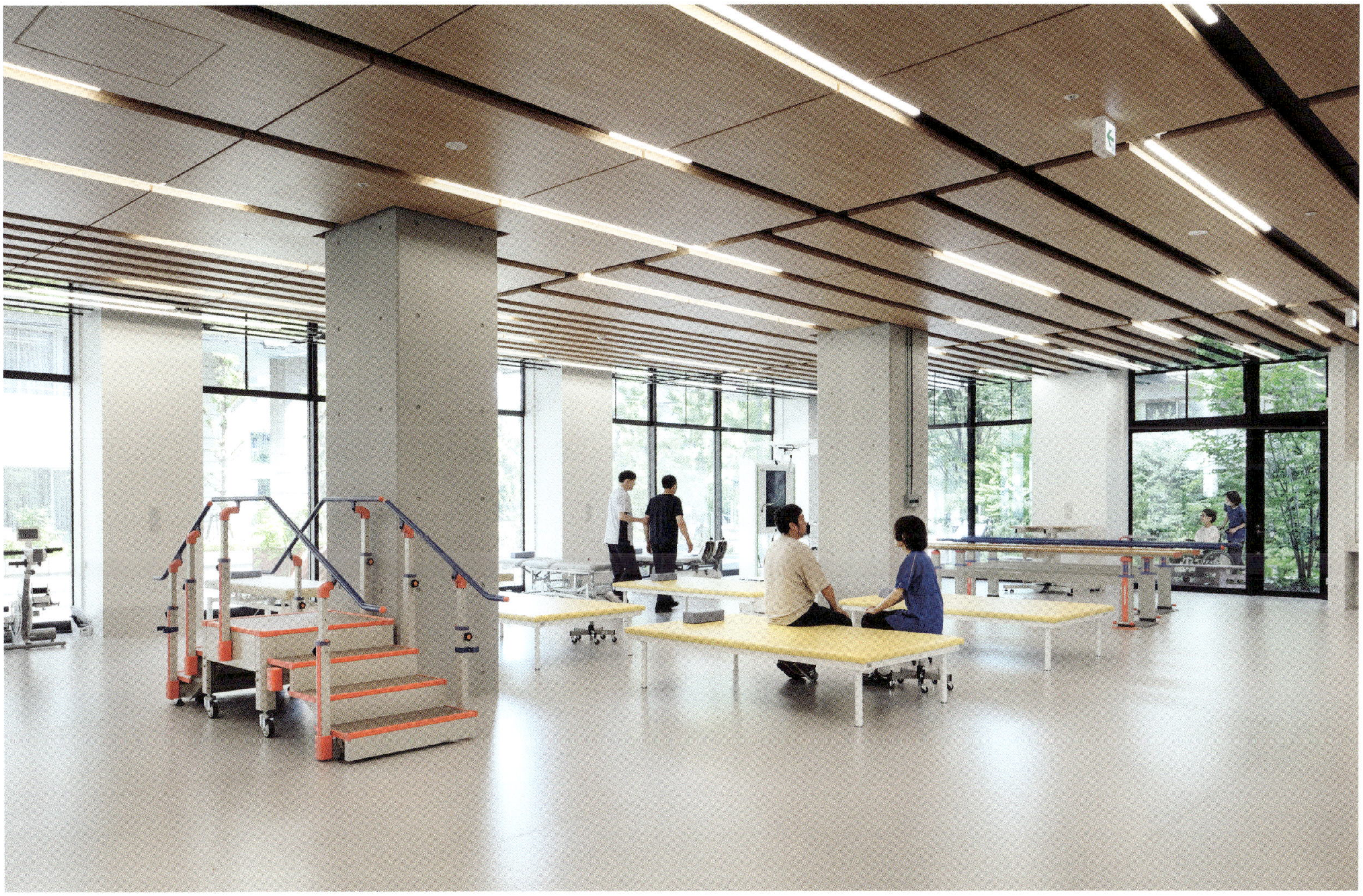

Interior view of the ground floor rehabilitation room.

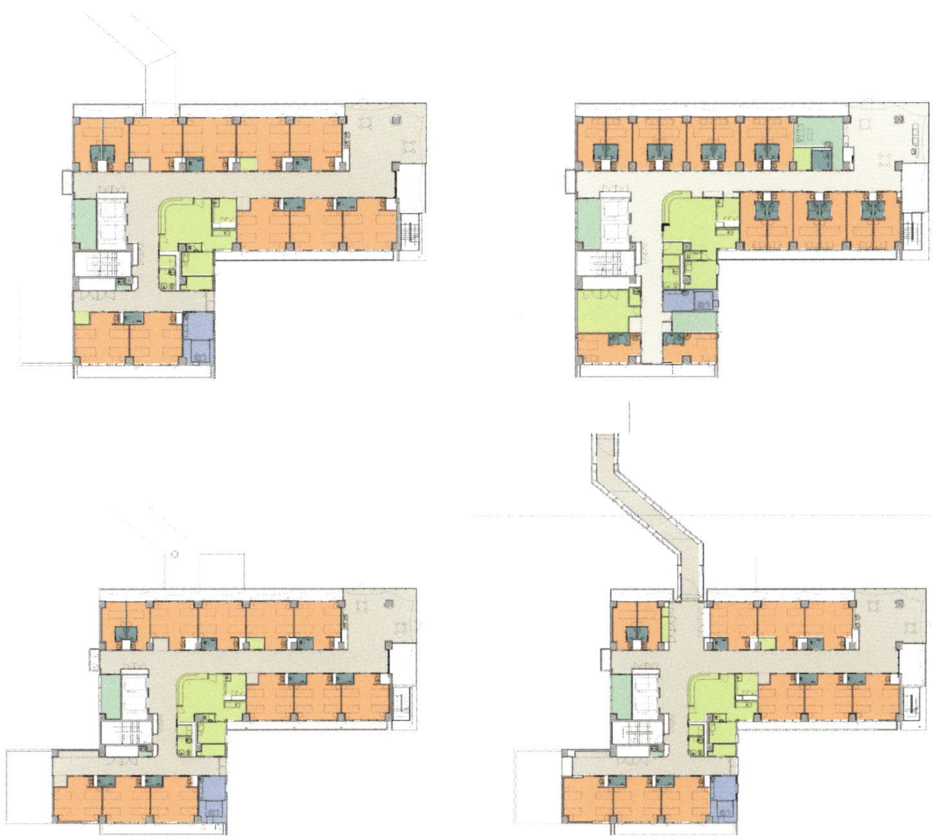

Third, fourth, first and second floor plans.

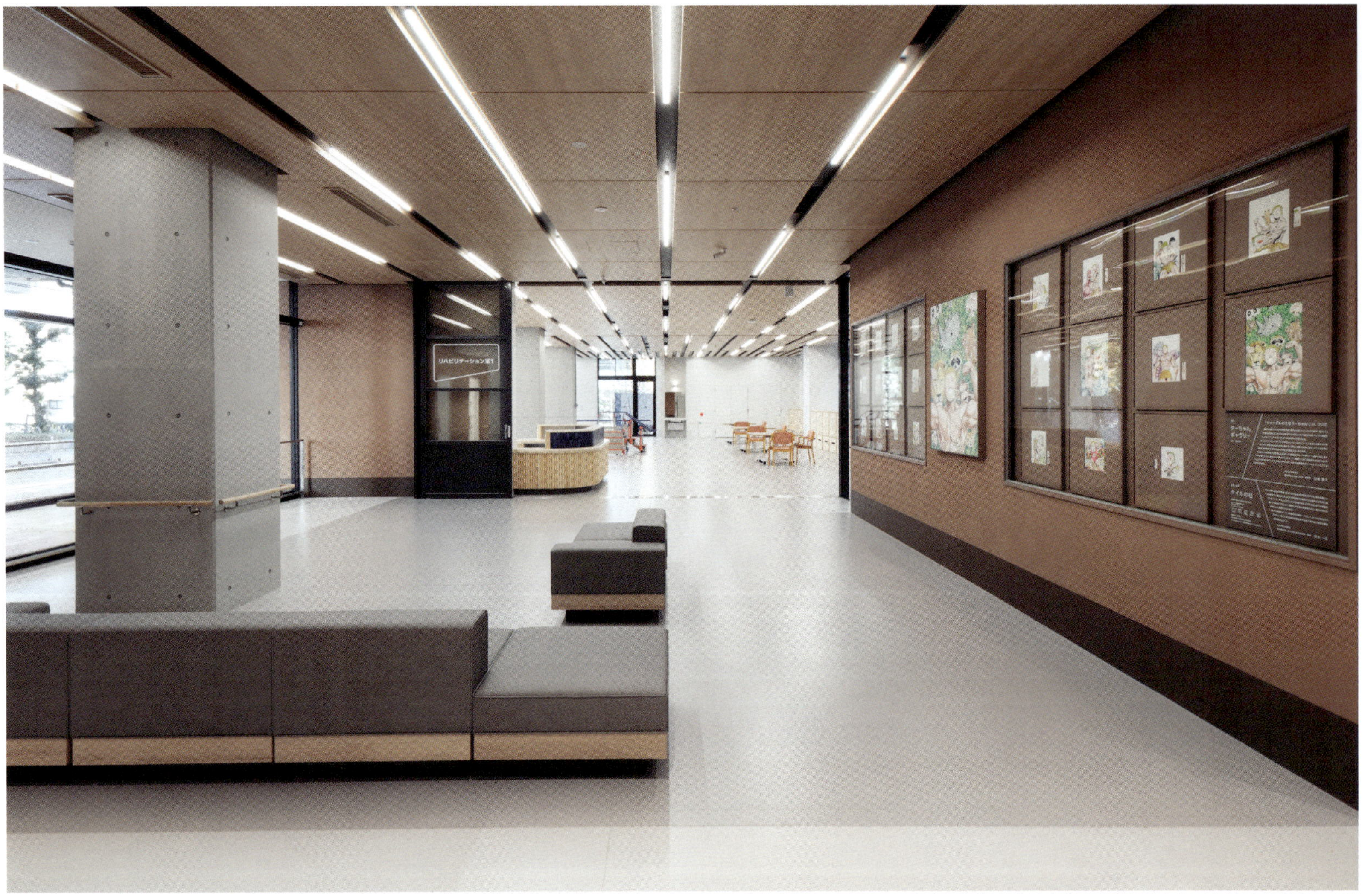

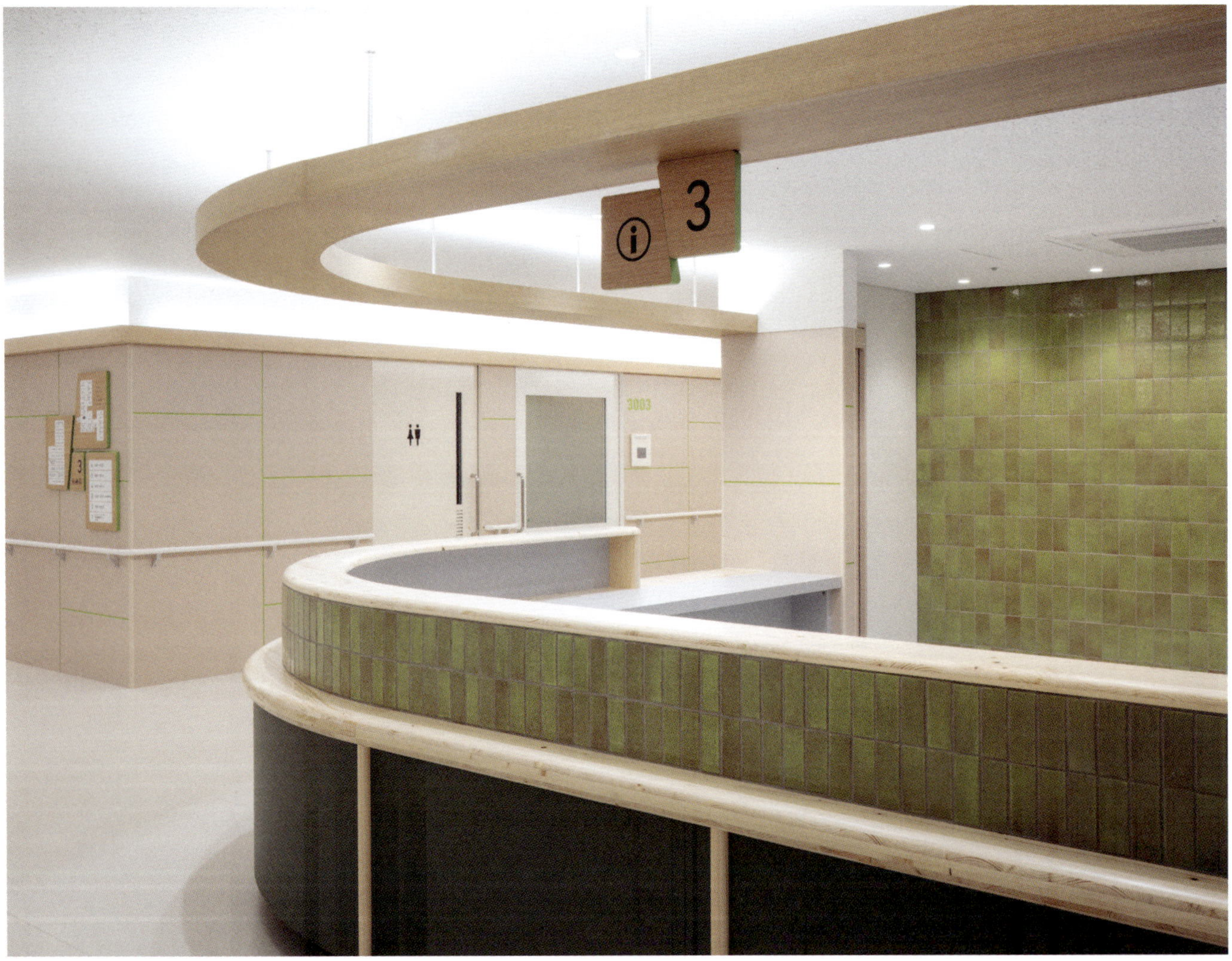

Interior view of the ground floor entrance hall and rehabilitation room.

The reception area and common corridor in the third-floor rehabilitation ward.

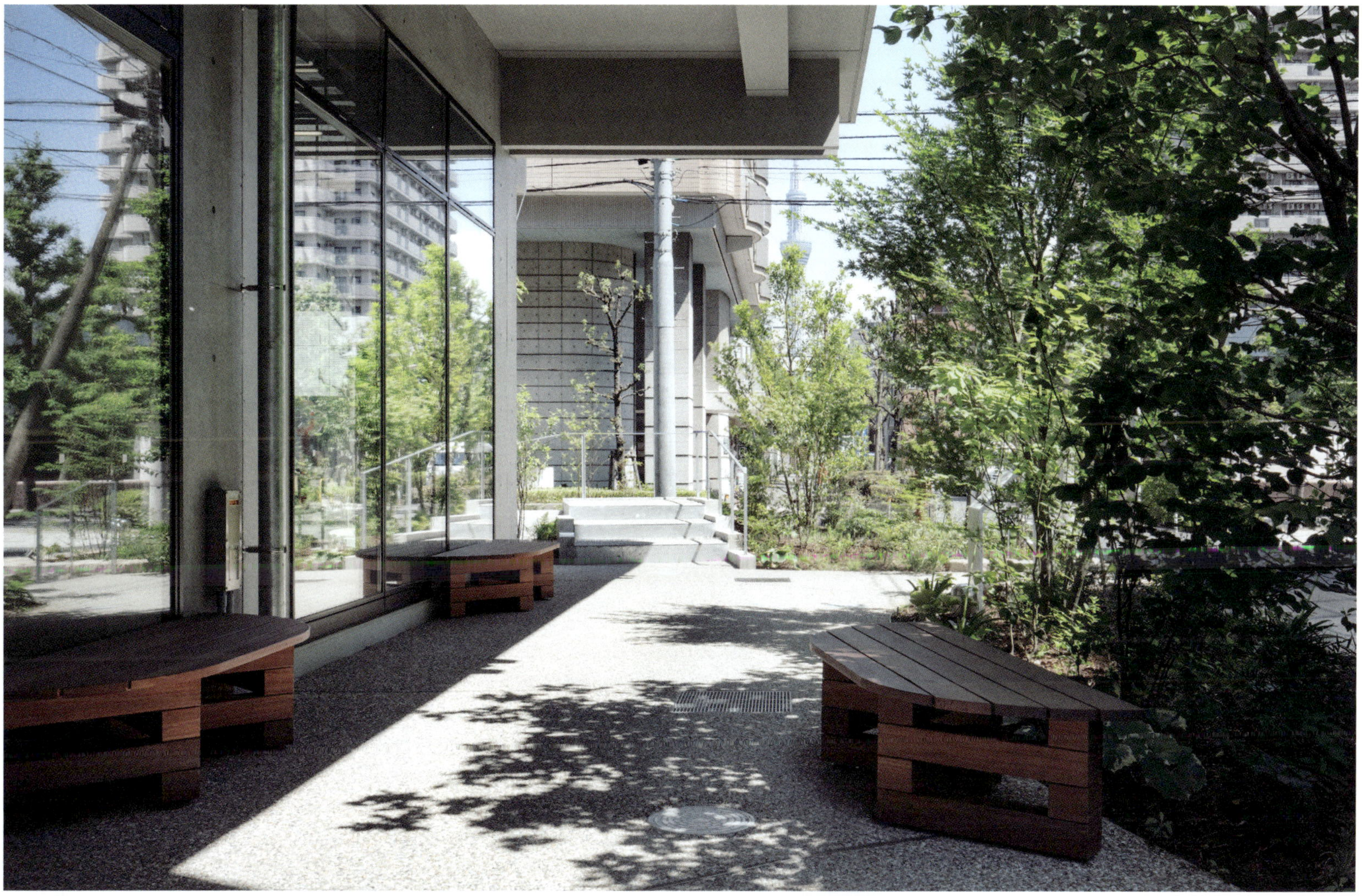

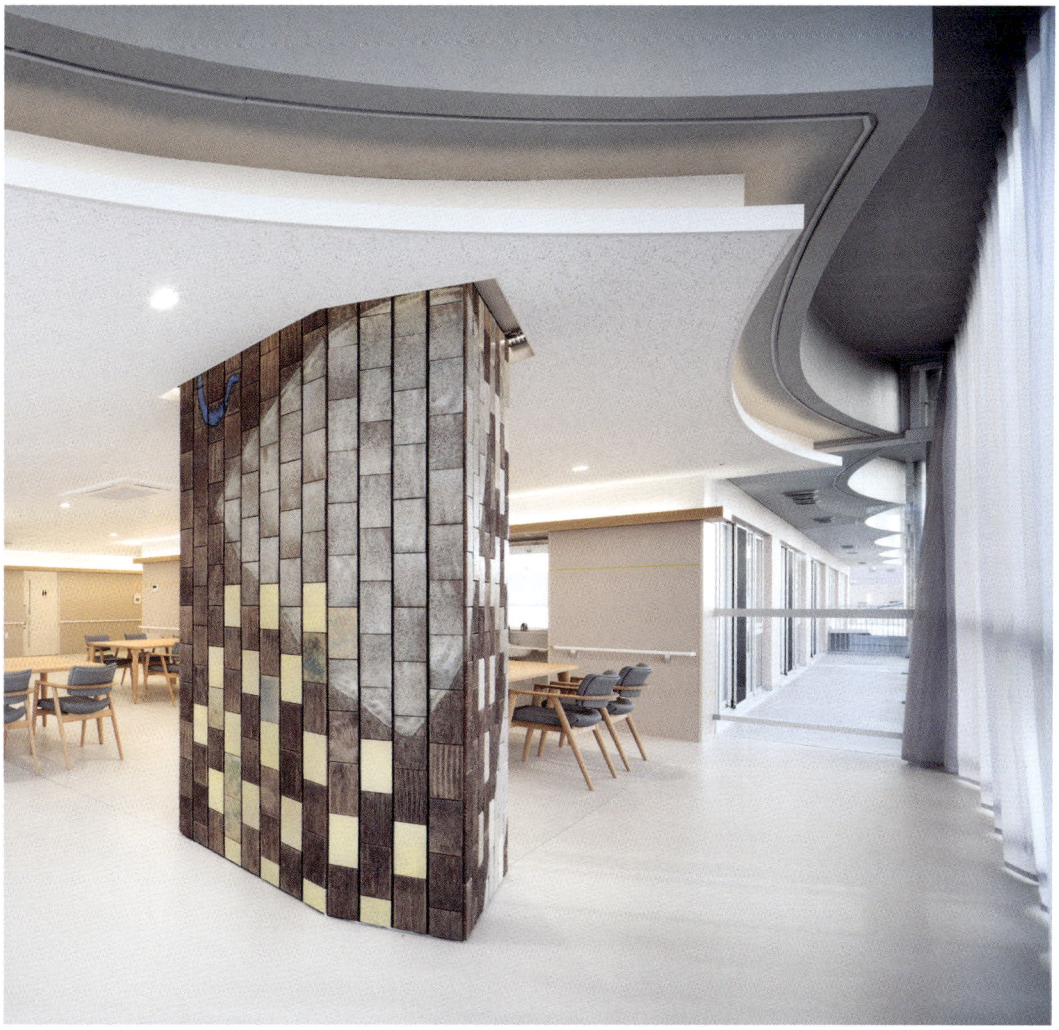

A walking path and benches, open to the community and also used for patient rehabilitation.

The dining and lounge in the rehabilitation ward, taken from the window side.

Schnittger Architekten + Partner

Kiel
Germany

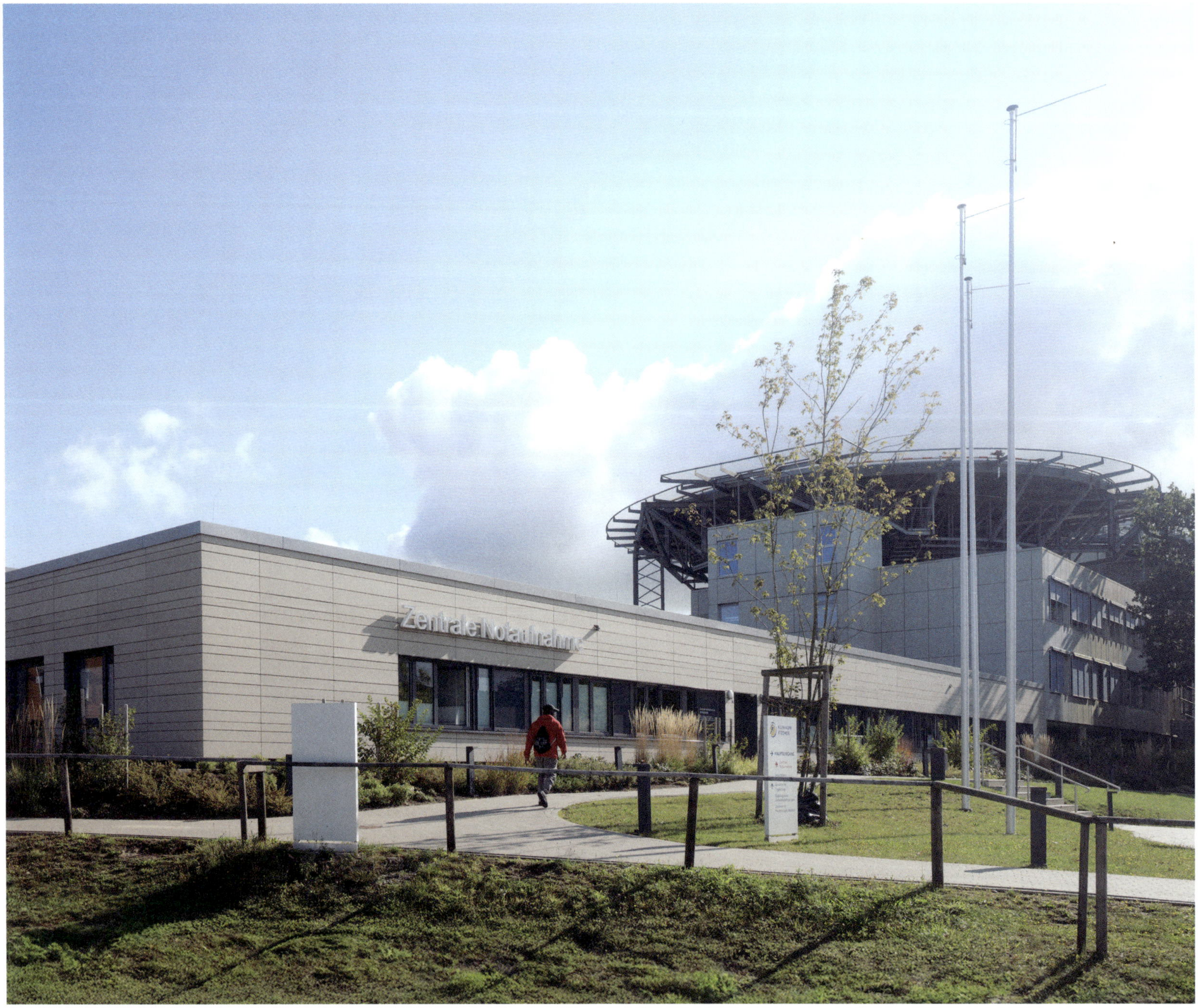

Entrance of the new emergency department.

Back view of the emergency department.

Close-up of its façade with signage.

Itzehoe Hospital Emergency Department

Located in northern Germany the central emergency department at Itzehoe Hospital was expanded to ensure a modern, future-proof patient intake process. The new building creates a clear patient flow and a walk-in clinic that optimizes synergies and filters out unnecessary patient movement from the emergency department. Besides the walk-in clinic it includes a stretcher ramp, an entrance for ambulatory patients, a triage zone, and a patient registration area with waiting zones. The wayfinding within the existing building has been adapted. In addition, a new shock room and a CT room with adjacent ancillary spaces were implemented. Furthermore, multifunctional office workspaces were positioned in the façade area, along with four examination rooms. The construction project was carried out in three phases while the hospital remained in operation.

Address: Robert-Koch-Straße 2, 25524 Itzehoe, Germany | **Client:** Itzehoe Hospital | **Completion:** 2023 | **Size:** 1,708 m² | **Sector:** other | **Specialization:** emergency department | **Number of treatment rooms:** 17 | **Landscape design:** Siller Landschaftsarchitekten

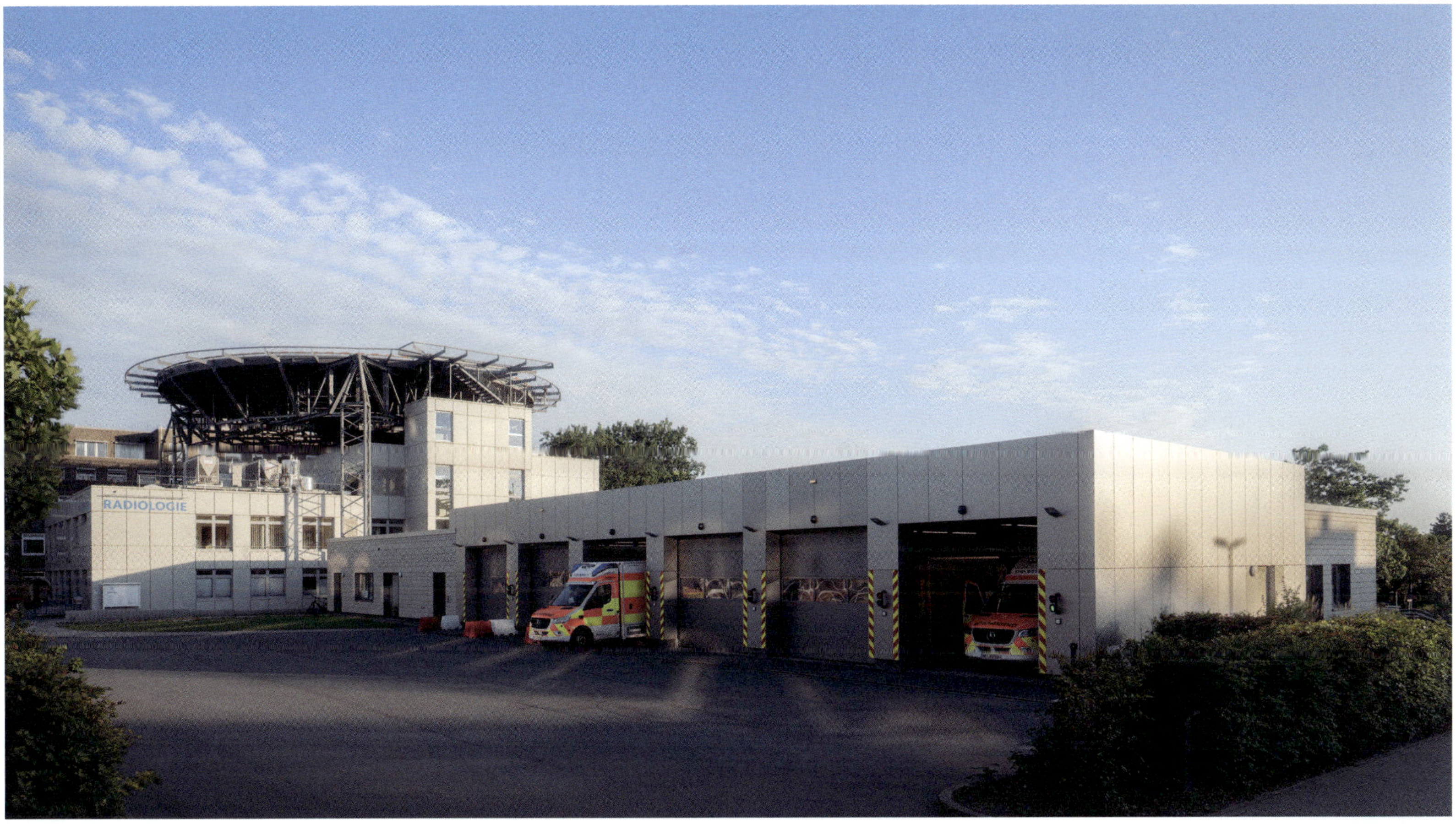

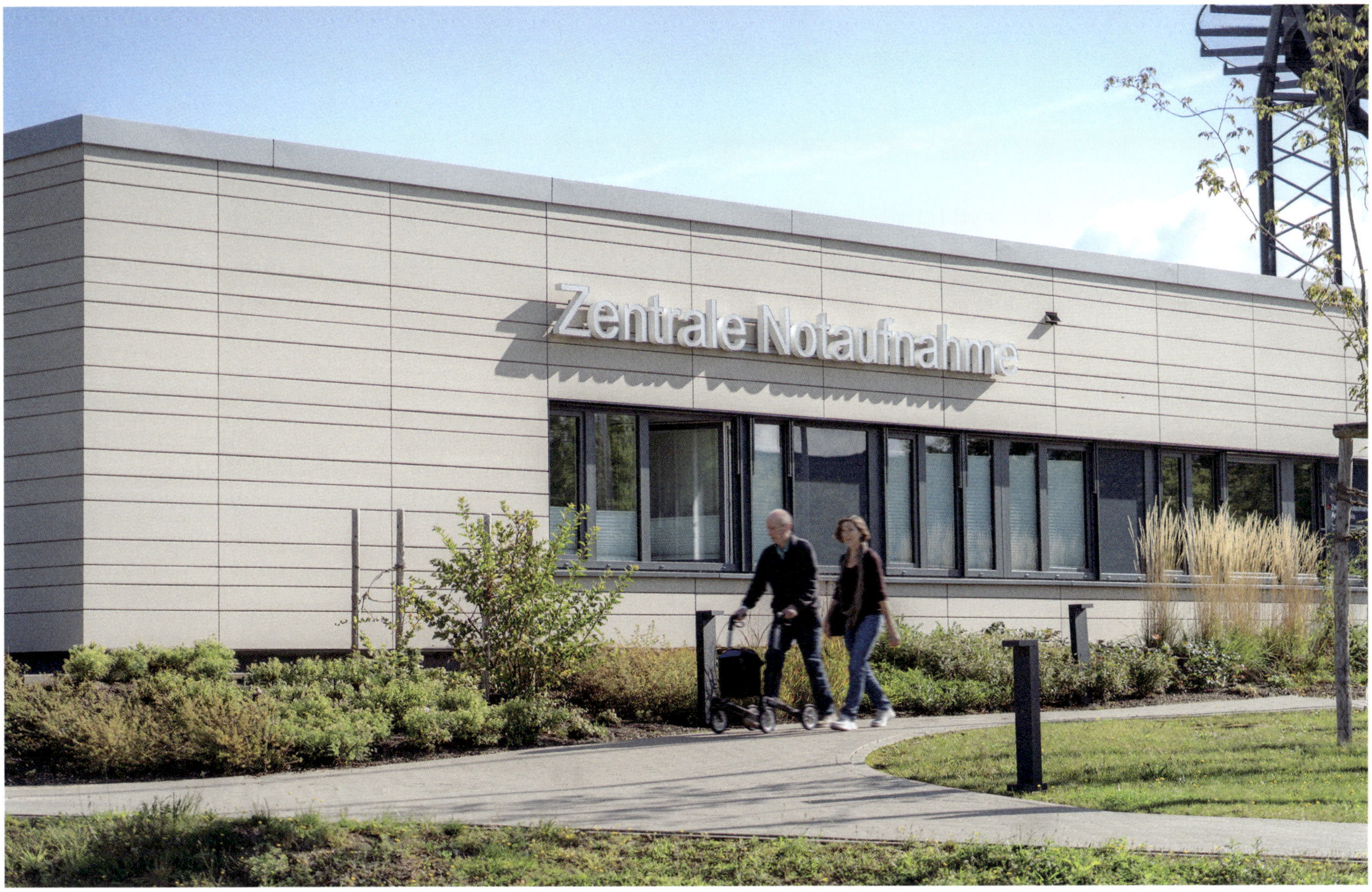

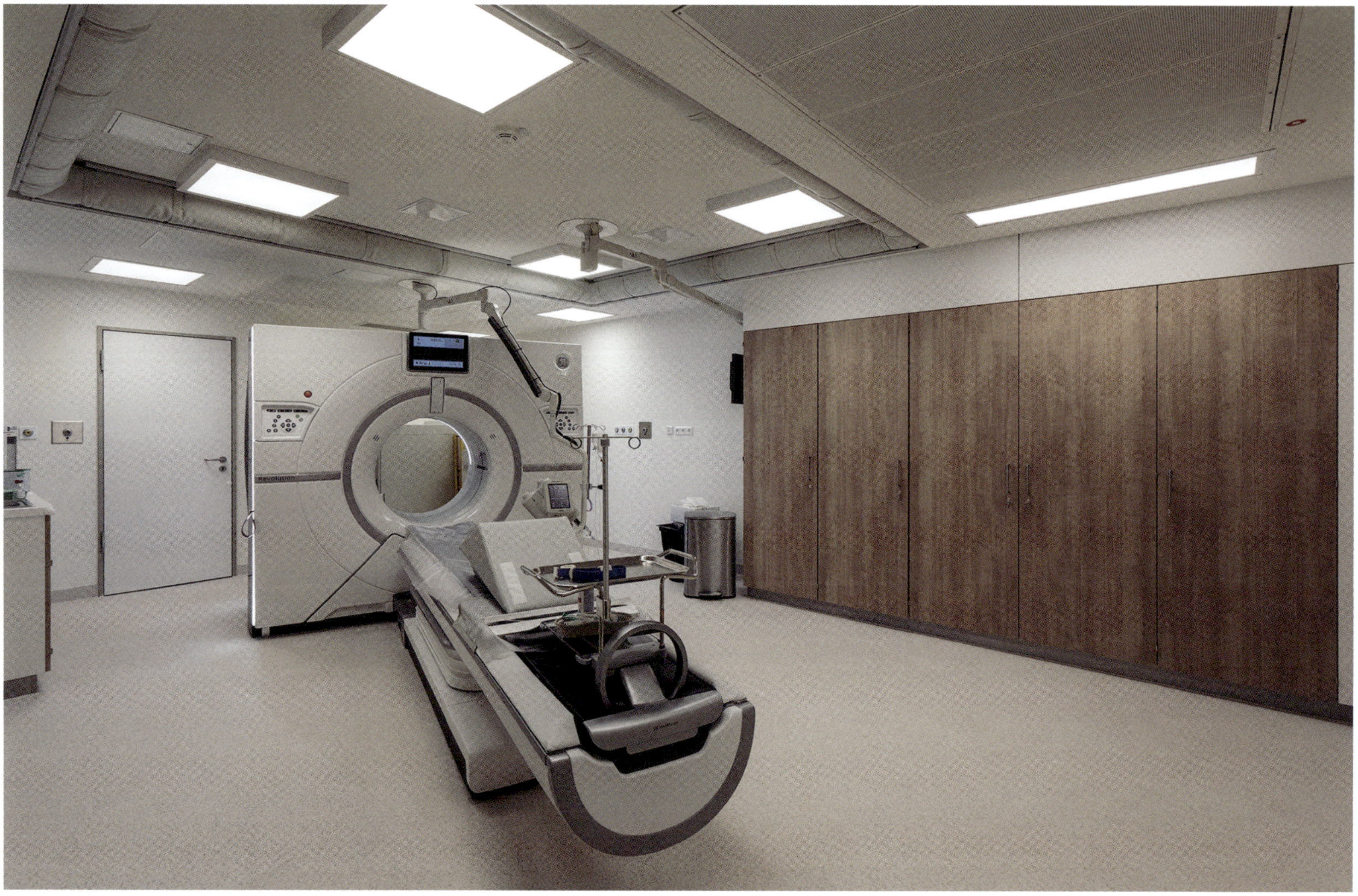

Interior view with CT scan.

Floor plan of the new constructed building.

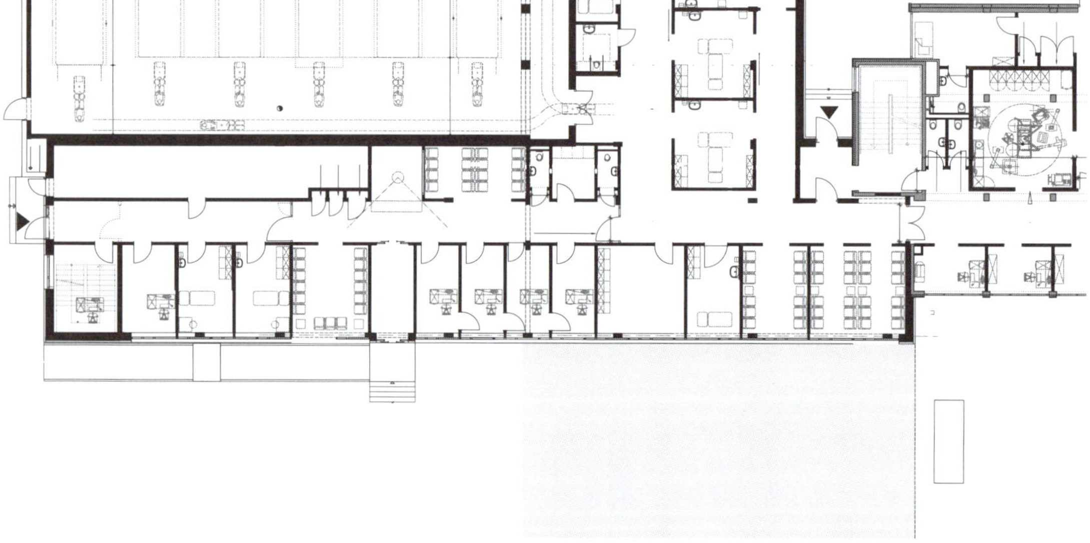

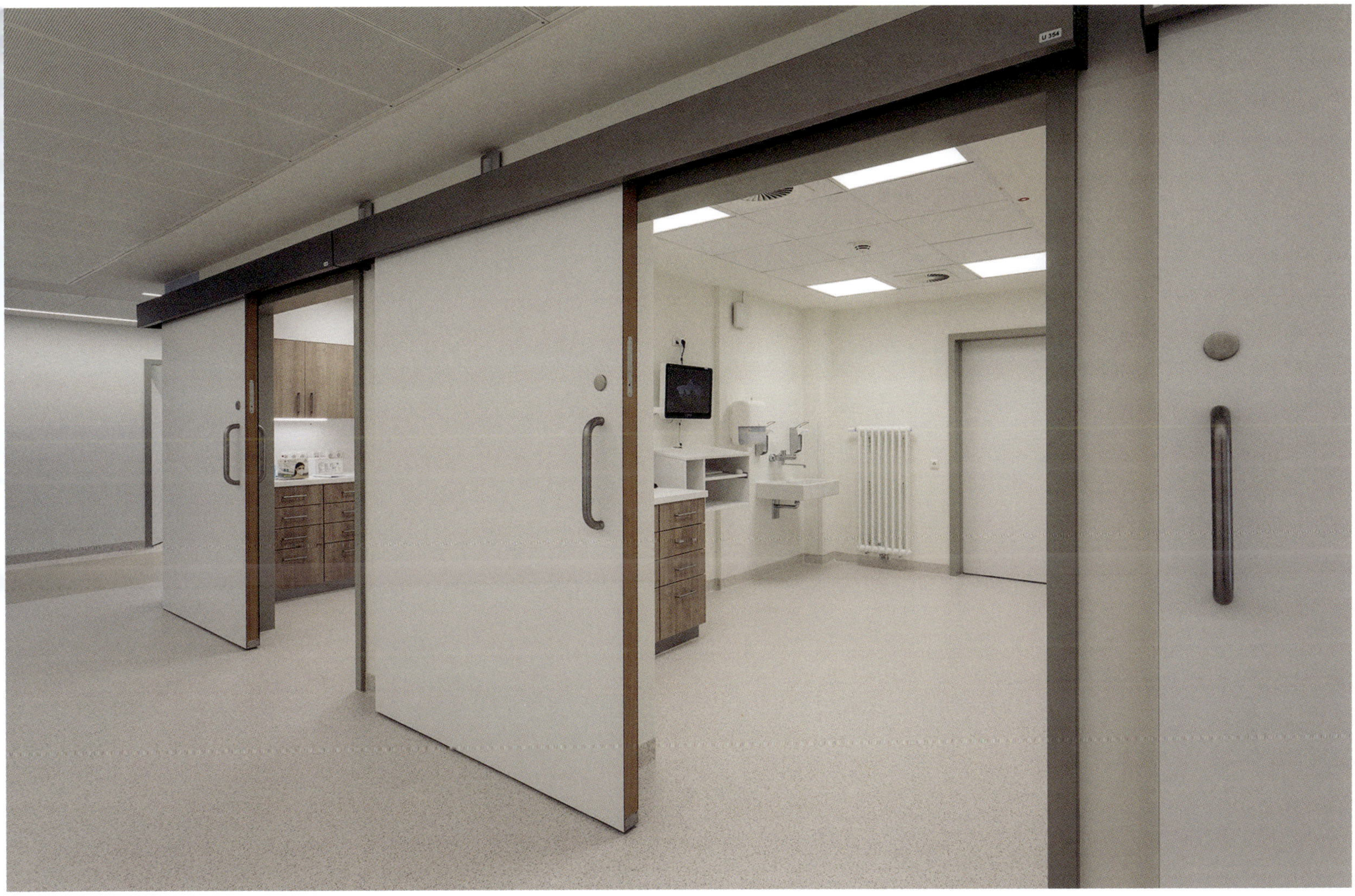

Interior view of the examination rooms.

Floor plan of the renovated existing building.

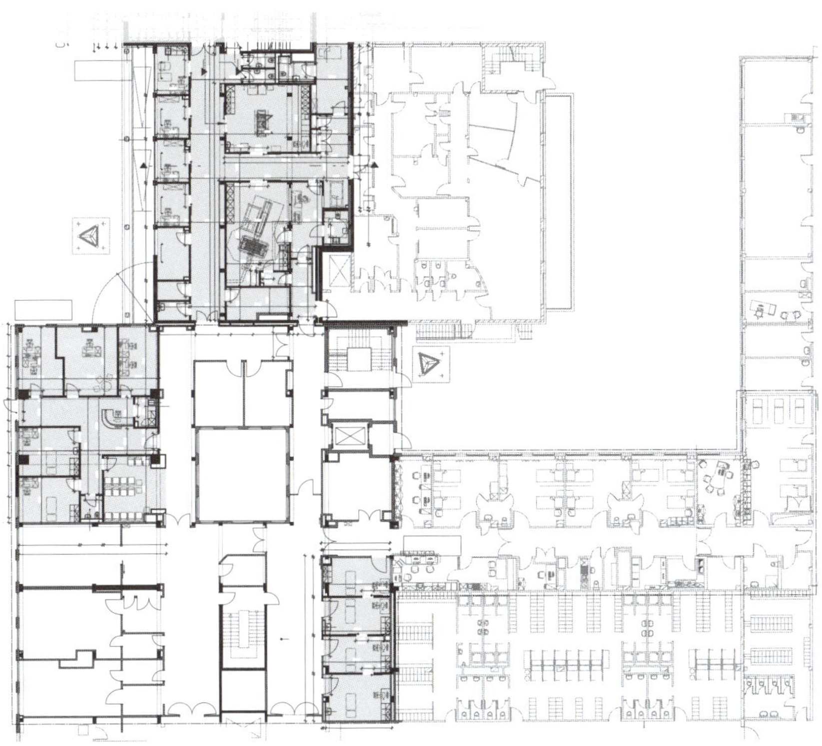

Wiegerinck

Hilversum
The Netherlands

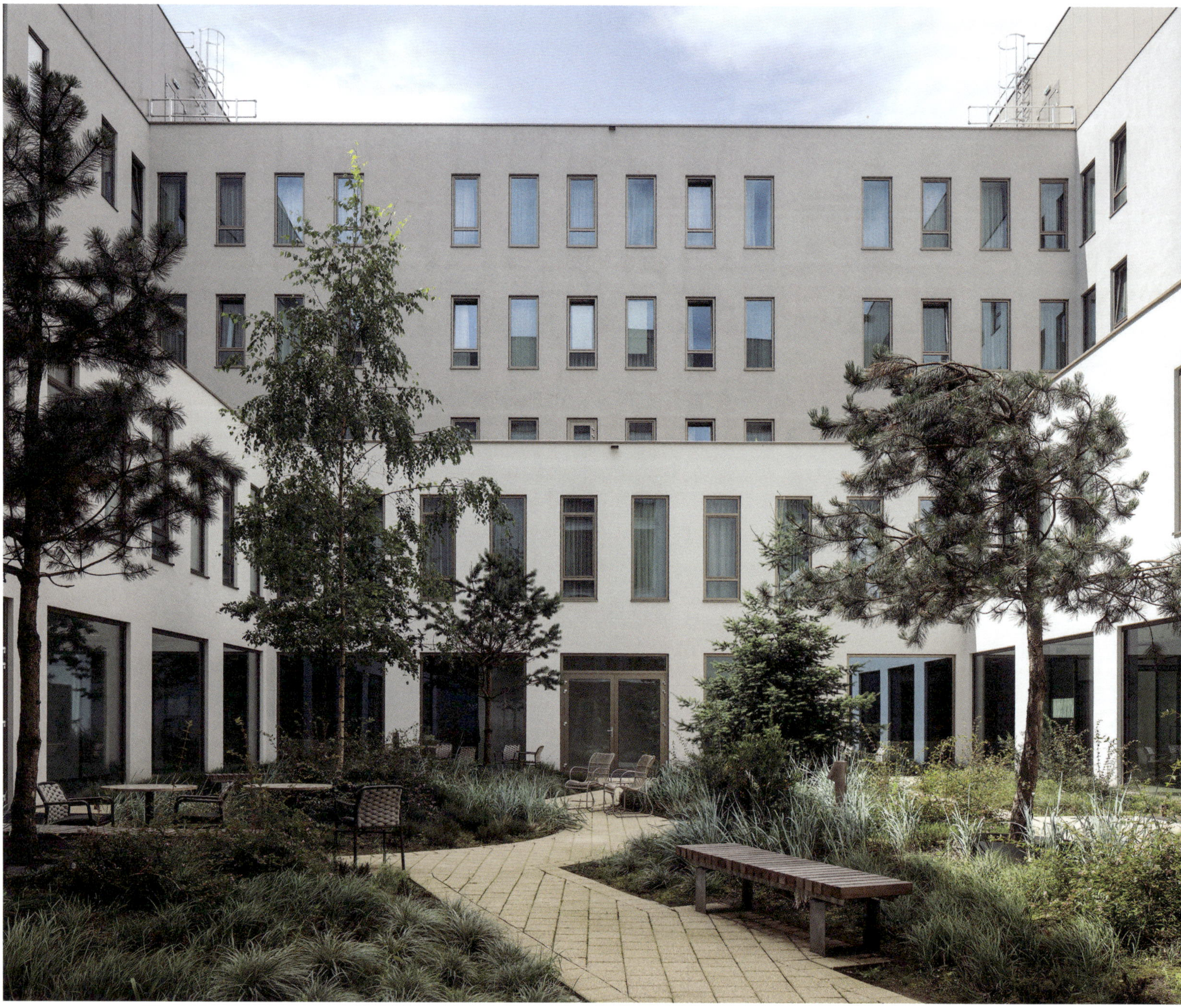

Green spaces harmoniously connect all sections of the hospital.

Main entrance of the hospital.

Entrance area and façade.

Tergooi MC

From 2023, Tergooi MC provides all acute, intensive, and clinical care at one central location in Hilversum. The new hospital offers a soft, calming, and open environment for patients and staff. Nature and daylight play an important role in the design. The building features numerous windows overlooking the beautiful green surroundings. Hidden in the trees are four seemingly separate building sections. On the ground floor and the first floor, however, the hospital feels like one continuous whole due to wide, light, transparent corridors. For patients and visitors in the central hall, the passage gives a sense of direction. It runs like a spine through the entire complex. At the transition from one part of the building to the other, one passes through conservatory-like corridors that gives the feeling of stepping outside. Each section also has a large patio, which ensures ample light and connection with the outside world.

Address: Laan van Tergooi 2, 1212 VG Hilversum, The Netherlands | **Client:** Tergooi MC| **Completion:** 2023 | **Size:** 55,000 m^2 | **Sector:** public | **Number of treatment rooms:** 250 | **Number of patient rooms:** 280 | **Interior design:** Wiegerinck | **Landscape design:** Bosch Slabbers

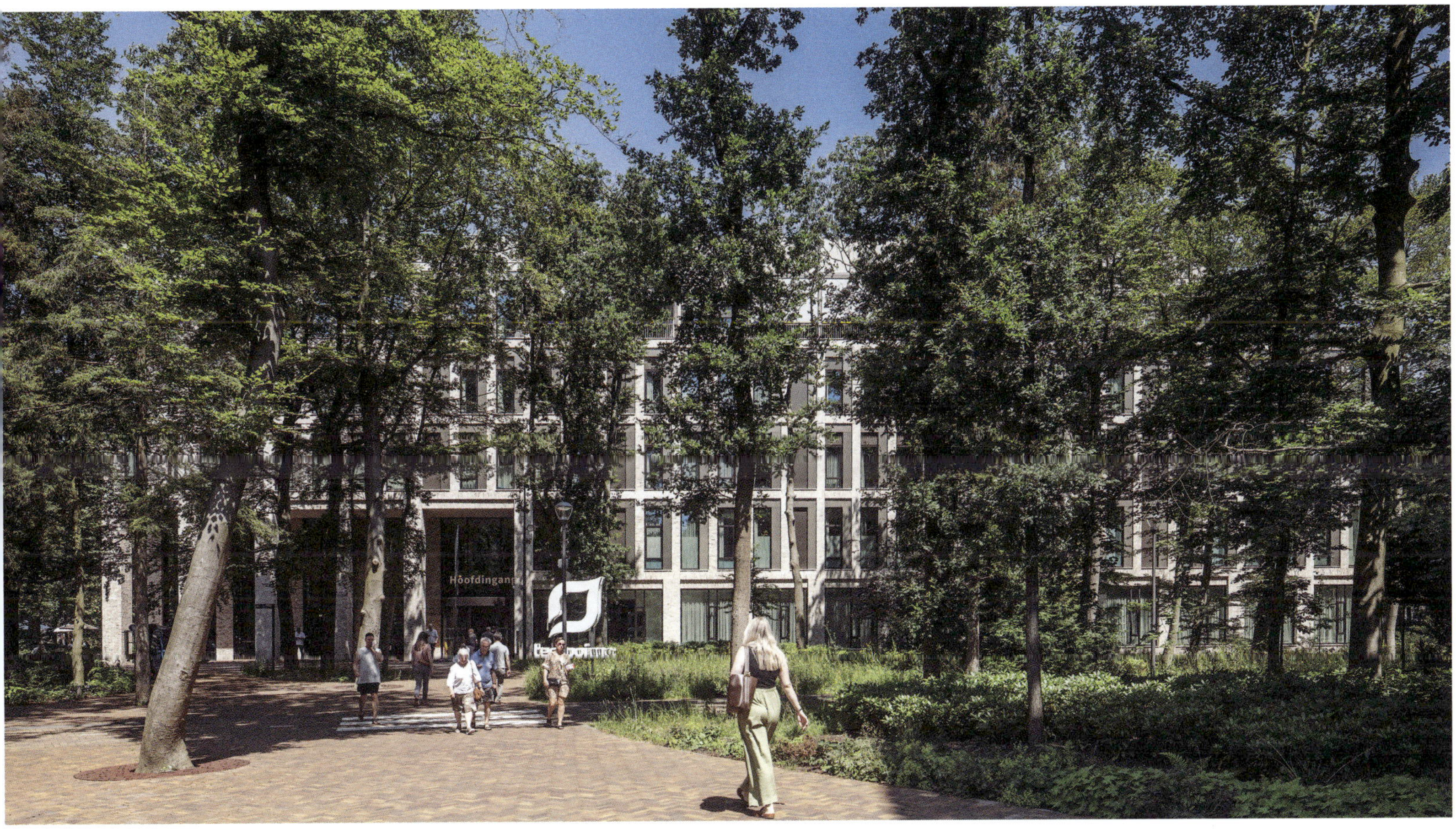

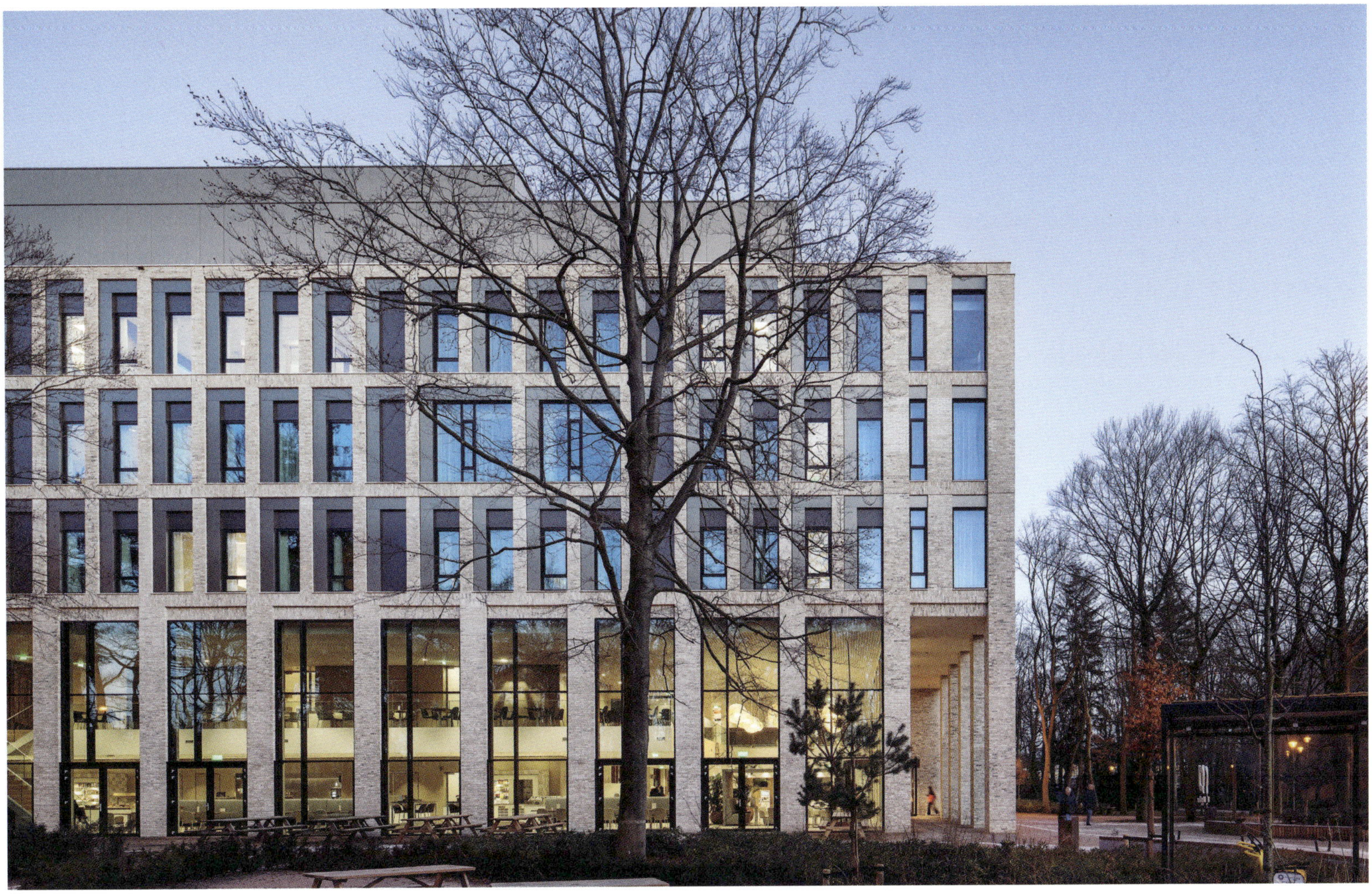

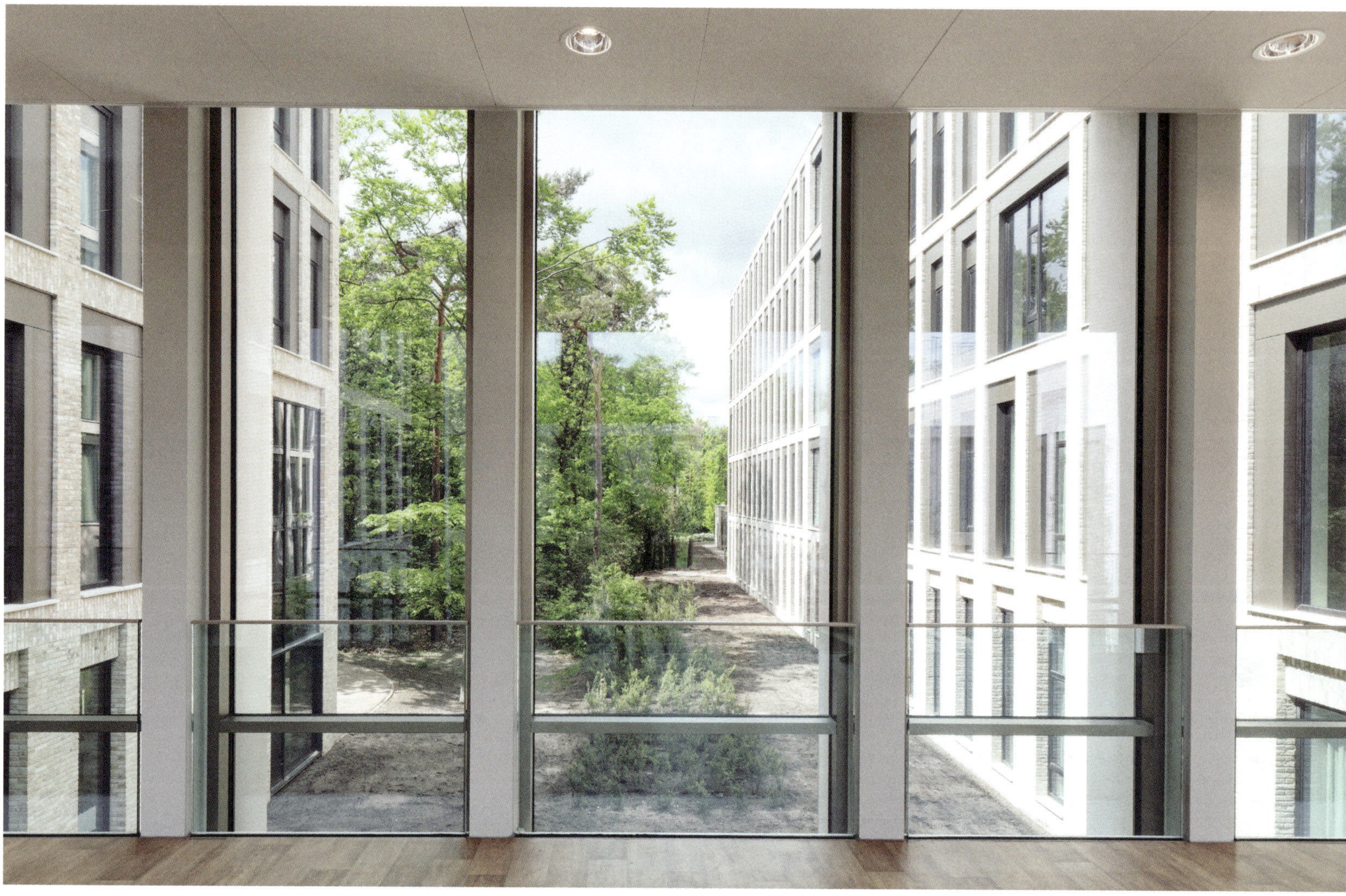

One of the conservatory-like corridors in the passage.

First floor plan.

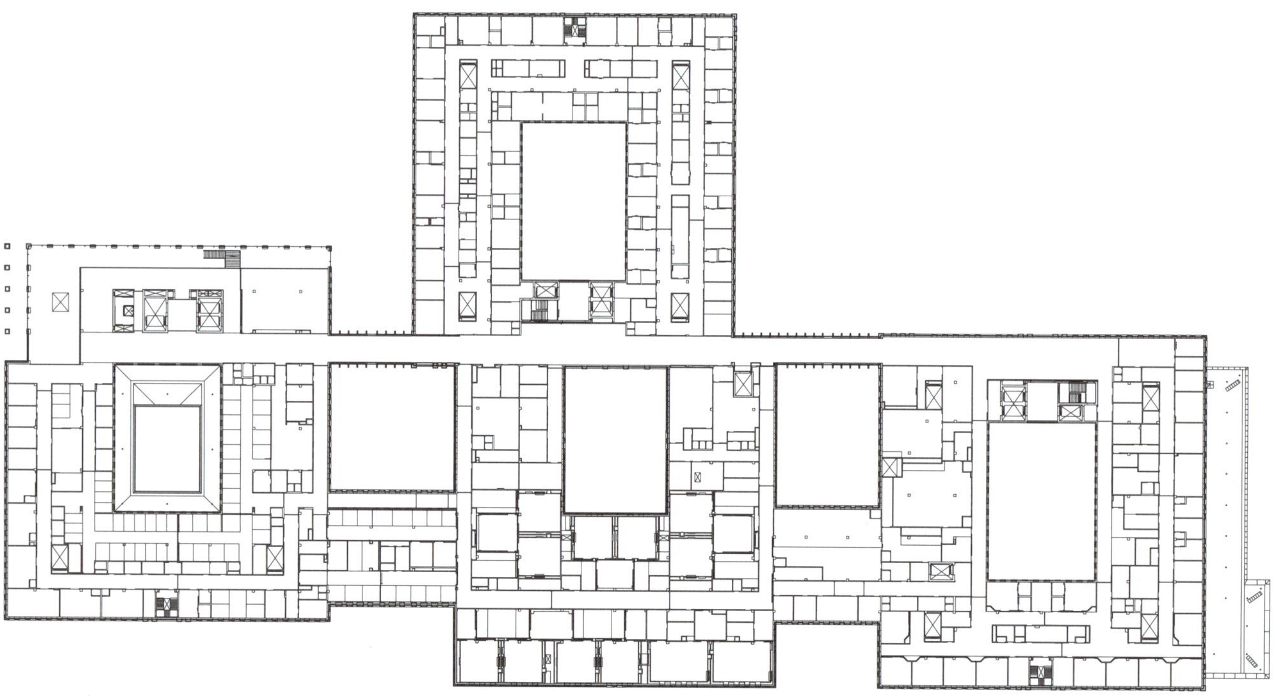

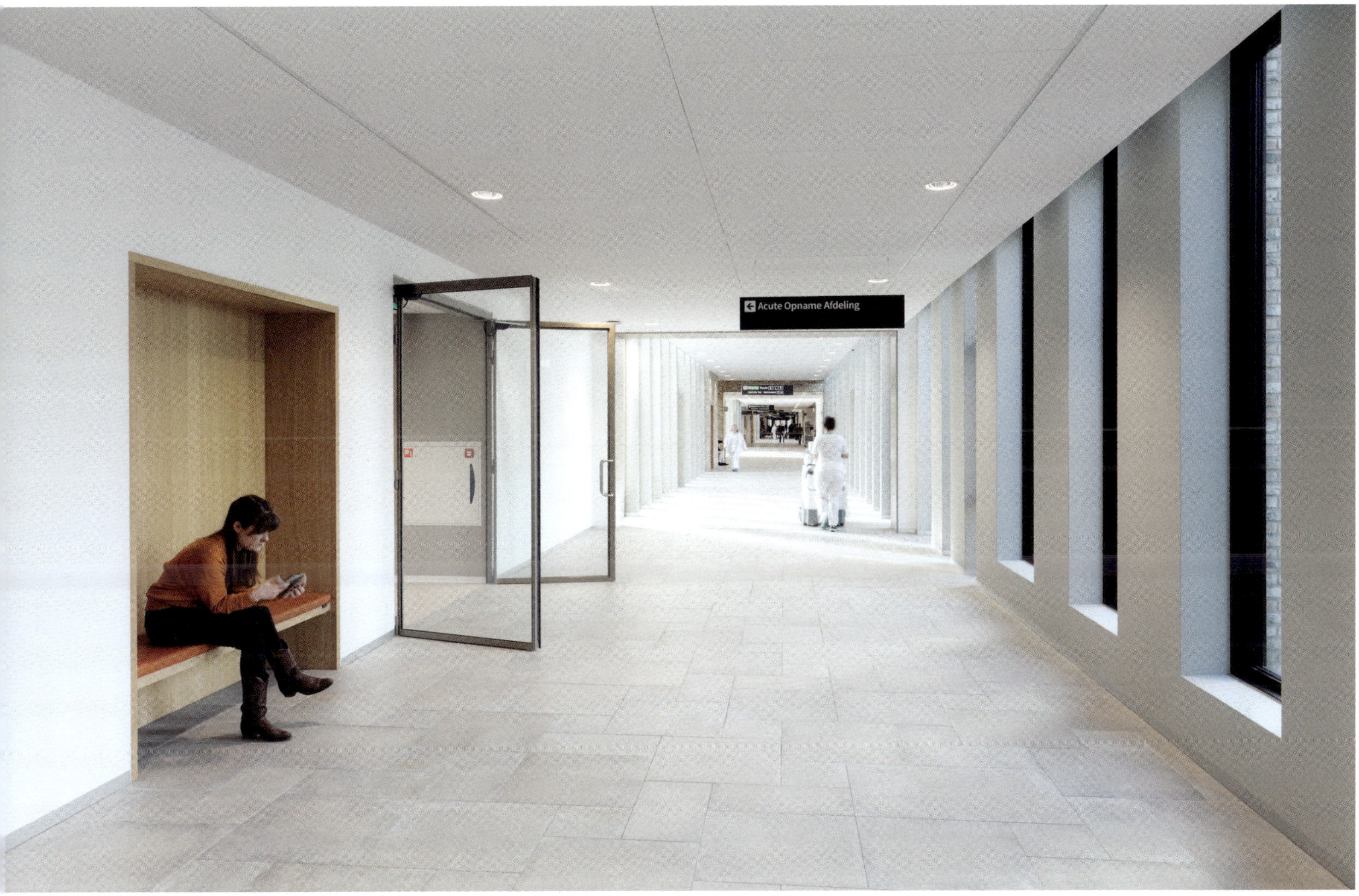

A central corridor runs through the complex, guiding visitors.

Situation.

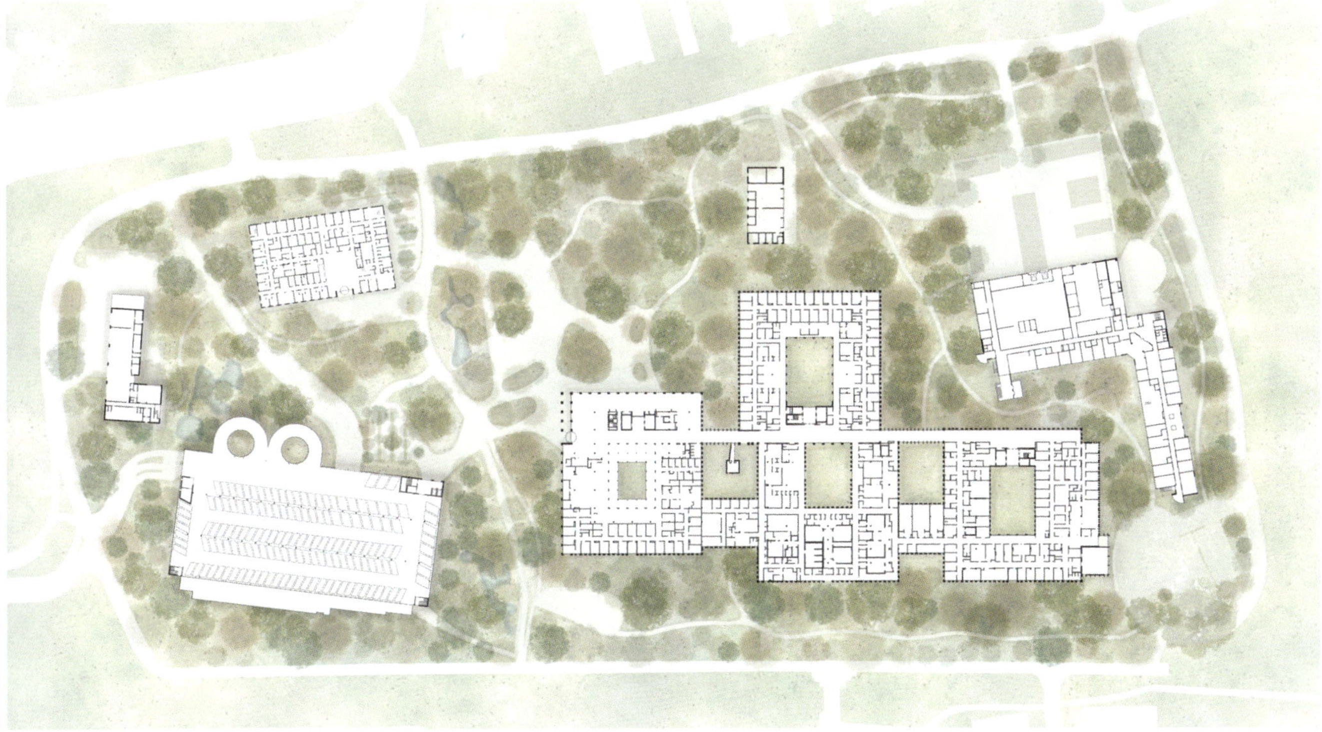

Verstas Architects

Rovaniemi
Finland

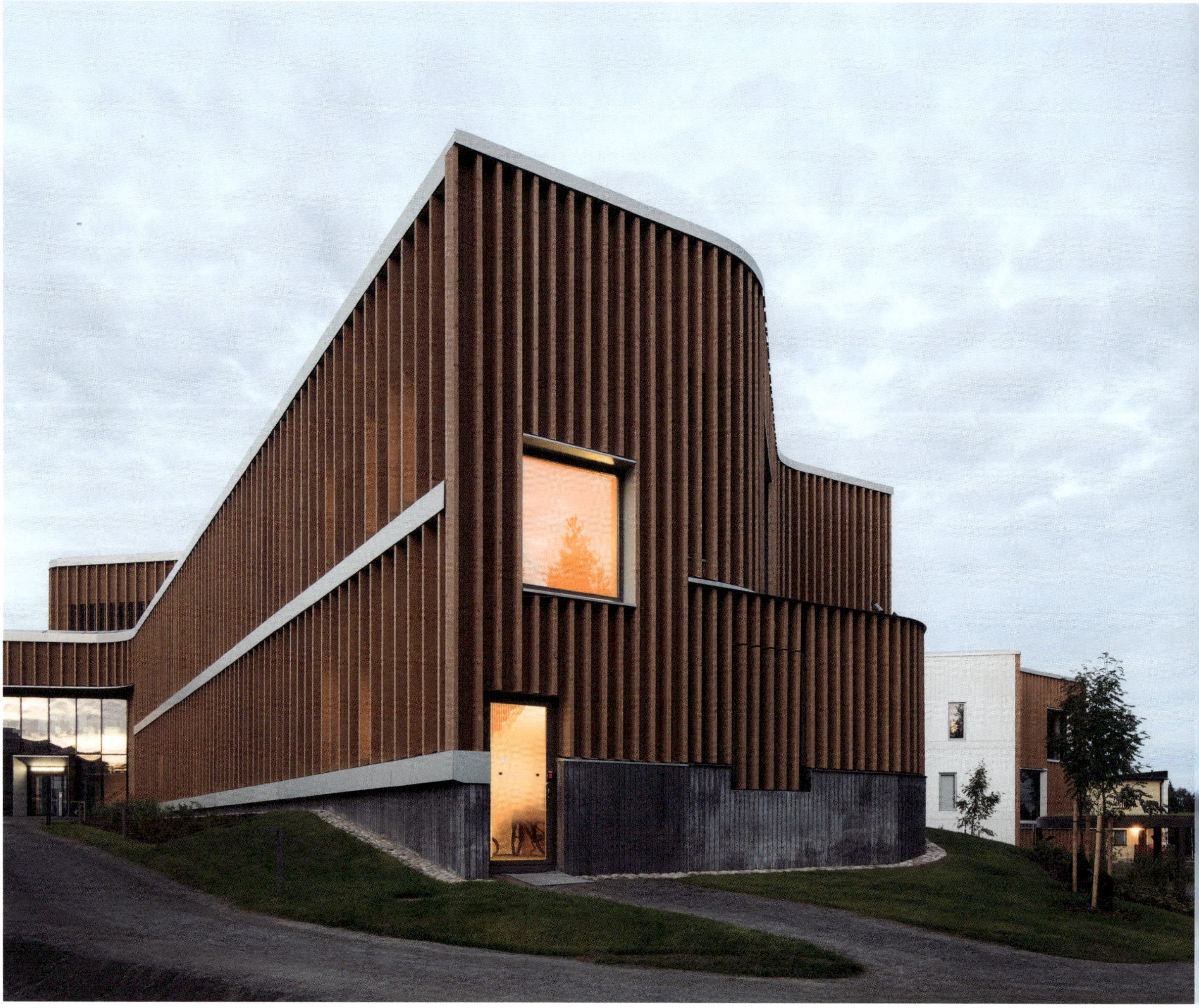

Psychiatric hospital patient wards and outdoor yard.

The new section of Hot Hospital and the parking facility.

Hot Hospital's main entrance canopy.

Lapland Central Hospital Extension

Lapland Central hospital extension turns the 1980s hospital by architect Reino Koivula into a patient-centered campus that supports active rehabilitation and healing. The new efficient hospital is a public building integrated into the living city, moving away from the concept of an isolated institution. The extensions double the current premises of the hospital, including emergency outpatient clinic, observation ward, operation rooms, psychiatric wards, and facilities for several supporting functions. The extensions create conditions for extensive synergy of operations, transforming the whole campus into a more integrated and efficient whole. The buildings share a clear and consistent architectural language, using materials, spatial design, and natural light to create a calm, healing environment. The psychiatric hospital's wooden façade slats soften the building's appearance while allowing light to gently filter through.

Address: Ounasrinteentie 22, Rovaniemi, Finland | **Client:** Wellbeing Services County of Lapland | **Completion:** 2023 (1st phase) | **Size:** central hospital extension 29,840 m² | **Original building:** Reino Koivula, 1988; Arkkitehtitoimisto Tähti-Set, 2006 | **Sector:** state | **Number of treatment rooms:** 47 | **Number of patient rooms:** 46 | **Landscape and interior design:** Verstas Architects

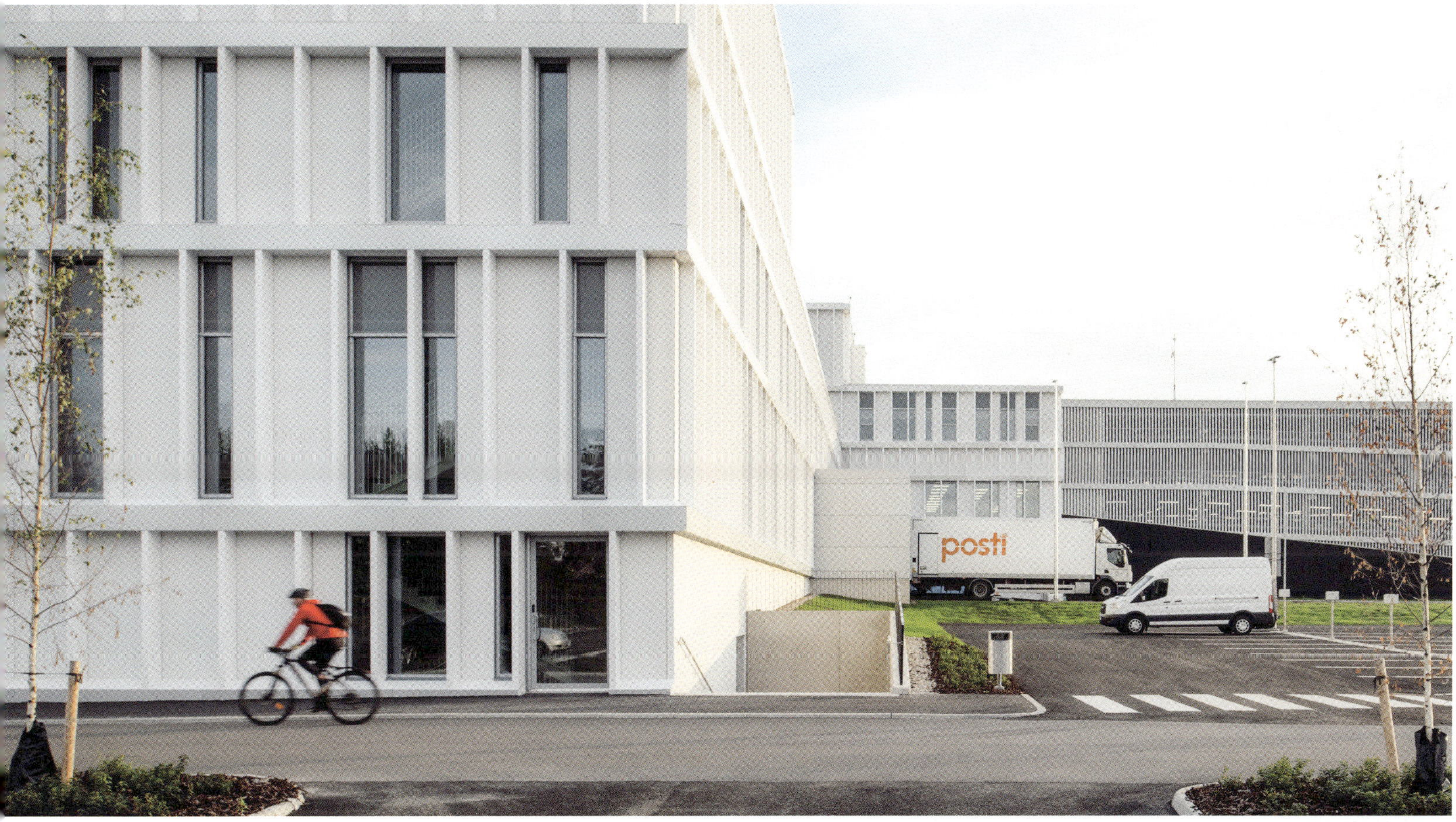

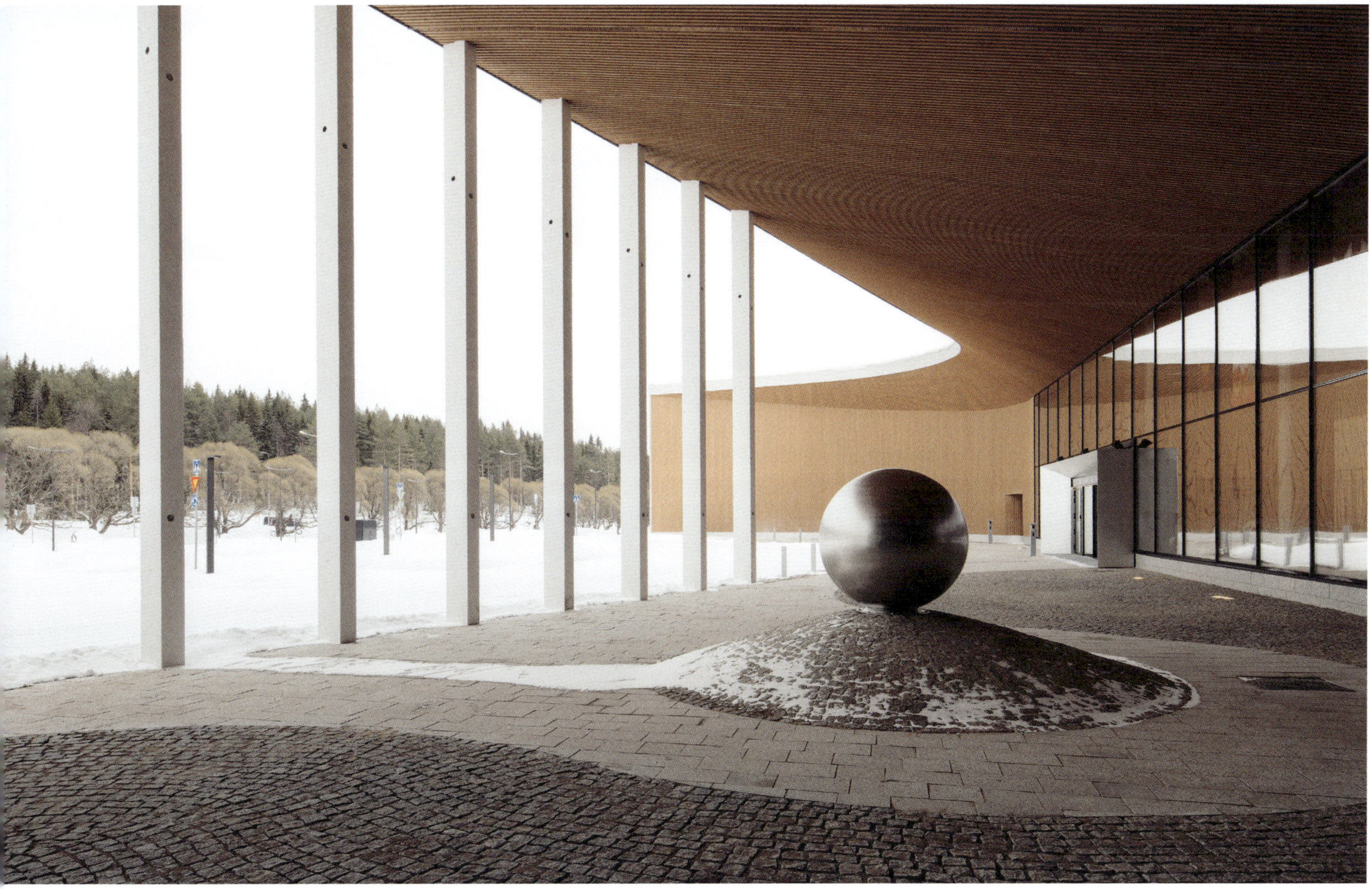

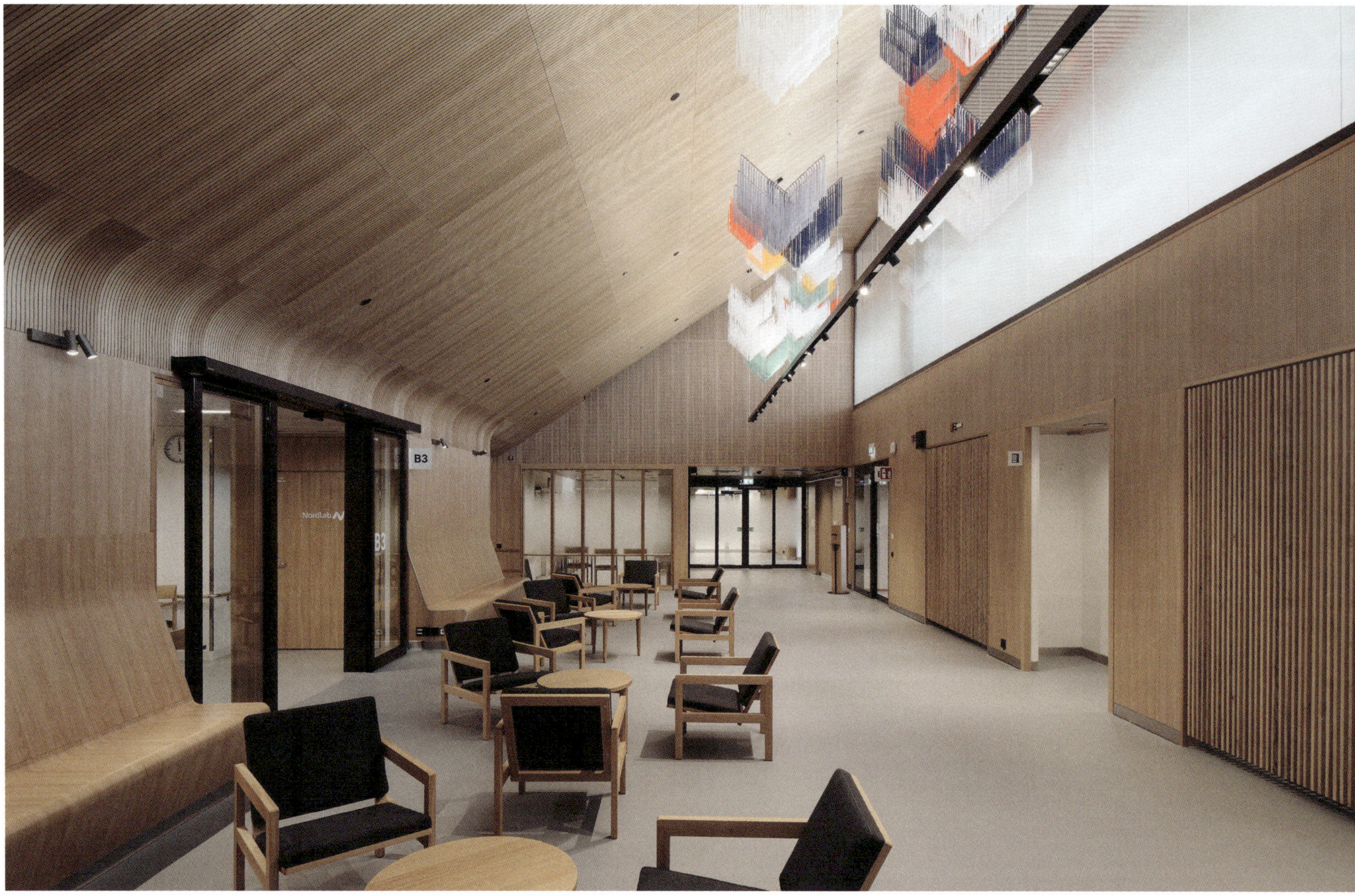

Emergency department's waiting area.

Combined first and second floor plan.

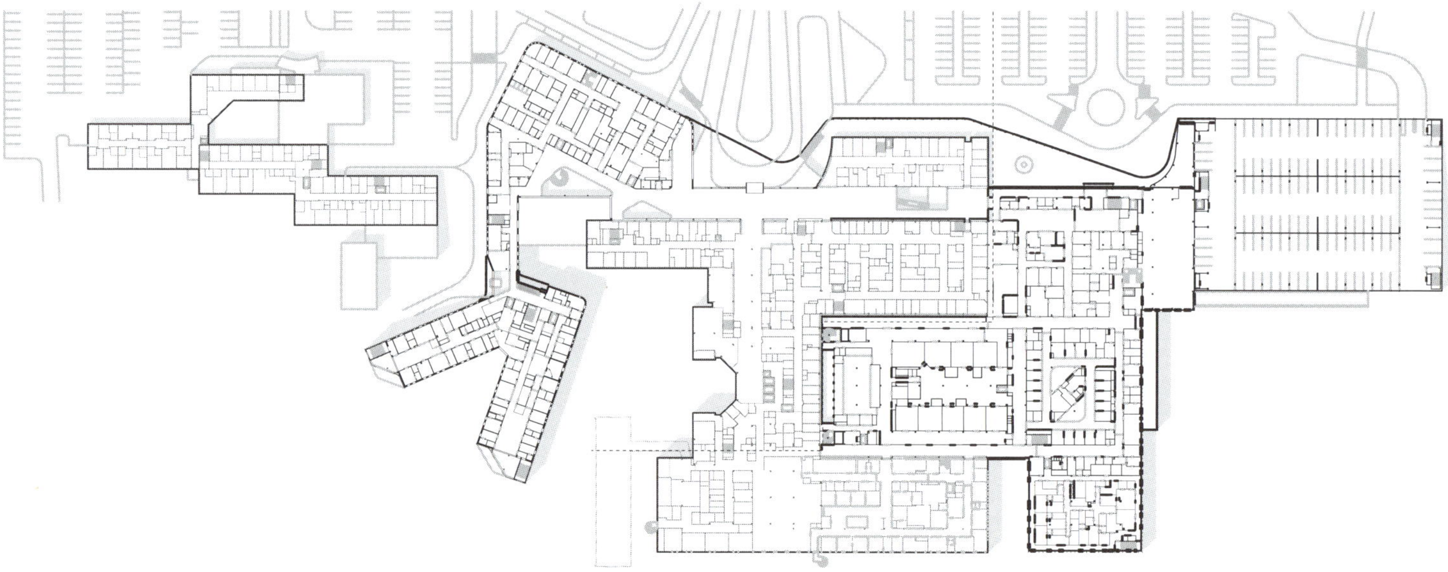

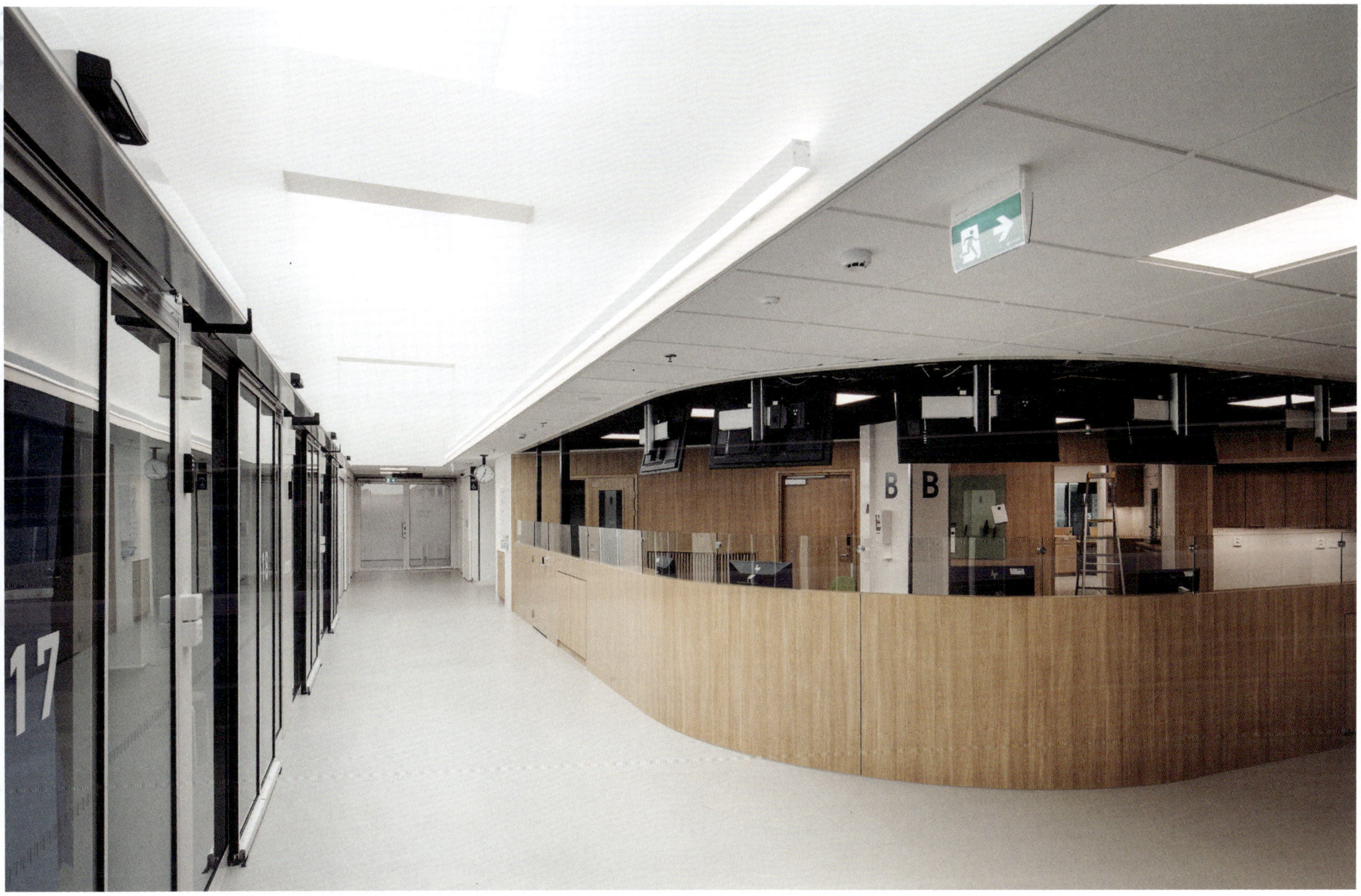

Nurse's desk at the observation ward.

Section.

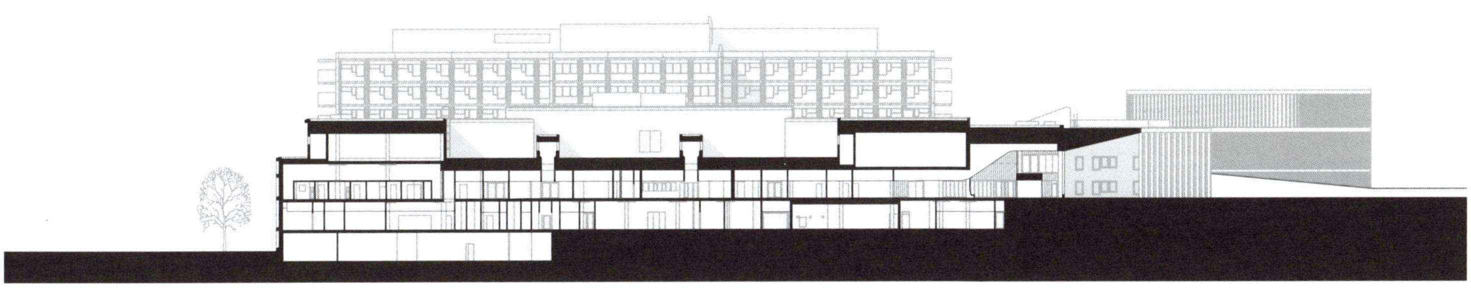

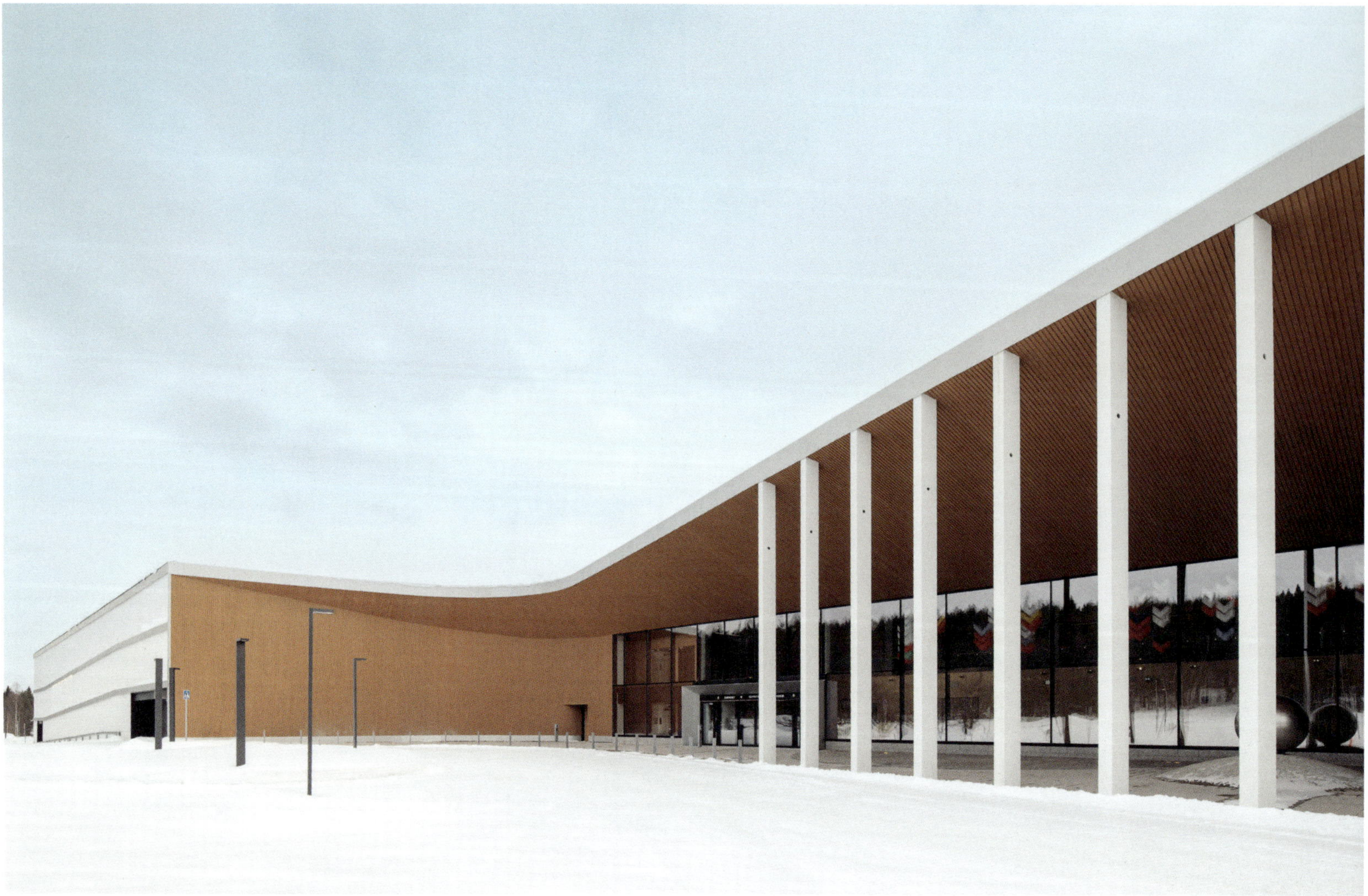

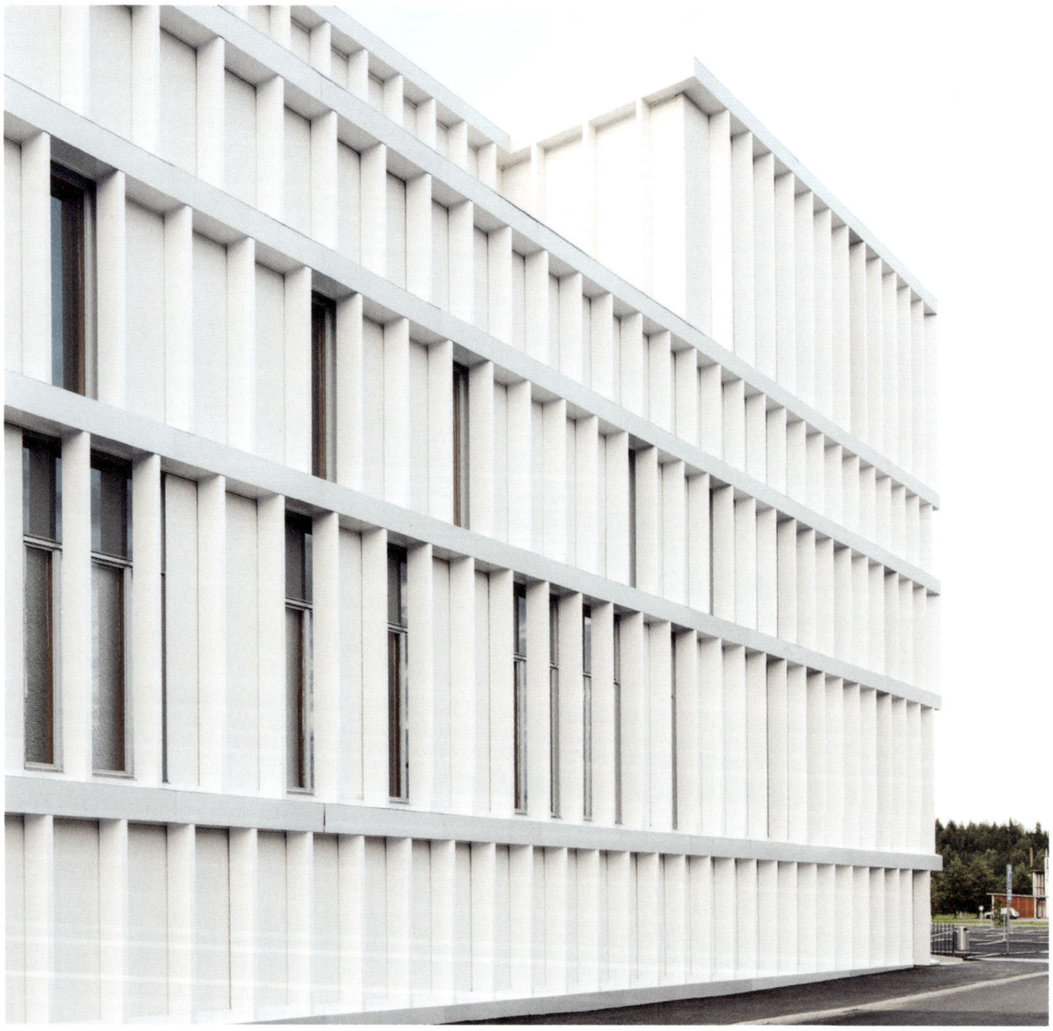

The main entrance area of the extension.

The façades of the Hot Hospital feature white concrete and aluminum.

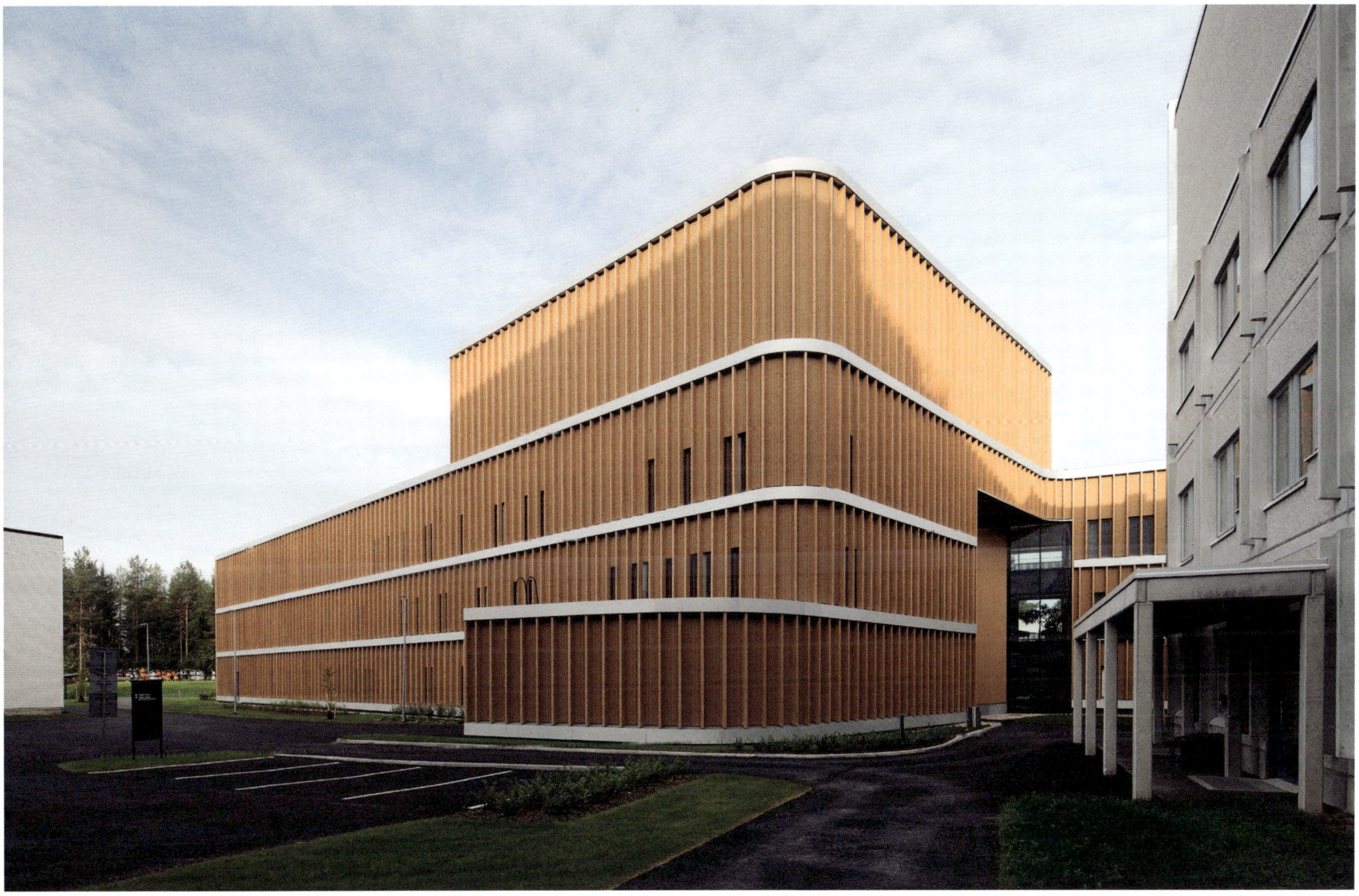

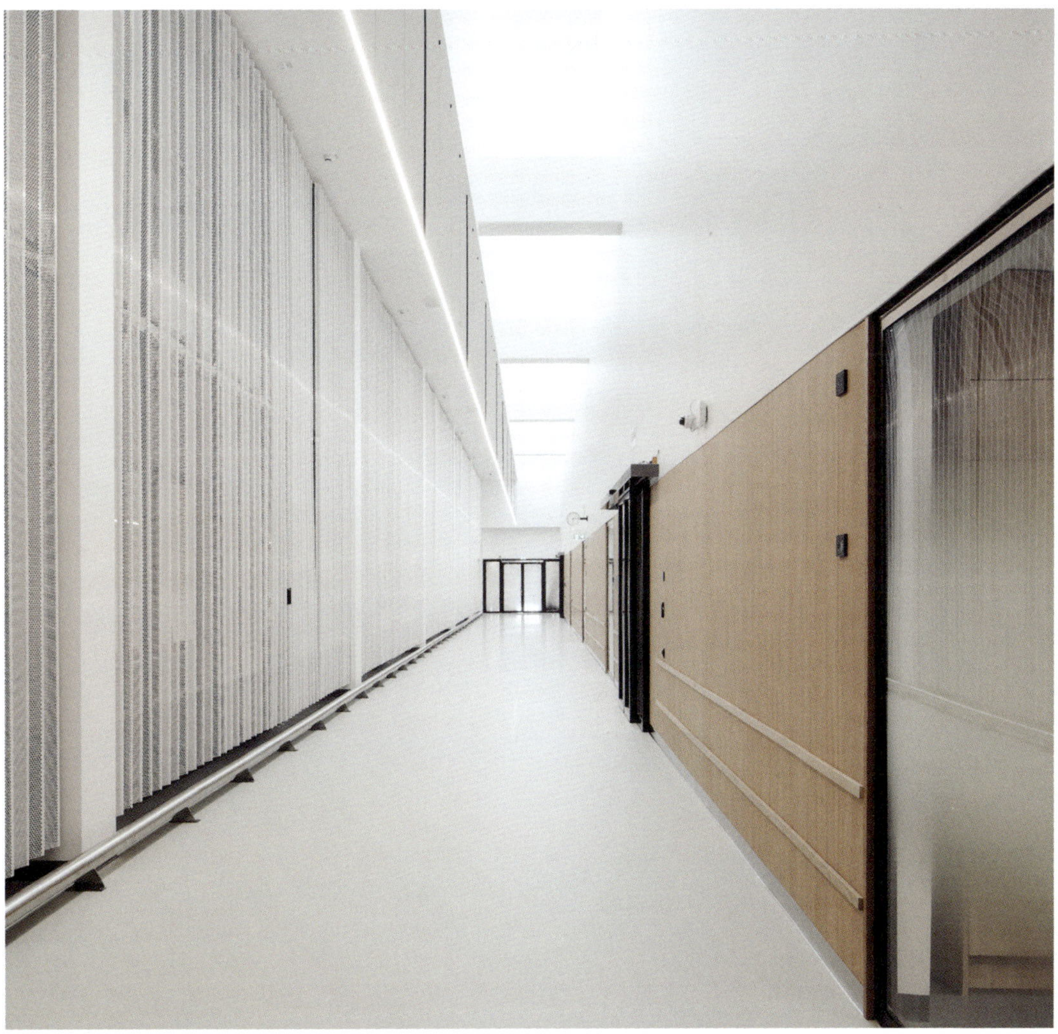

Façade of the psychiatric hospital.

Brightly lit corridors link the existing building with the extension.

HOK
Reddy Architecture + Urbanism

Limerick
Ireland

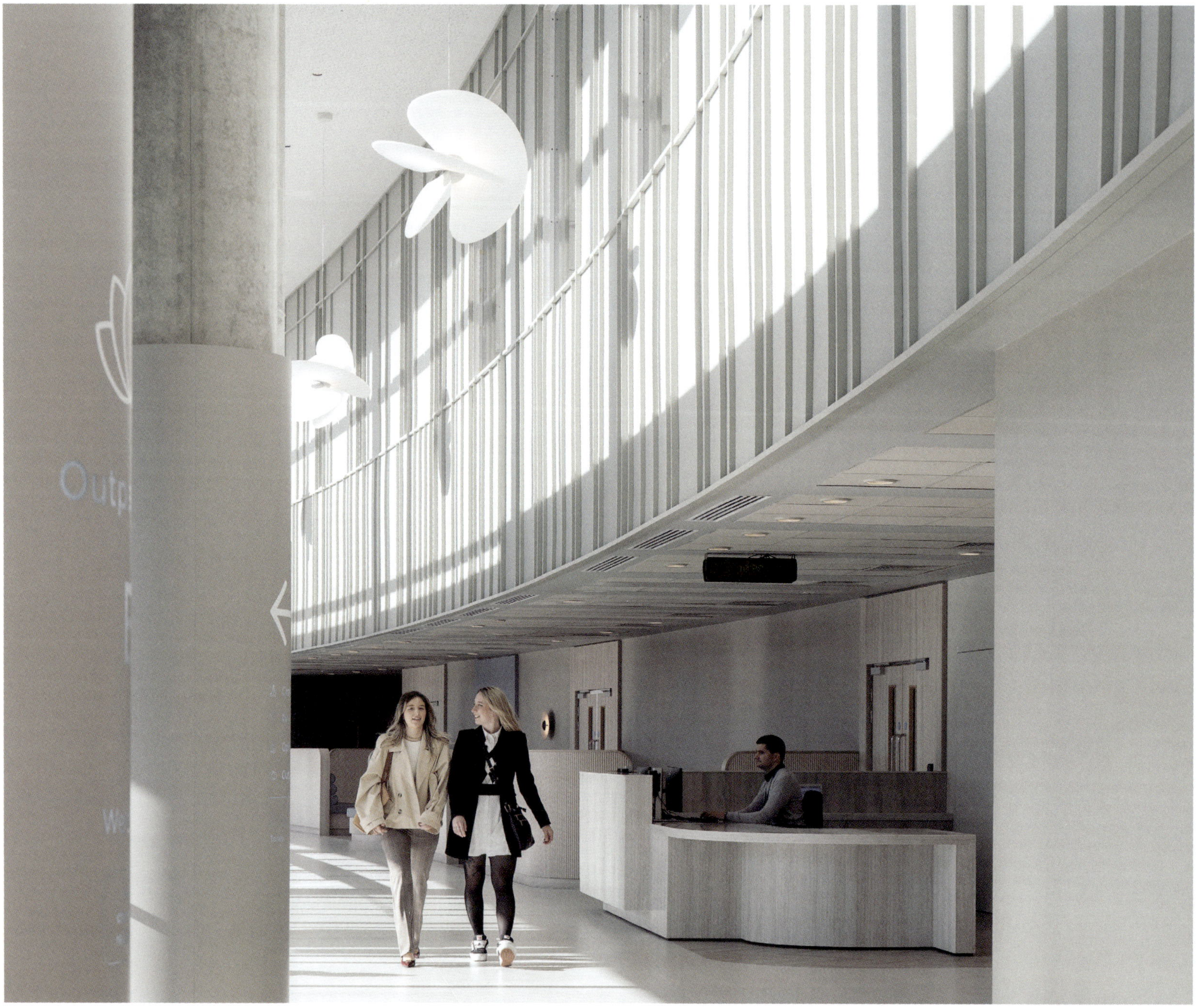

Shared spaces, including the welcoming concourse, support well-being.

The curved block serves as a welcoming gesture.

The biophilic design includes a roof garden accessible from inpatient floors.

Bon Secours Hospital Limerick

HOK, in collaboration with Reddy Architecture + Urbanism, designed the Bon Secours Hospital Limerick – the first new acute hospital to open in Ireland in nearly 20 years. The 23,050-square-meter, 99-bed facility in Ballysimon addresses a critical gap in medical services for Limerick's growing population, with capacity to serve 50,000 patients annually across general medicine, specialty care and day-case surgery. The design organizes the program across two buildings linked by glazed bridges and separated by external courtyards. Person-centered care principles and biophilic design, including a double-height welcoming concourse, a rooftop patient garden, and nature-inspired interiors, support healing throughout. The hospital is Bon Secours' most sustainable to date, incorporating heat pump technology, natural ventilation, high-performance building systems, and robust multimodal site access.

Address: Towlerton, Limerick, V94 9D36, Ireland | **Client:** Bon Secours Health System | **Completion:** 2025 | **Size:** 23,050 m^2 | **Sector:** private | **Number of treatment rooms:** 20 | **Number of patient rooms:** 99 | **Contractor:** Sisk | **Medical and clinical planning:** HOK's London Studio and Reddy Architecture + Urbanism | **Architecture:** HOK's London Studio and Reddy Architecture + Urbanism | **Interior design:** HOK's London and Chicago Studios and Reddy Architecture + Urbanism

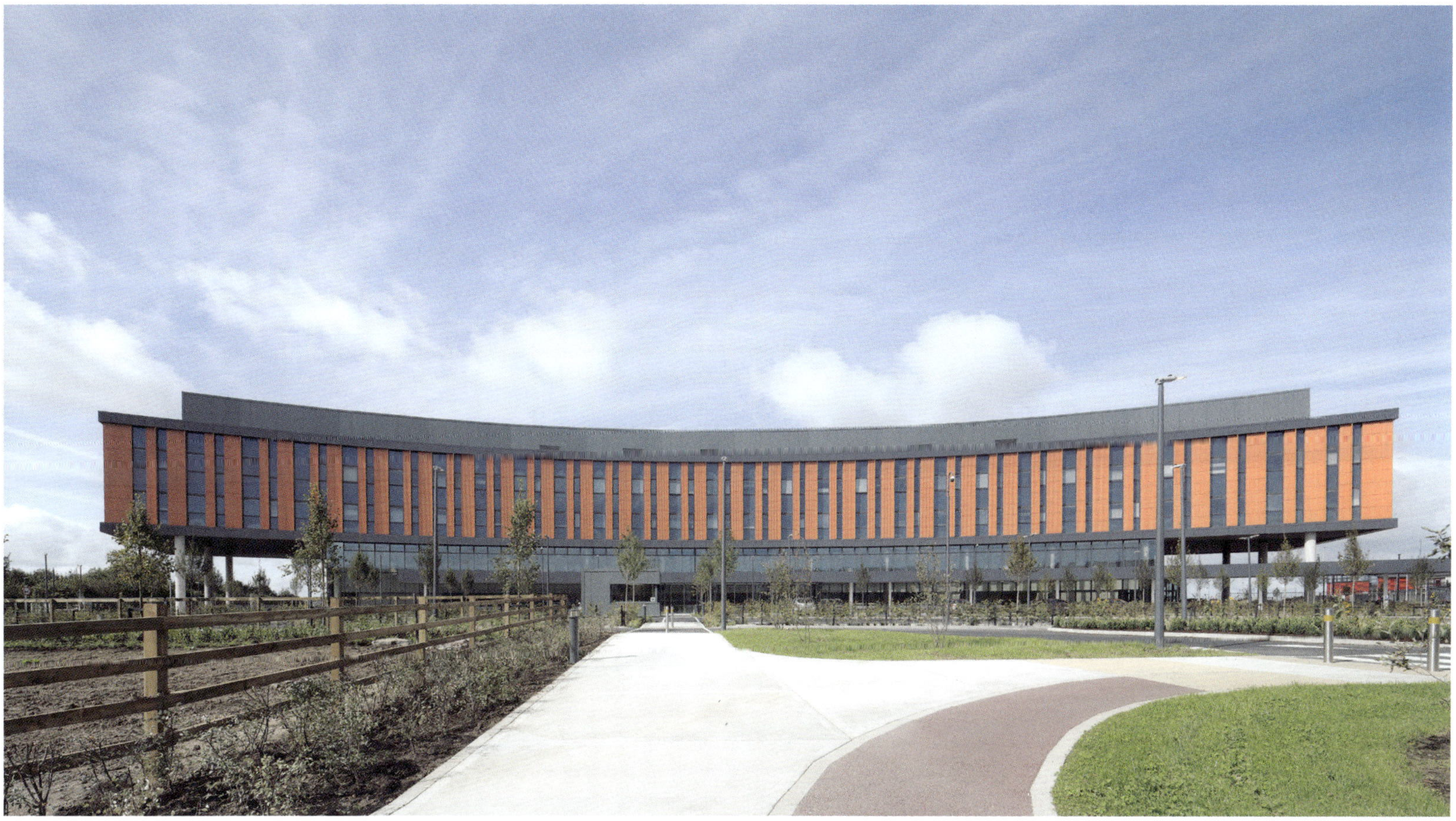

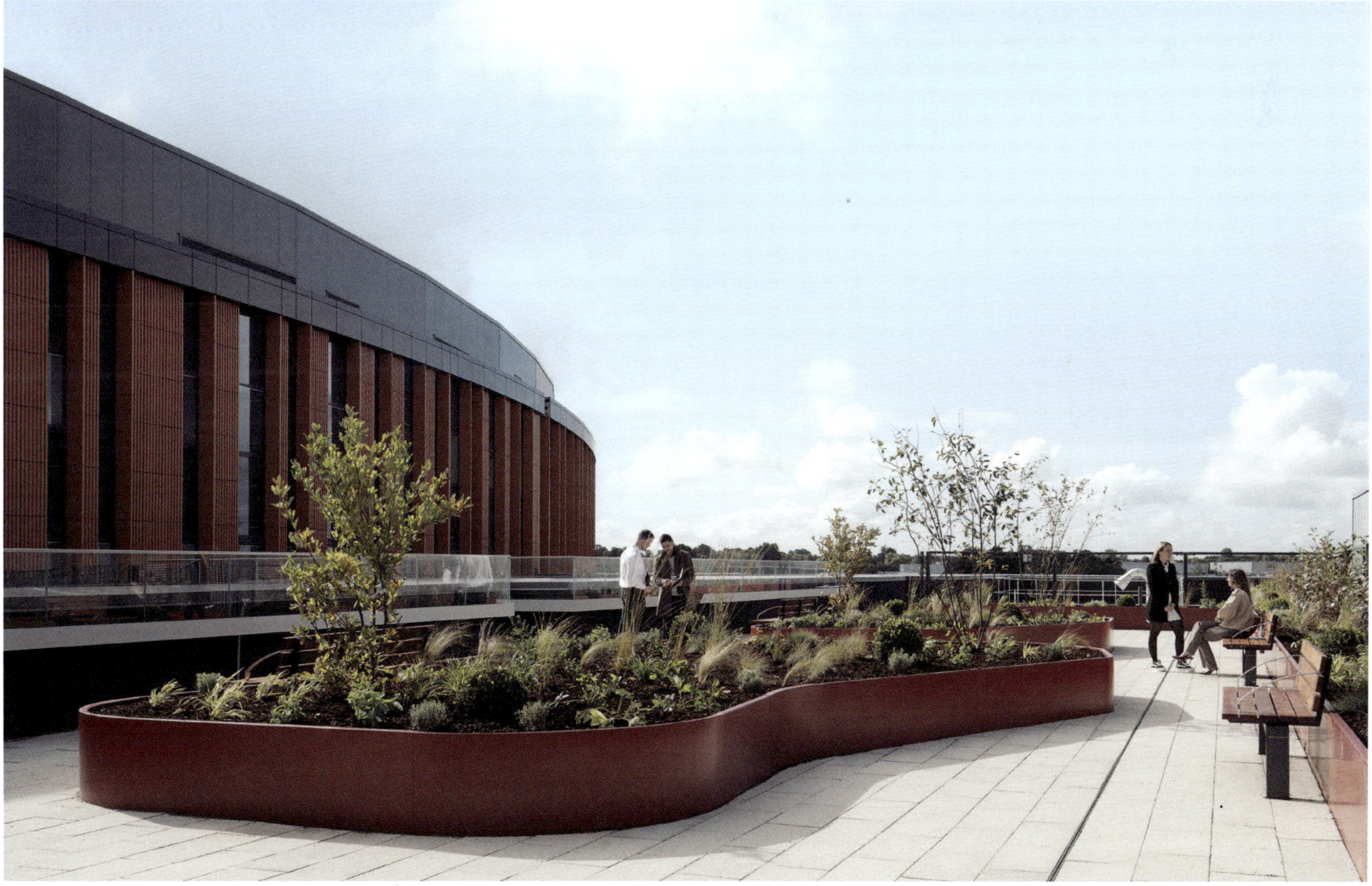

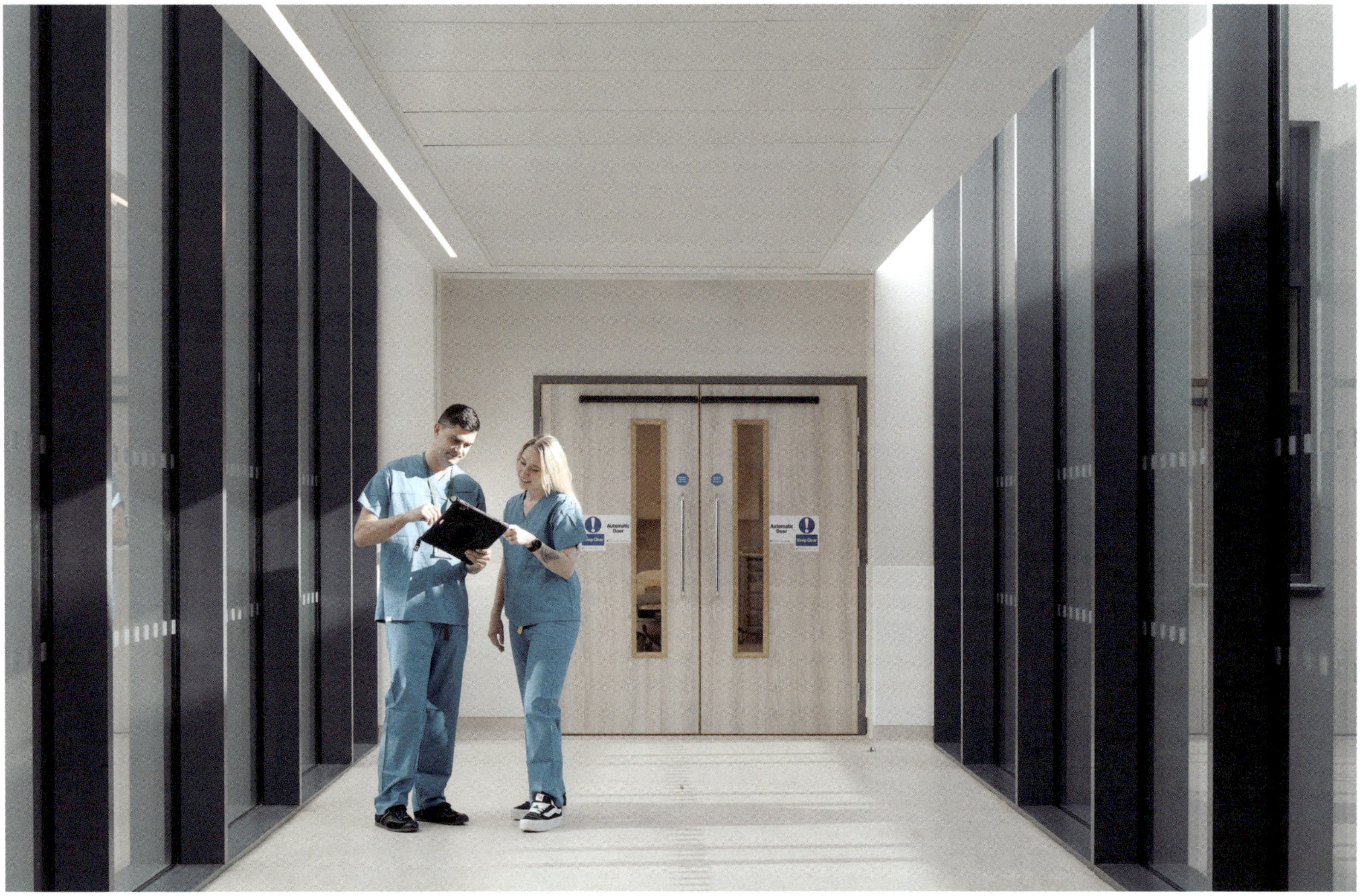

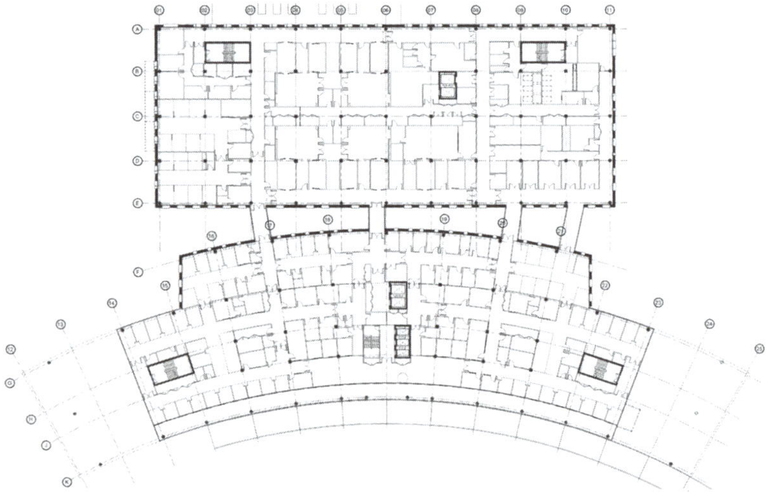

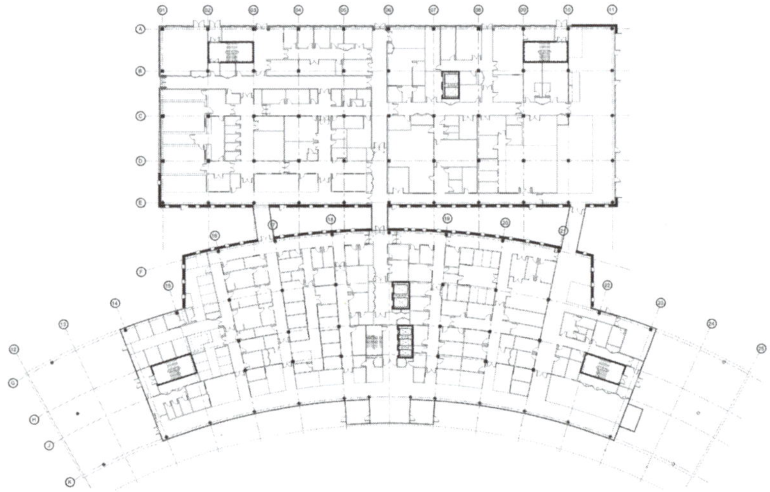

The inpatient wards corridor is flanked by private patient rooms, each with an en-suite bathroom.

First and ground floor plans.

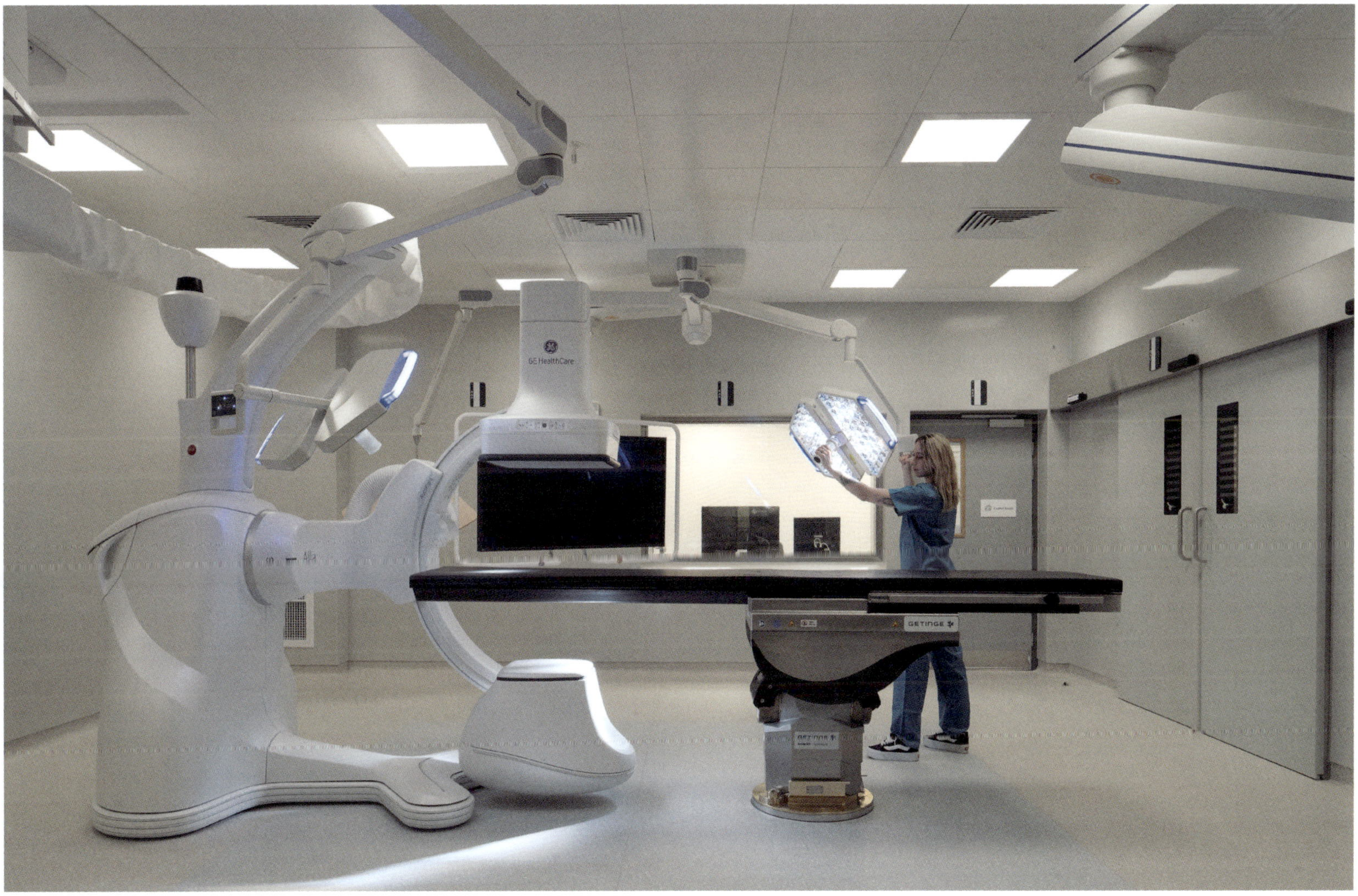

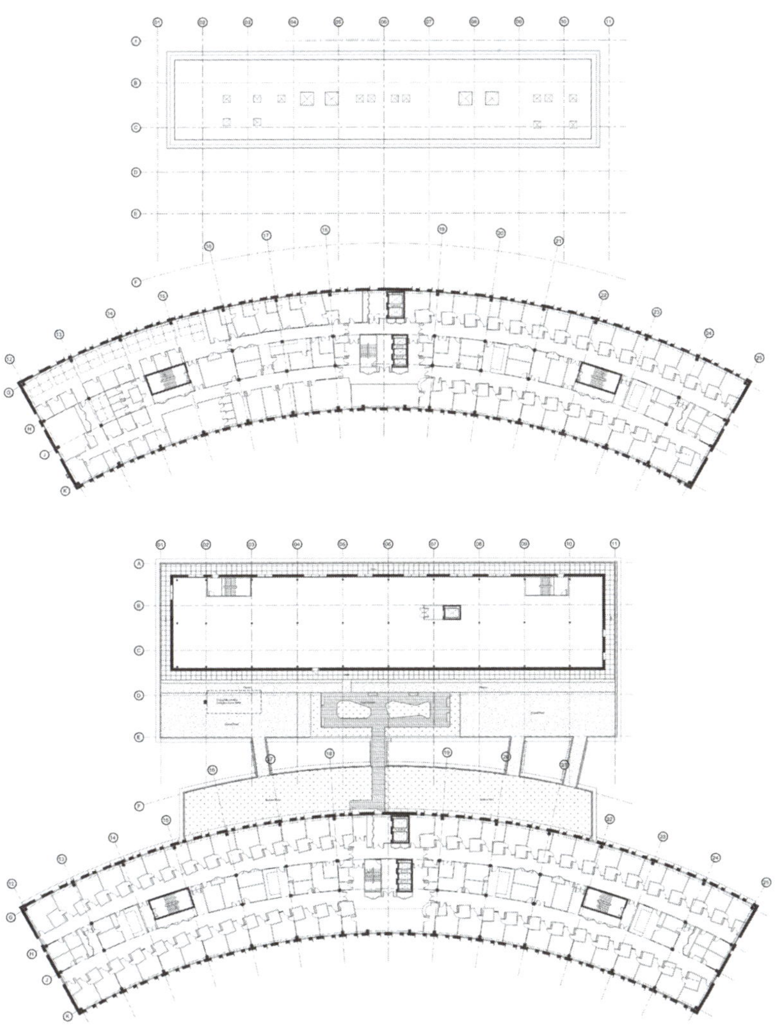

The state-of-the-art cardiac catheterization lab supports minimally invasive, image-guided procedures.

Third and second floor plans.

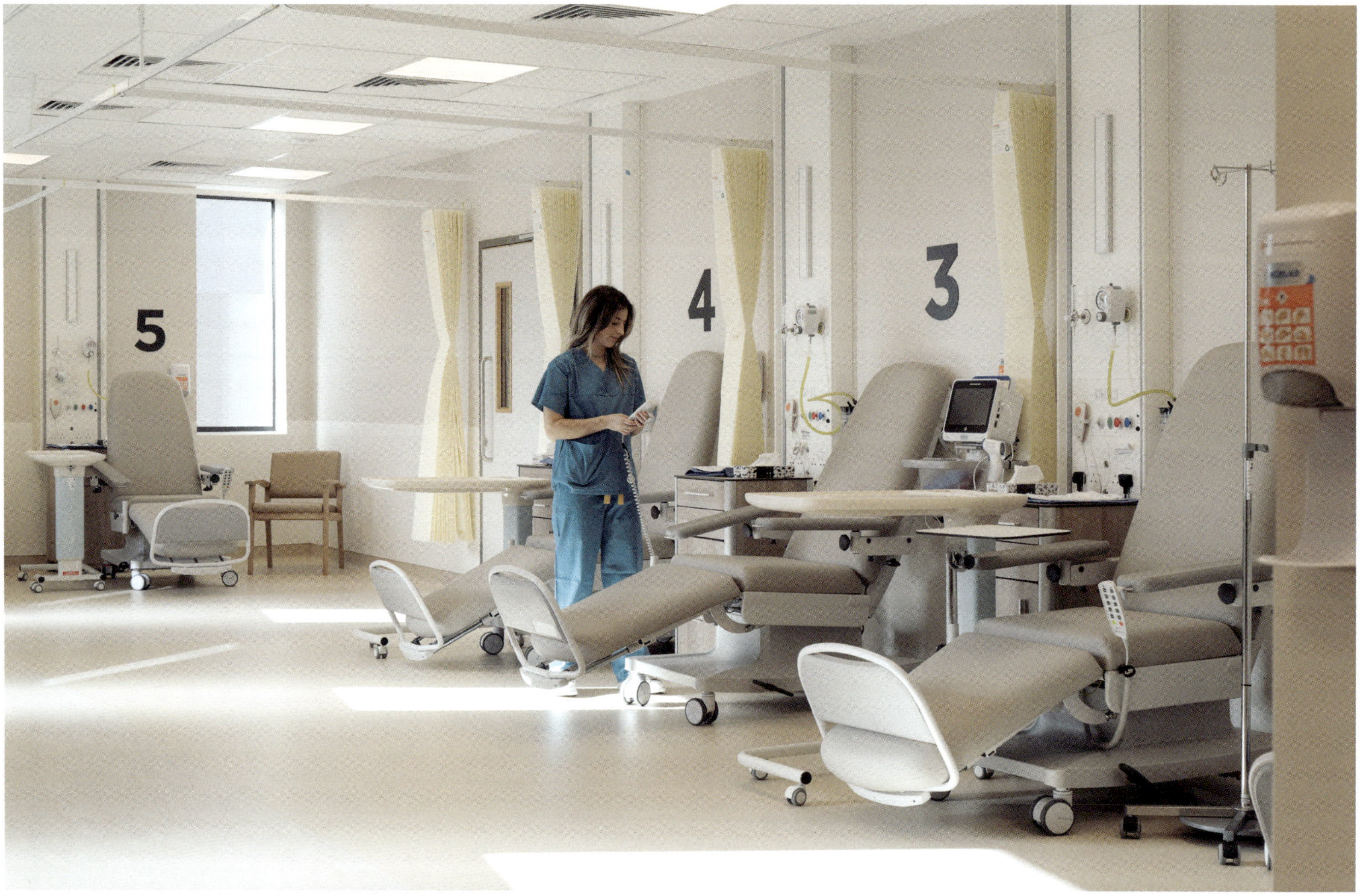

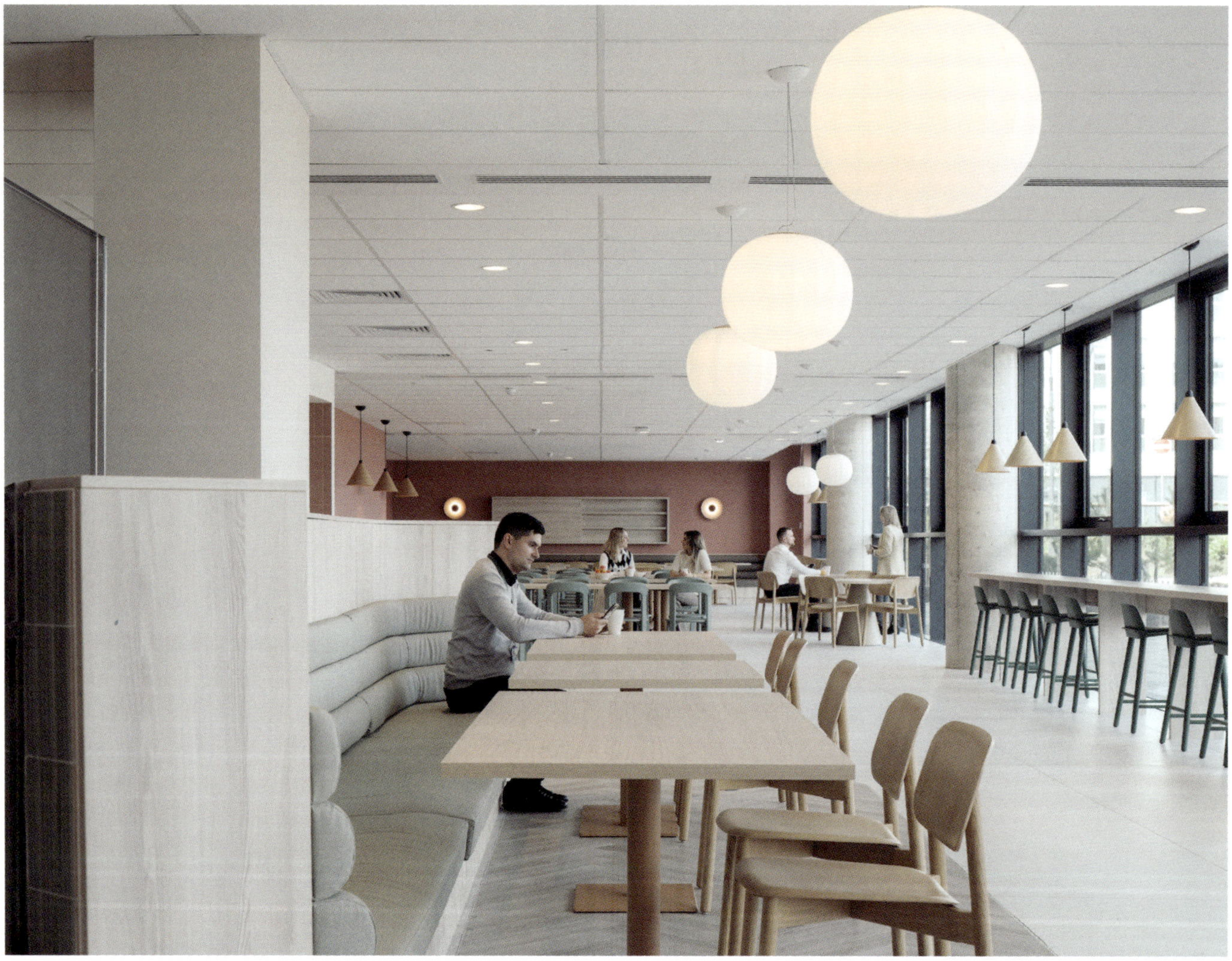

The 27-bay day-case surgery suite features semi-private stations.

The on-site restaurant opens out toward the garden and chapel.

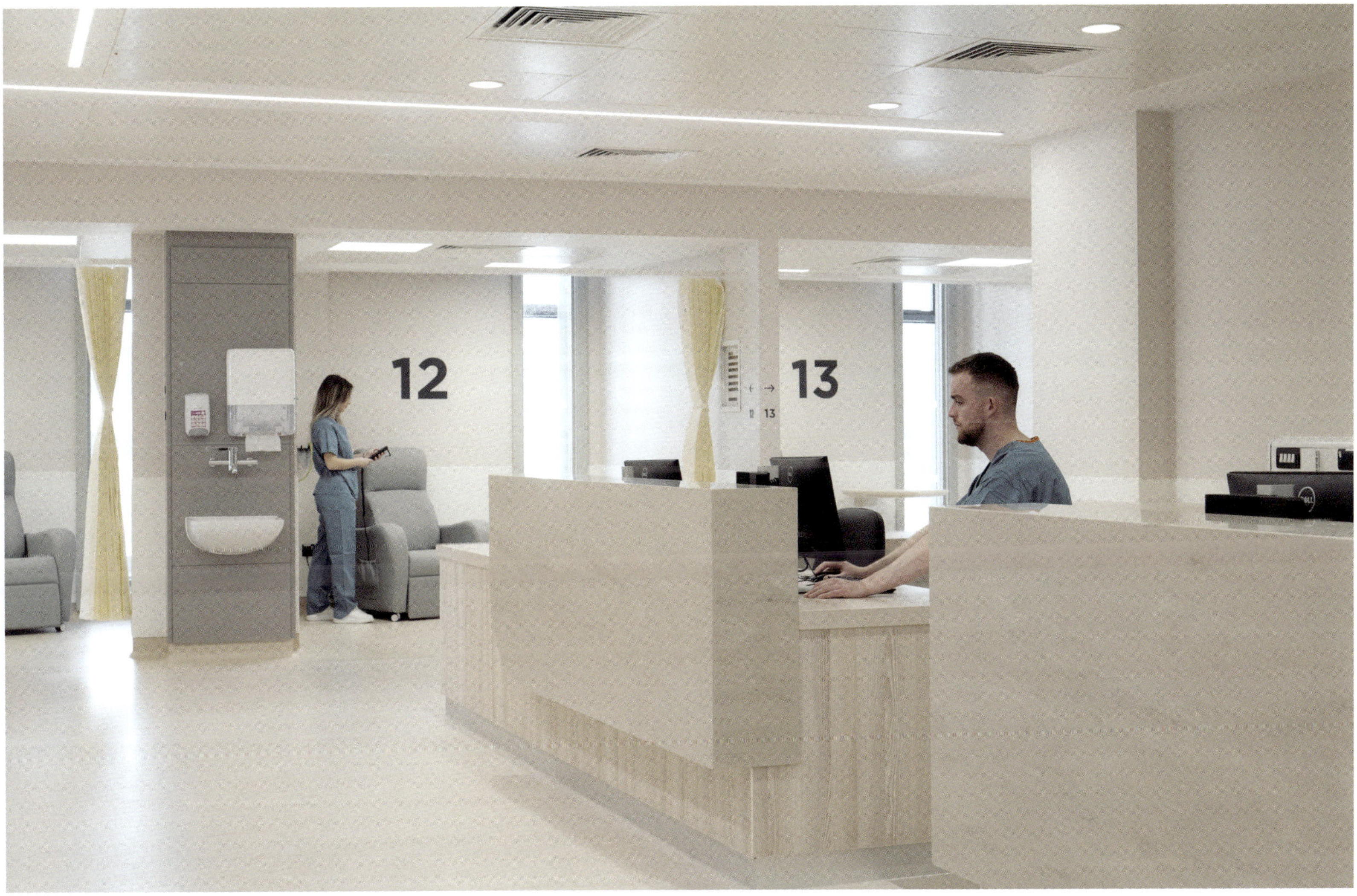

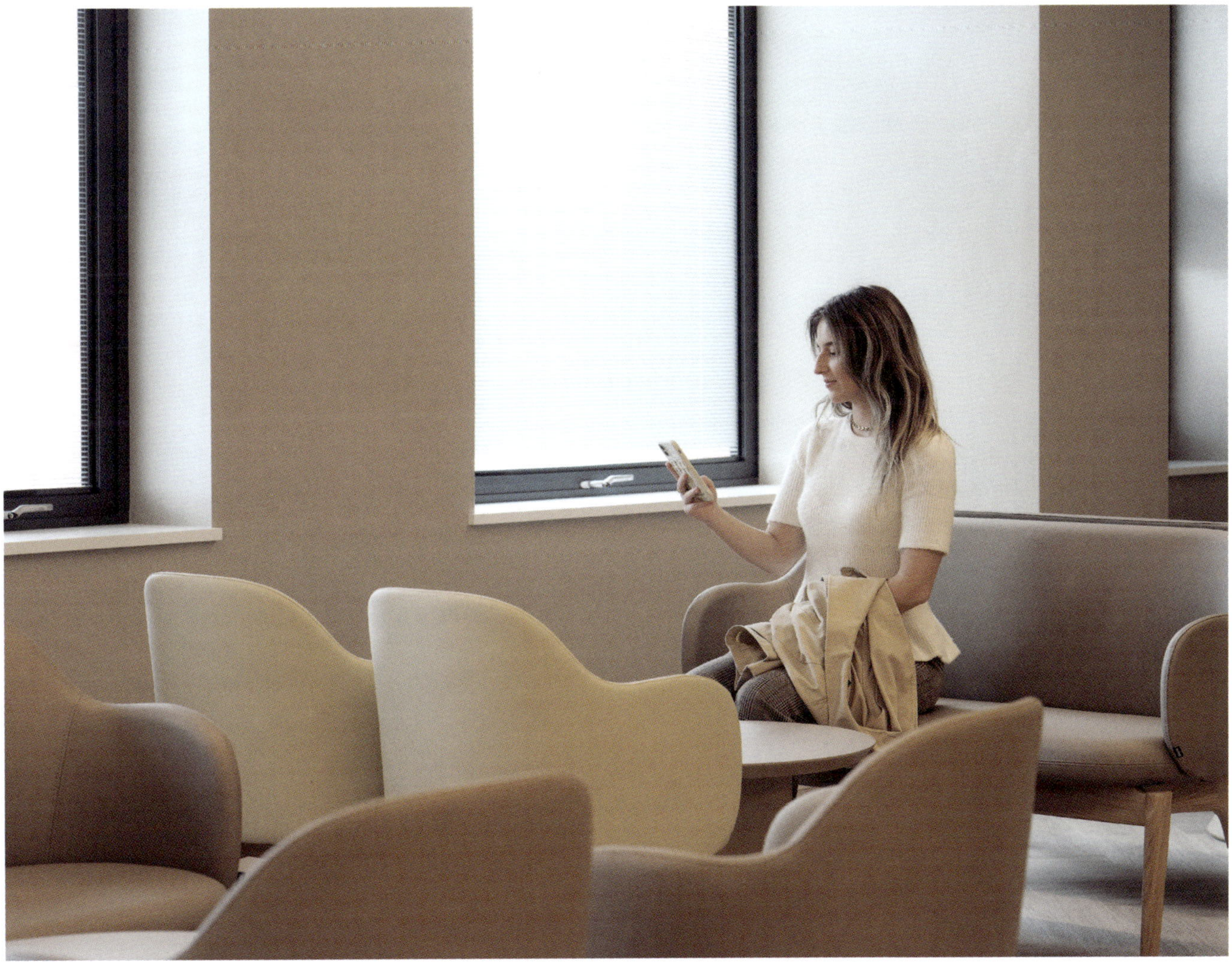

The day surgery unit offers patients a comfortable, light-filled space for recovery.

Calming color palettes imbue waiting areas with tranquility.

Atelier Martel

Issy-les-Moulineaux
France

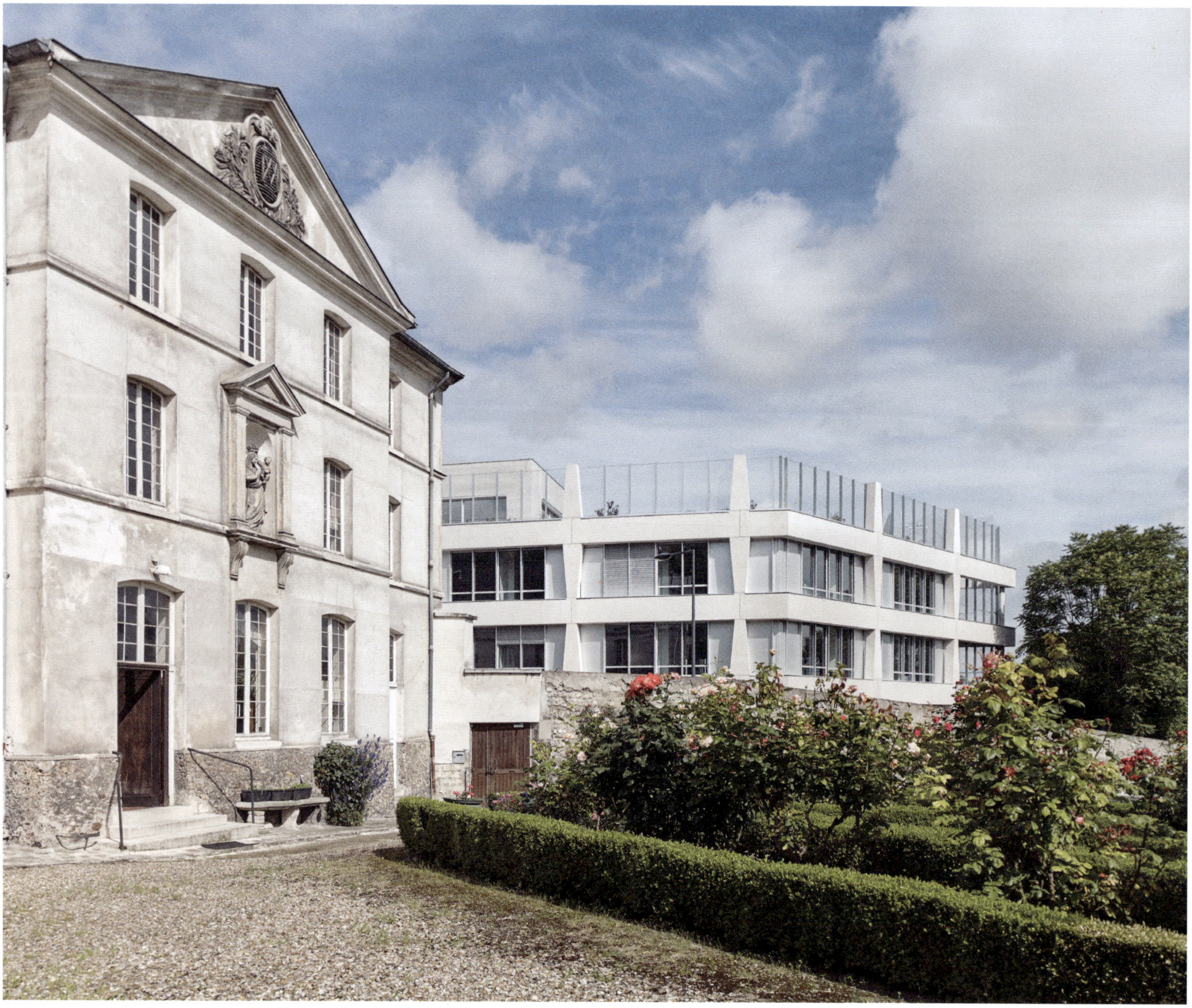

The new wing seen from the Jean Paul II parc.

The structure of the extension echoes the one of the original part of the building.

The new wing stitching with the original building on the left of the picture.

Restructuring and Extension of the Hôpital Suisse de Paris

The extension and restructuring of the Hôpital Suisse de Paris redefine the functionality and identity of this rehabilitation and physiotherapy institution on the hillsides of Issy-les-Moulineaux. Over time, successive additions had fragmented the site and disrupted its circulation and coherence. The project restores clarity by reorganizing patient flows, improving accessibility, and creating new shared spaces dedicated to care and well-being. Designed in dialogue with the original late-1960s modernist building, the extension follows the structural logic of the existing concrete exoskeleton while simplifying its architectural expression. This continuity reinforces the unity and adaptability of the institution. New facilities include a covered entrance forecourt and a rooftop belvedere garden with a restaurant overlooking Paris and the surrounding parks, contributing to a calm therapeutic environment.

Address: 10, rue Minard, 92130 Issy-les-Moulineaux, France | **Client:** Association de l'Hôpital Suisse de Paris | **Completion:** 2016 | **Size:** 2,600 m² | **Original building:** Jacques and Pierre Delaire architects, 1970 | **Sector:** private | **Specialization:** physiotherapy | **Number of treatment rooms:** 40 | **Number of patient rooms:** 119

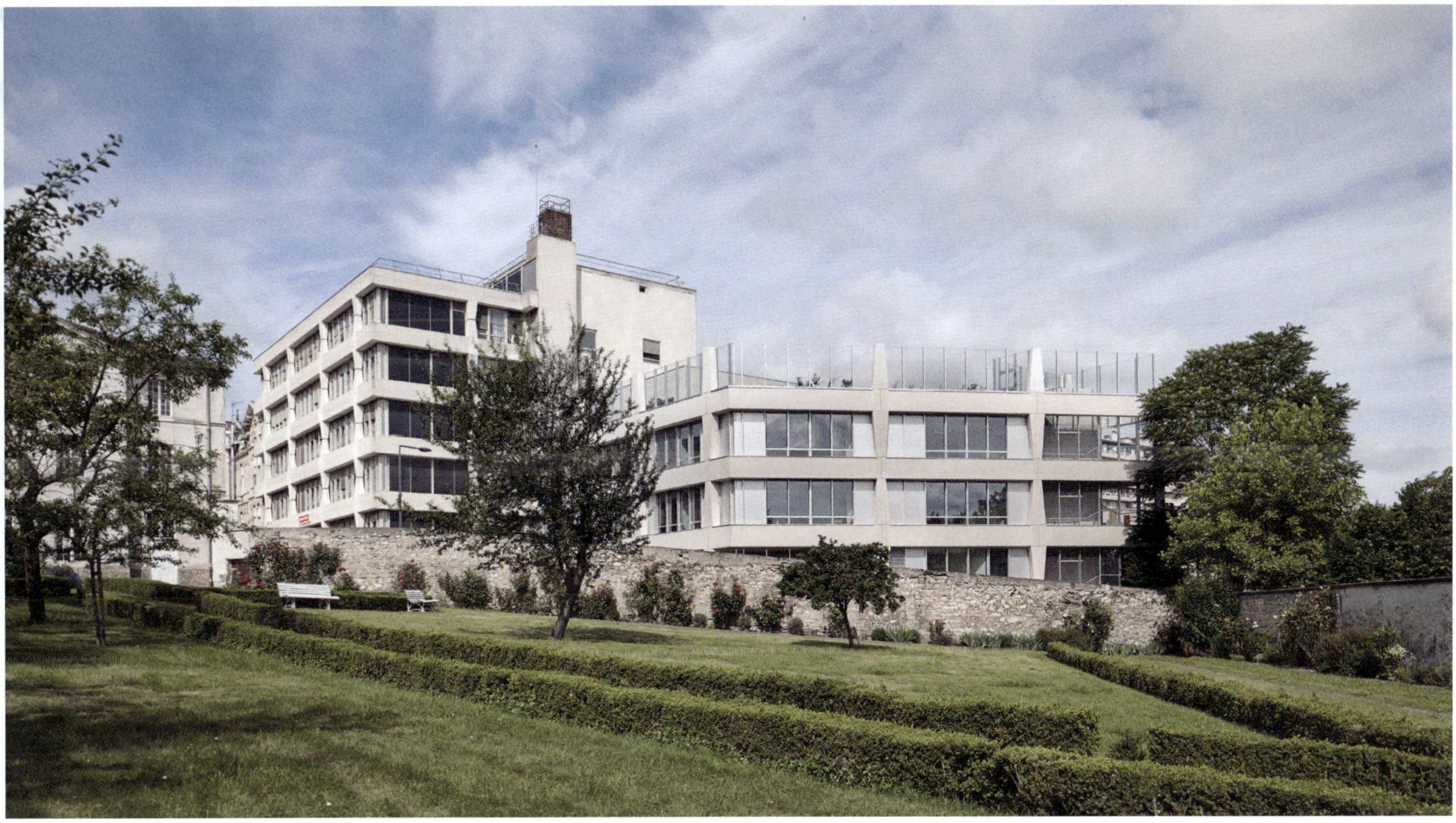

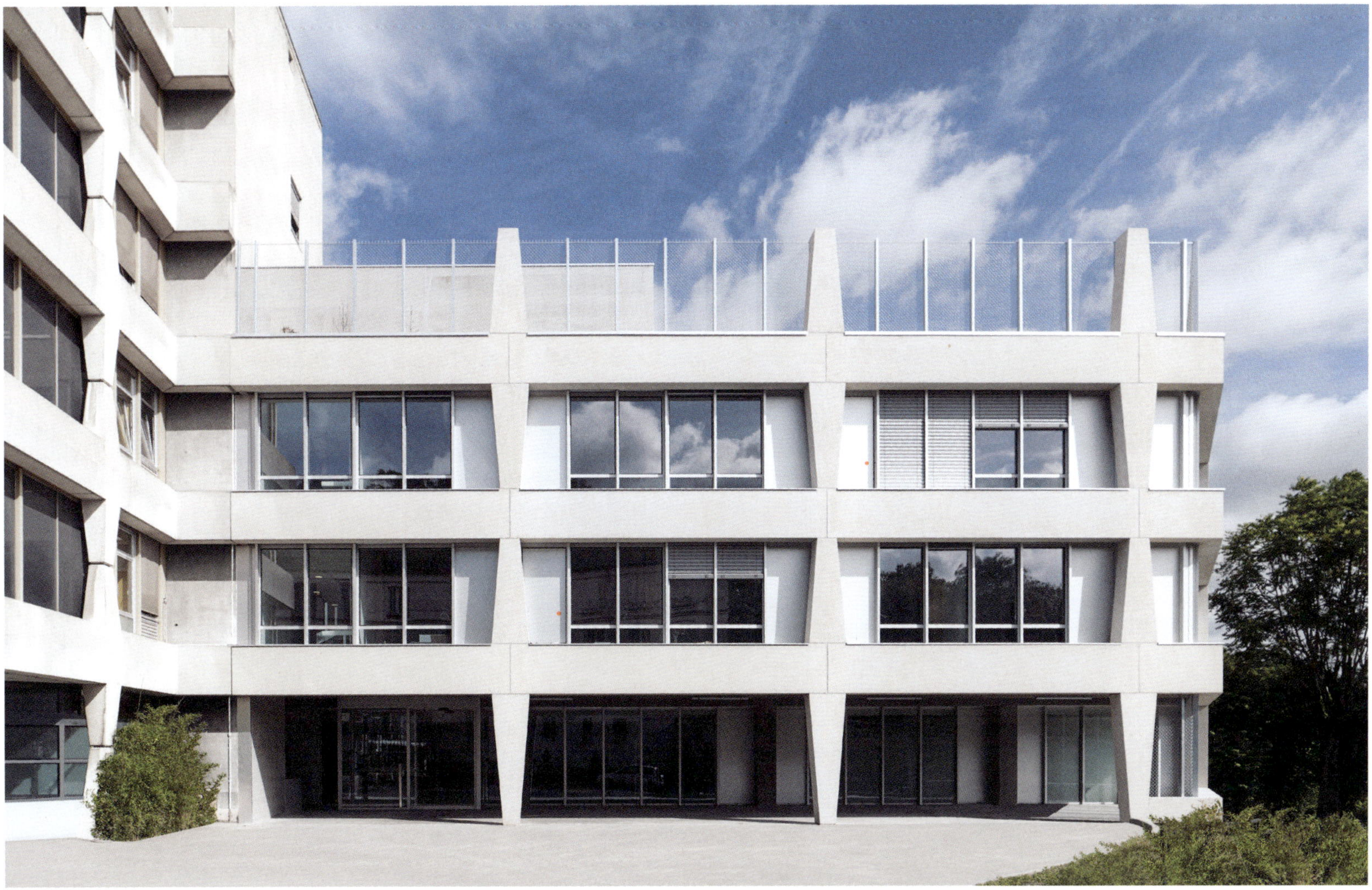

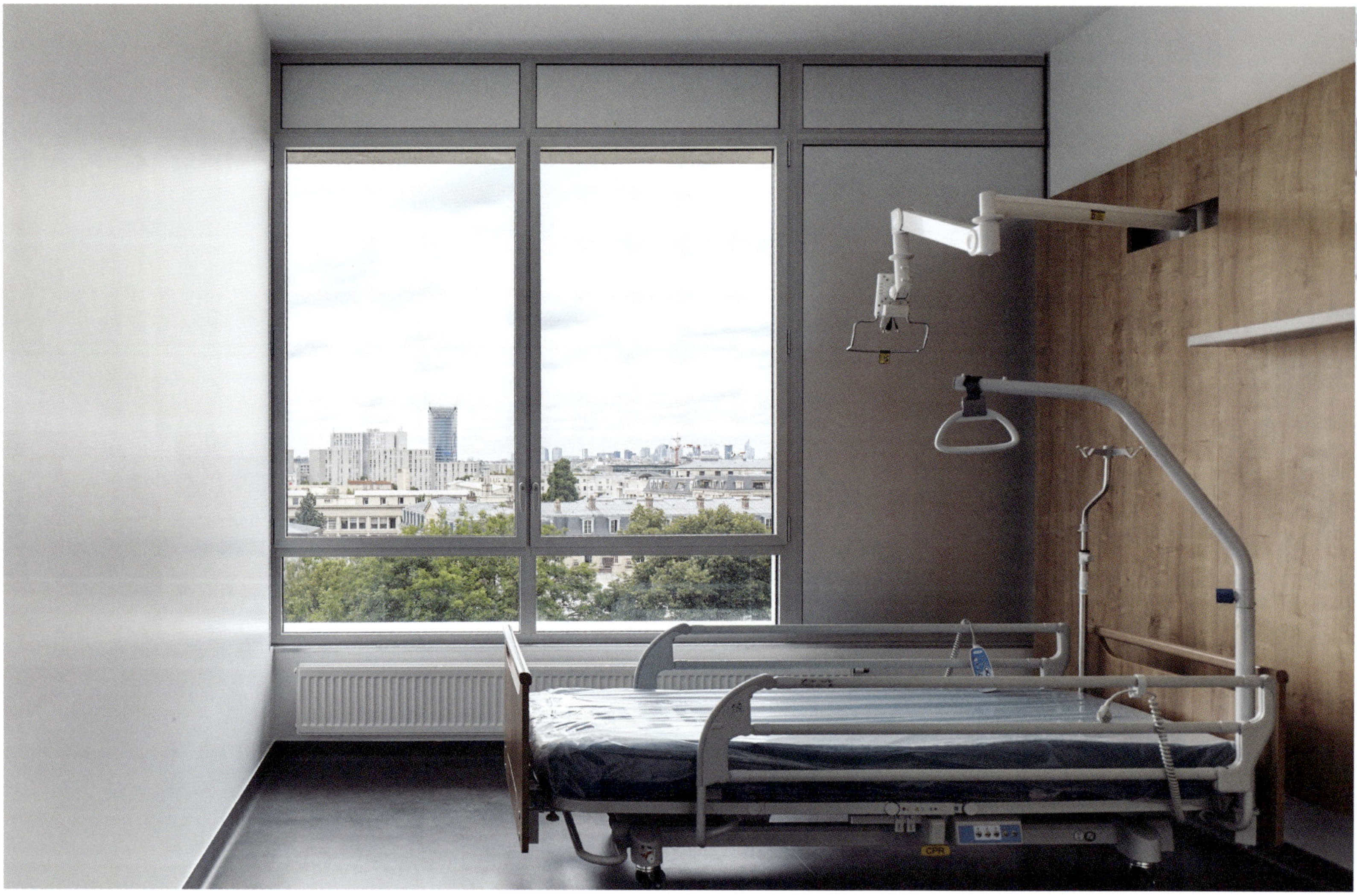

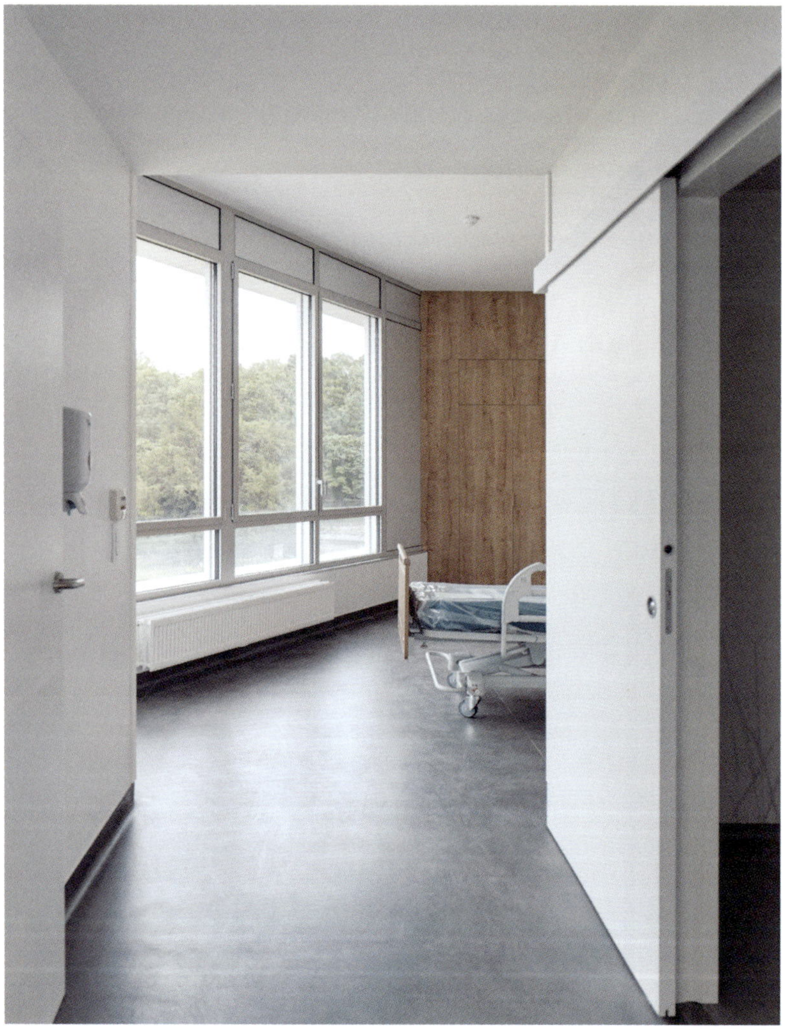

Patients room with view over Paris.

Entrance to a room with view of the park.

Cross section through the extension.

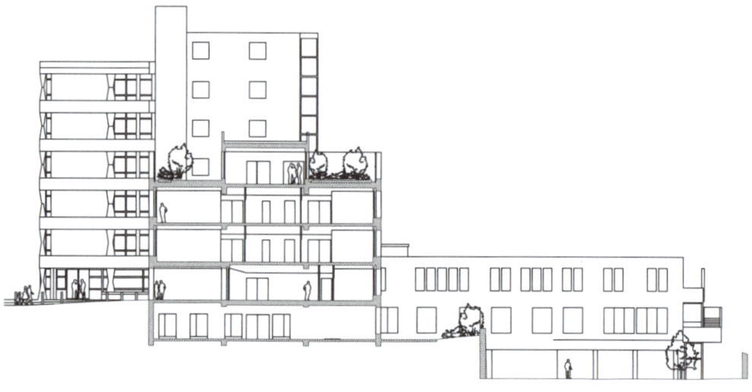

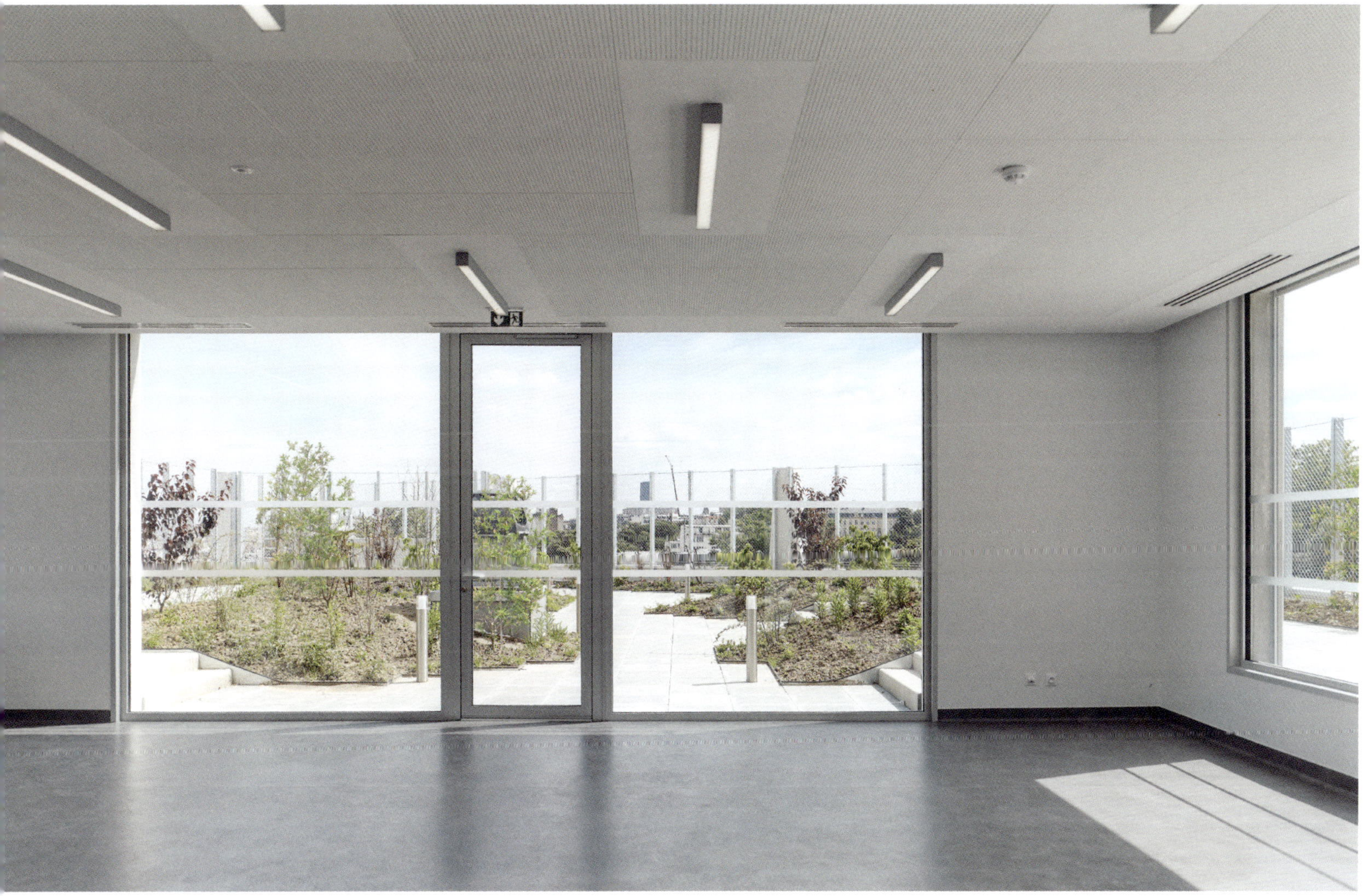

Relaxation room opening onto the roof terrace.

Ground and second floor plan.

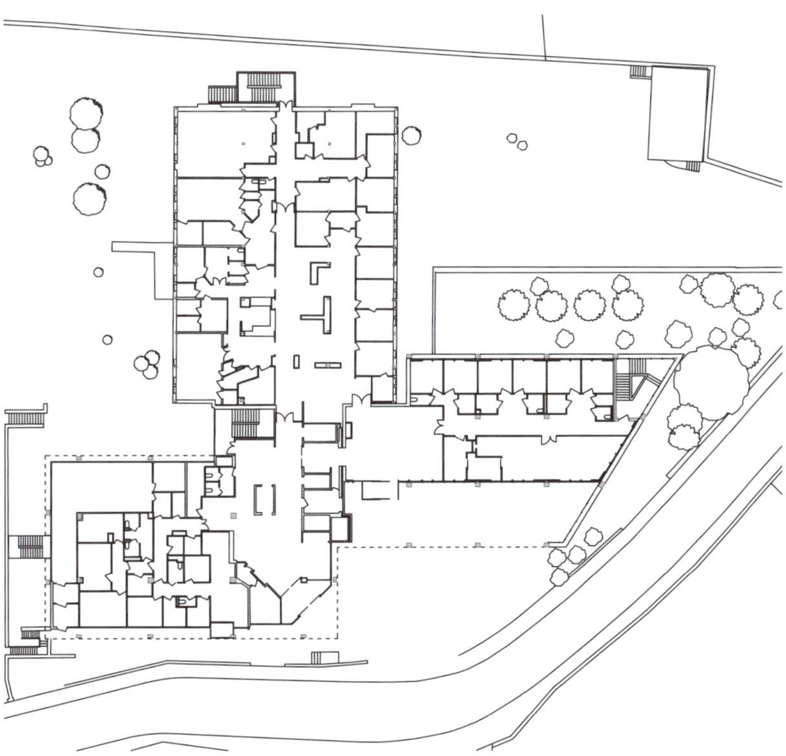

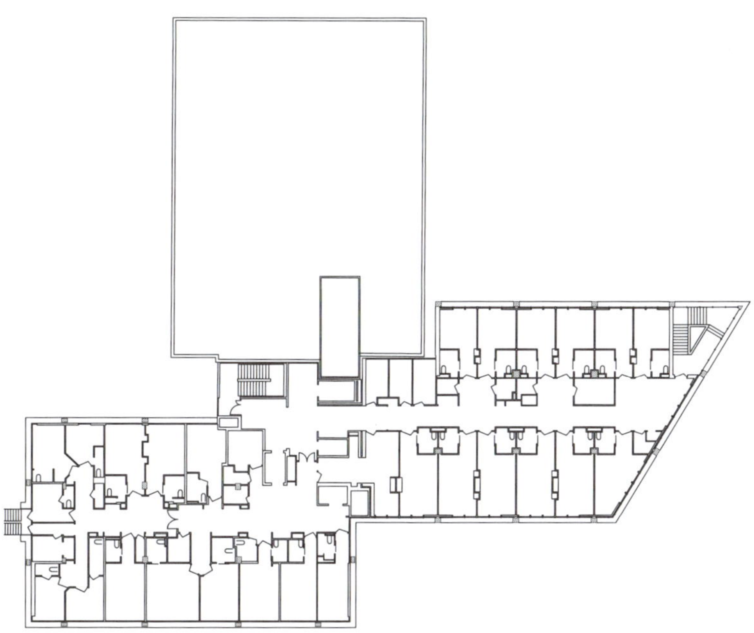

tsj-architekten

Lüneburg
Germany

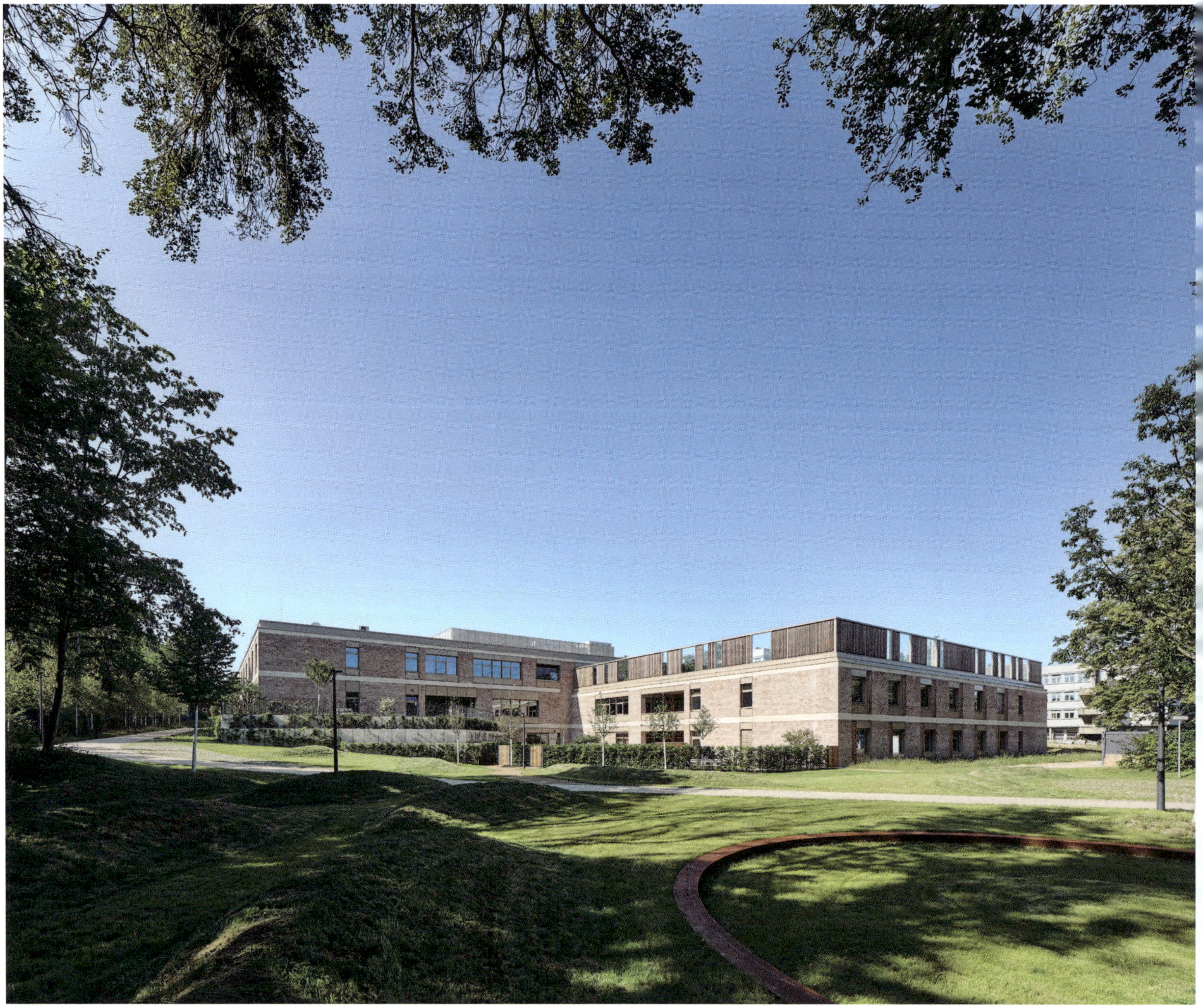

View of the hospital nestled within the green campus.

Hospital's central staircase.

Lüneburg Psychiatric Clinic

The new building brings together the adult and geriatric psychiatry units – previously scattered across the park-like hospital grounds – into two interlocking structures. The four wards are arranged along a circular route around bright inner courtyards. A spacious rooftop garden extends the landscape park, connects the building to the adjacent southern forest garden of the city, and offers a harmonious environment that invites to take a stroll and pause for reflection. The first construction phase is a milestone for health-oriented architecture that goes beyond structural functionality. The design conveys serenity, confidence, and openness and fosters the healing journey of patients suffering from mental illness within a protective space. Respectful coexistence forms the foundation of the building and is simultaneously expressed through thoughtful spatial solutions that strengthen self-determination and well-being.

Address: Am Wienebütteler Weg 1, 21339 Lüneburg, Germany | **Client:** Psychiatrische Klinik Lüneburg | **Completion:** 2024 | **Size:** 11,862 m^2 | **Sector:** state | **Specialization:** psychiatric and psychotherapeutic hospital | **Number of treatment rooms:** 13 | **Number of patient rooms:** 48 | **Number of patient beds:** 96 | **Landscape design:** lad+ landschaftsarchitektur

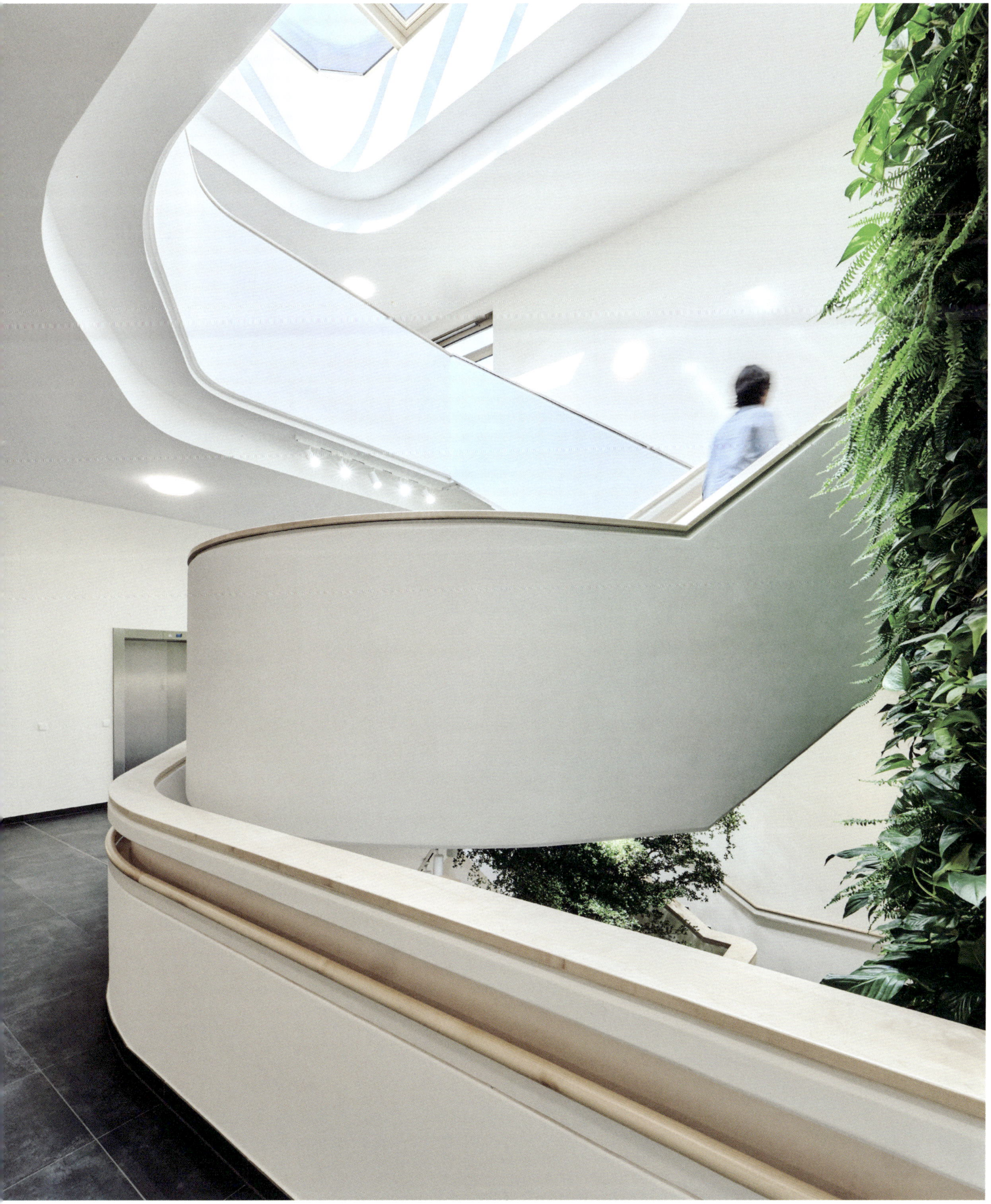

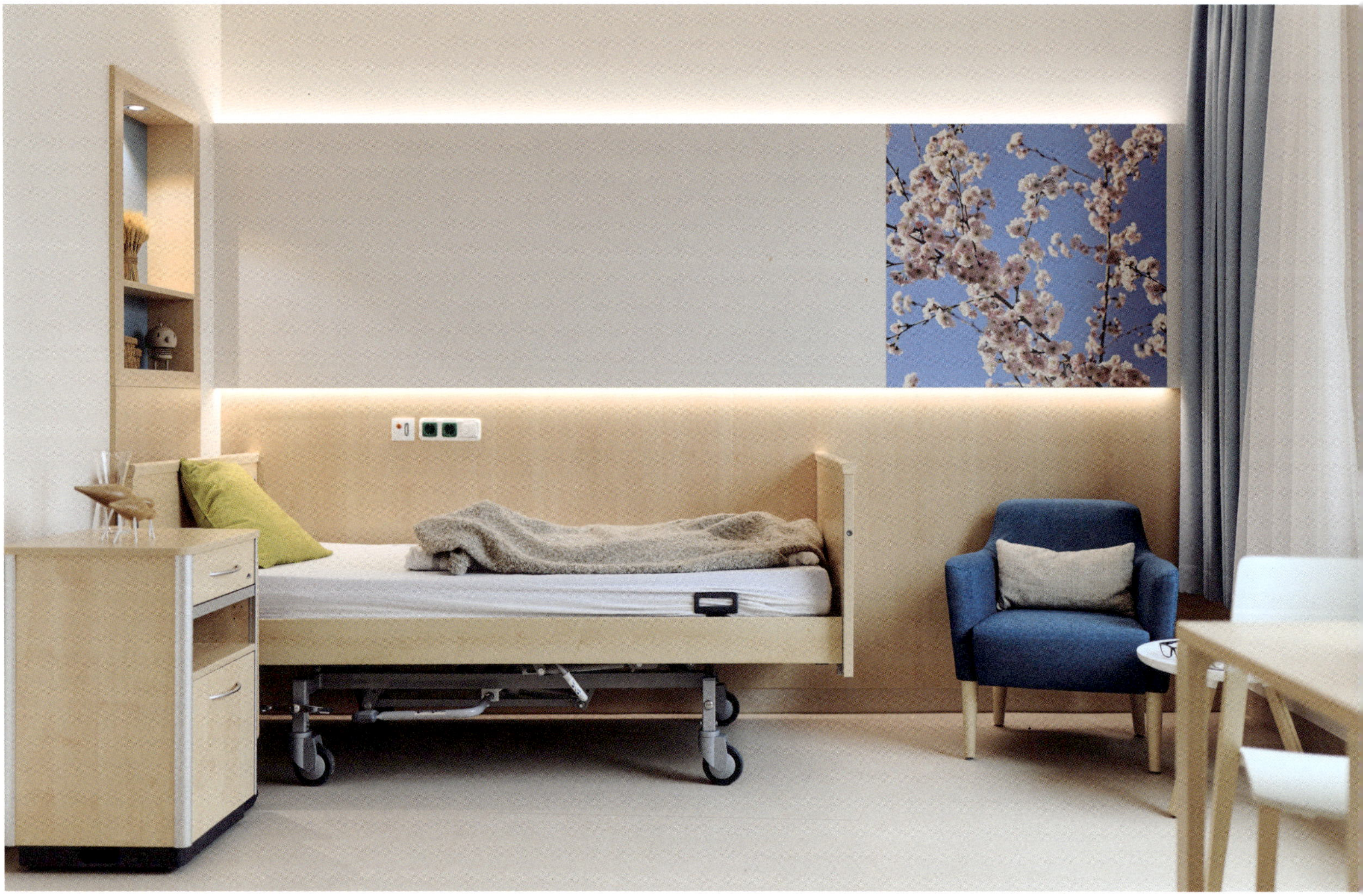

Adequately designed patient room.

Site plan.

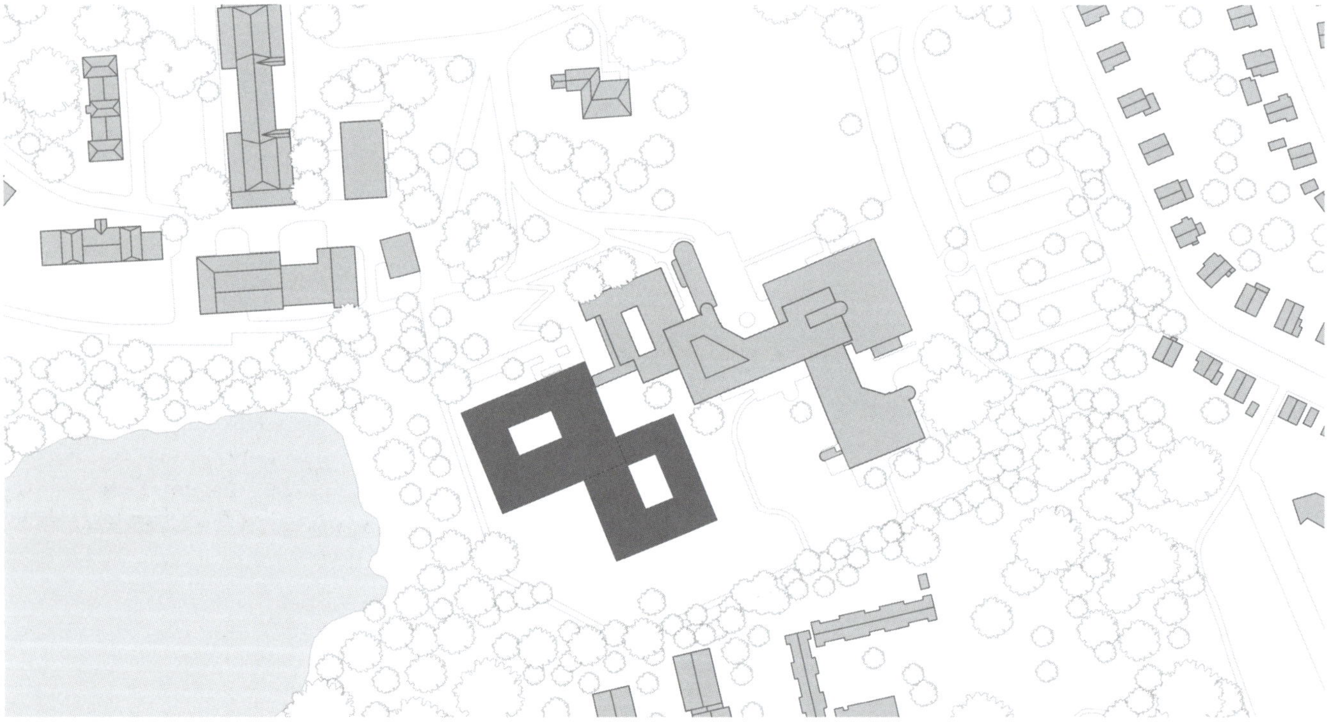

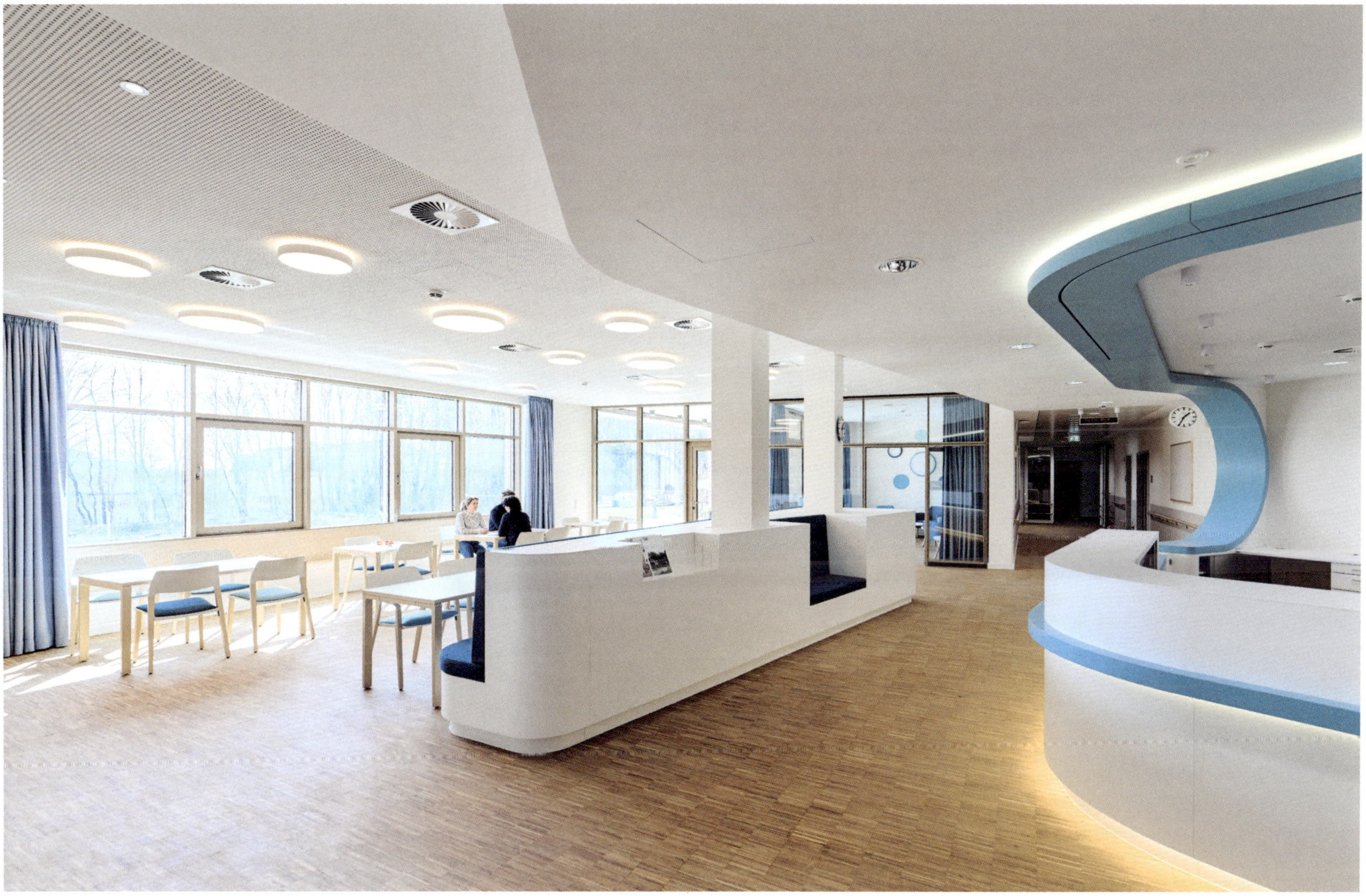

Nursing station and dining area of the ward.

Ground floor plan.

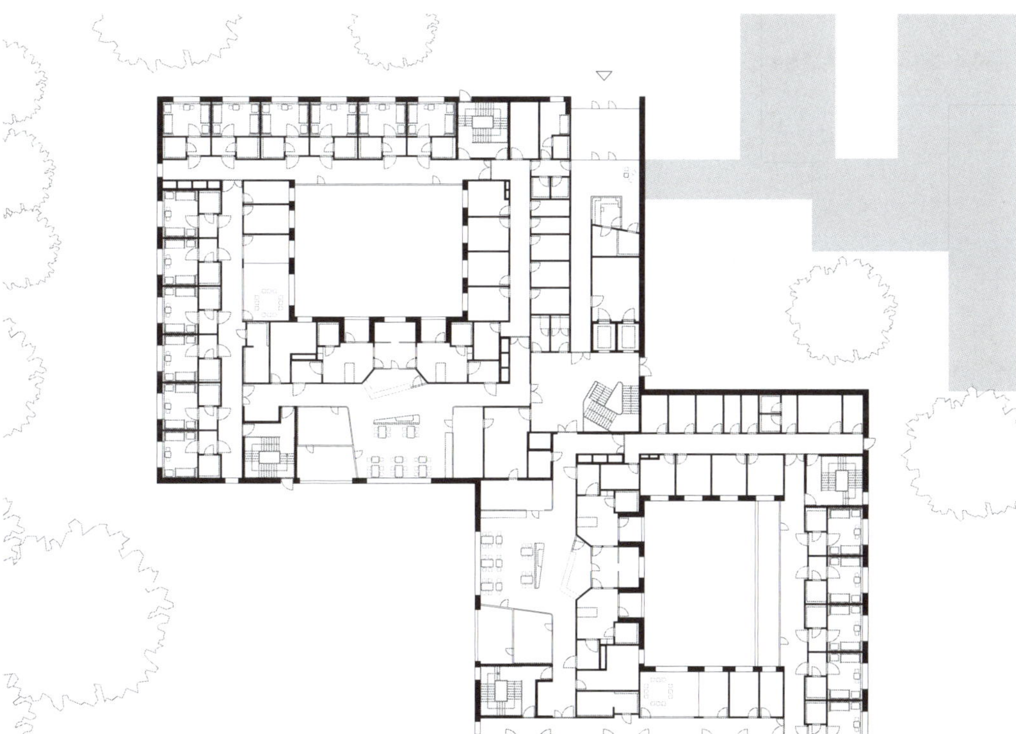

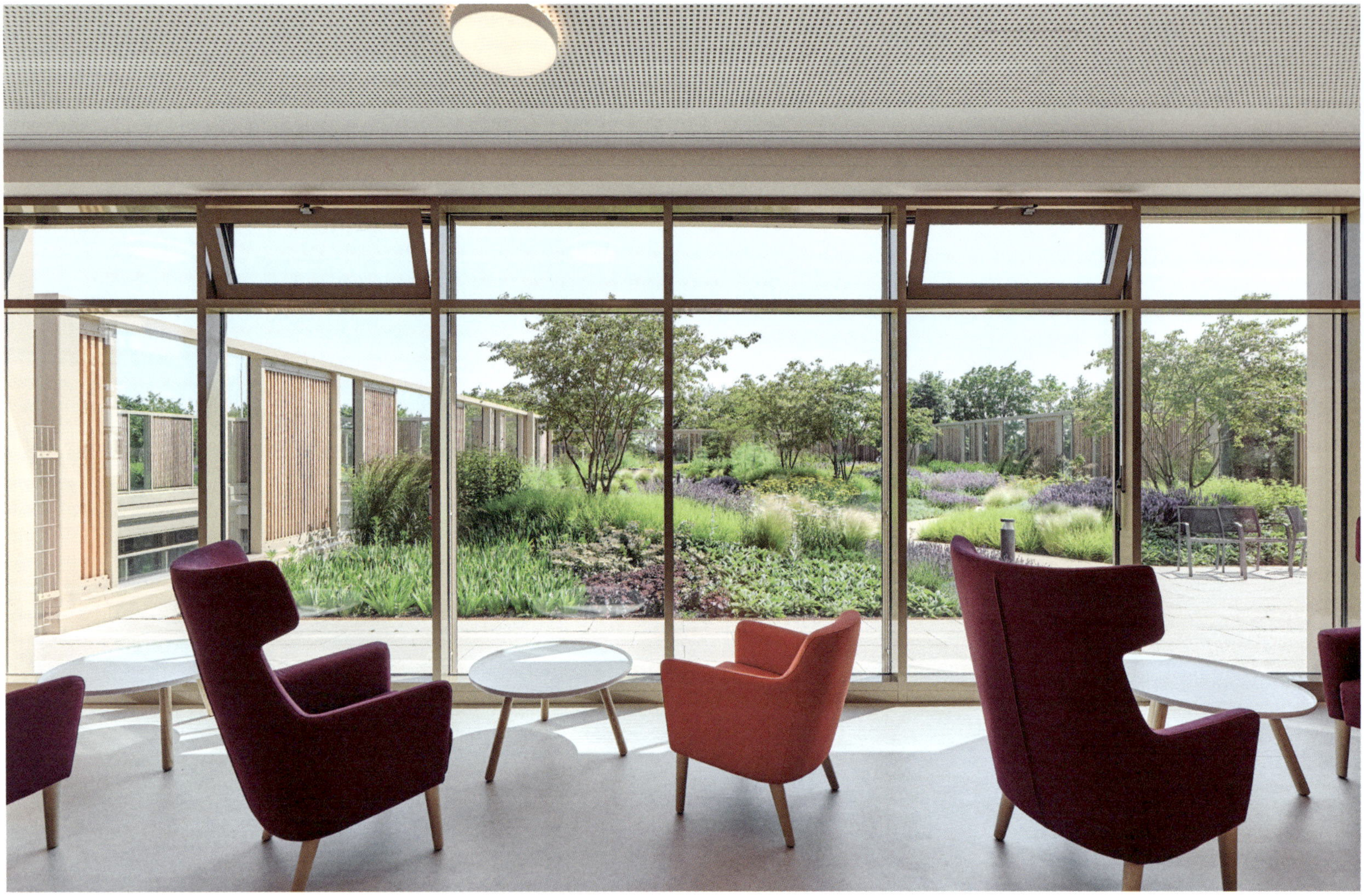

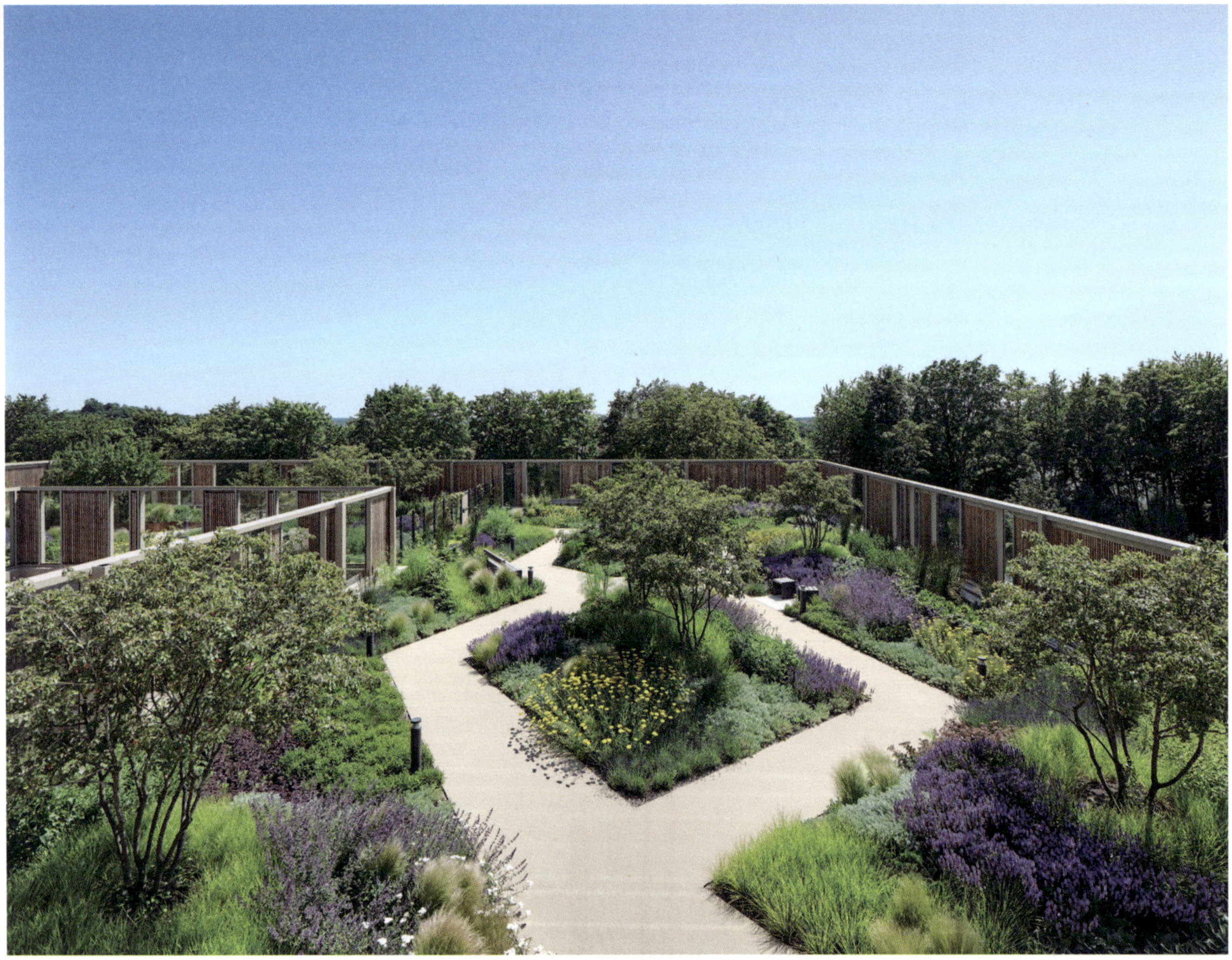

View of the rooftop garden from the lounge area.

The rooftop garden offers patients a green oasis of tranquility.

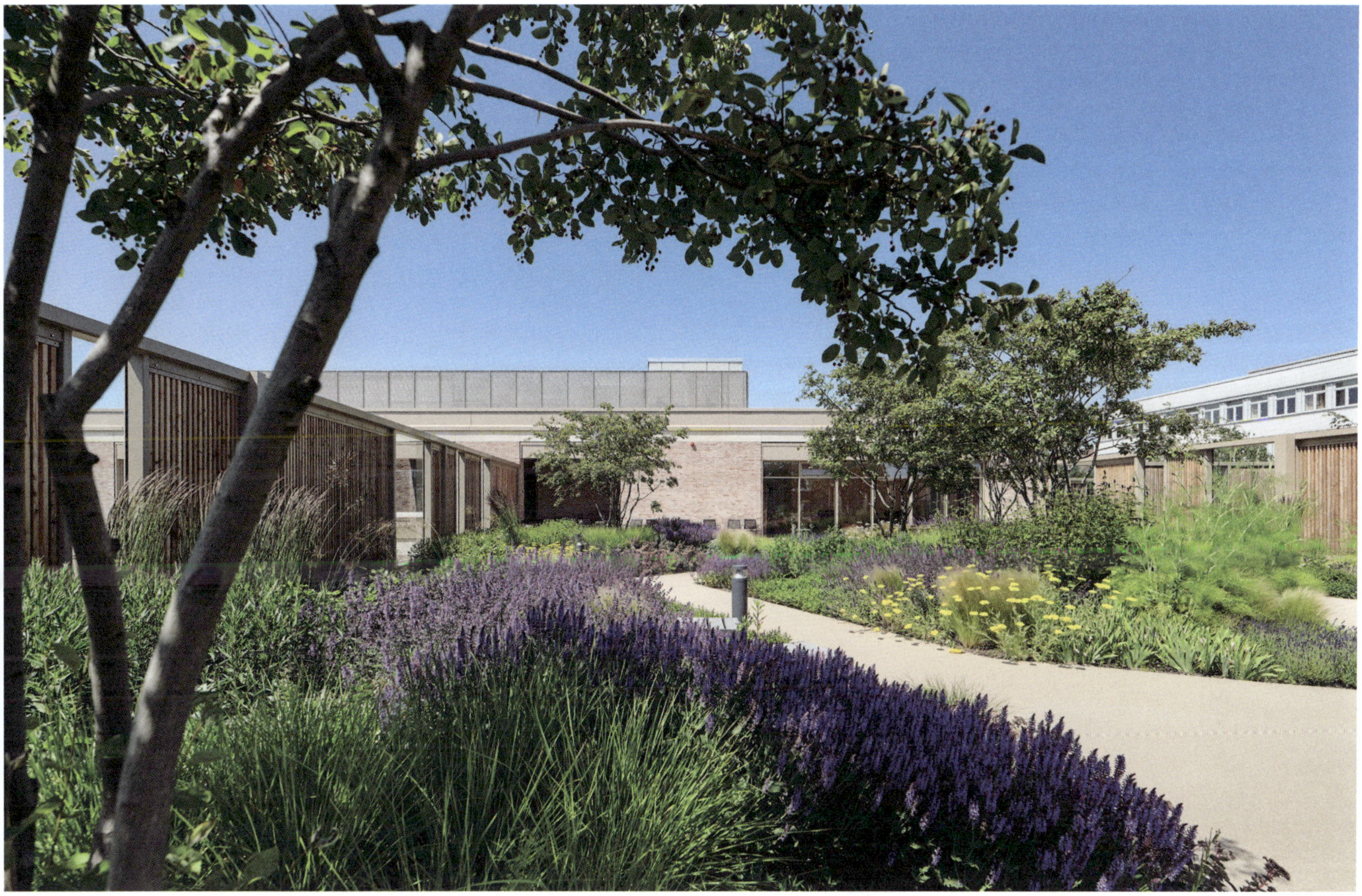

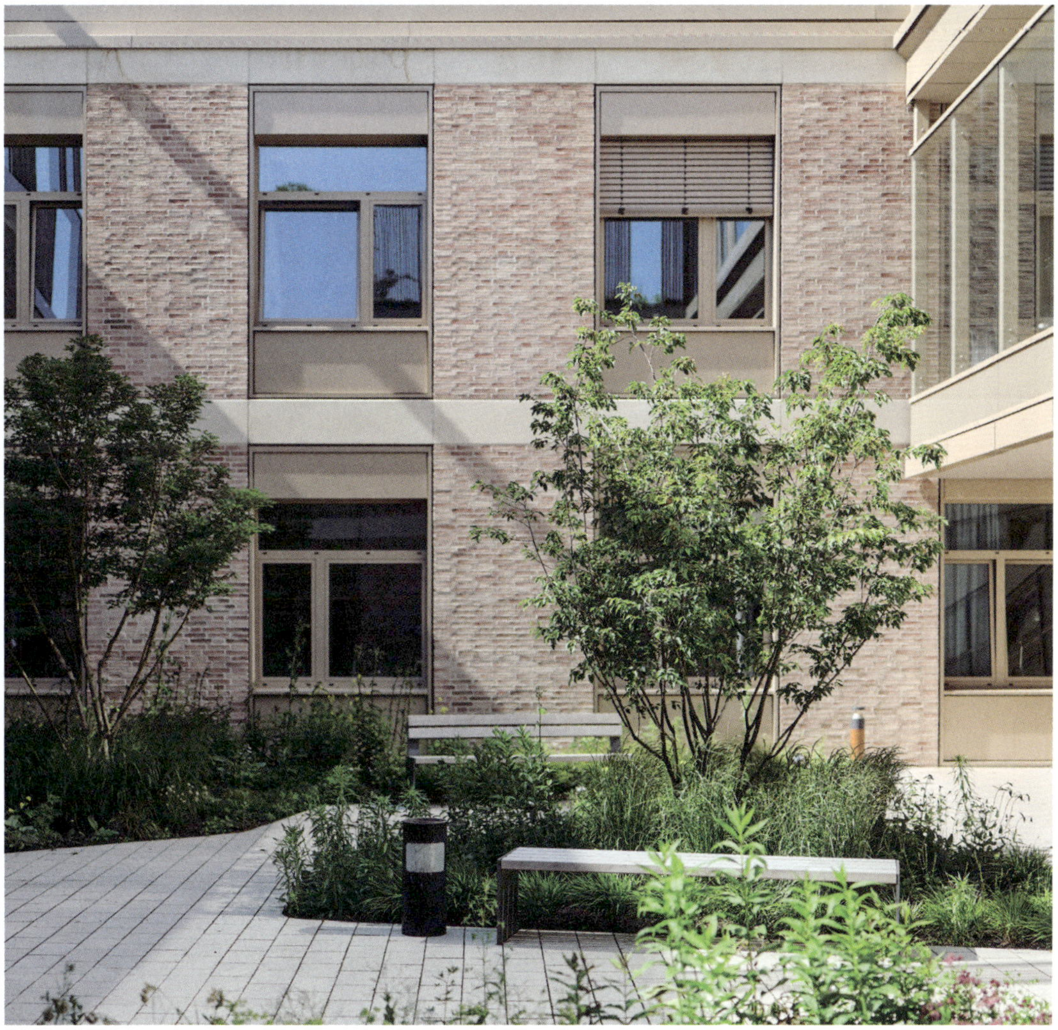

Illuminated paths wind through the diverse rooftop landscape.

The courtyard is divided by a variety of plantings.

Ernst Giselbrecht + Partner

Leoben
Austria

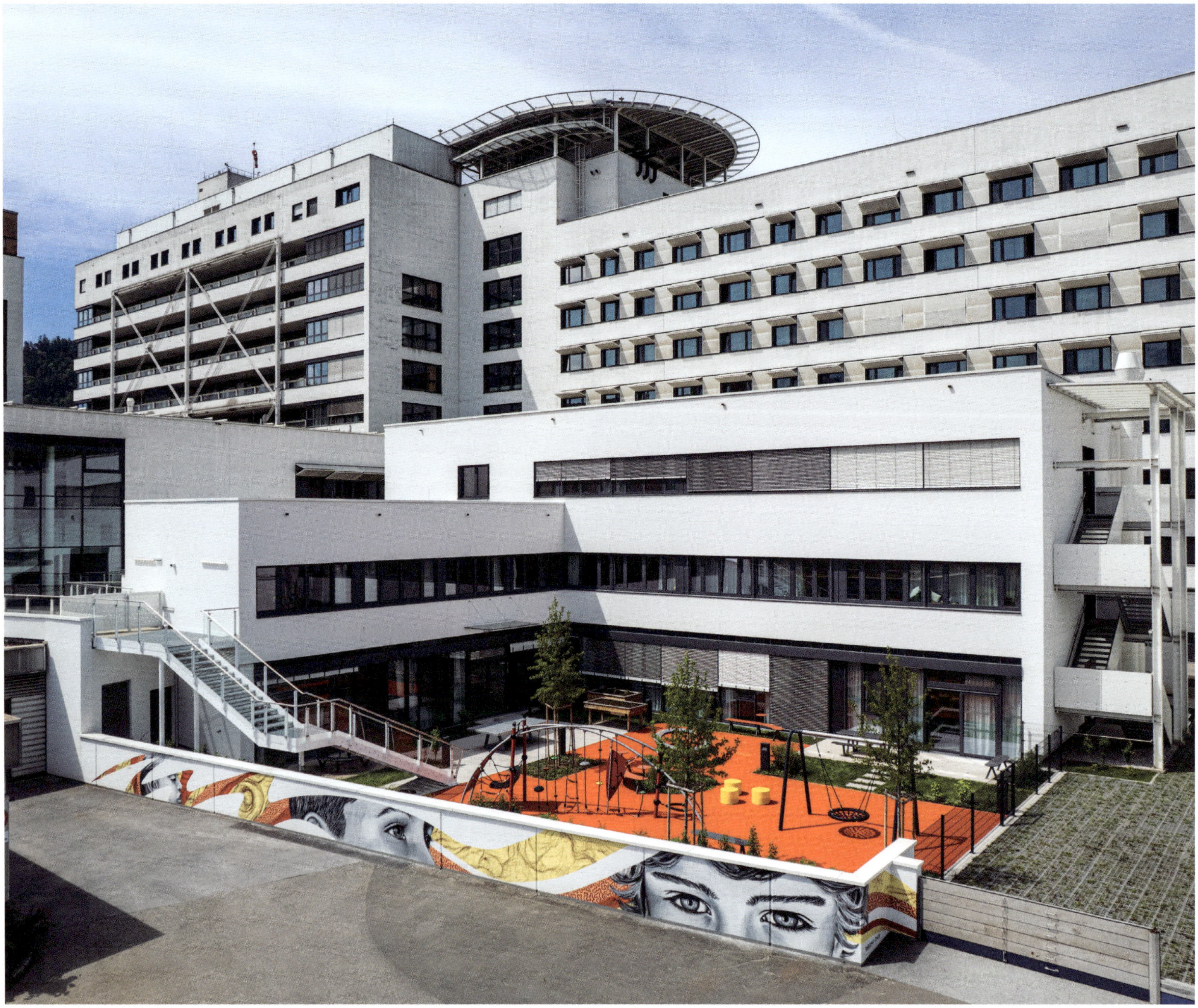

Façade of the hospital building.

Courtyard with a play area for the children.

The wall graffities.

Leoben Regional Hospital – Pediatric Outpatient Clinic

The new clinic has been completed as a standalone building on the east side of the hospital. The location offers better accessibility, more natural light, and will allow for future expansion into a Children's House. The clinic is directly connected via the east-west corridor, for short walking distances. A particularly thoughtful wayfinding system featuring colorful balloon ceiling lights guides children to the ward and helps alleviate their fears. Eight examination rooms surround the reception area and waiting room. Playful drawings on glass surfaces transform medical equipment into friendly figures. Directly below the pediatric outpatient clinic, new areas for physical therapy, speech therapy, occupational therapy, and special education for children have been created. The second basement level houses the child and adolescent psychiatry department, which includes an outpatient area and a day clinic with six beds.

Address: Vordernberger Straße, 8700 Leoben, Austria | **Client:** Steiermärkische Krankenanstalten GmbH KAGes | **Completion:** 2021 | **Size:** 2,556 m² | **Sector:** state | **Specialization:** pediatric outpatient clinic, child and adolescent psychiatry | **Number of treatment rooms:** 24 | Landscape architect: Koala Landschaftsarchitektur | **Graffities / Wall Art**: Gernot Passath

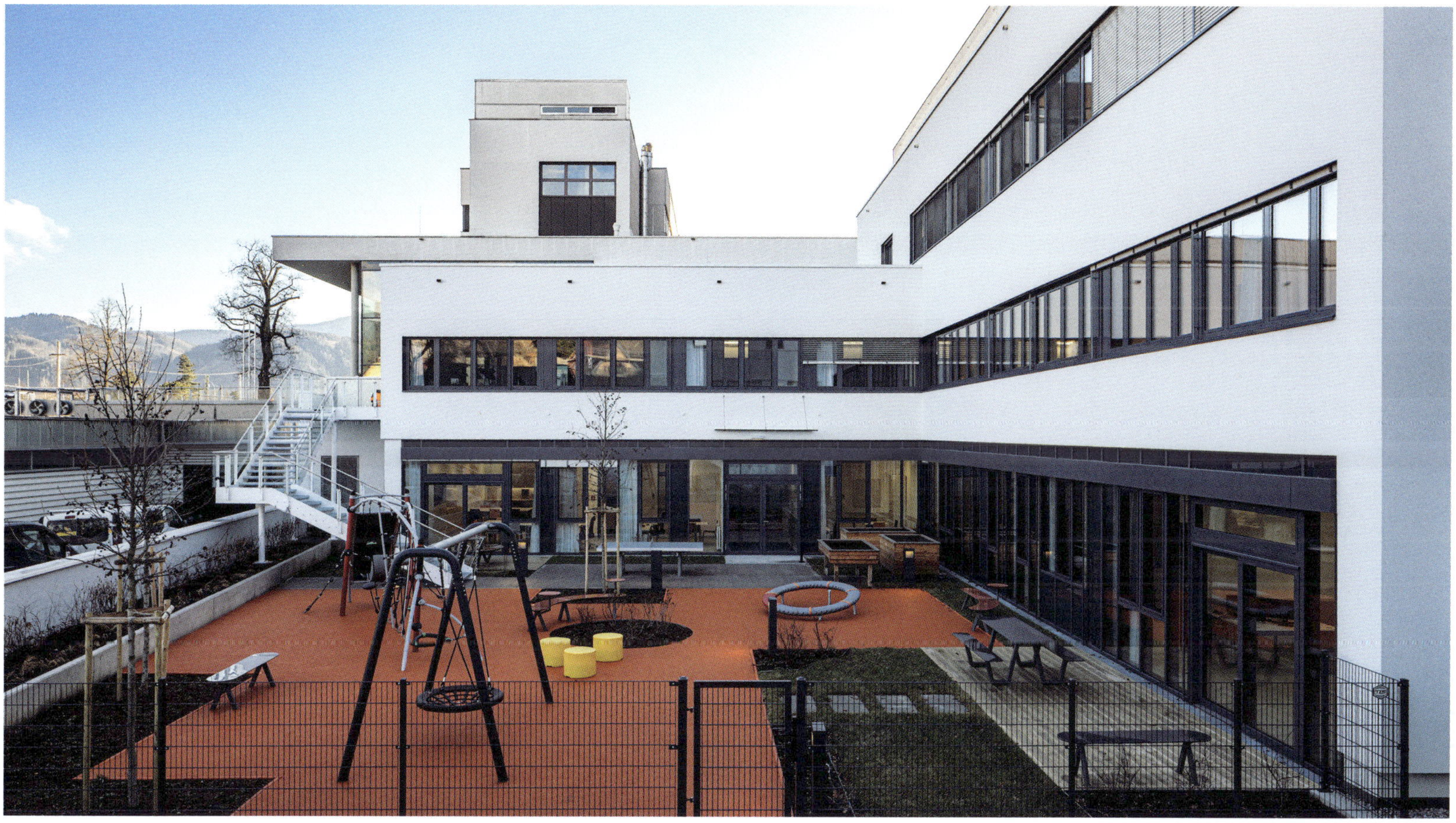

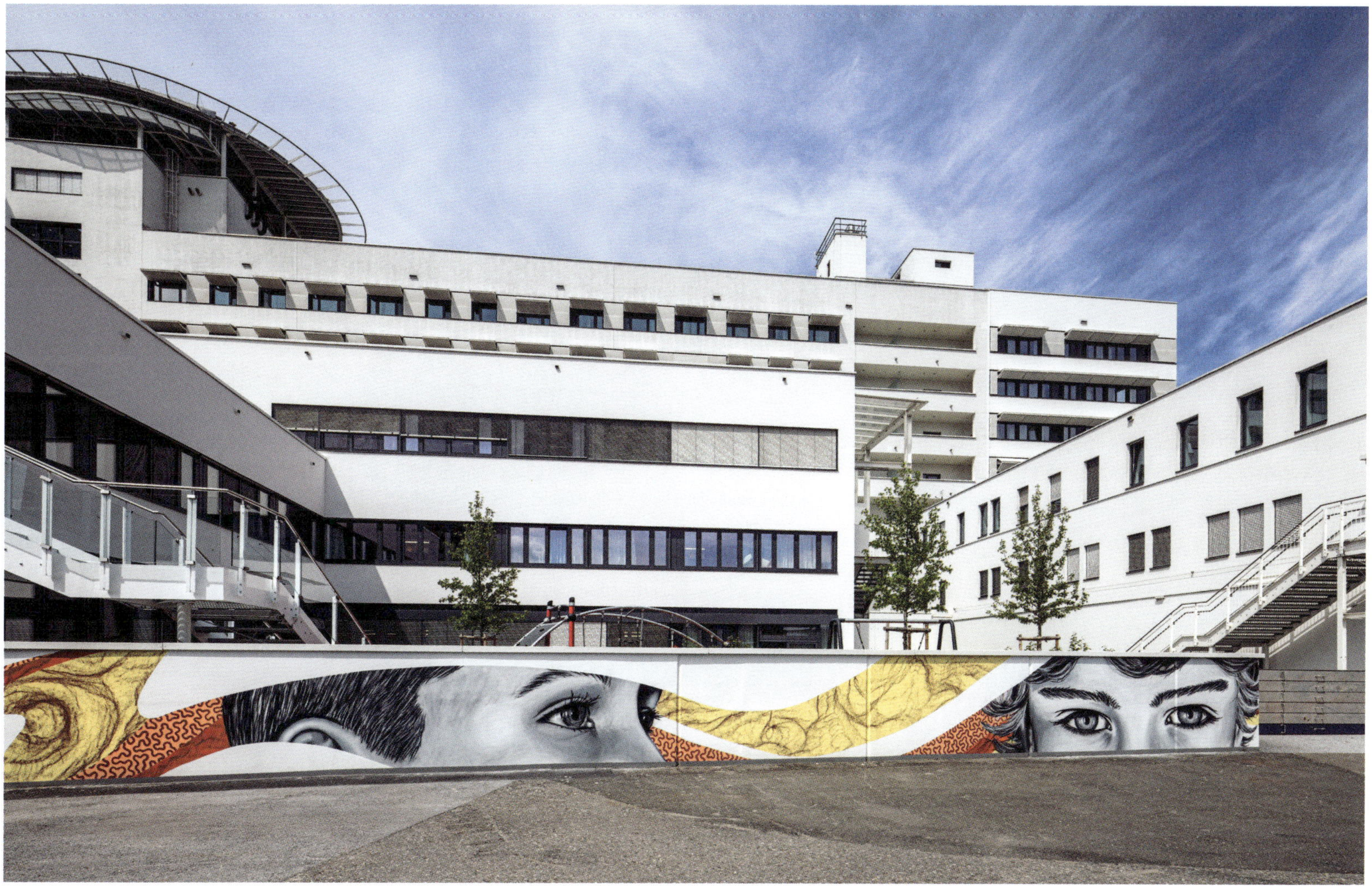

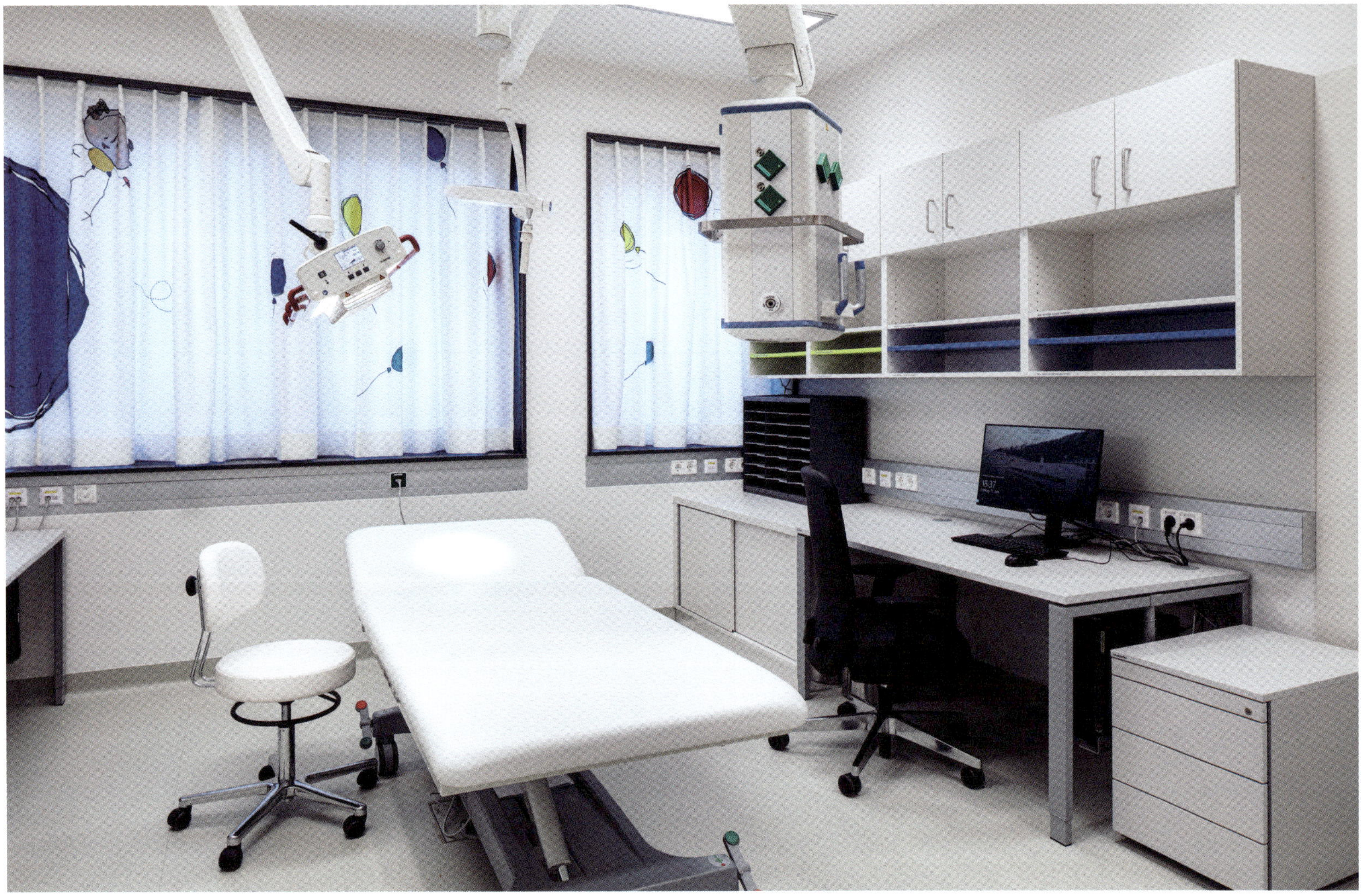

Hospital's examination room.

Typical floor plan.

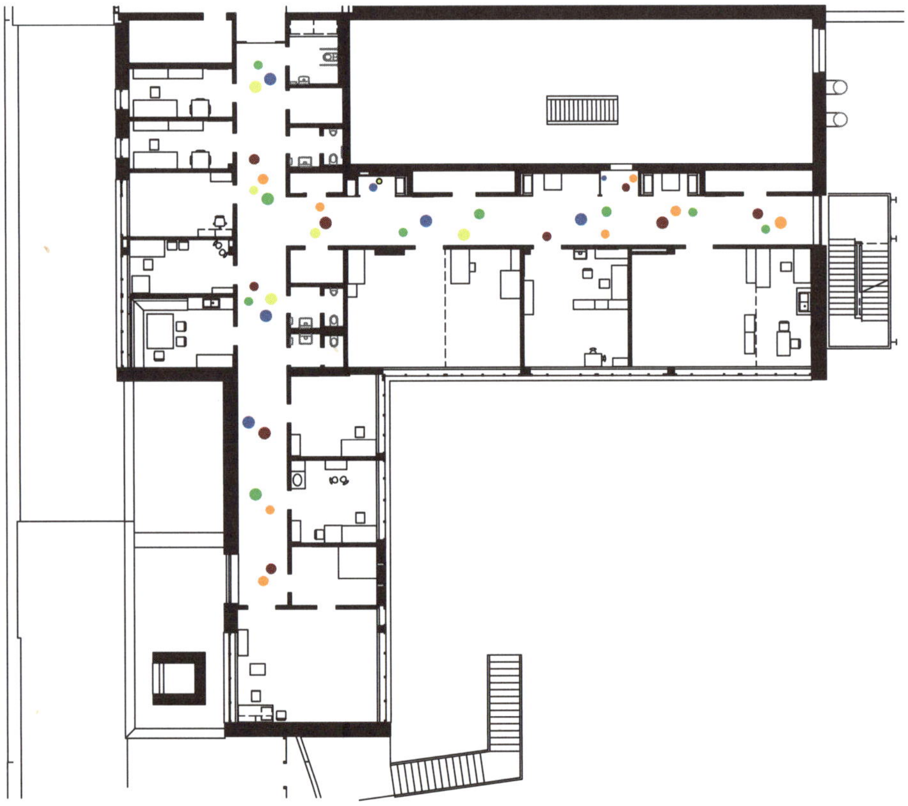

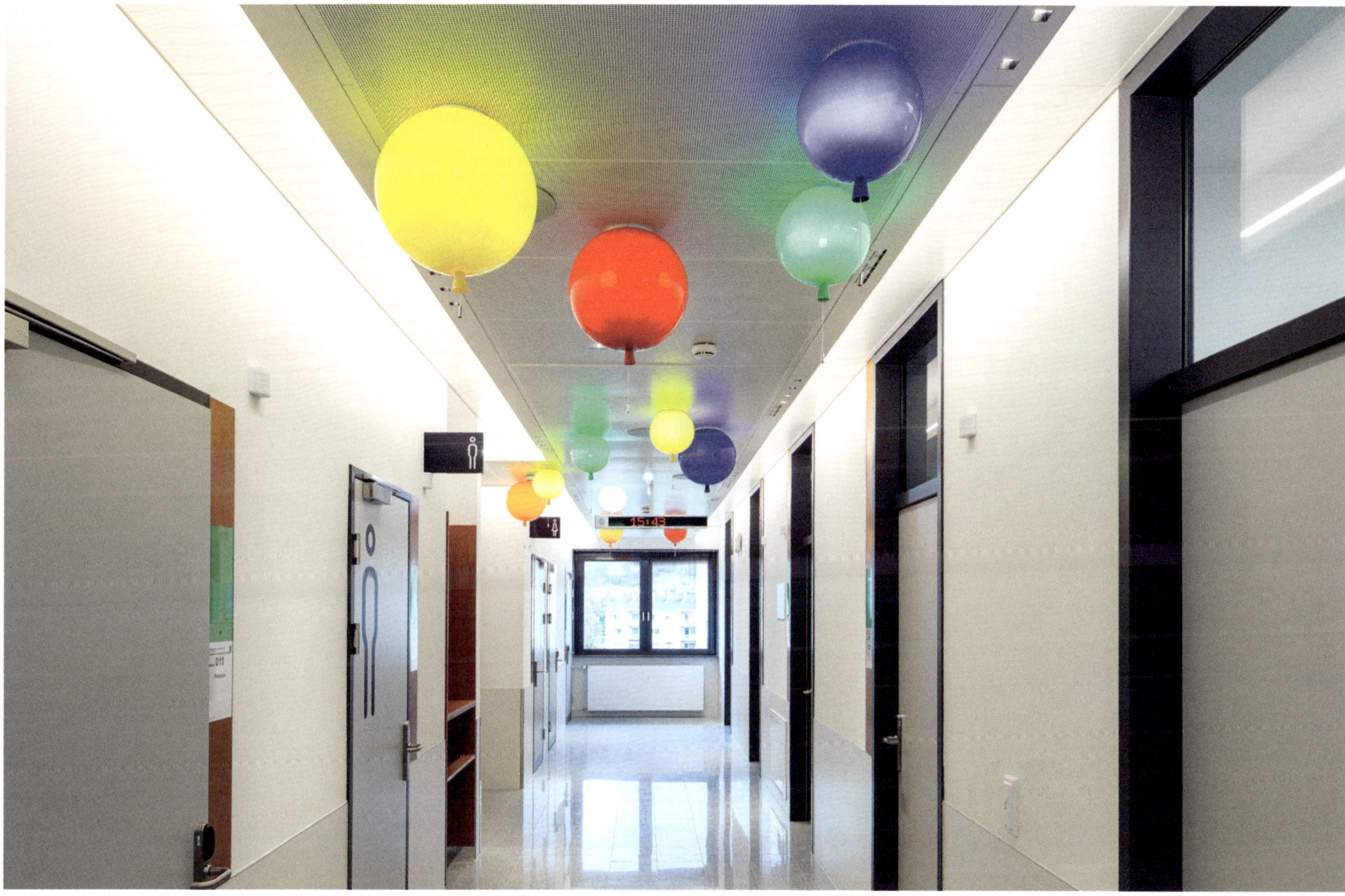

Spacious corridor with ample natural light.

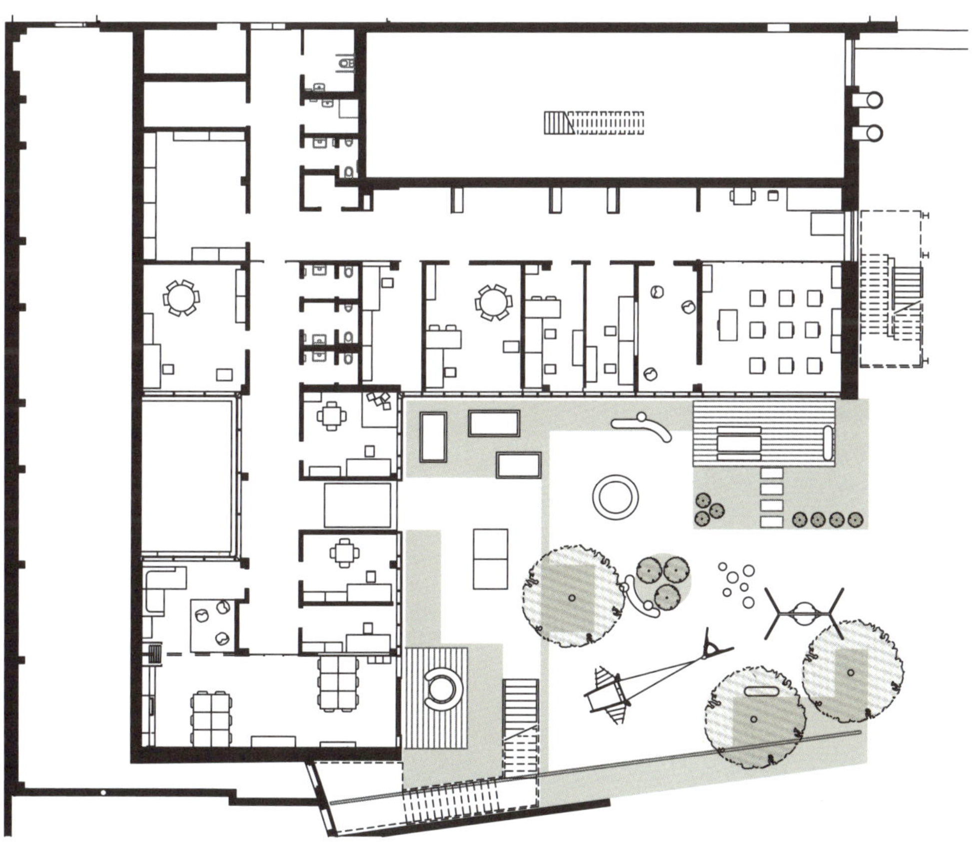

Ground floor plan with courtyard.

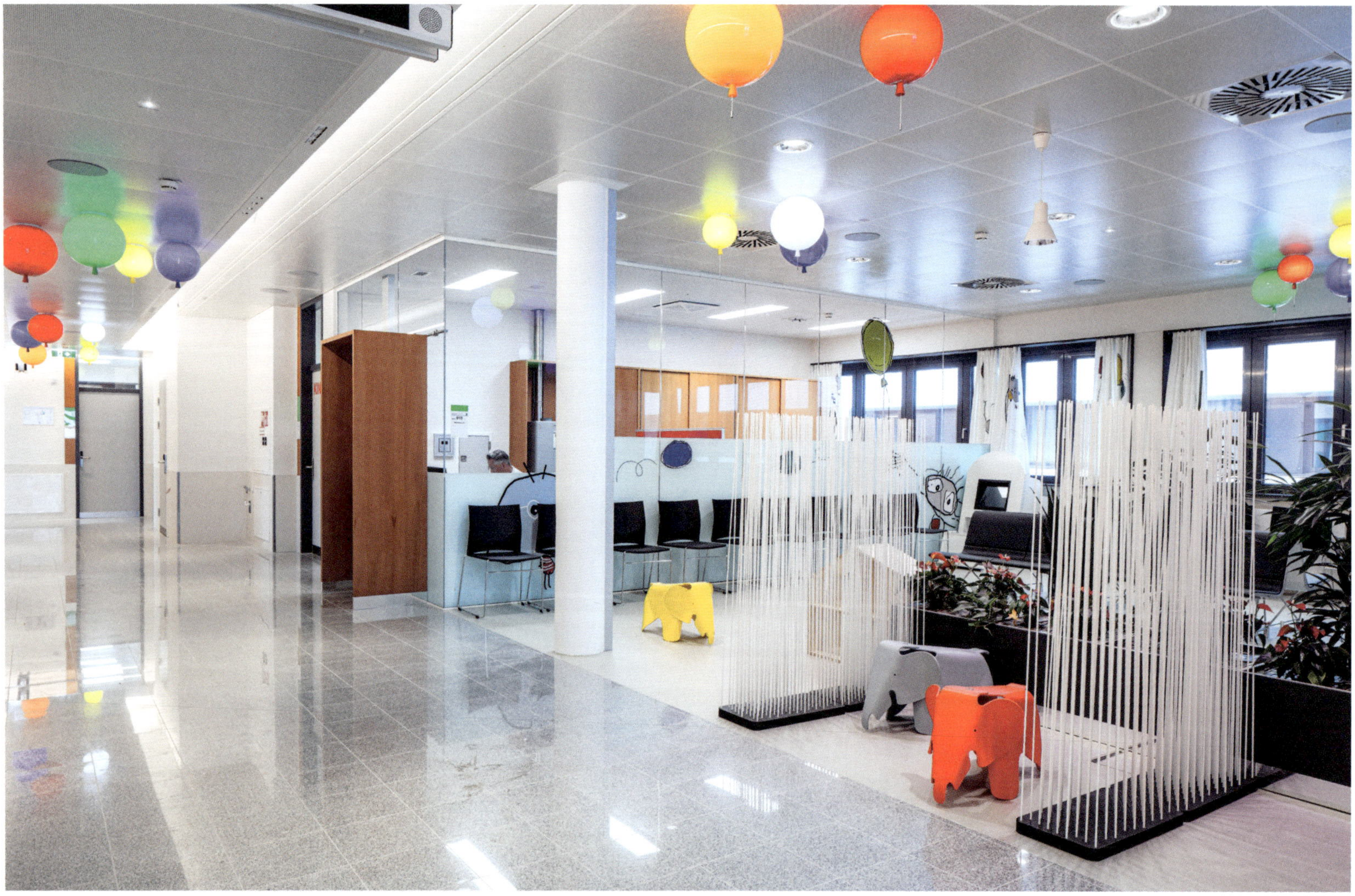

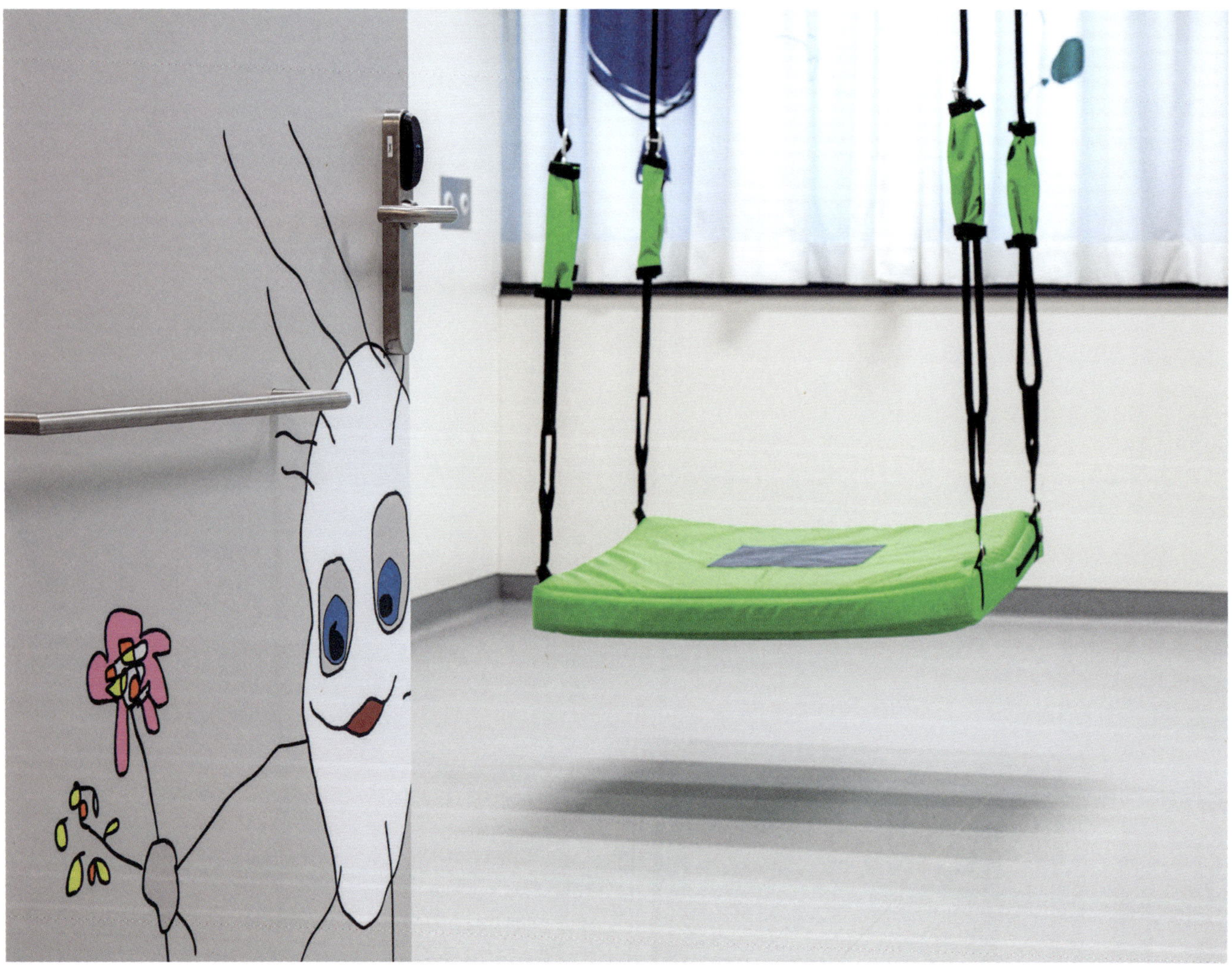

Playful waiting room and reception area with wood, glass, and good acoustics for a calm atmosphere.

Examination room with a swing for the children.

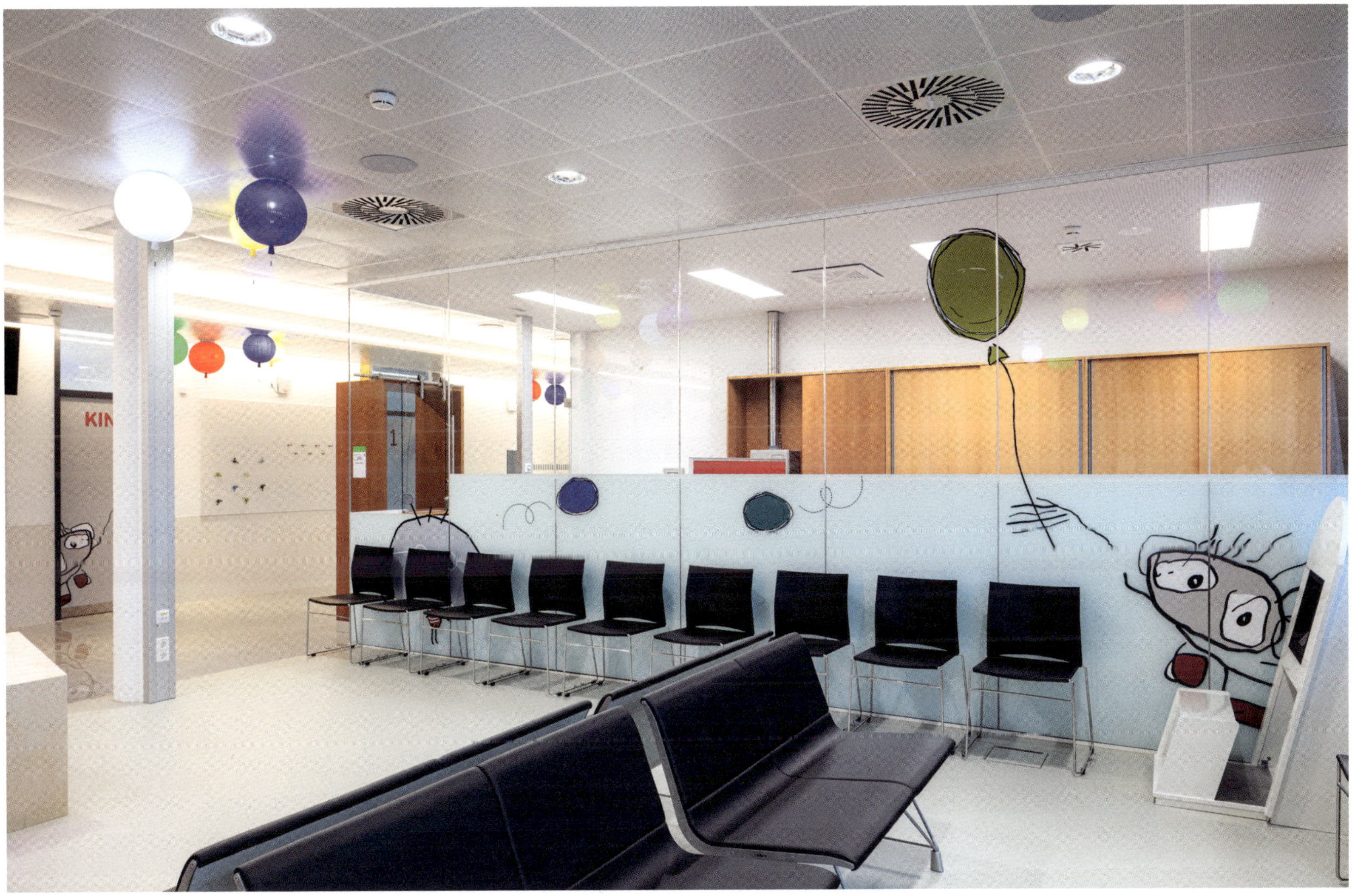

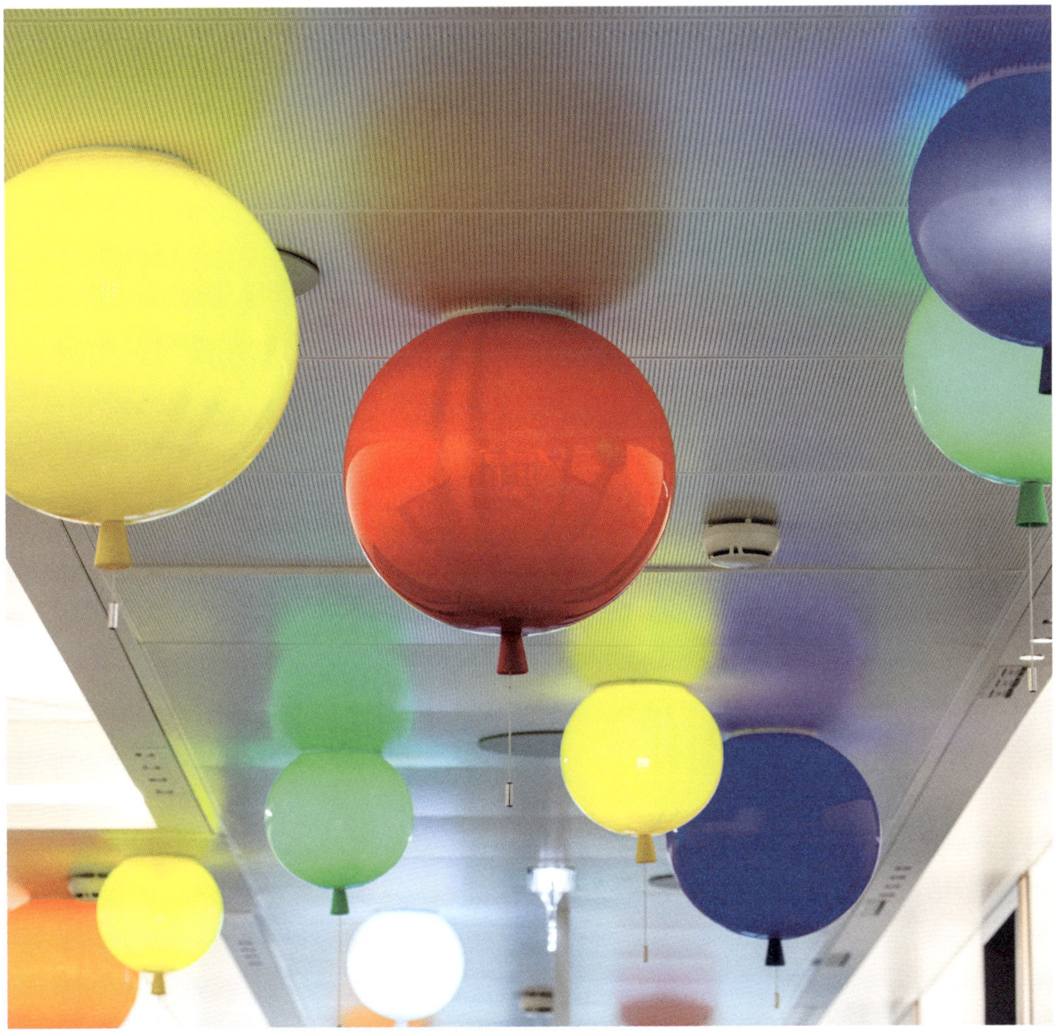

Waiting room with playful drawings on glass surfaces.

Colorful balloon-like guiding lights to alleviate children's fear.

EGM architects

Nijmegen
The Netherlands

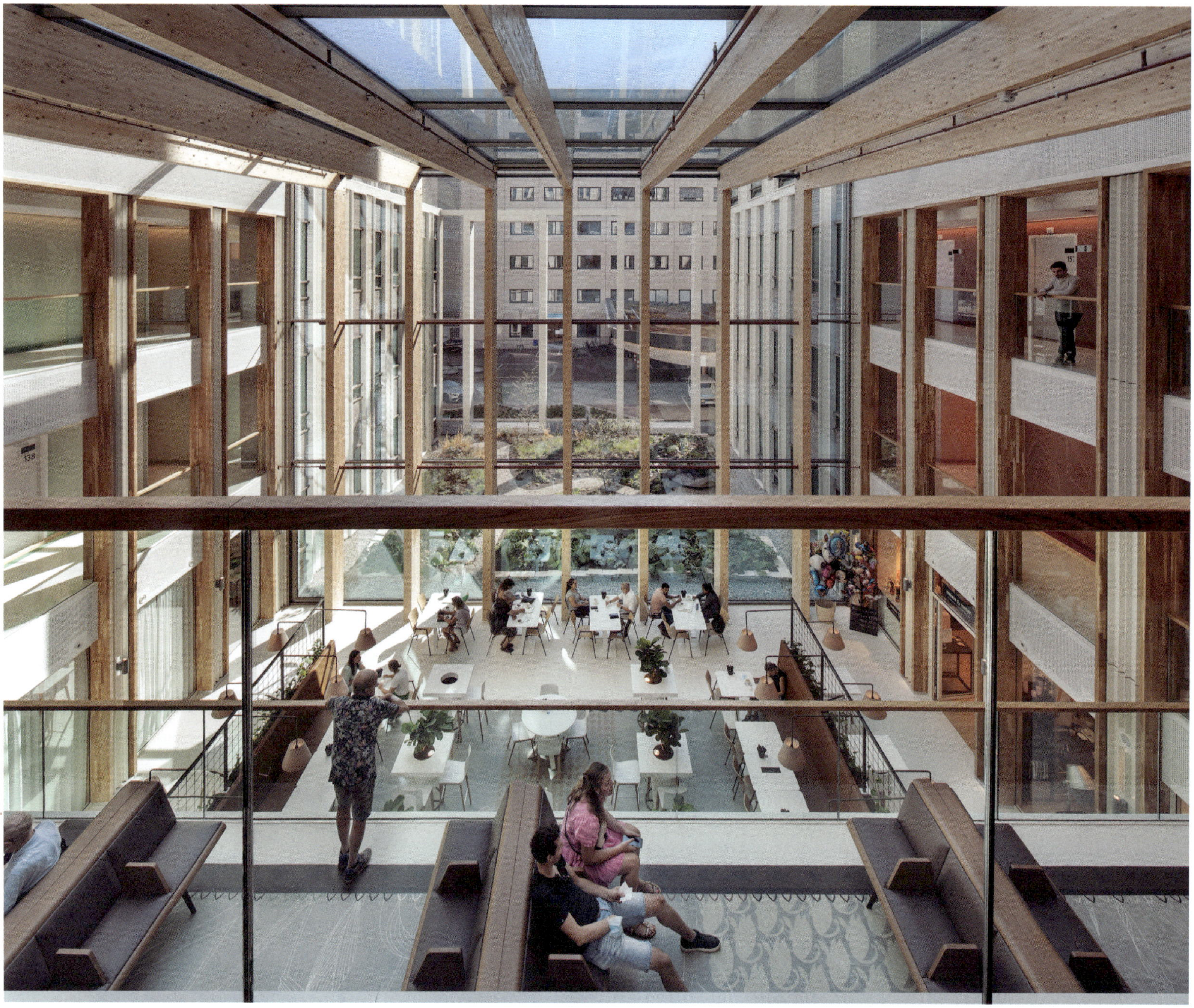

One of two atria with a wooden structure.

Covered courtyard with elevators.

Radboudumc Main Building

The Radboudumc Main Building embodies the principles of healing architecture through a carefully orchestrated balance of light, nature, and human-centered design. As the new heart of a compact and sustainable campus, the building integrates generous daylight, open views, and surrounding greenery to create a calm and restorative environment. Patient rooms and public spaces are designed to reduce stress, offering privacy, quietness, and a sense of control, while social areas encourage encounter and connection. Biophilic strategies, natural materials, and a hotel-like atmosphere further soften the clinical setting. By combining adaptability, sustainability, and sensory comfort, the hospital supports recovery not only medically, but spatially and emotionally. At its opening in 2022 the hospital was the first university medical center in The Netherlands to be awarded the BREEAM Excellent certificate.

Address: Geert Grooteplein 10, 6525 GA Nijmegen, The Netherlands | **Client:** Radboudumc | **Completion:** 2022 | **Size:** 46,300 m² | **Sector:** public | **Number of patient rooms:** 150 | **Interior design:** Suzanne Holz Studio | **Landscape design:** Copijn

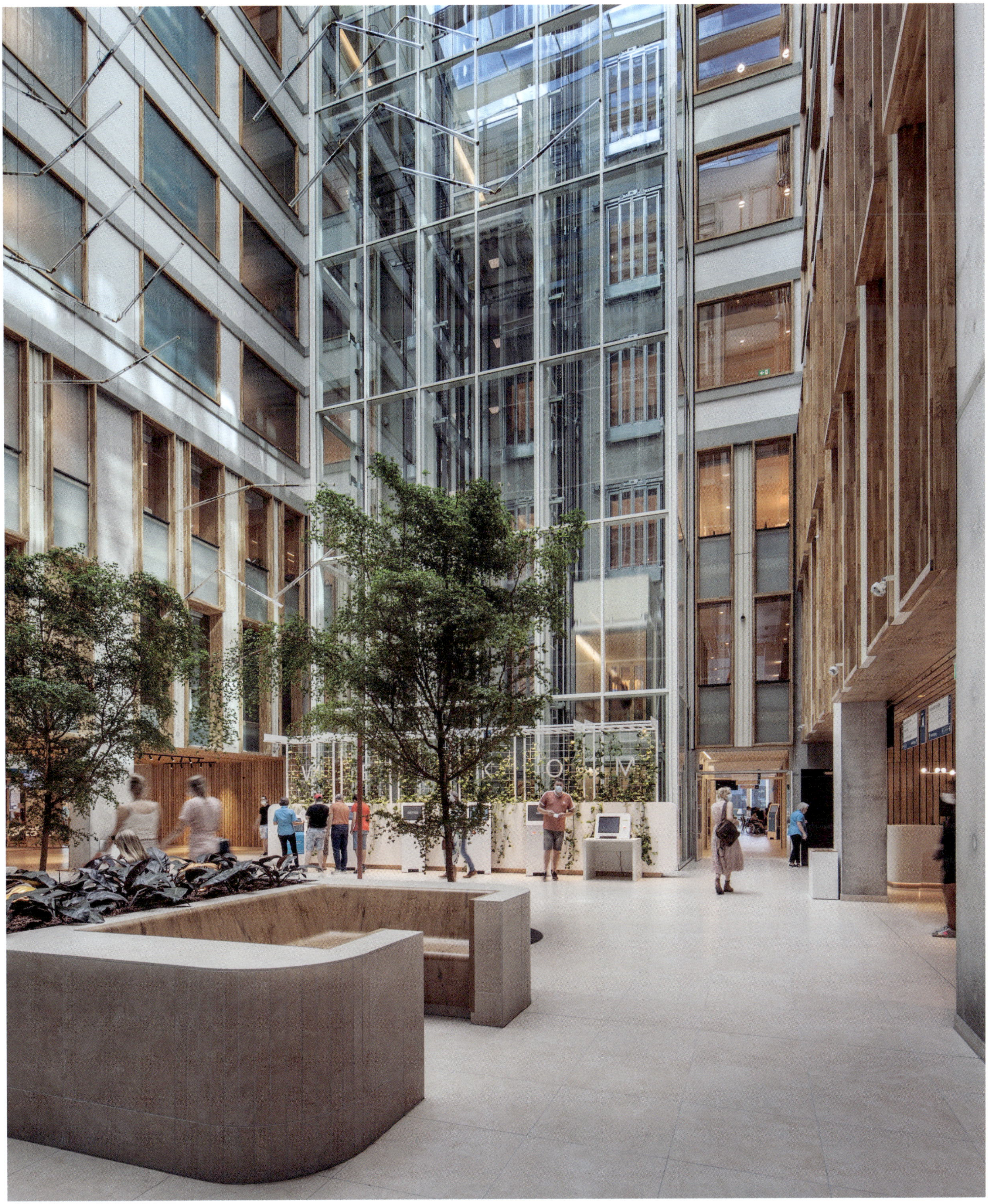

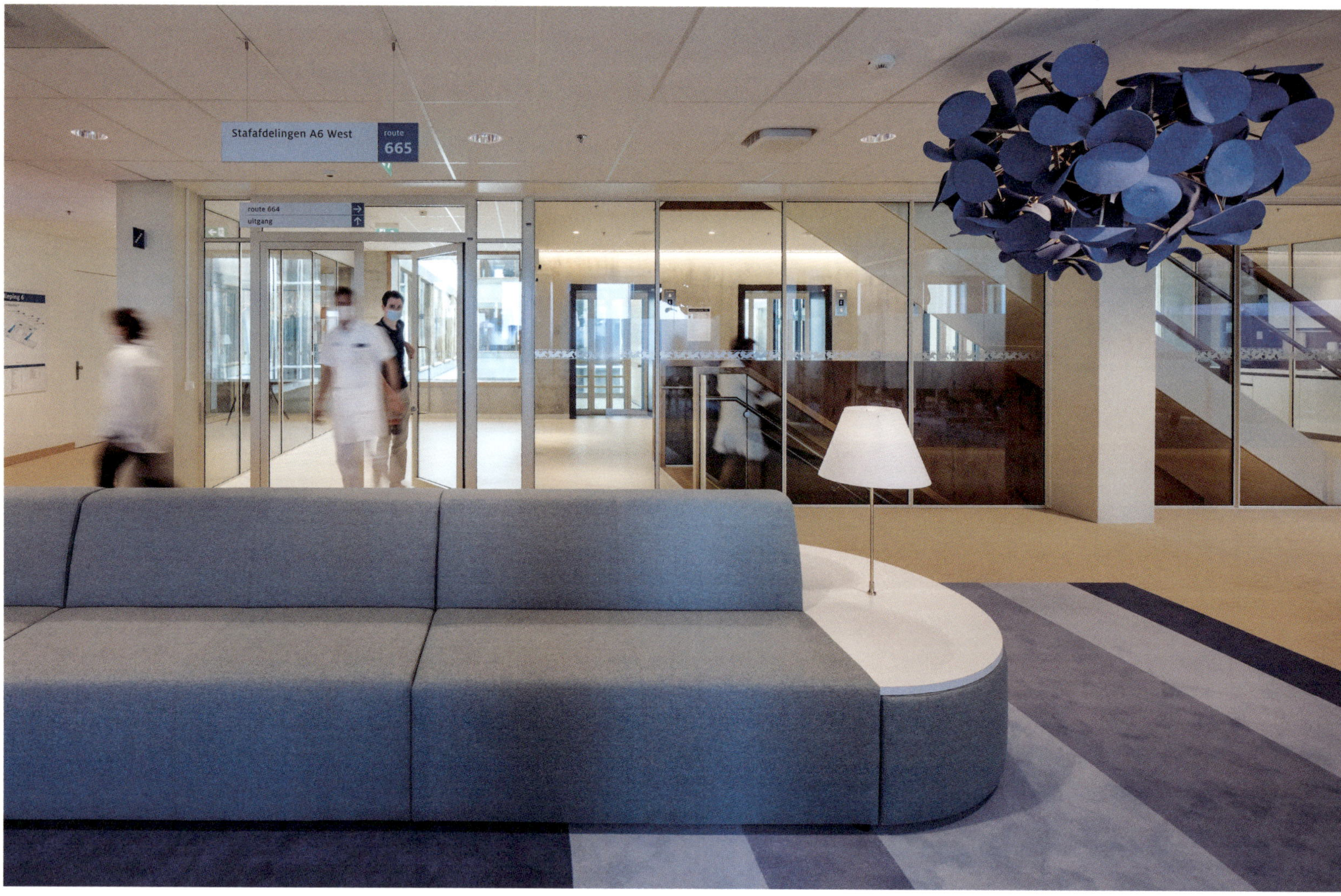

Informal meeting area at staff department.

Ground floor plan.

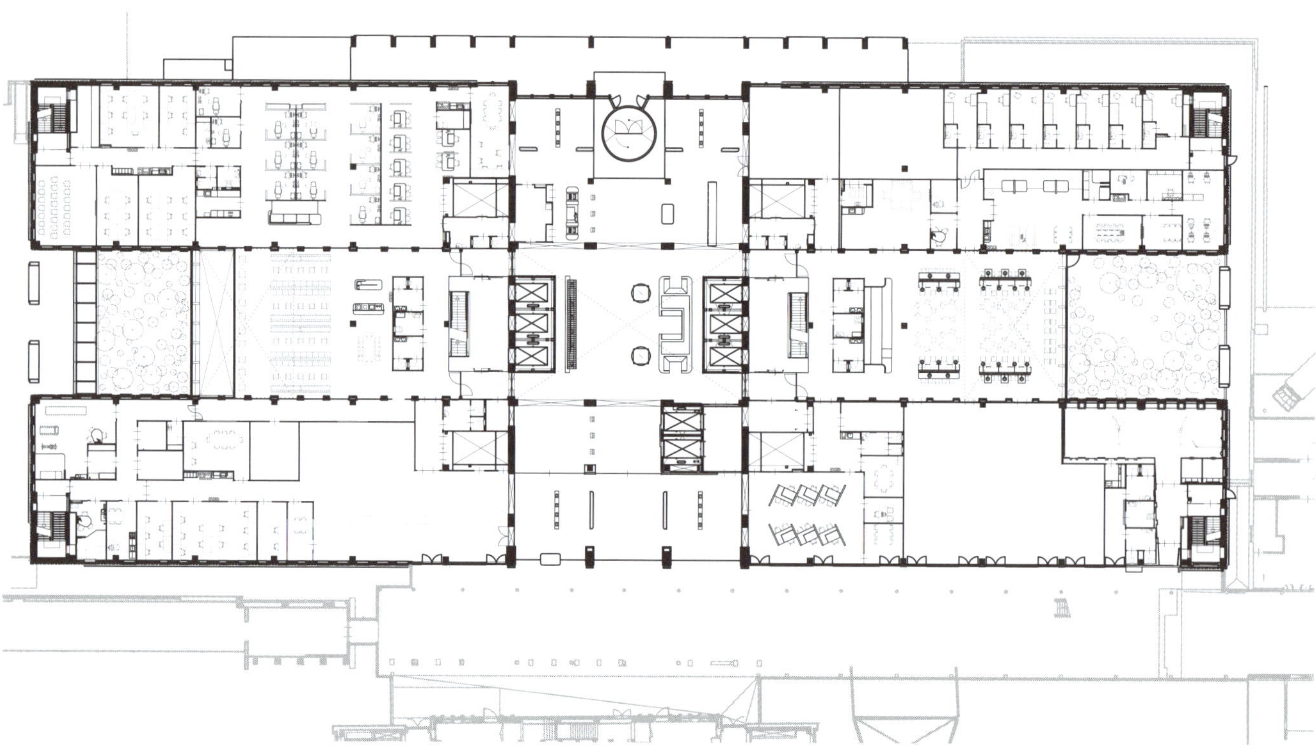

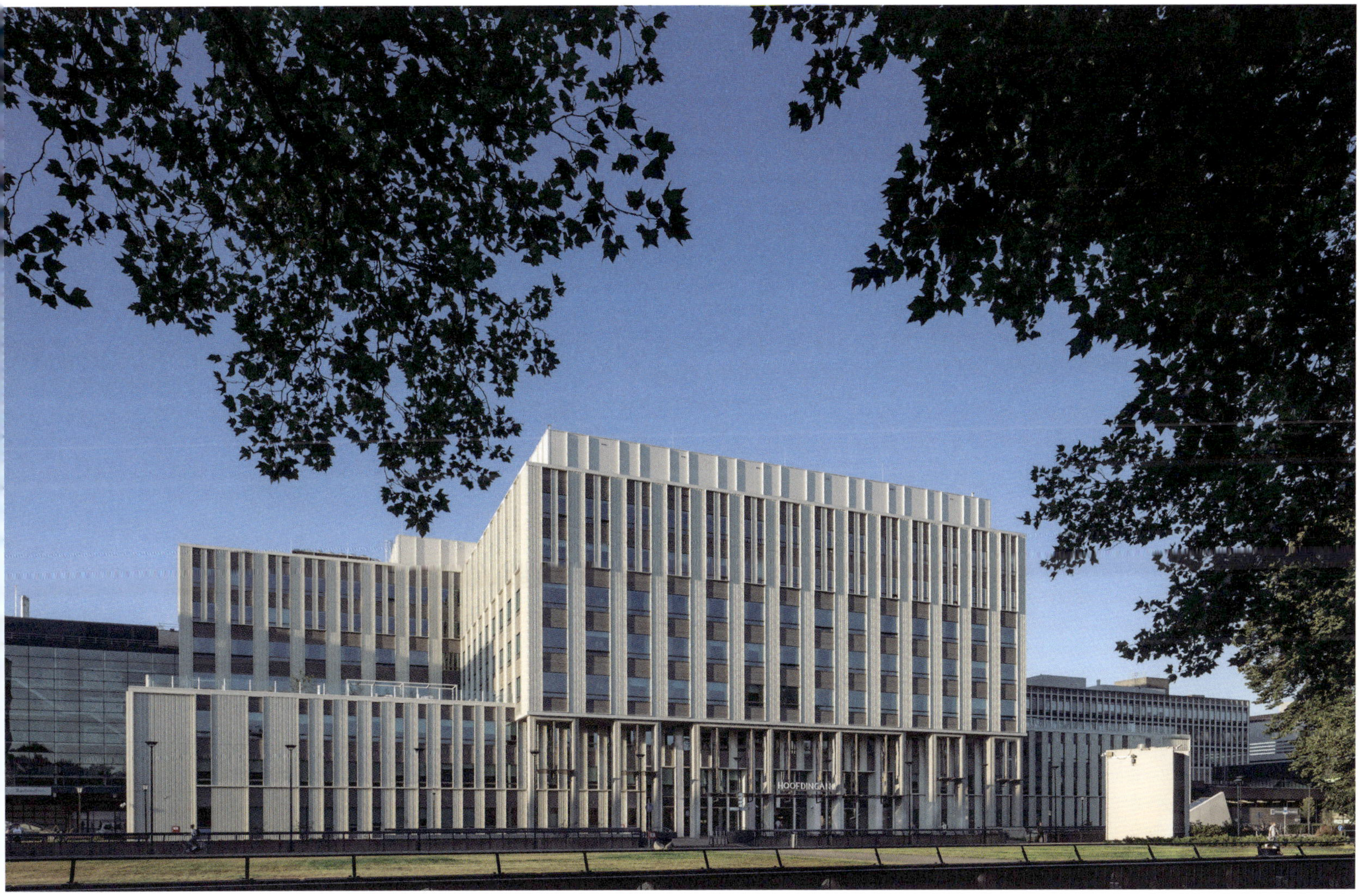

Exterior view of the main entrance.

Conceptual pictograms to the human scale approach (left) and light (right).

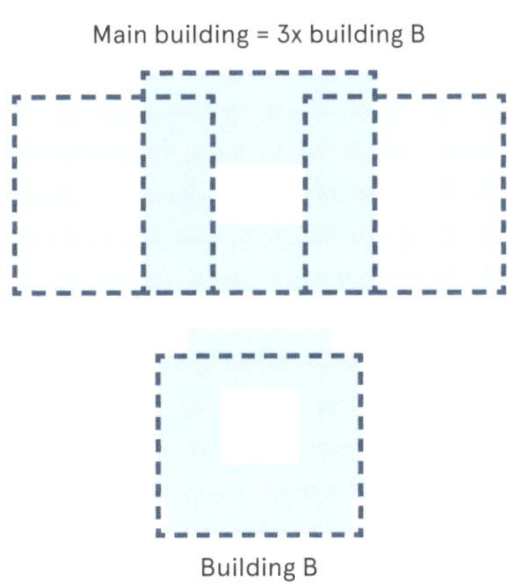

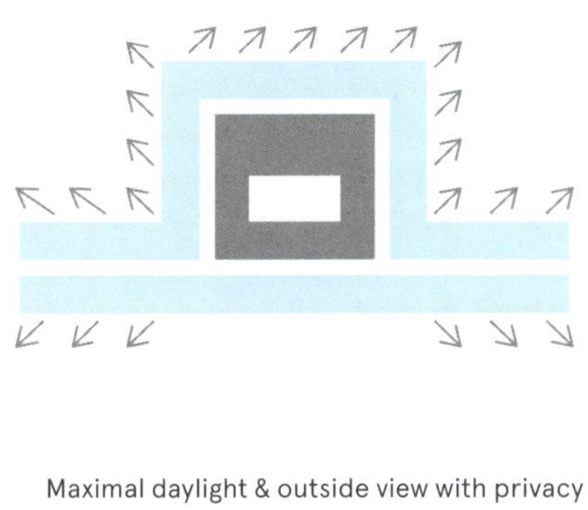

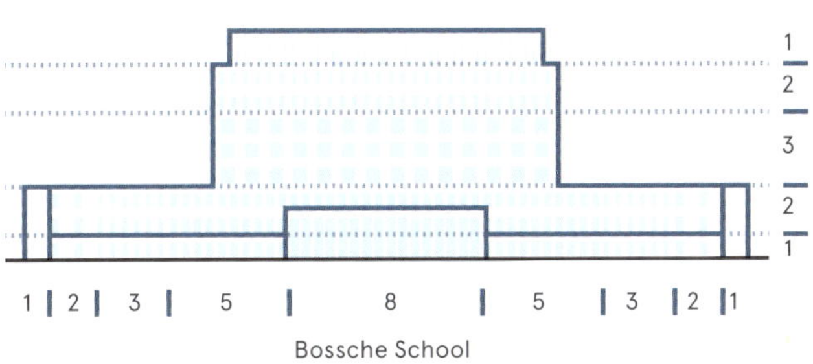

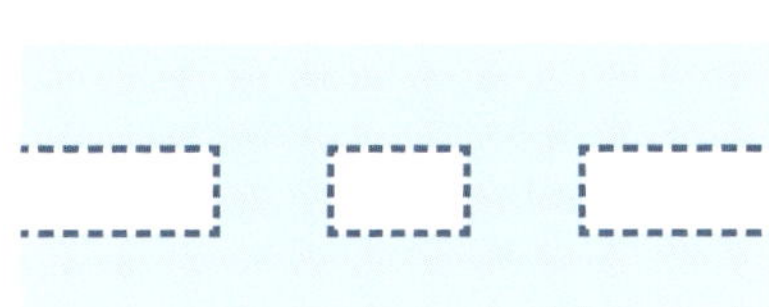

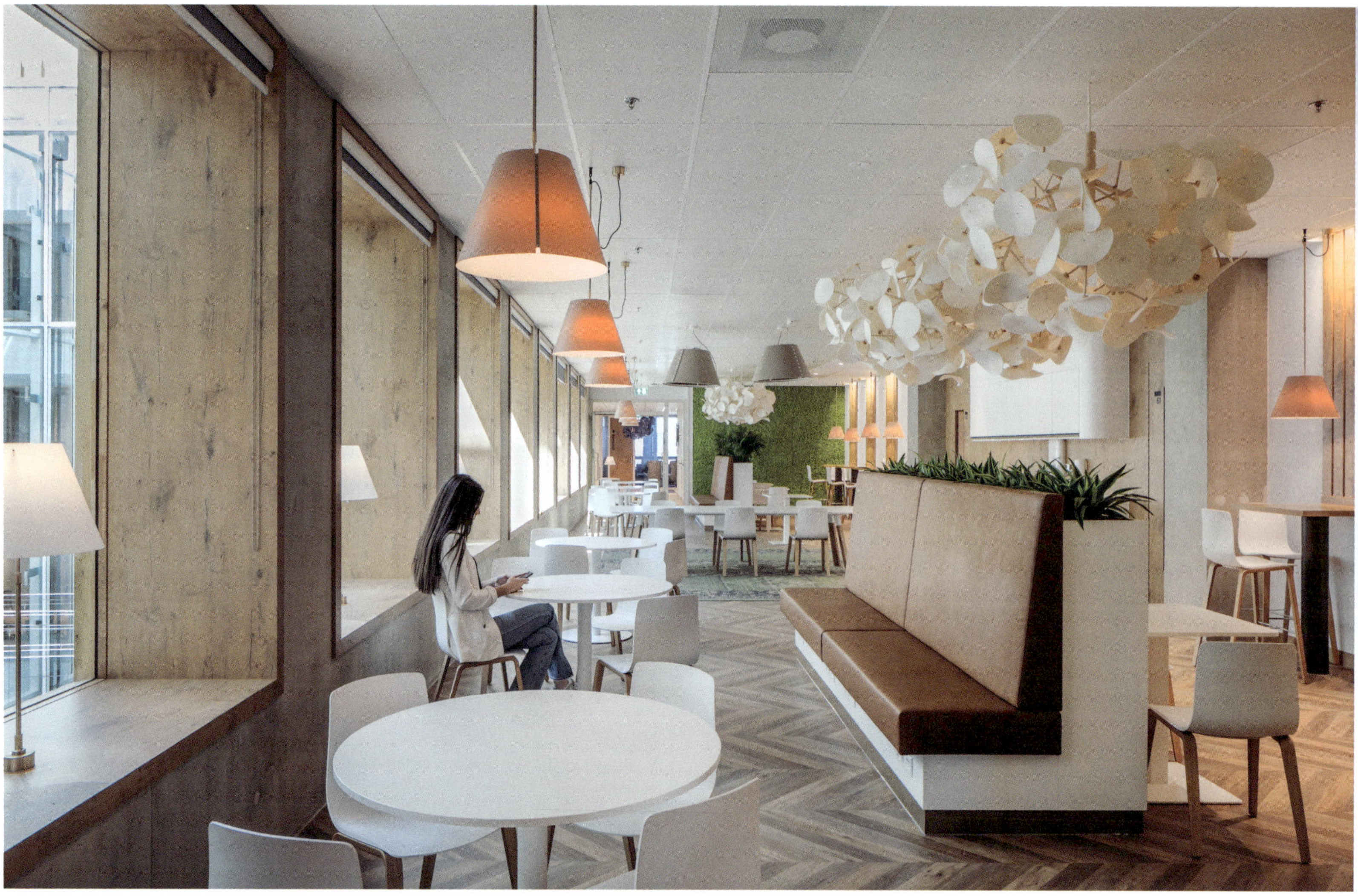

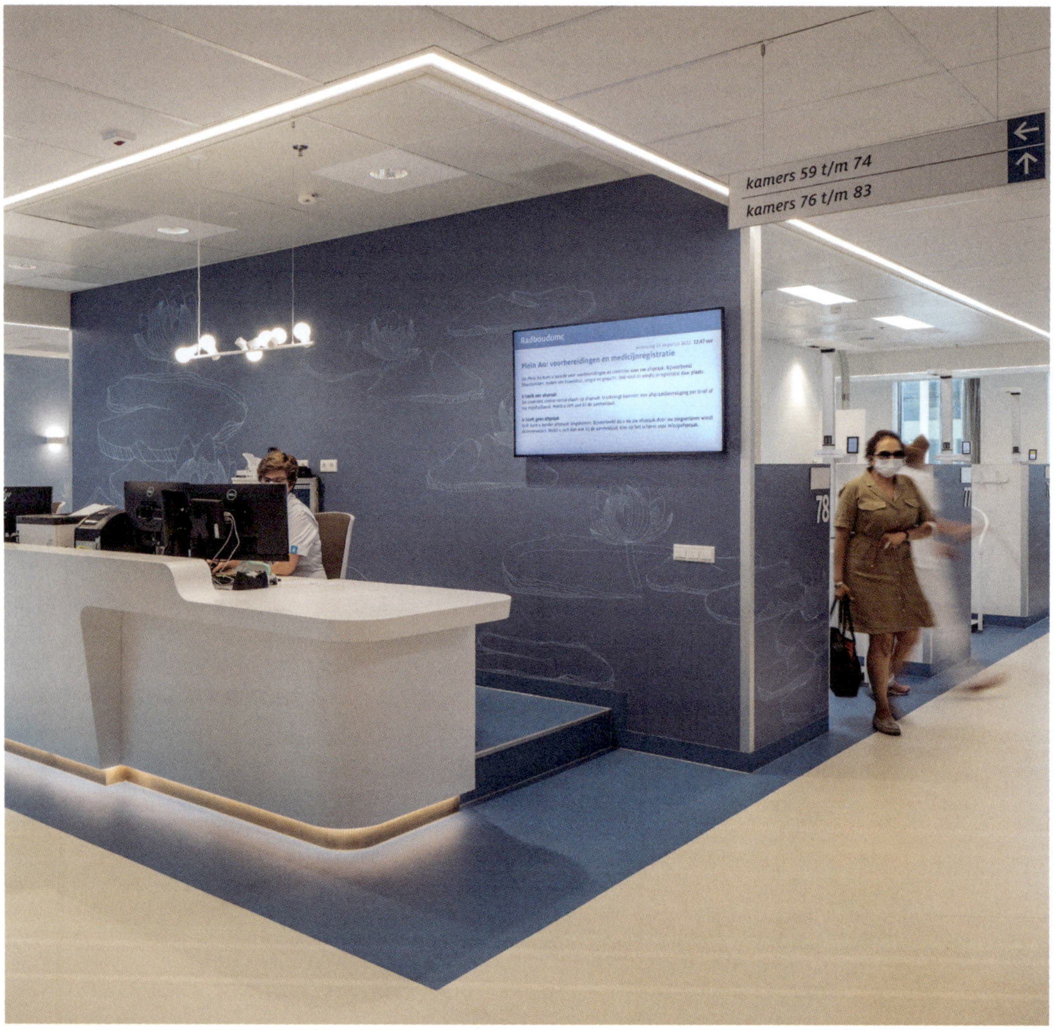

Lounge area with soft and warm color scheme.

Blood collection.

Isometric drawing.

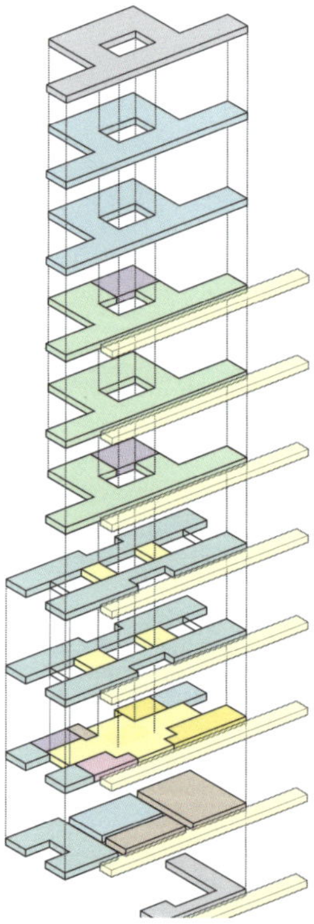

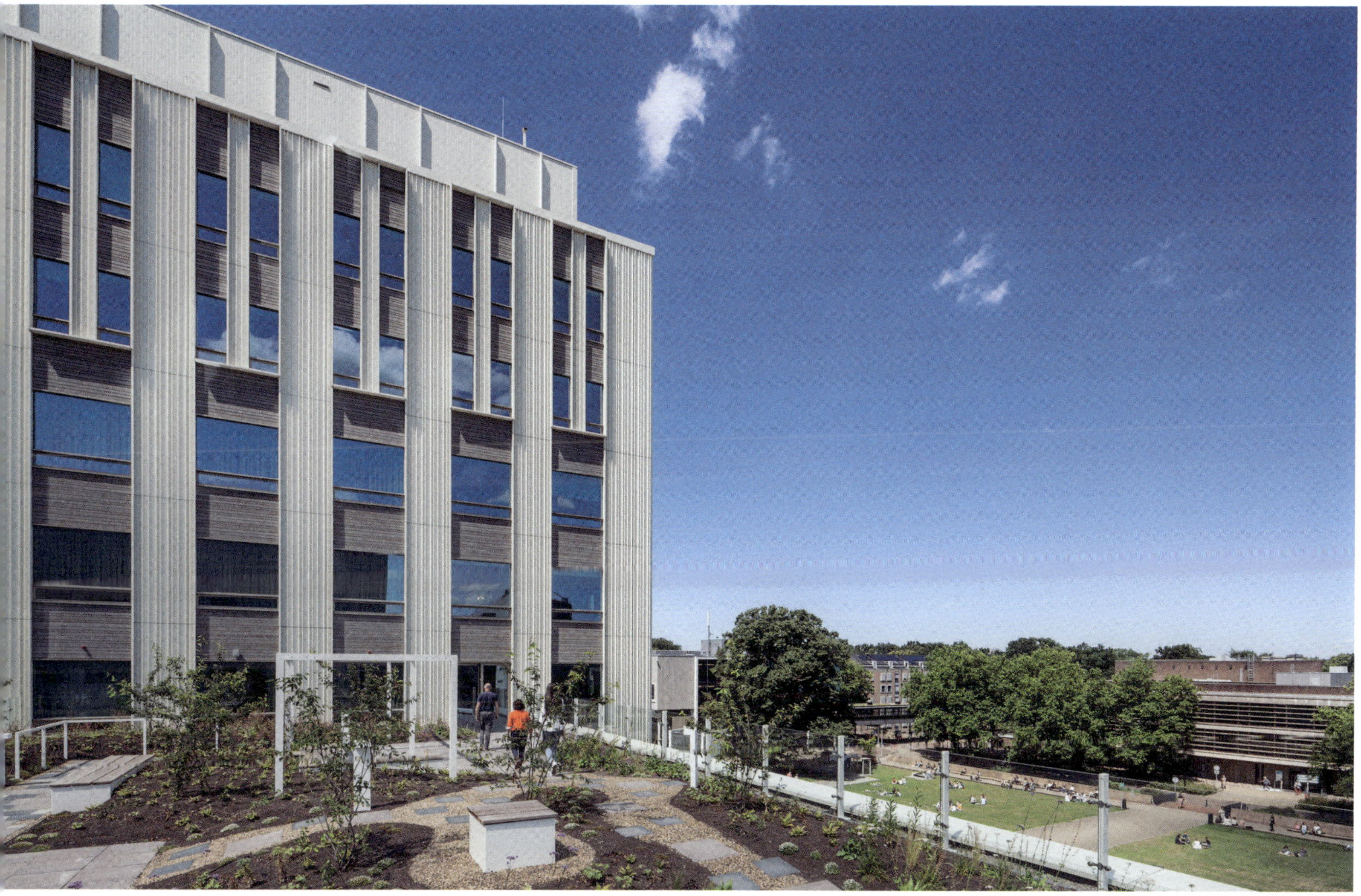

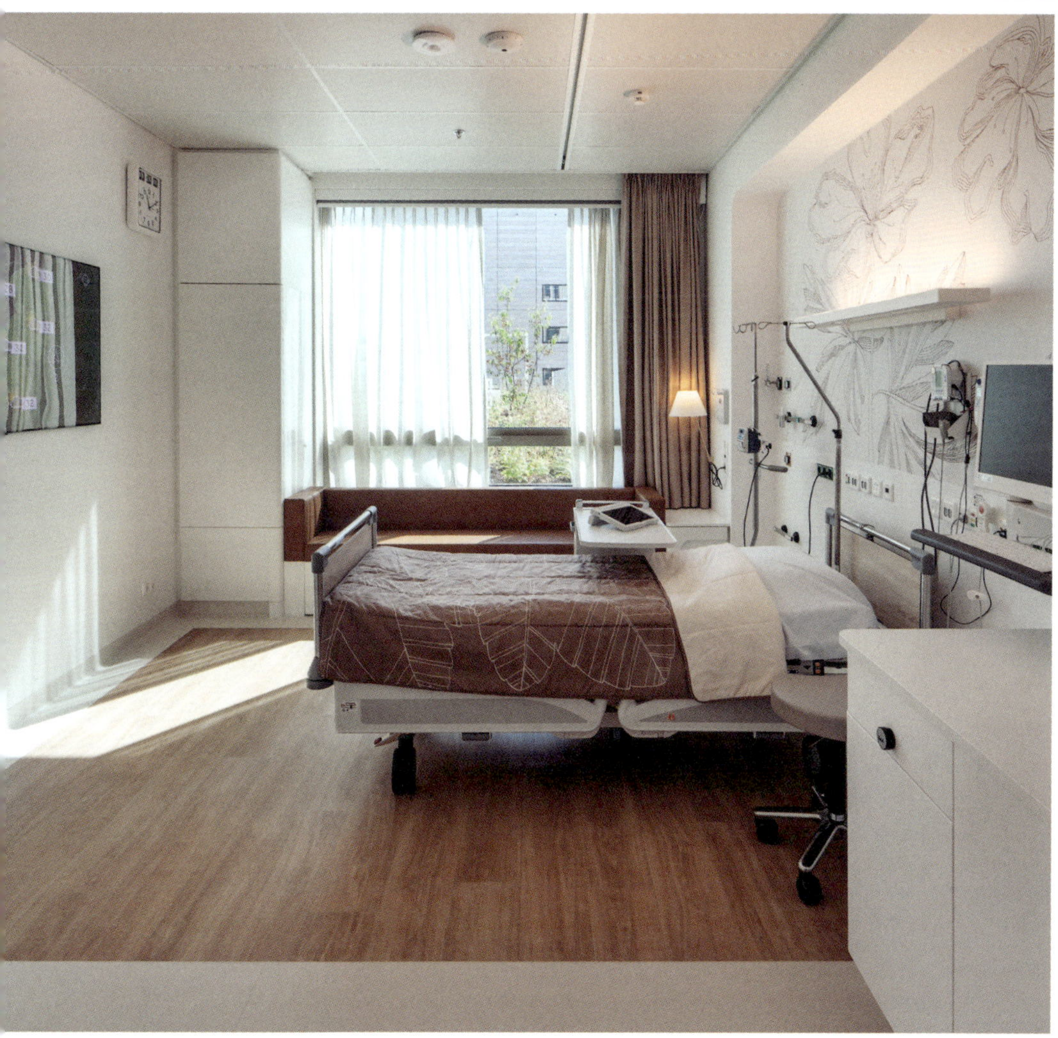

Roof garden for patients.

Patient room.

wörner traxler richter

Münster
Germany

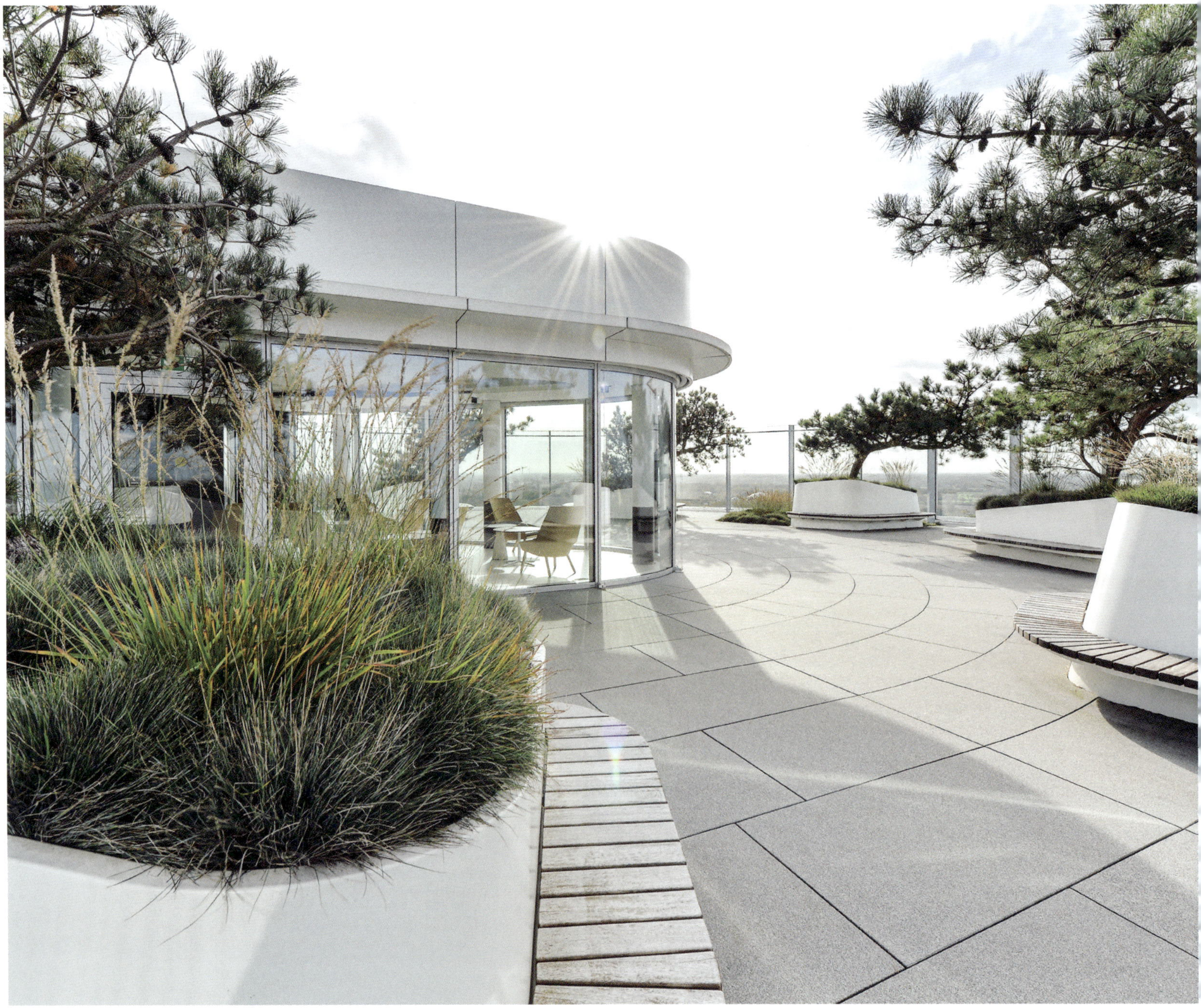

Outdoor area of the new café on the rooftop terrace.

Patient room terrace of the extension.

University Hospital Münster – Interdisciplinary Expansion

For nearly 20 years, the University Hospital of Münster has been successfully carrying out renovation and expansion projects at the Central Hospital. The most recent construction project involved the renovation and expansion of the multi-story base building to include numerous functional areas. The defining central corridor was preserved as the heart of the facility, continuing to serve as a circulation route, while now offering diverse and innovative spatial experiences. The landmarks of the University Hospital – its two patient towers – were each raised by one additional floor. A café was added, providing patients and staff with a welcome break from daily hospital routine. The goal was to use the expansion of the existing structure to create clinical operations that are just as functional, forward-looking recovery spaces, and, at the same time, respectful work environments as new buildings would.

Address: Albert-Schweitzer-Campus, Gebäude D5, 48149 Münster, Germany | **Client:** UKM Infrastruktur Management | **Completion:** 2023 | **Size:** 27,000 m^2 | **Original building:** University Hospital, Weber, Brand & Partner | **Sector:** public | **Interior design:** Haverkamp Interior Design | **Landscape design:** Rehwald Landschaftsarchitekten

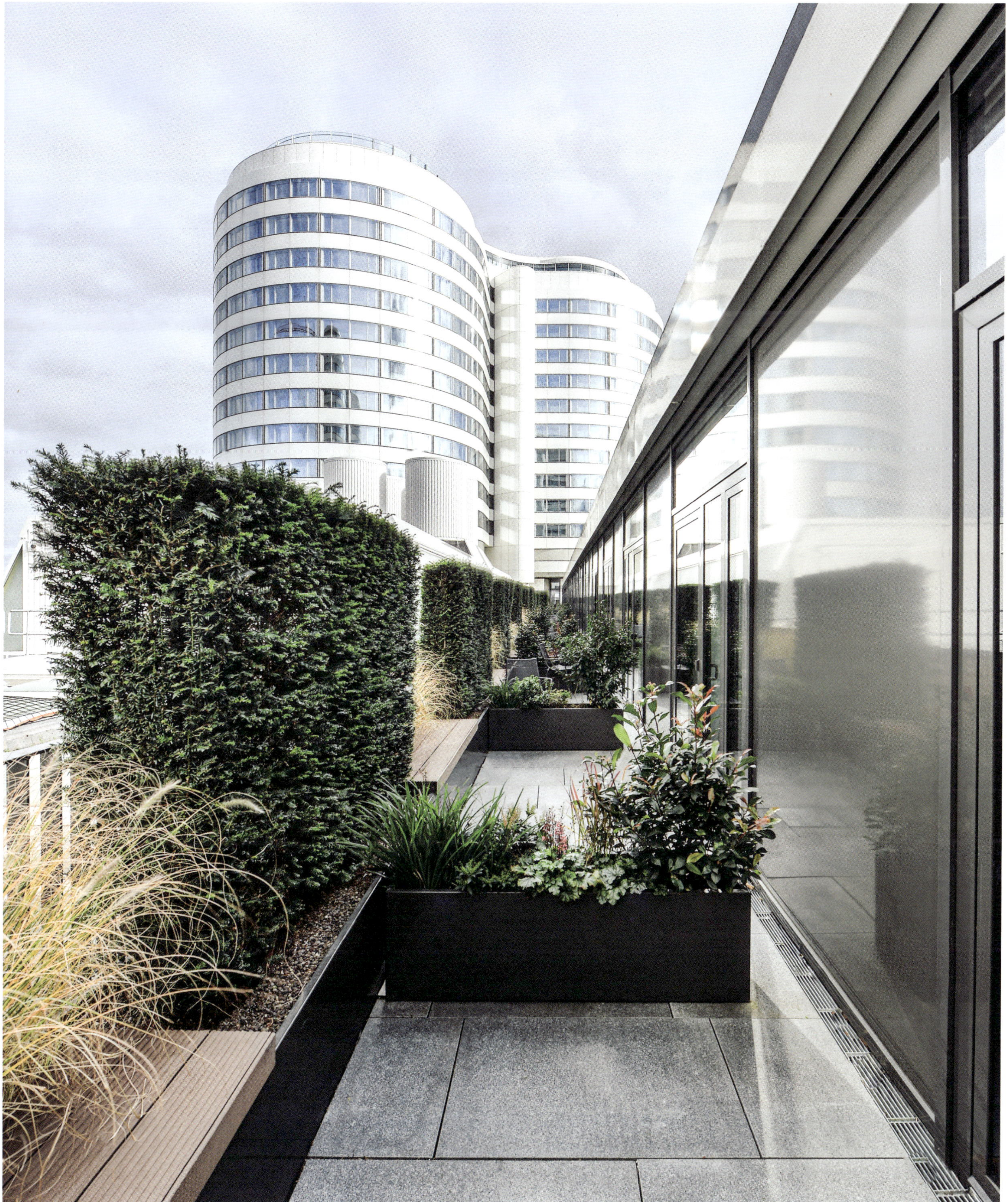

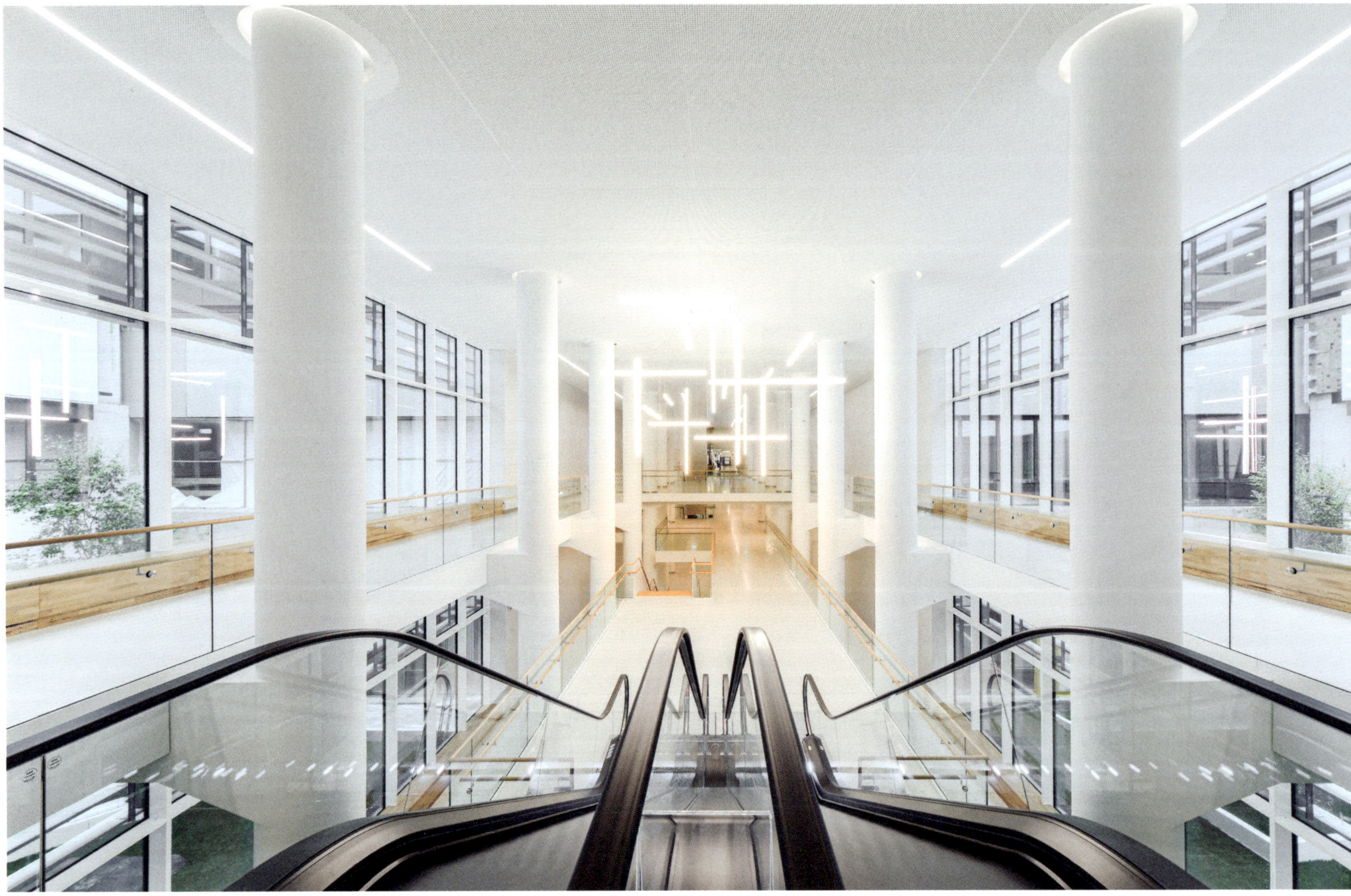

View of the extended, new central corridor.

Fifth floor plan showing the expansion with its extension of the central corridor.

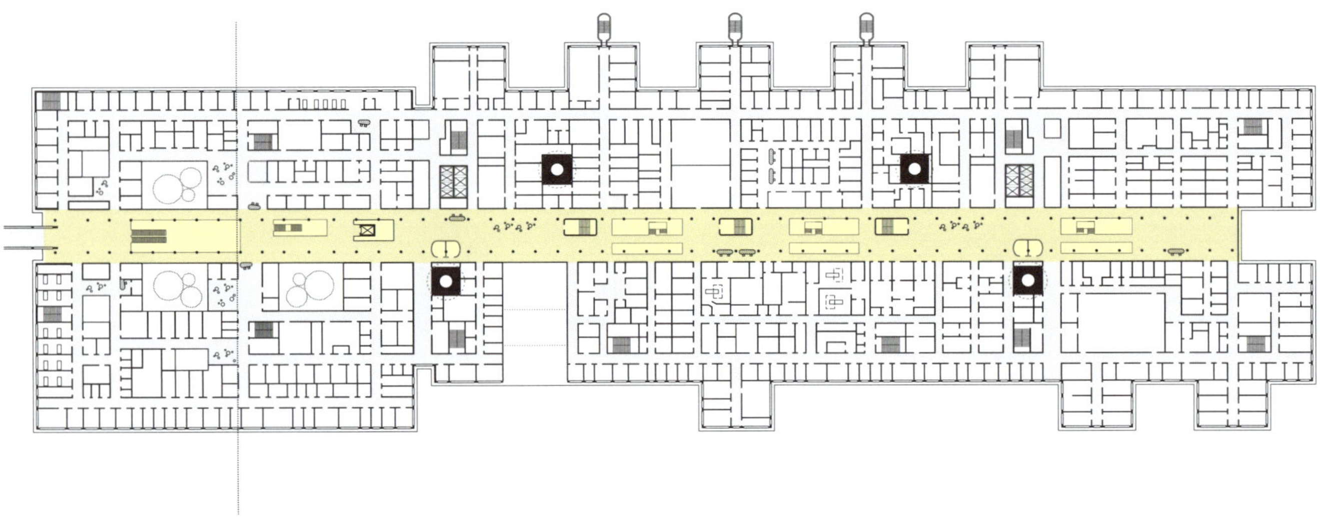

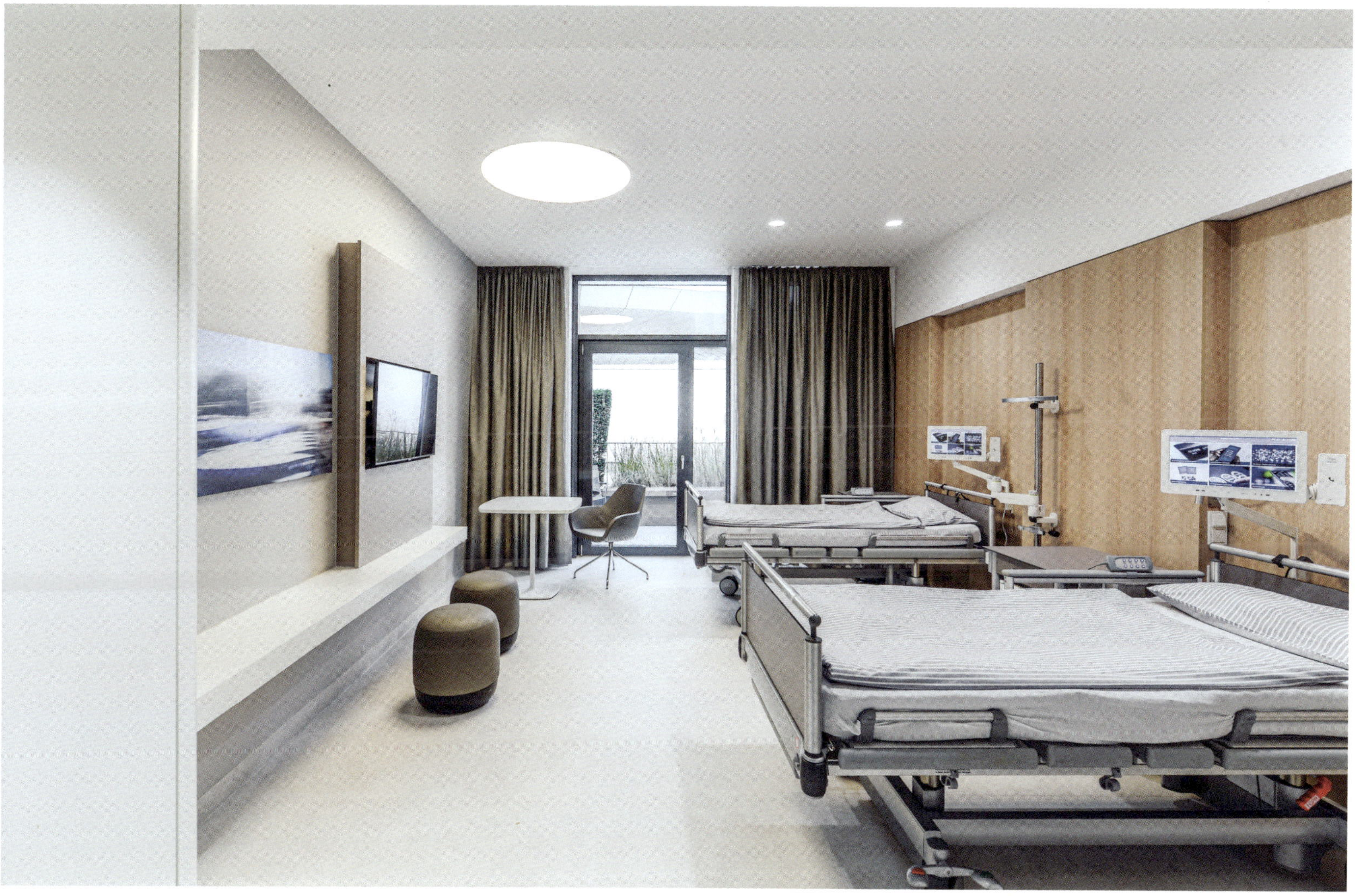

Interior design of a patient room.

Seventh floor plan showing patient rooms and terraces.

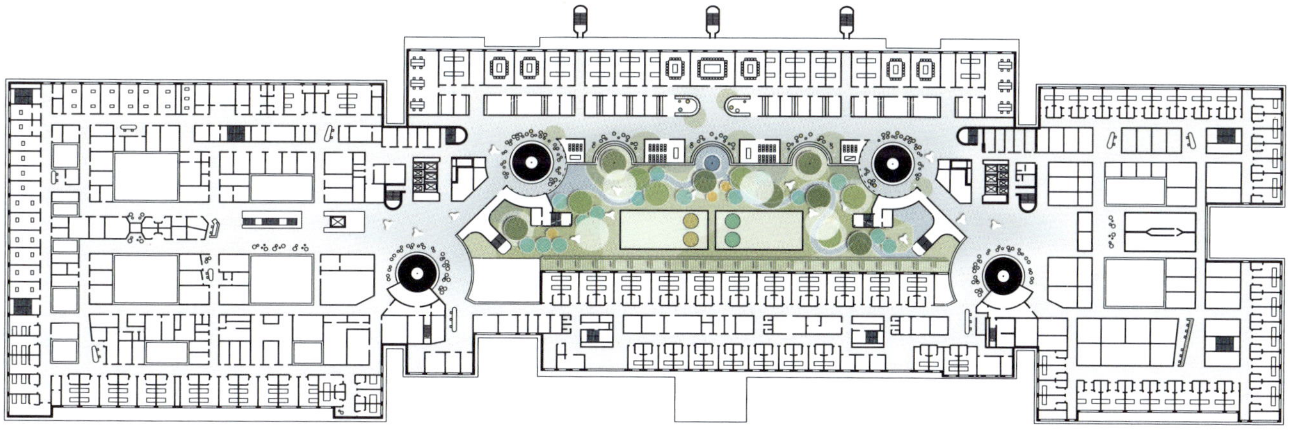

Moloney O'Beirne Architects
O'Connell Mahon Architects

Dublin
Ireland

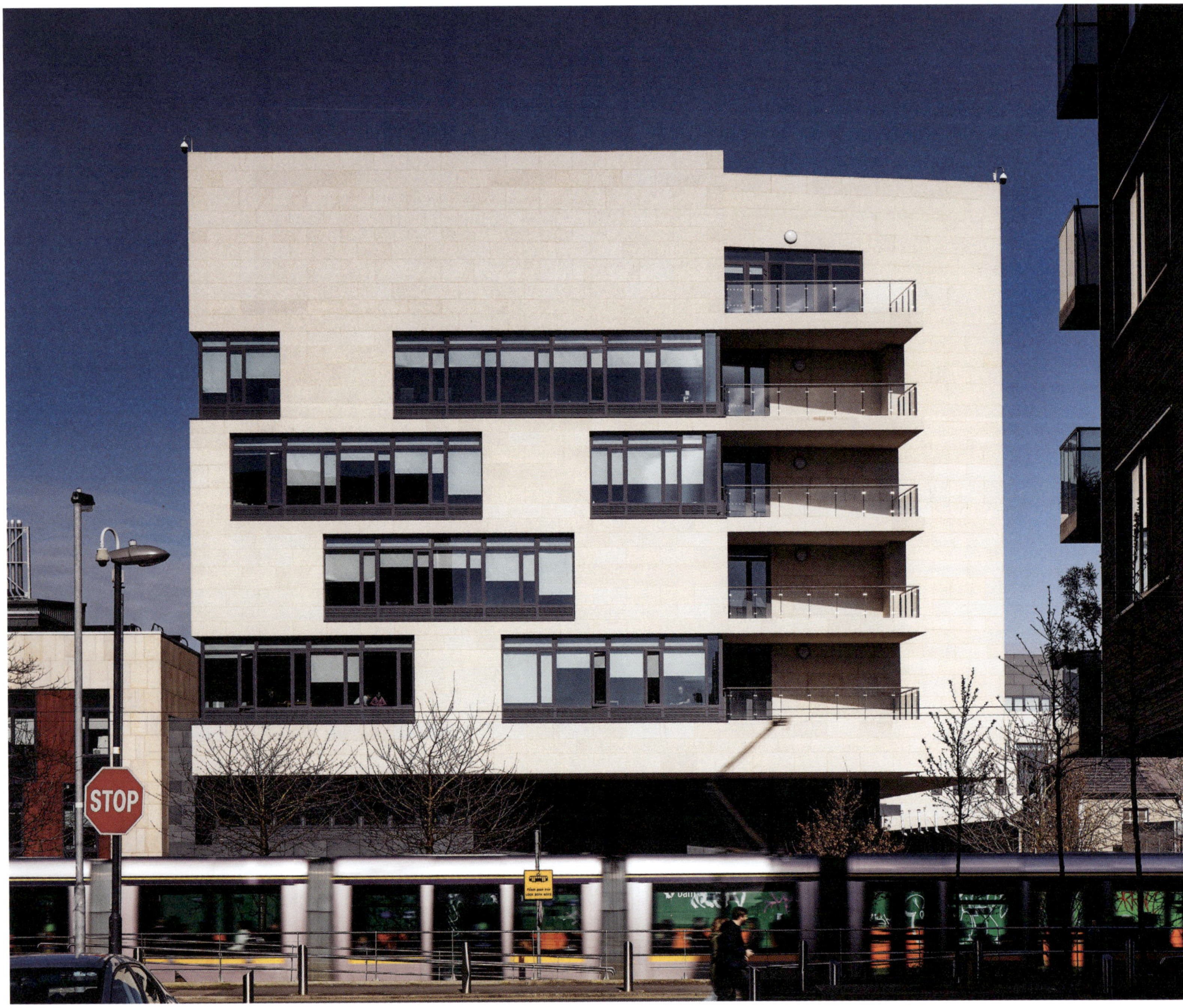

Mercer's Institute for Successful Ageing at St. James's Hospital (MISA)

Conceived as an integrated model for elderly care, MISA combines clinical services, research, teaching, and creative activity within a single healthcare environment. Occupying a constrained site on the St. James's Hospital campus, the building responds to complex functional and contextual requirements. Daylight, views, and orientation are central to the spatial concept, supporting patient wellbeing throughout the facility. Inpatient wards are arranged along a north-south axis, while south-facing lounges and protected balconies offer views across Dublin and connections to the surrounding landscape. A central courtyard brings natural light and greenery into outpatient areas, enhancing waiting spaces and the two-story concourse. Natural ventilation is used wherever possible. The architectural expression responds to both the site context and the building's care-focused program.

The south elevation is defined by a stone-clad envelope and a carefully composed window arrangement.

A distant view of the building within the St James's Hospital campus.

Entrance area with large glazed walls, filled with natural light and defined by clear spatial composition.

Address: James's Street, Dublin 8, Ireland | **Client:** Board of Managers, St. James's Hospital | **Completion:** 2018 | **Size:** 14,800 m^2 | **Sector:** other | **Specialization:** elderly care | **Number of treatment rooms:** 10 | **Number of patient rooms:** 92

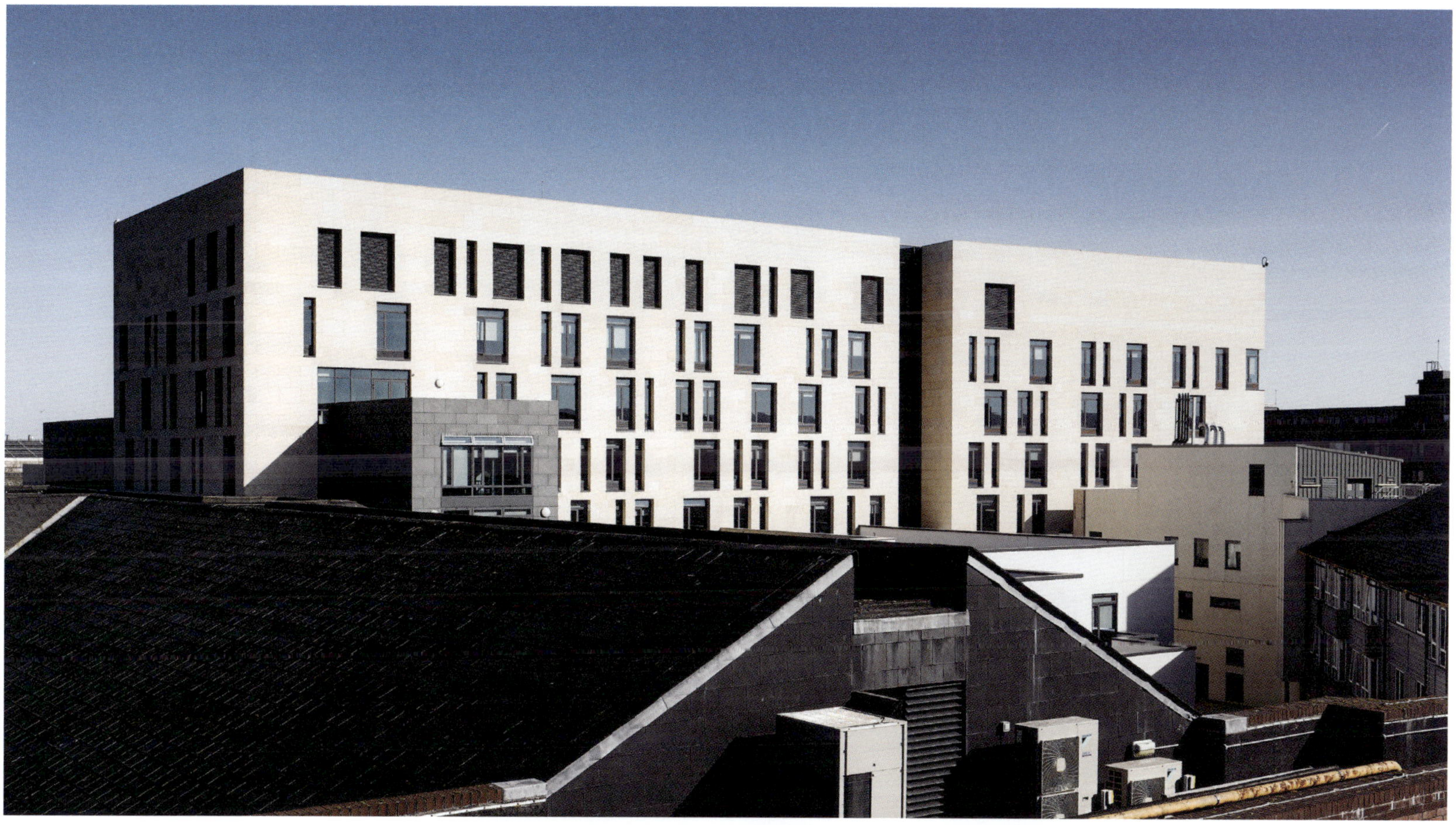

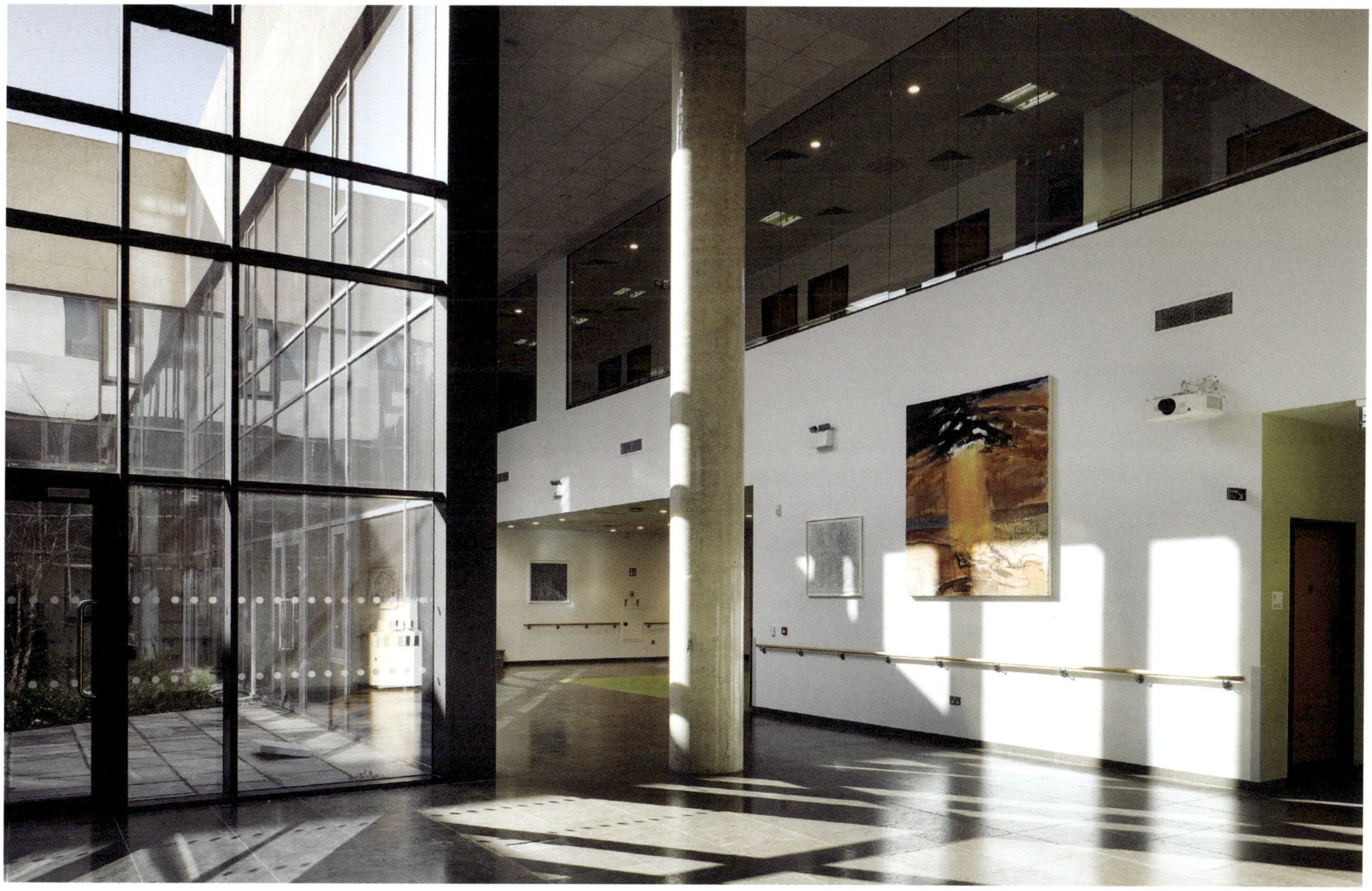

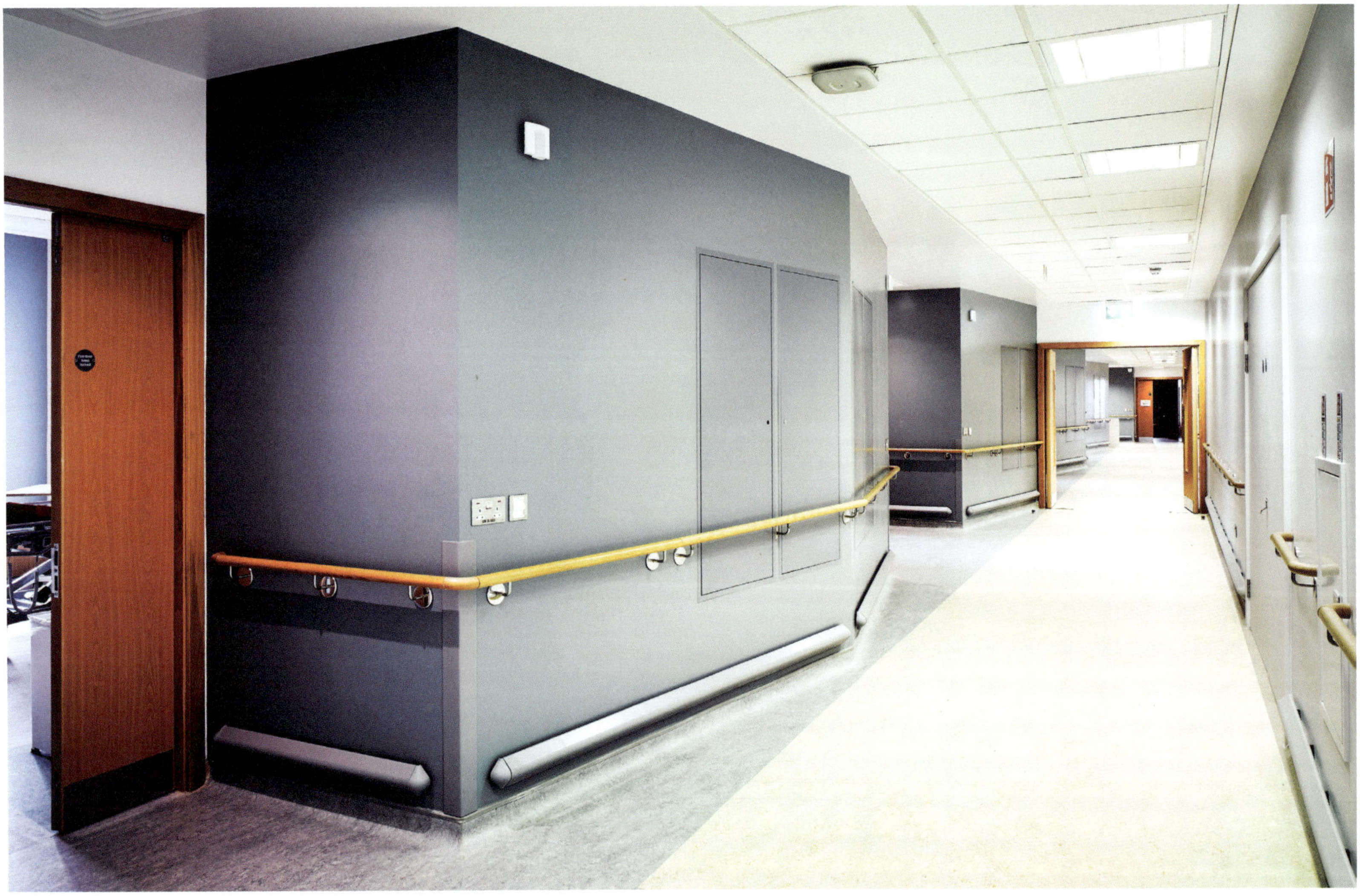

Corridor with grey walls, warm yellow-orange accents, and timber room door, designed for a visual comfort.

Façade elevation drawing.

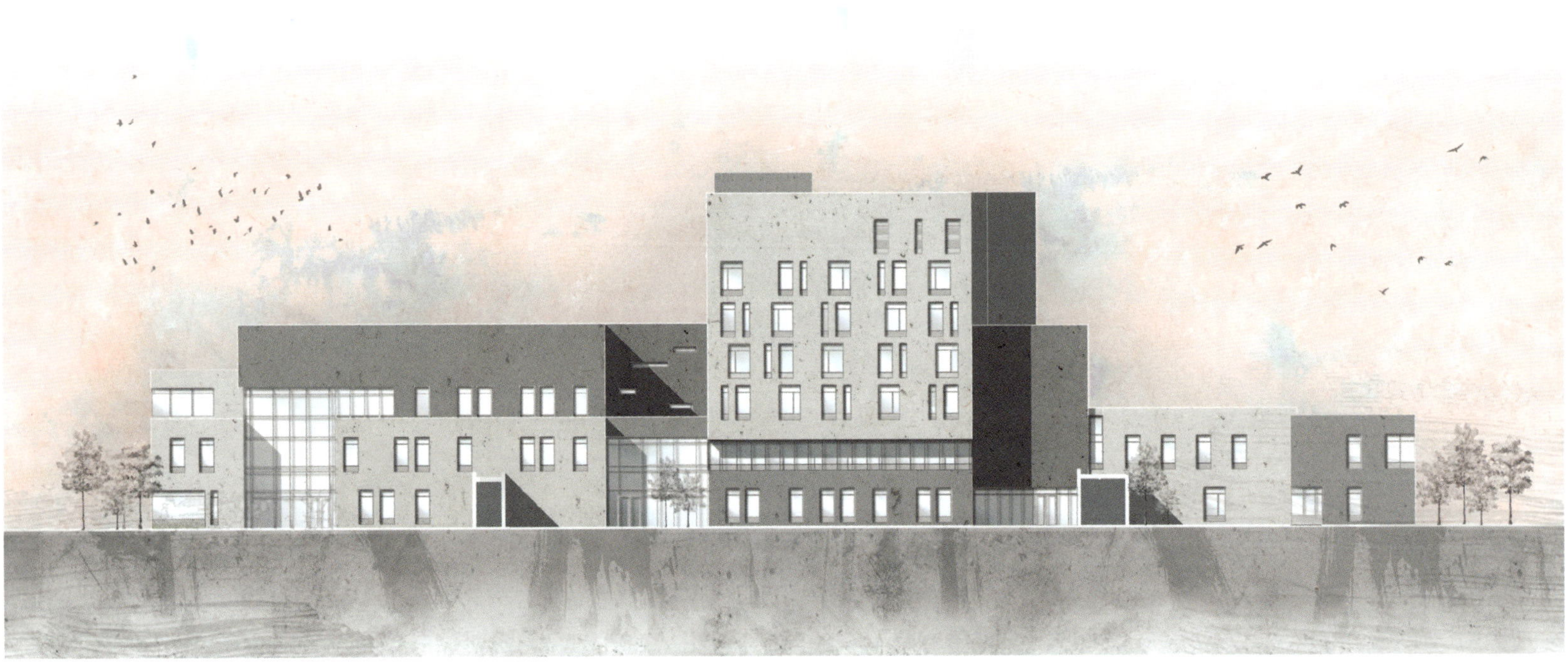

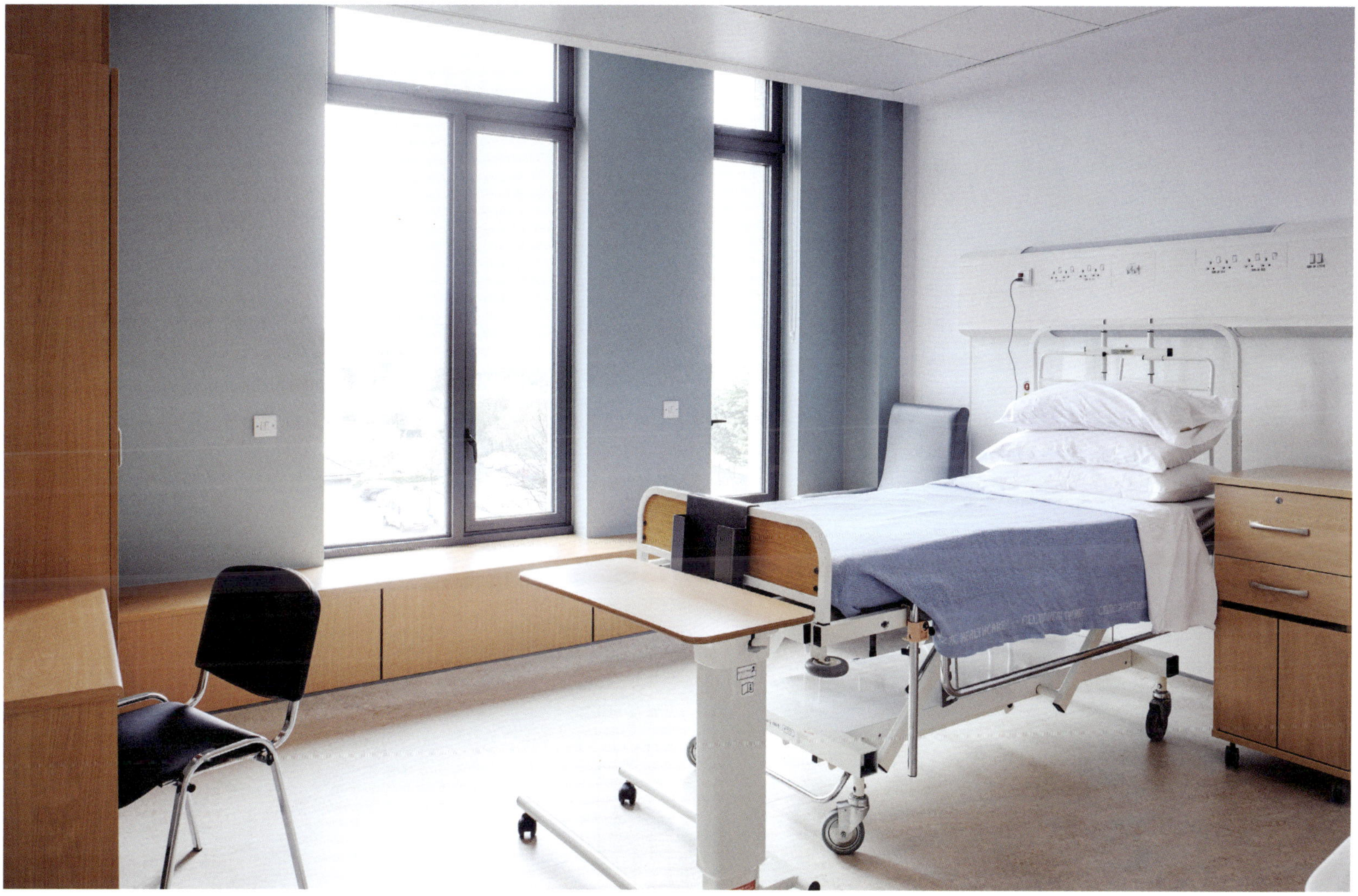

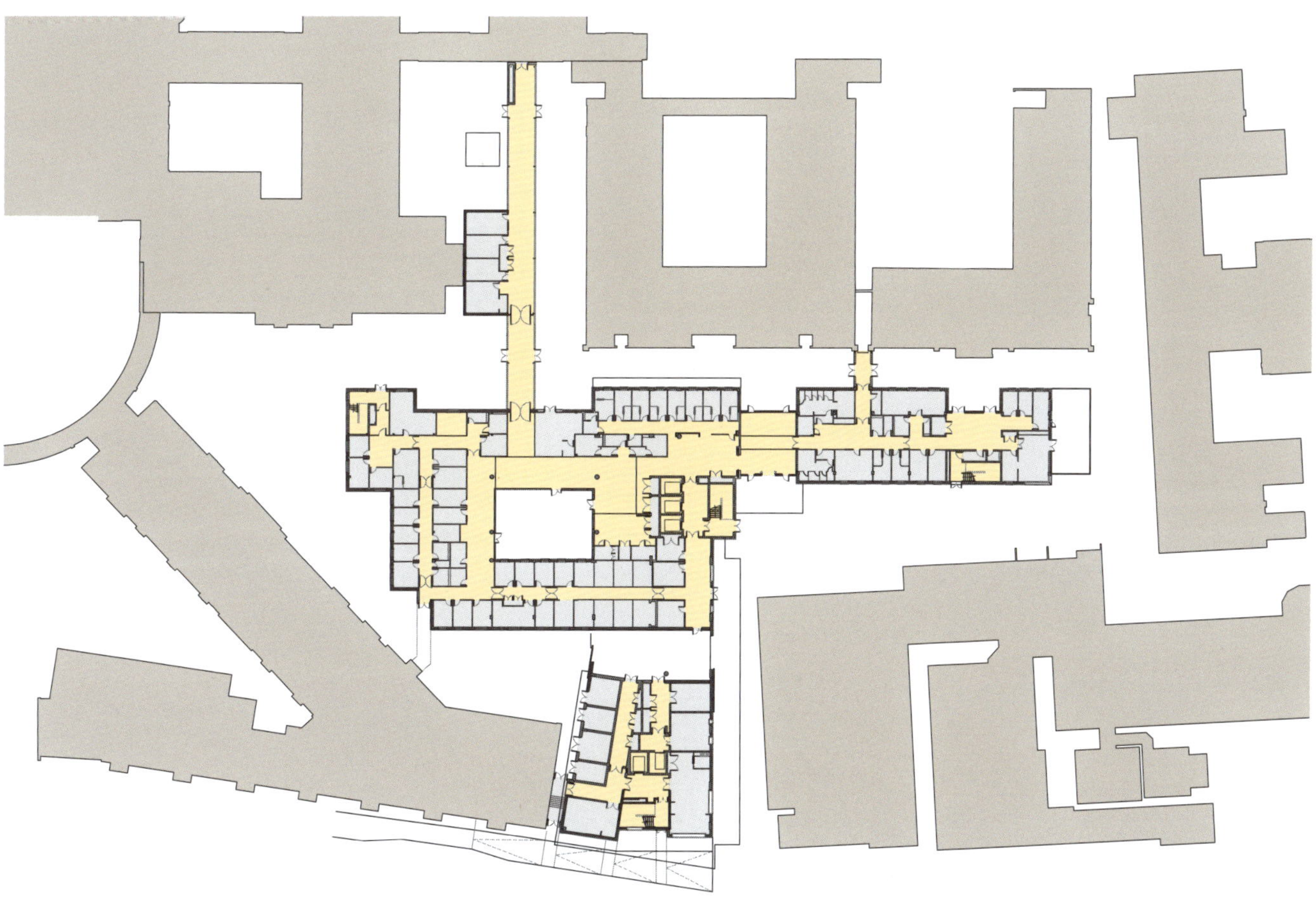

Patient room with large windows, timber elements, and professional equipment, creating a safe and inviting environment for patients.

Ground floor plan.

Archipelago with Gortemaker Algra Feenstra architects

Diest
Belgium

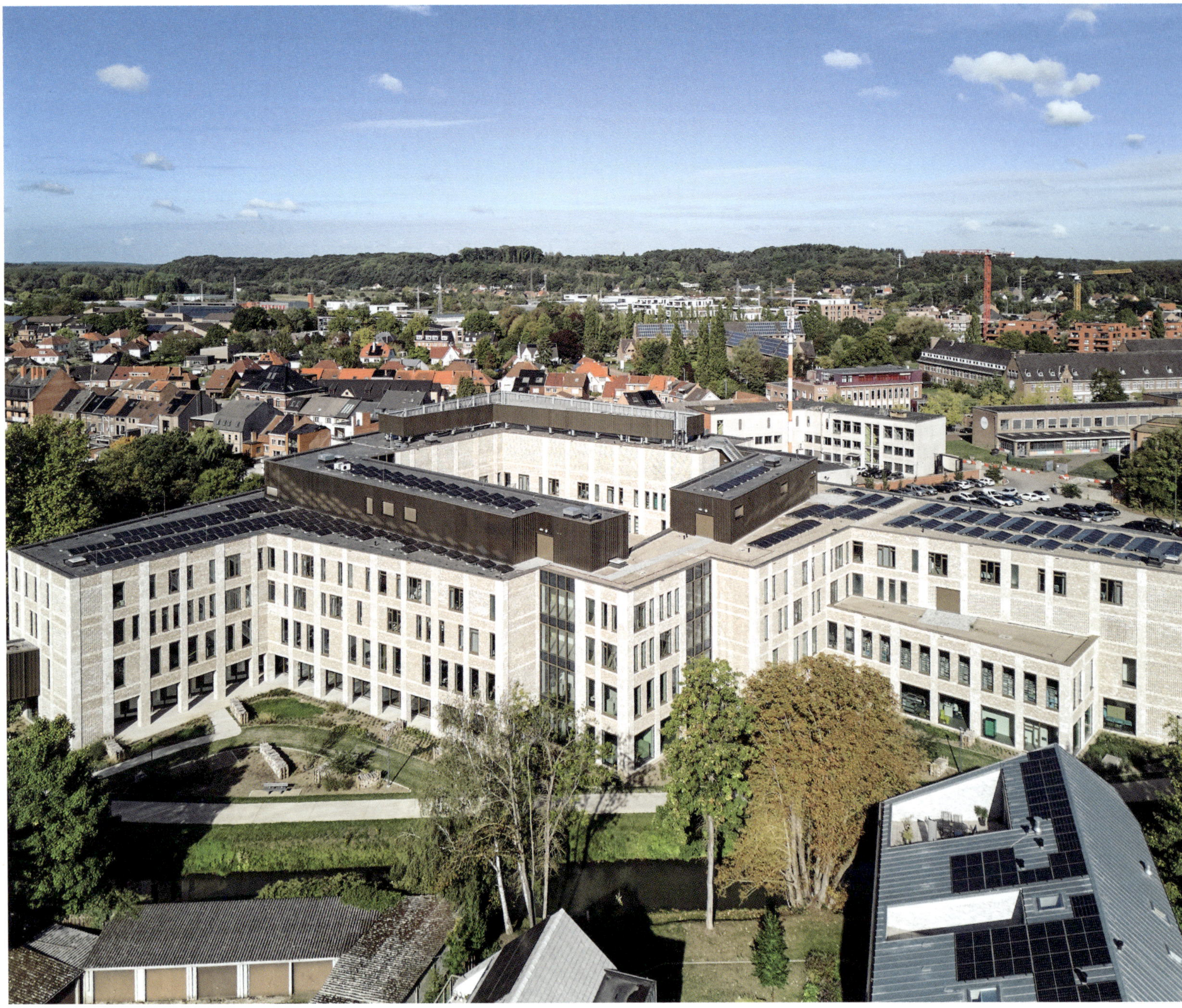

General Hospital Diest

The new General Hospital Diest is located on the historic brook De Demer.

The inviting courtyard allows patients and visitors to find their way around the hospital.

The care campus is situated in a park structure, offering patients a suitable location for their recovery.

This hospital brings all healthcare functions together on a single central campus in the heart of the city. The design creates a community hospital that connects care, city, and landscape, keeping in mind the human scale. A mineral axis connects the hospital with the train station and the city center, while views of the river and surrounding greenery support recovery. The façade is composed of three layers that combine aesthetics, daylight, and technical performance. An open arcade provides connectivity, above which is a middle section with large windows, and at the top a layer of perforated brickwork obscuring technical spaces. The design consists of three L-shaped parts. On the upper floor, the geriatric and rehabilitation departments are linked into an internal walking route, allowing patients with cognitive vulnerabilities to move freely and safely. A central lounge encourages social interaction and relaxation.

Address: Statiestraat 65, 3290 Diest, Belgium | **Client:** General Hospital Diest | **Completion:** 2025 | **Size:** 22,380 m² | **Sector:** private | **Number of treatment rooms:** 8 | **Number of patient rooms:** 86 | Landscape architecture: Ontwerpbureau Pauwels

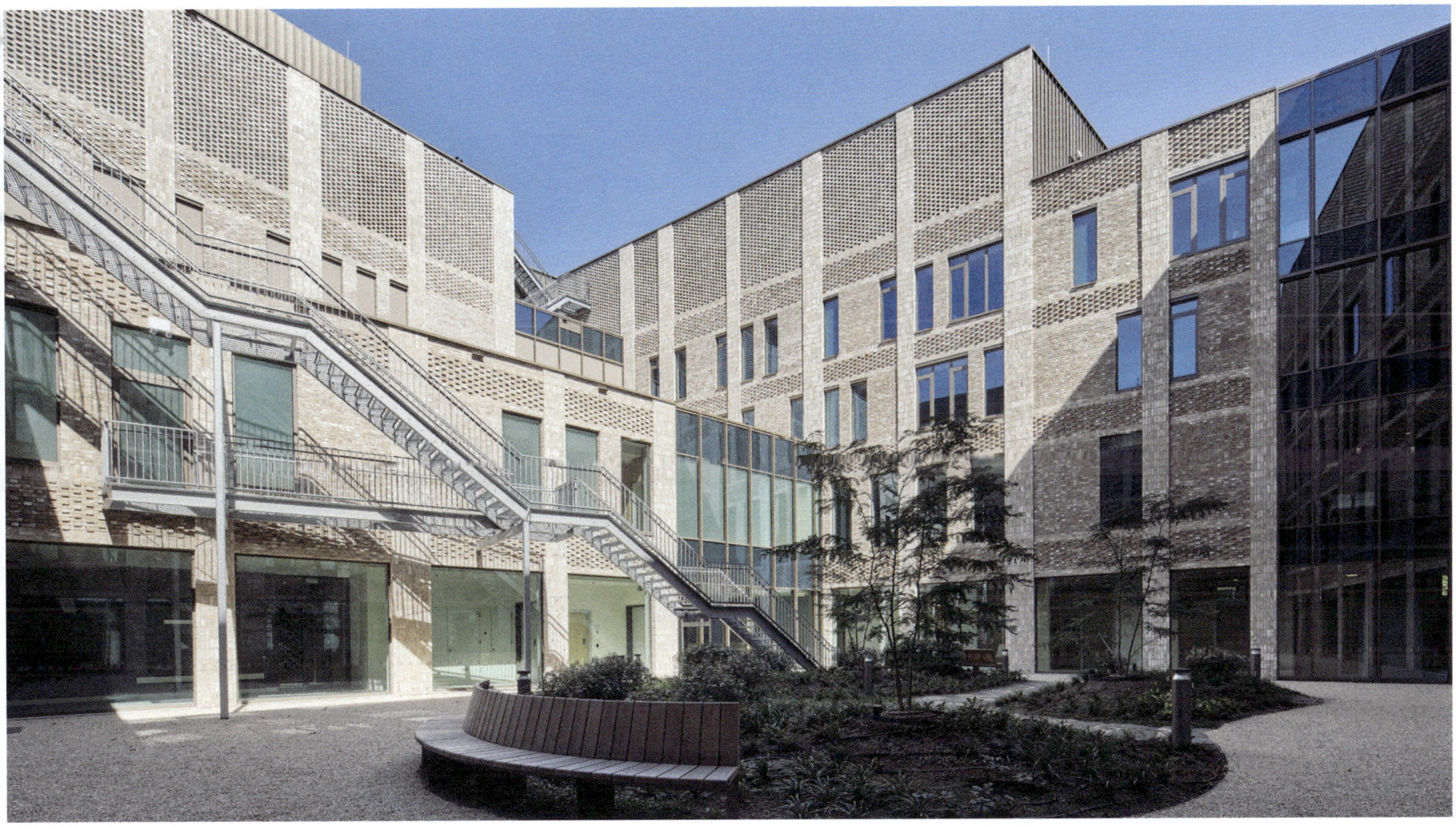

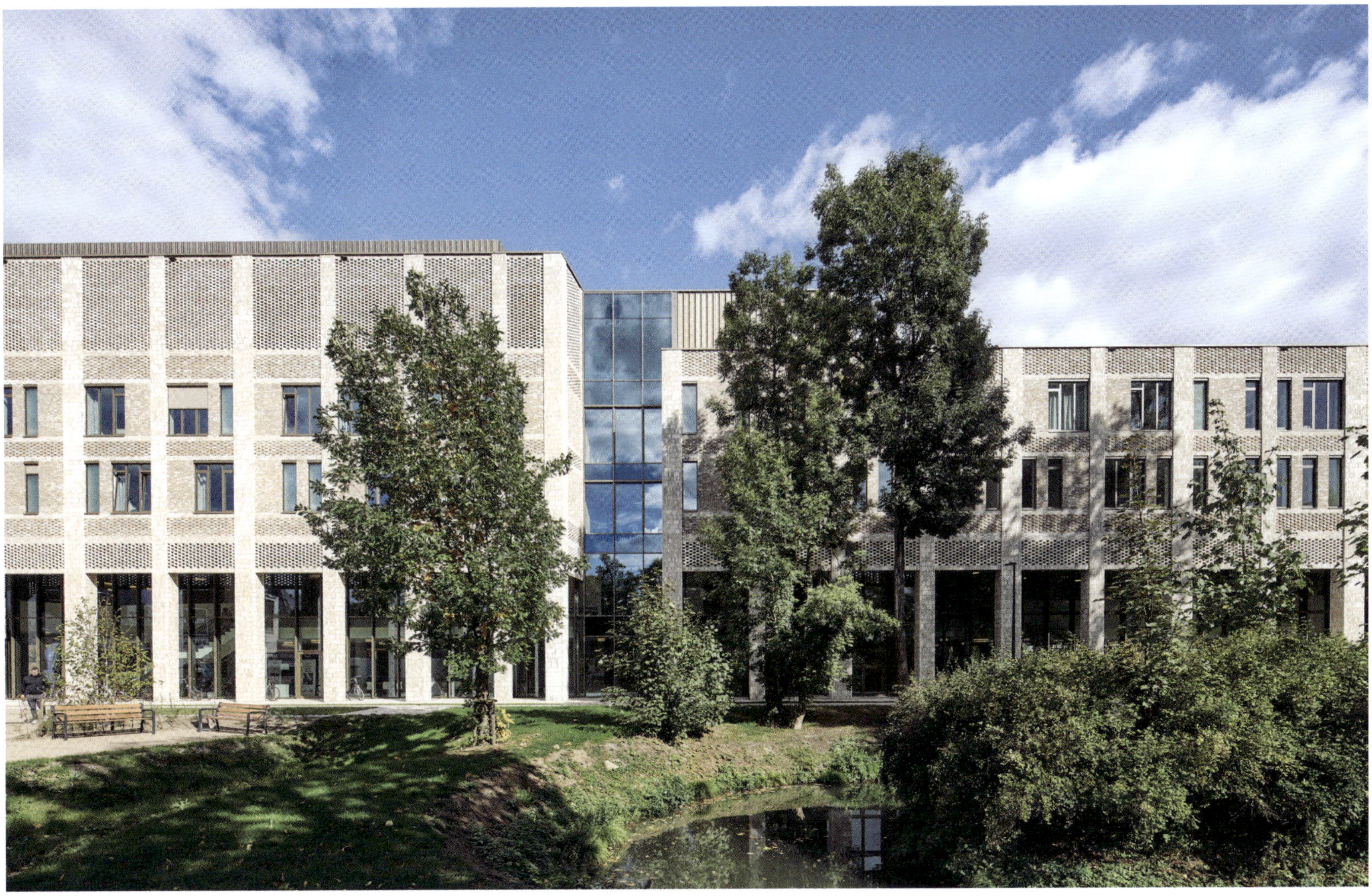

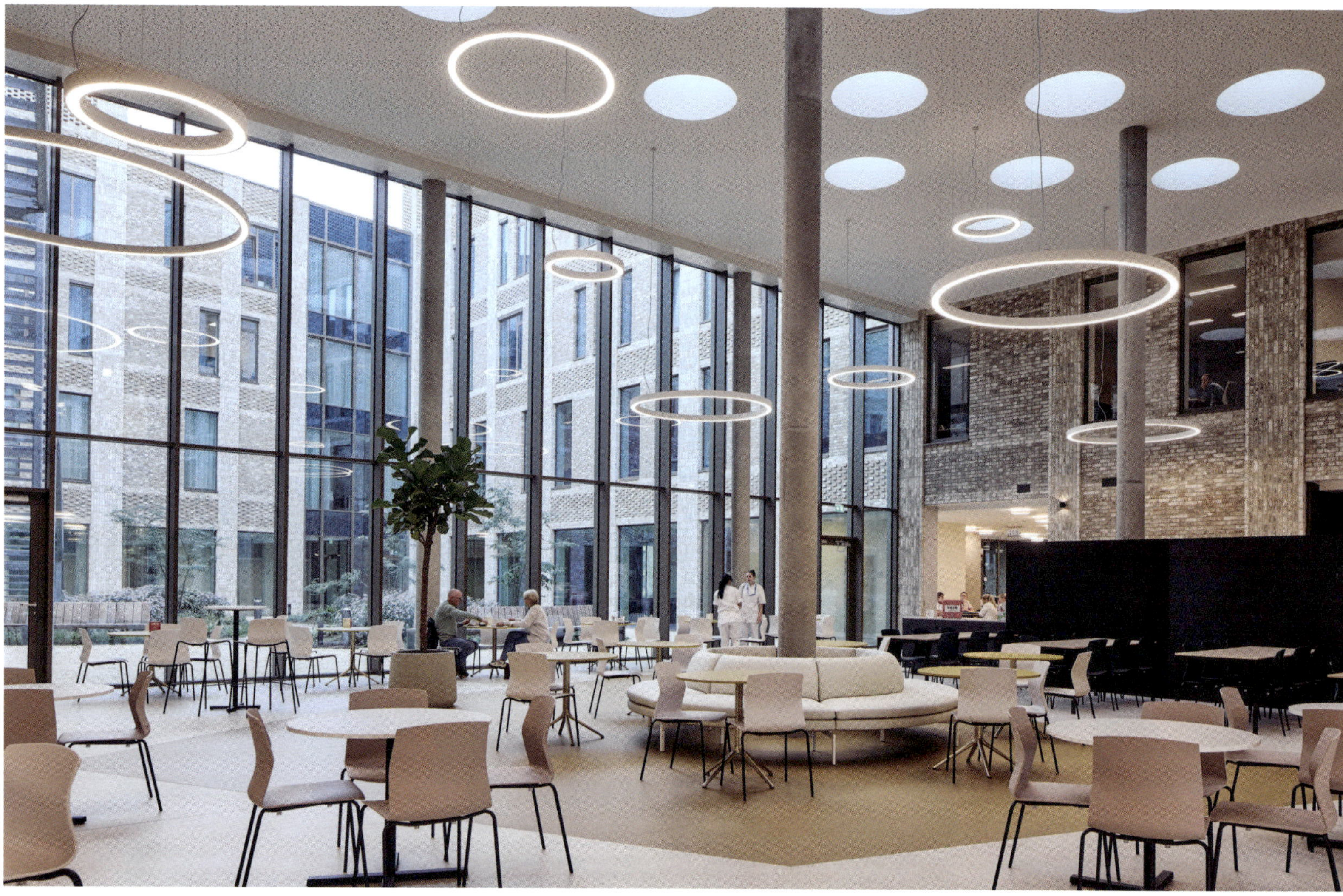

The restaurant features covered outdoor areas overlooking the park.

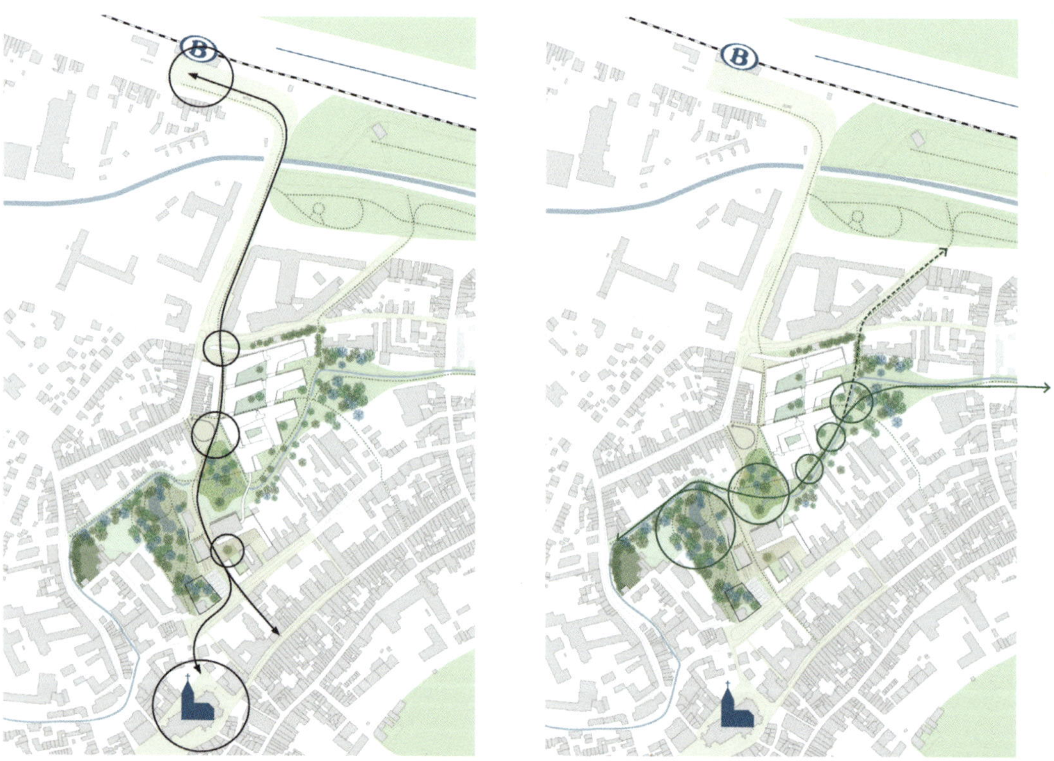

New building at intersection of green corridor and urban route.

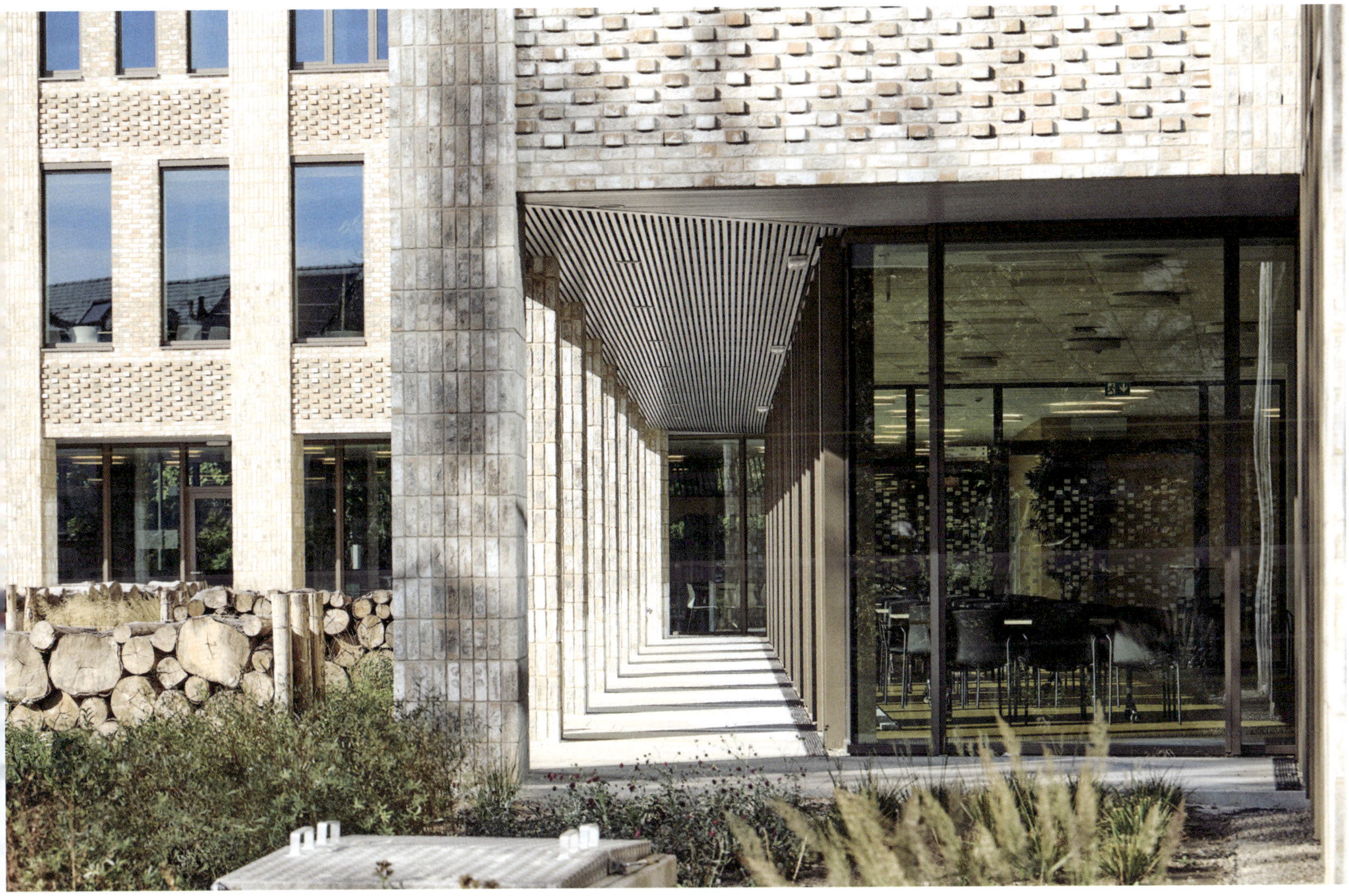

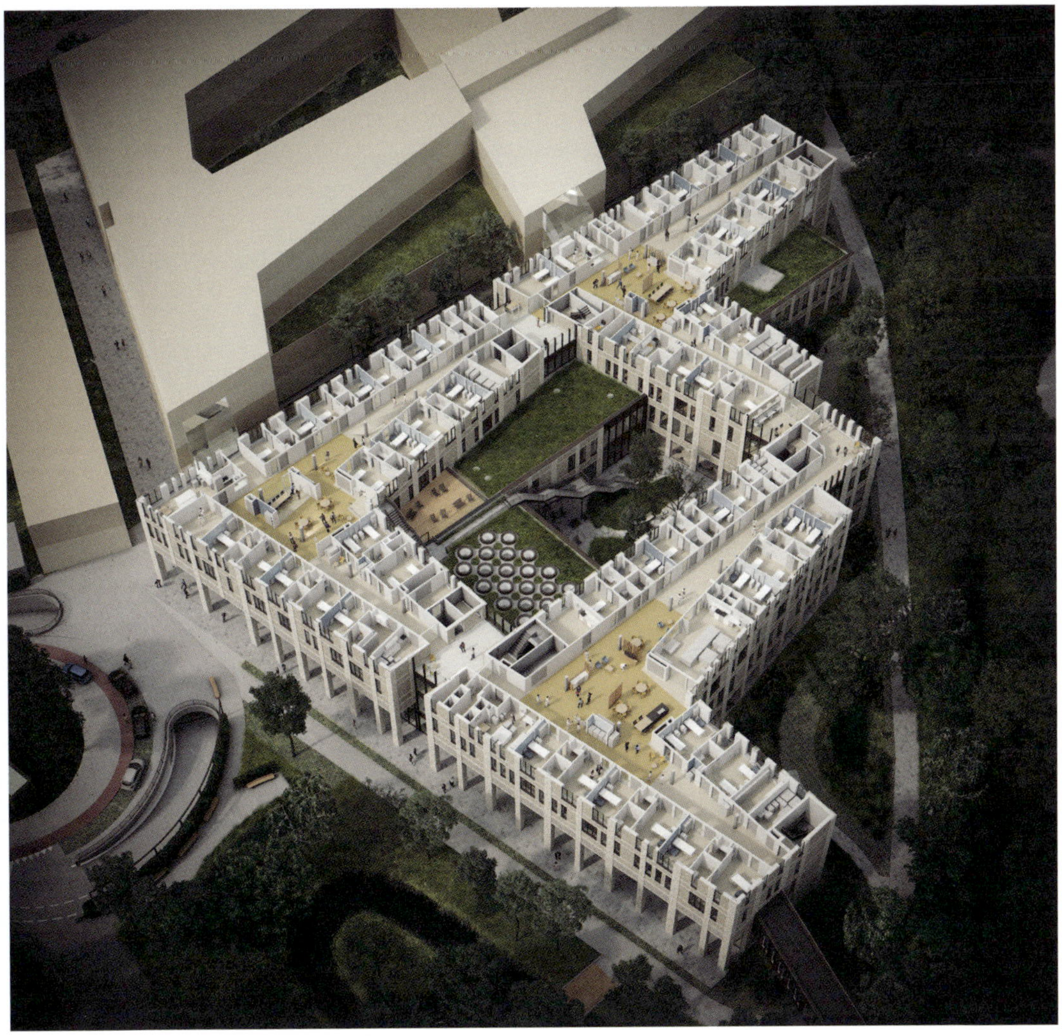

Central lounges encourage patients out of their rooms, creating a more open environment.

Rendering.

tsj-architekten

Sehnde
Germany

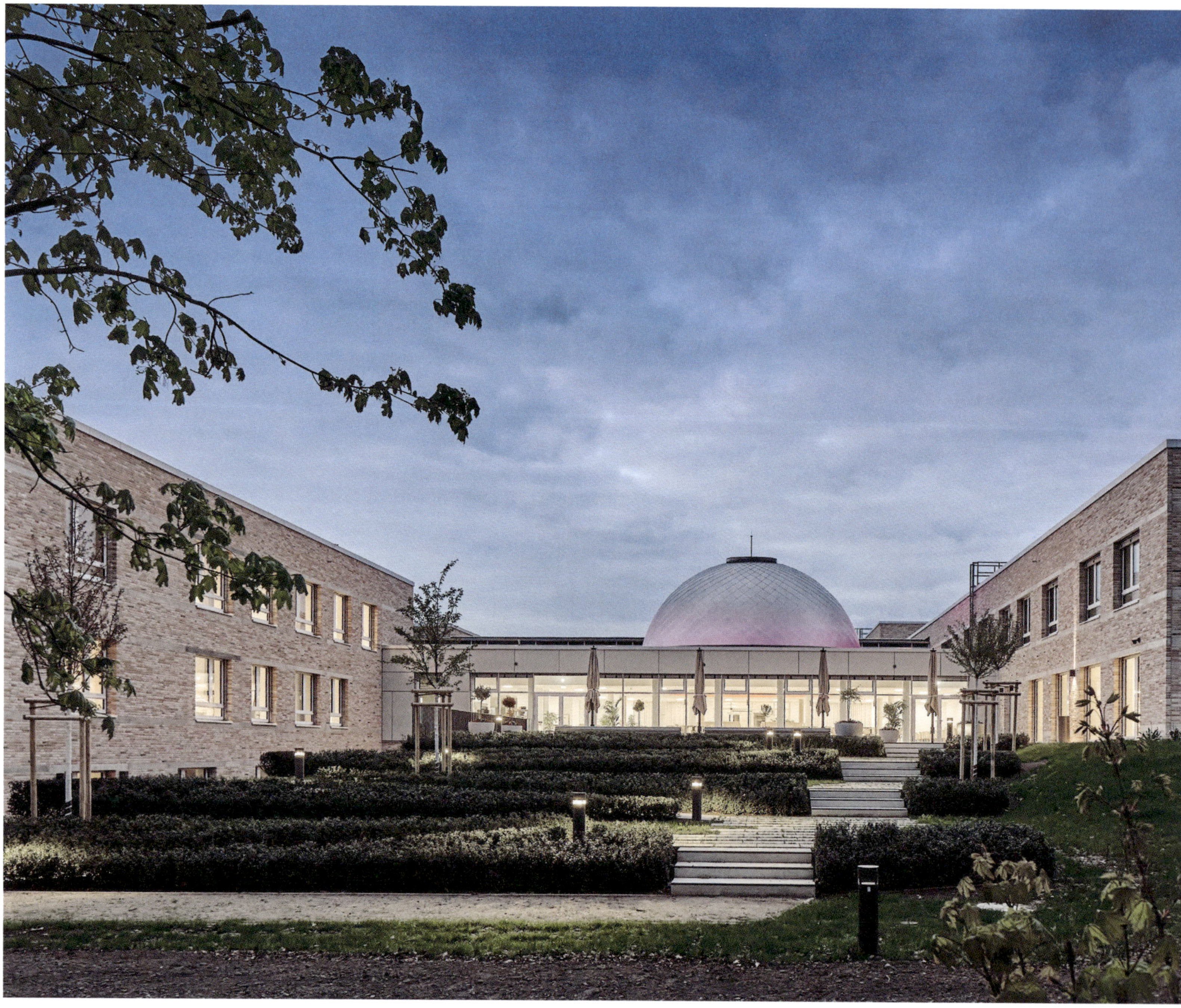

View of the terrace and the dining hall in twilight.

Hospital view from the west side.

Specialized Hospital for the Soul at the Wahrendorff Clinic

As a small, self-contained village the five buildings of the new Hospital for the Soul are grouped around a central courtyard, forming a cohesive and manageable unit. This inspiring temporary home offers a healing environment for body, mind, and soul, tailored to the diverse needs of its residents. Individual retreats and varied spaces with different degrees of privacy and publicness, where a wide range of social interactions as well as personalized therapy and leisure activities are possible, help ensure that the building is not perceived as a clinical institution, but rather as a loving embrace of its guests. The central dining hall – with its light installation by James Turrell – serves as a hub for communication. It radiates far beyond the clinic, inviting the outside world in, inspires wonder, and brings people into conversation with one another to break down barriers and reduce the stigmatization of people with mental health conditions.

Address: Matthias-Wilkening-Weg 6, 31319 Sehnde, Germany | **Client:** Klinikum Wahrendorff GmbH | **Completion:** 2023 | **Size:** 27,811 m² | **Sector:** private | **Specialization:** psychiatric and psychotherapeutic hospital | **Number of treatment rooms:** 30 | **Number of patient rooms:** 195 | **Number of patient beds:** 350 | **Interior design:** brandherm+kumrey interior architecture | **Landscape design:** lad+ landschaftsarchitektur

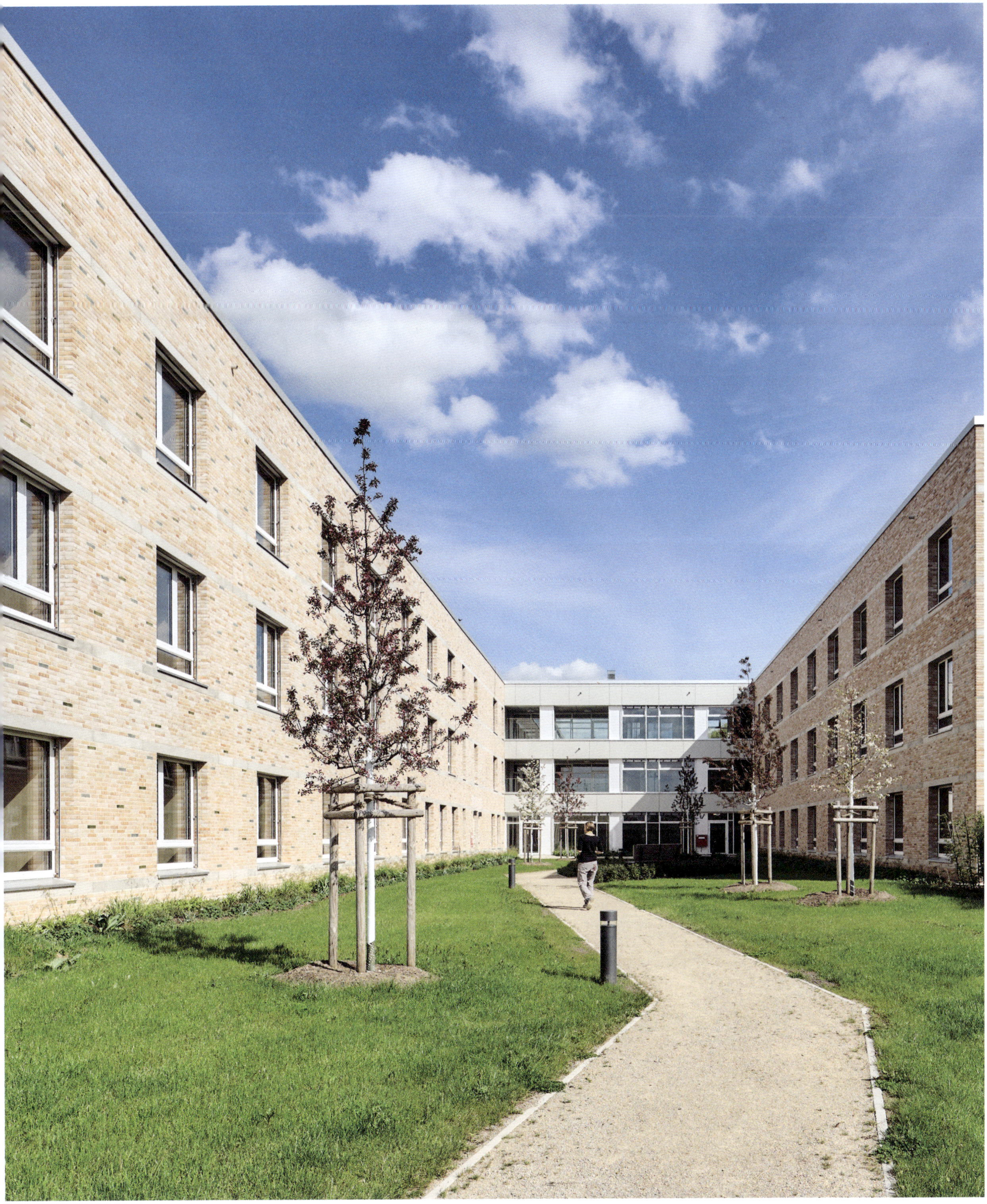

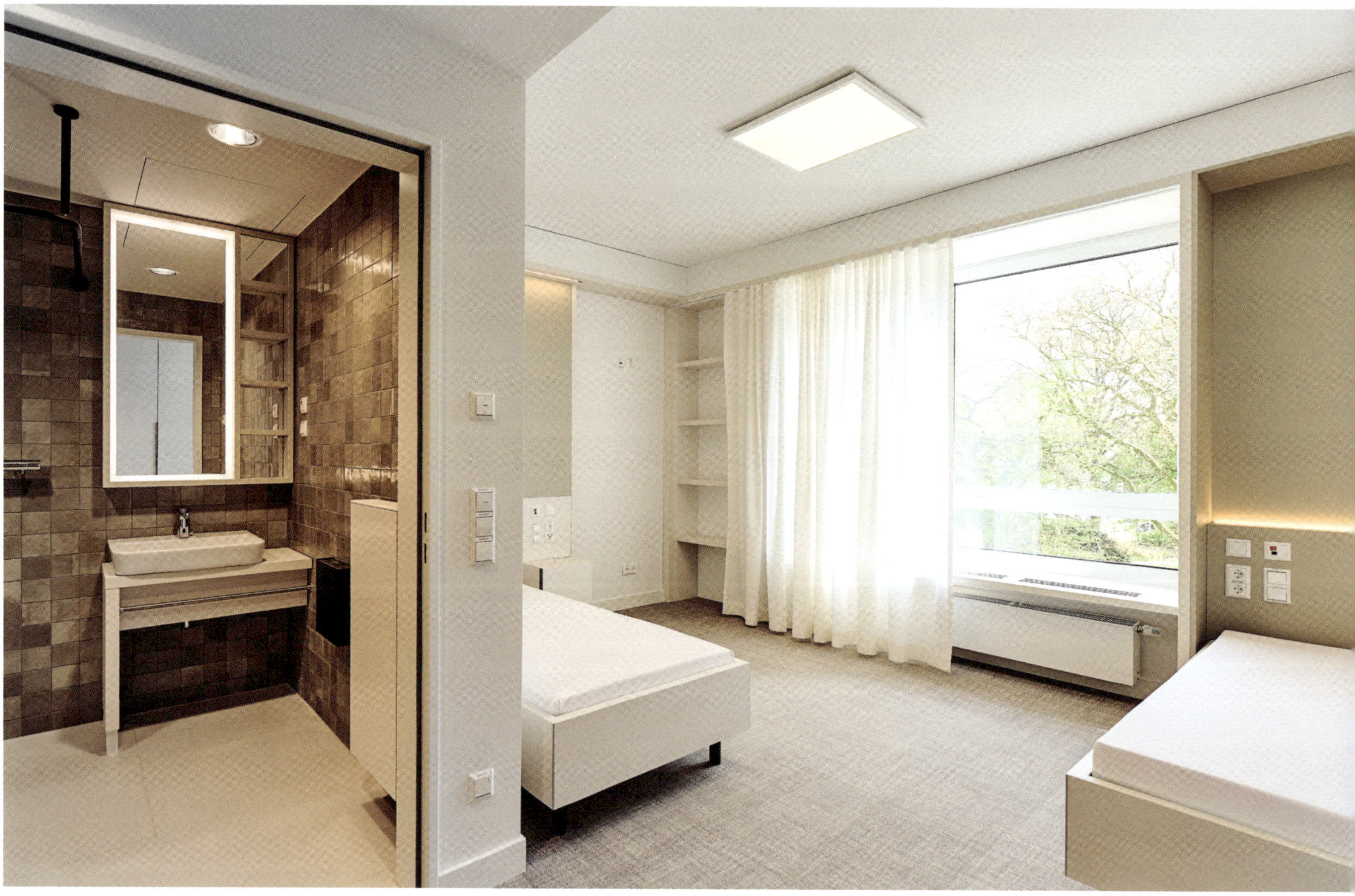

Two-bed patient room.

Site plan.

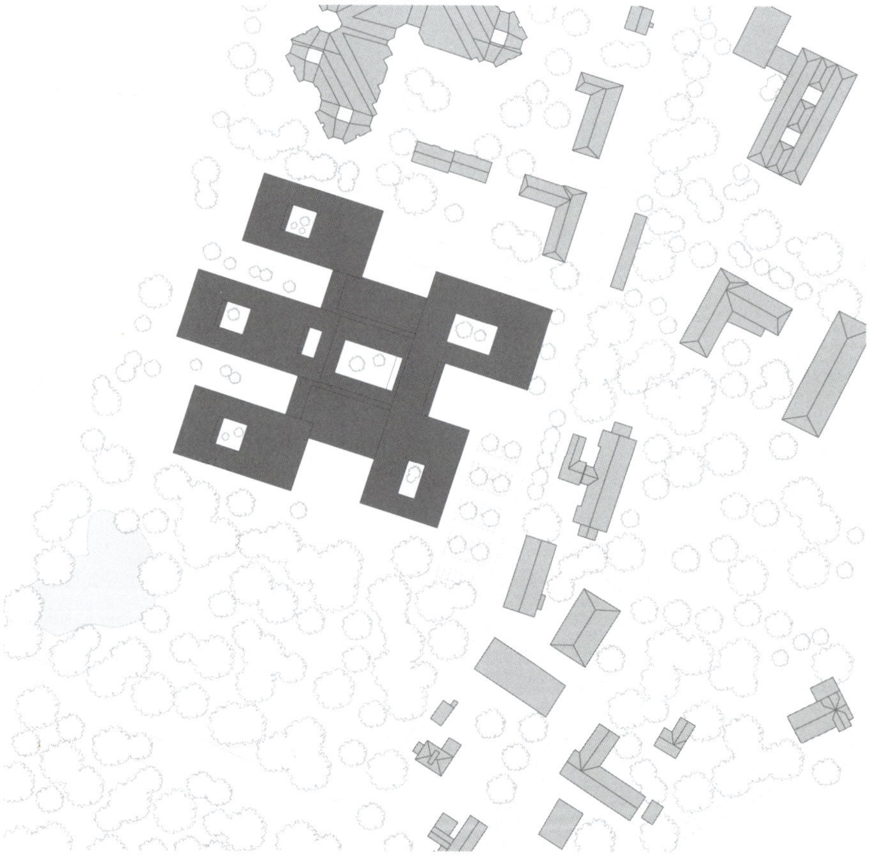

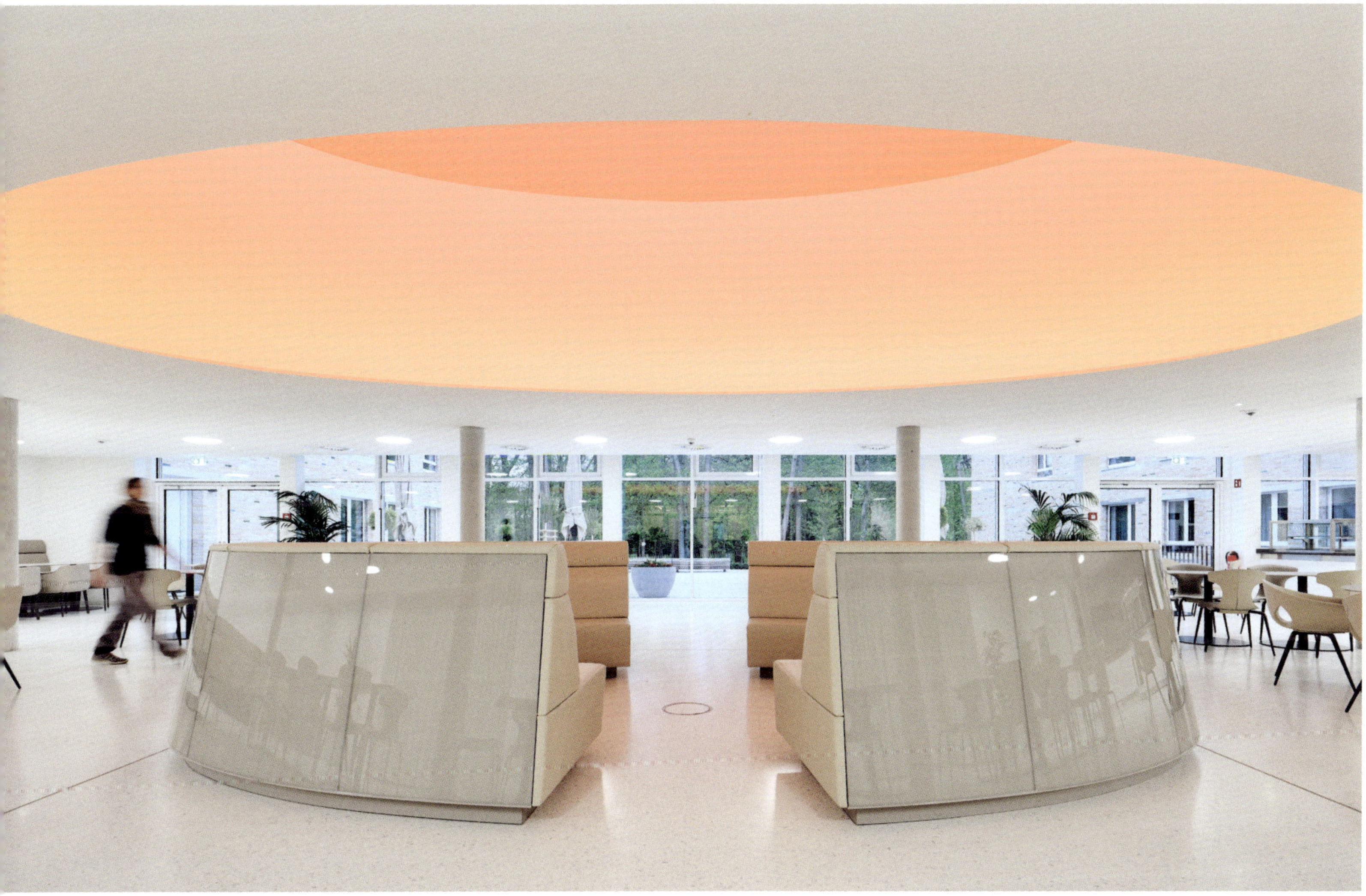

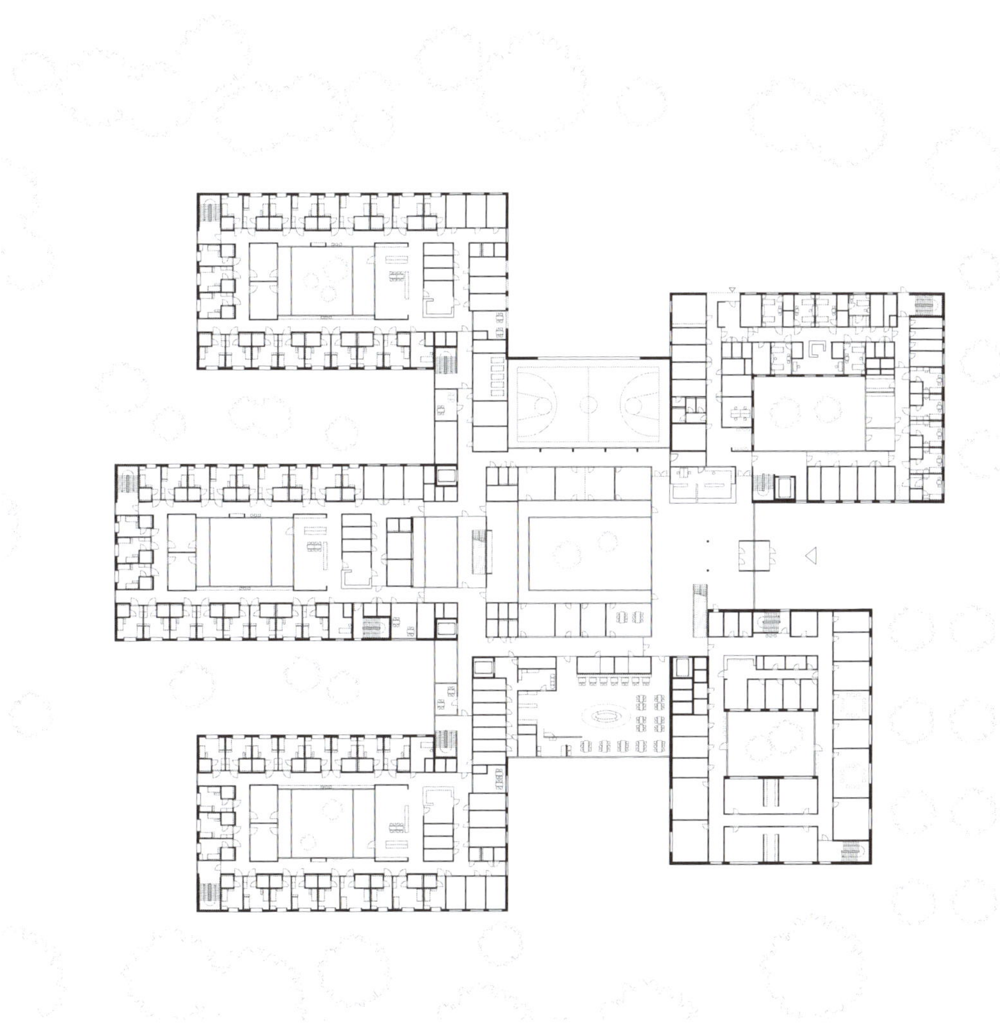

The ward corridor as a semi-public space for informal communication.

Ground floor plan.

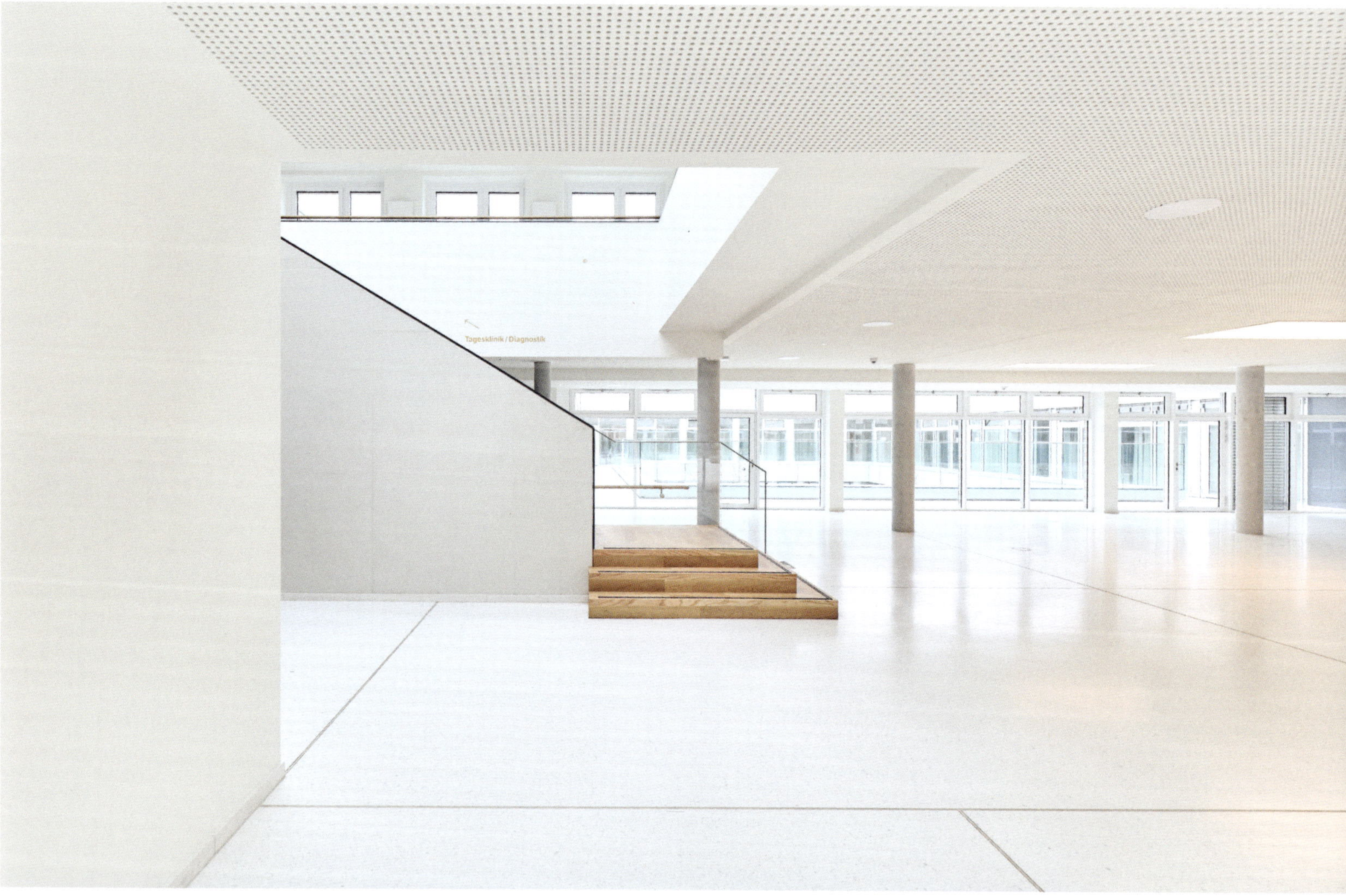

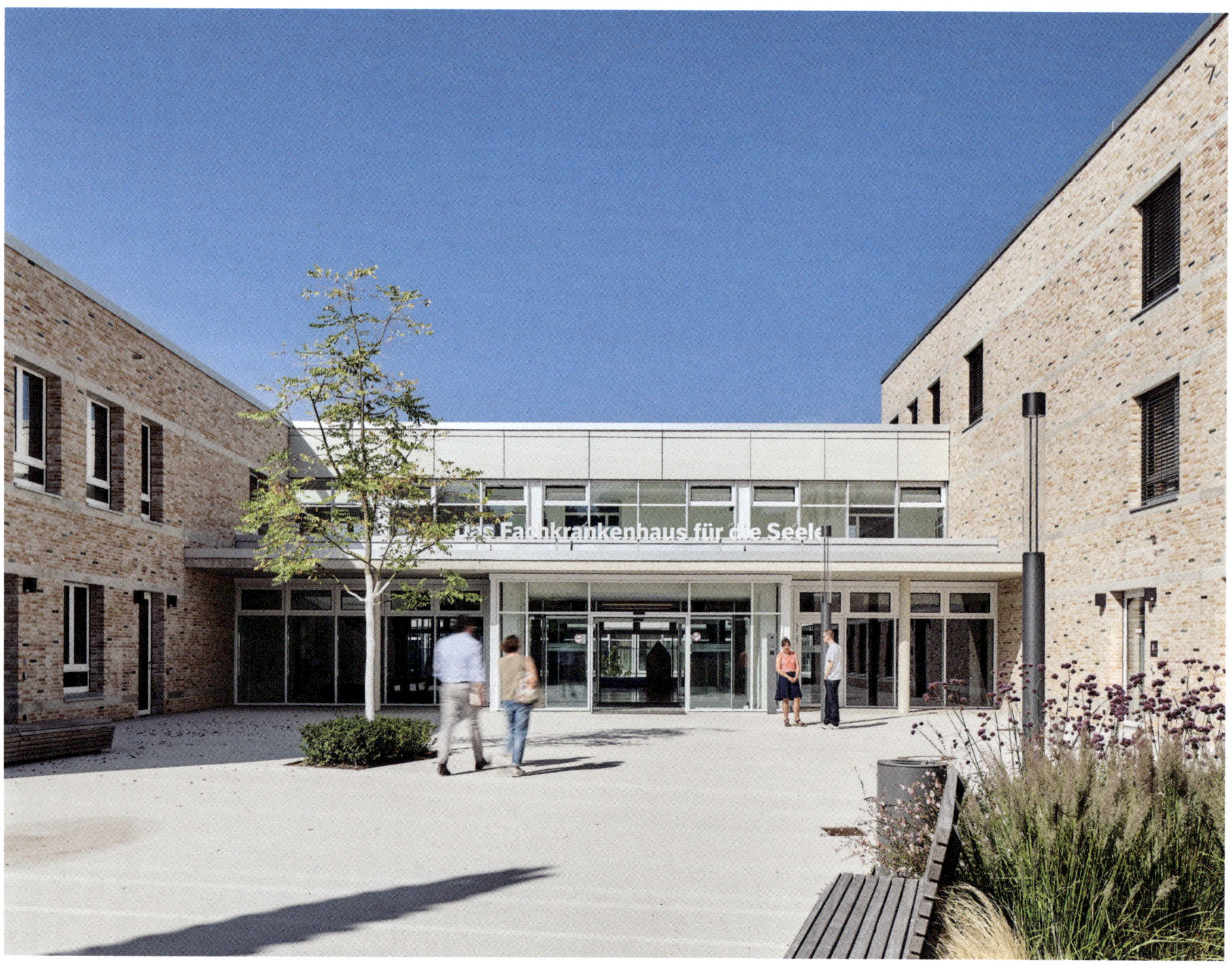

The light-filled foyer serves as a public space that invites people to gather.

The area in front of the building serves as a welcoming gesture.

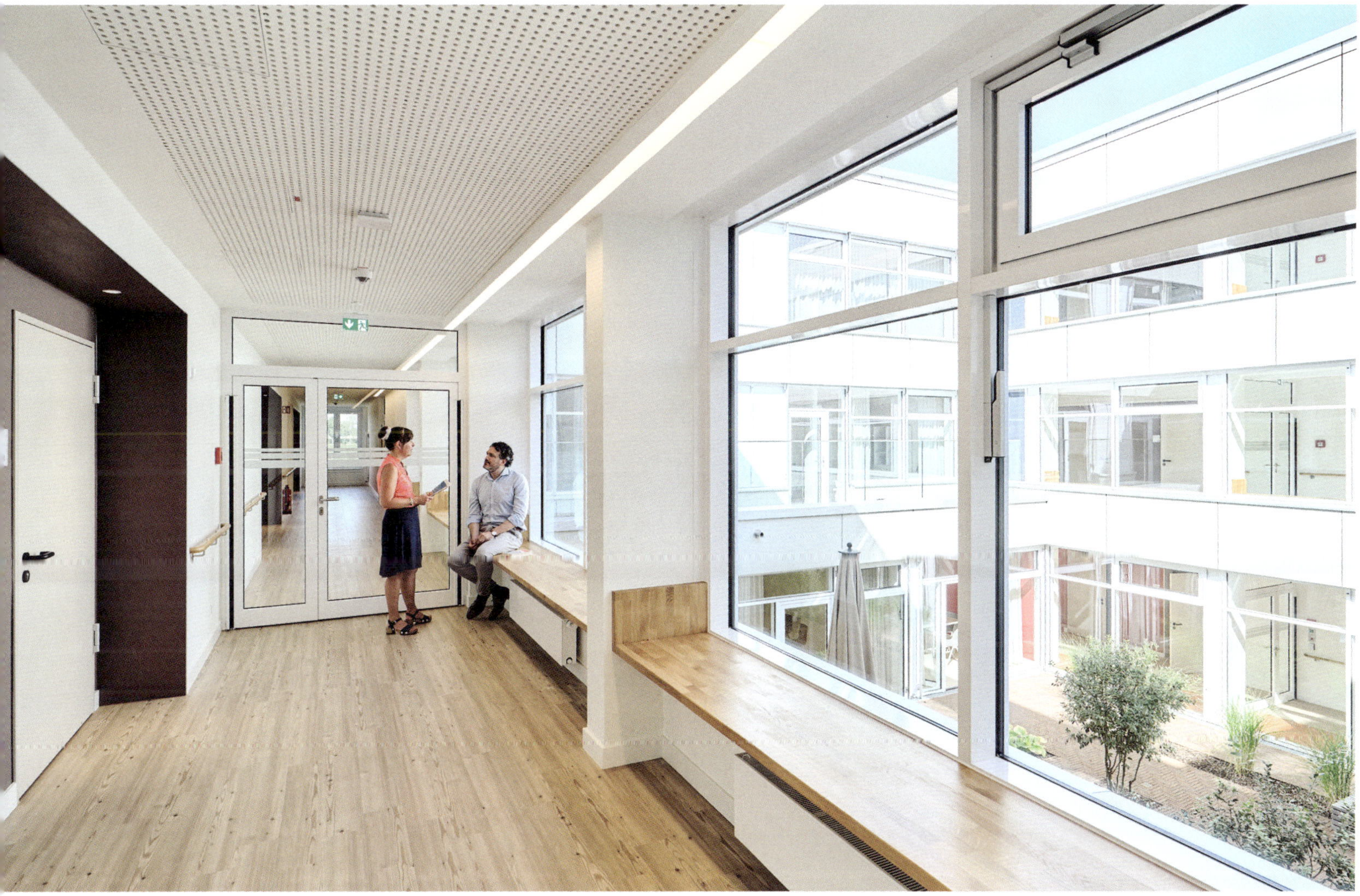

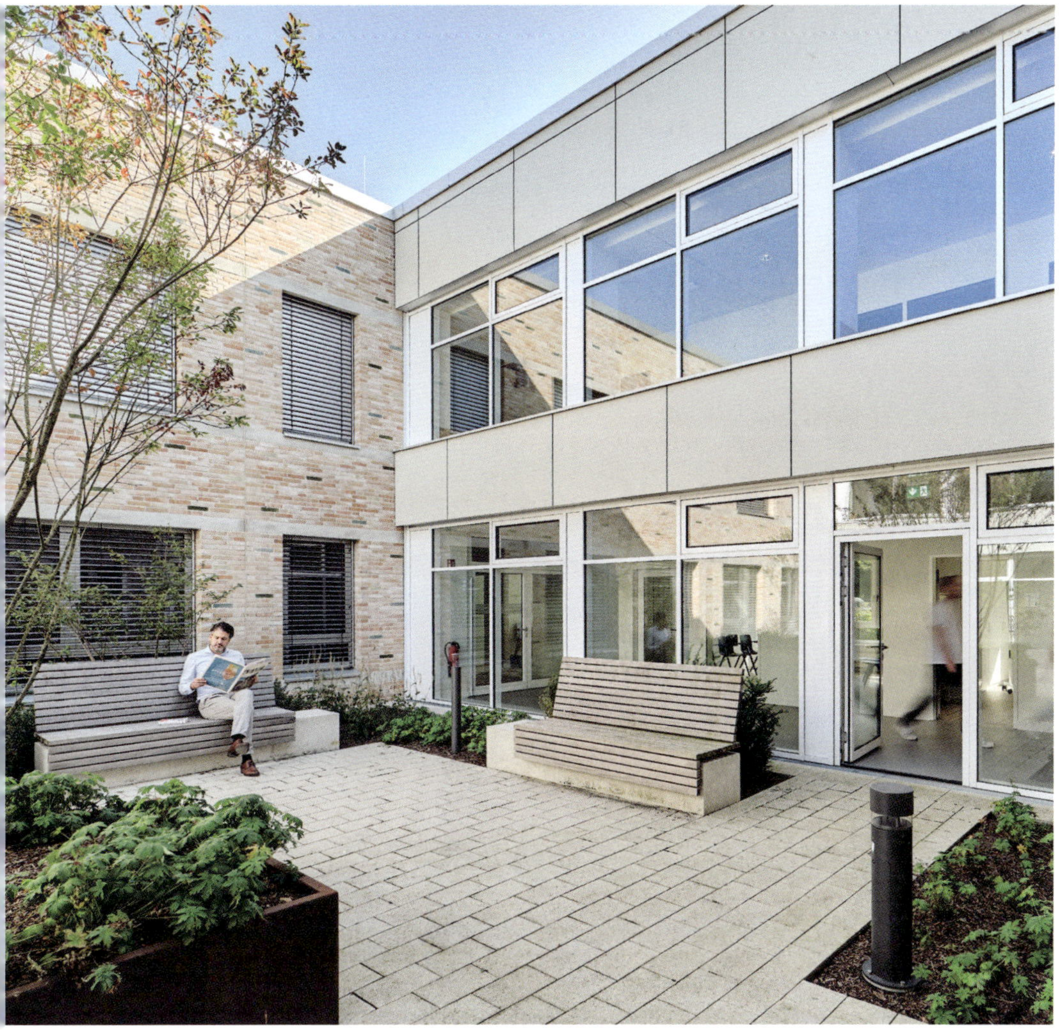

The ward corridor is a semi-public space for informal communication.

The sheltered, intimate courtyard of a station building.

brandherm + krumrey
interior architecture

Sehnde
Germany

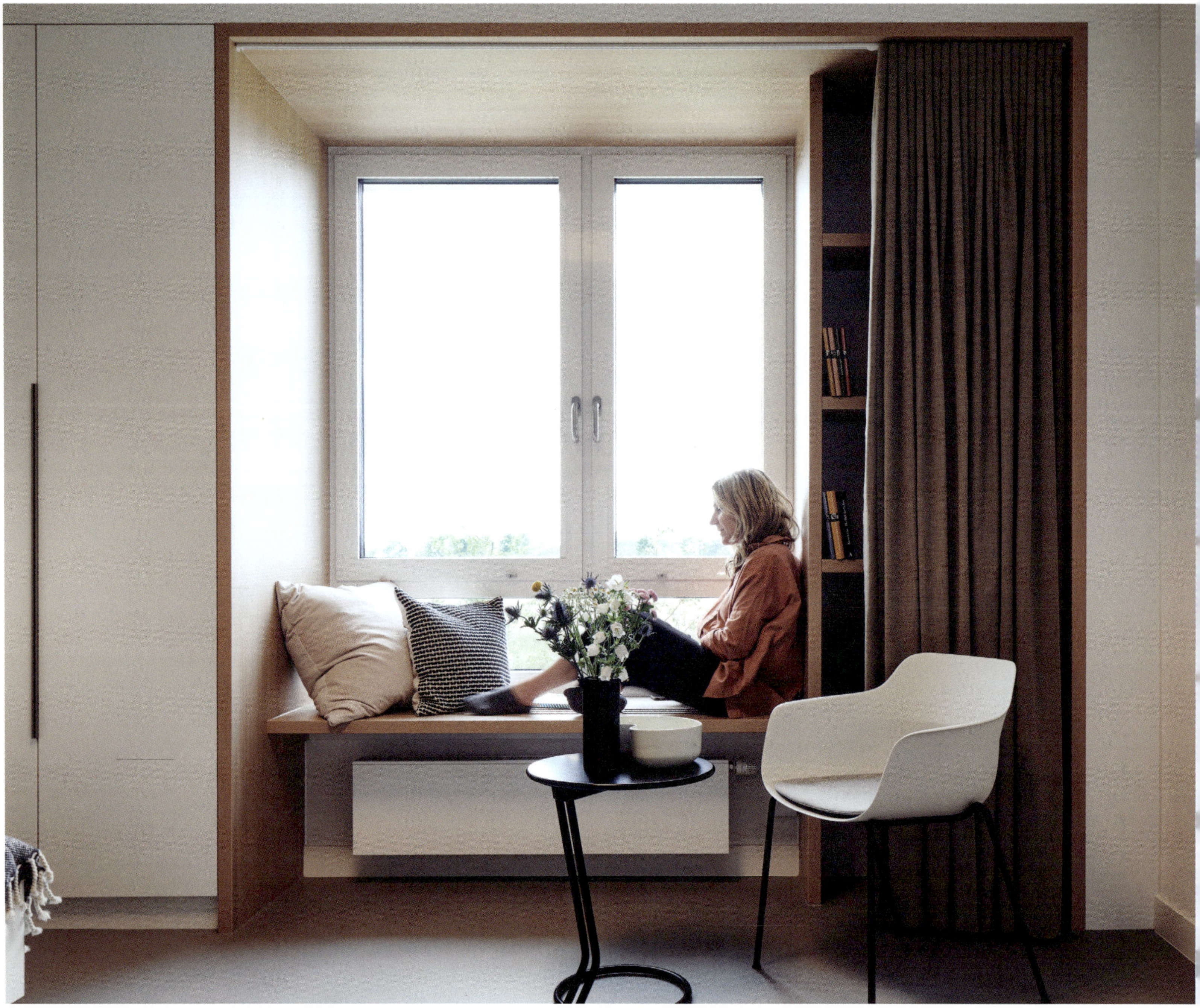

Cozy patient's room with beautiful and soothing interiors.

Hospital's main lobby.

Lobby-reception area.

Interior Architecture Wahrendorff Medical Center

The planning and construction of a new specialized psychiatric hospital required a sensitive approach. The largest new psychiatric facility in Northern Germany, spanning approximately 27,800 square meters, has been completed. The clinic comprises eleven treatment wards, 350 patient beds and 30 day-care spaces. A thoughtful design concept was developed for all patient rooms, including those in the geriatrics, secure psychiatry, psychosomatics, and private care departments. A monochromatic color scheme was developed for each of the three wards, which are distributed across three three-story wings. Shades of green, blue, and red accentuate each wing, facilitating orientation, and fostering a sense of identity. Textiles, wood surfaces, floor-to-ceiling curtains, and carpeted or vinyl flooring also serve as a recurring motif.

Address: Matthias-Wilkening-Weg 6, 31319 Sehnde, Germany | **Client:** Wahrendorff Clinic – Dr. Wilkening | **Completion:** 2022 | **Size:** 27,800 m² | **Sector:** state | **Specialization:** psychiatric and psychotherapeutic hospital | **Number of treatment rooms:** 30 | **Number of patient rooms:** 350 | **Architecture:** tsj-architekten | **Landscape design:** lad+ landschaftsarchitektur

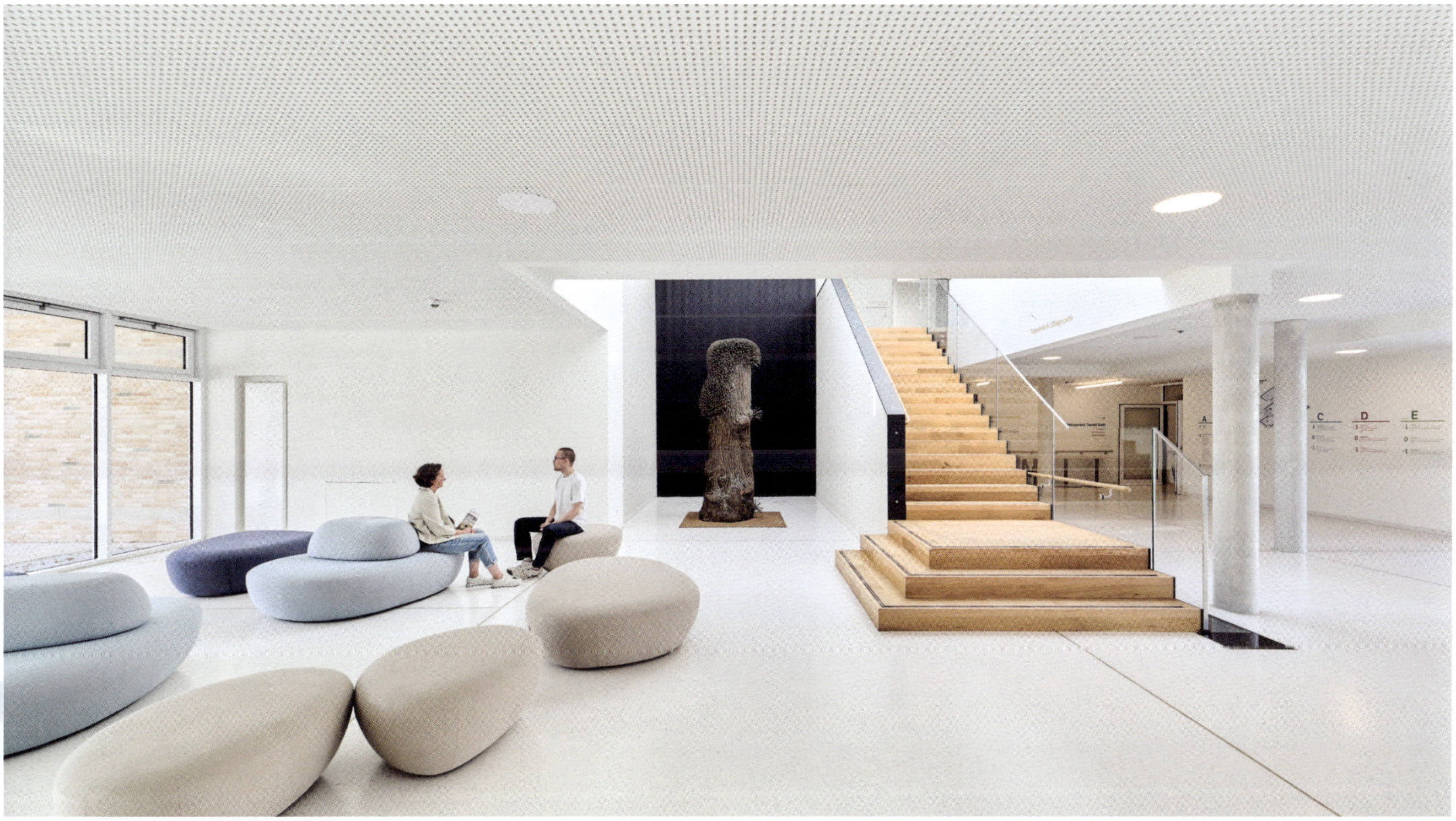

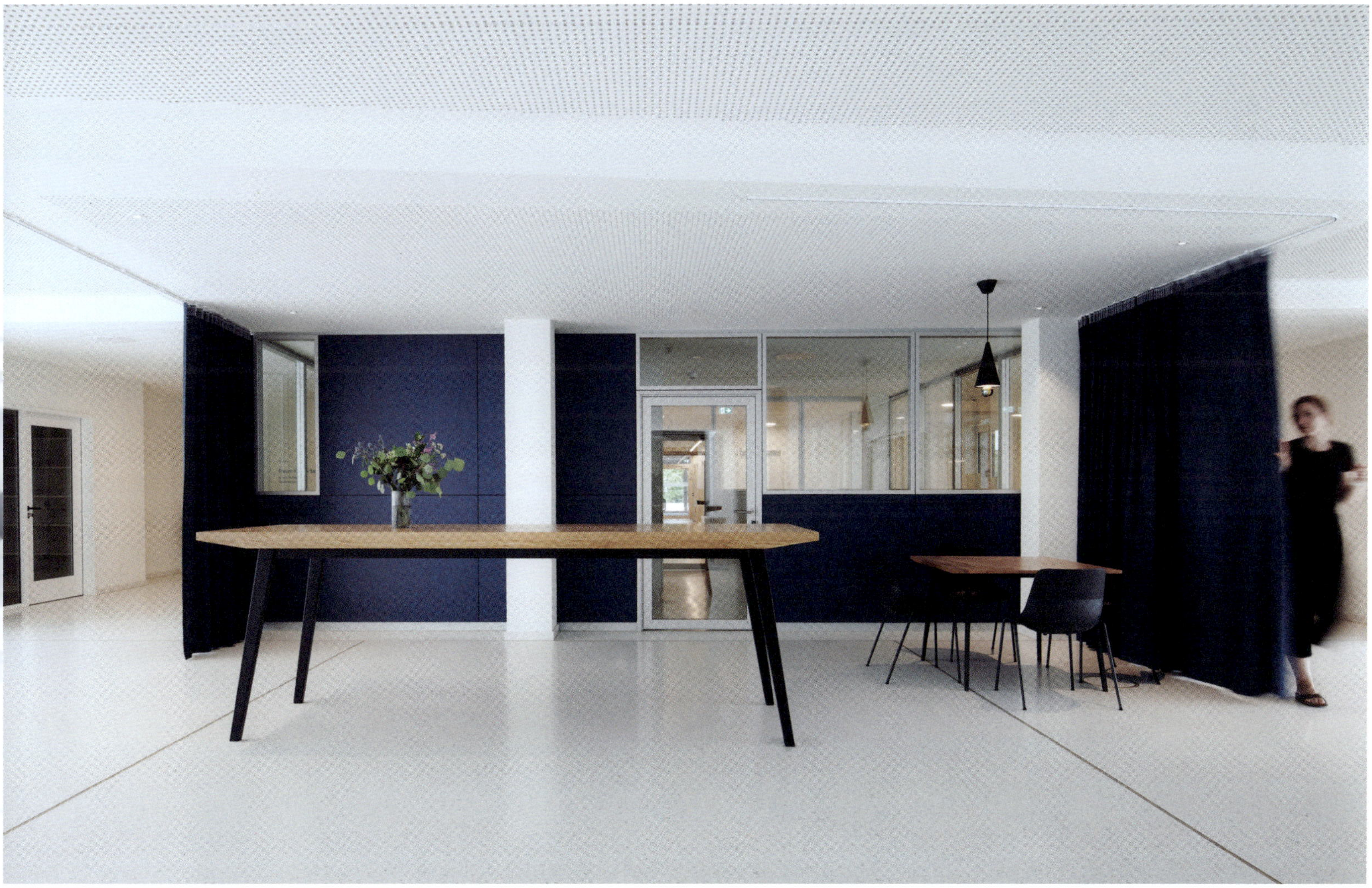

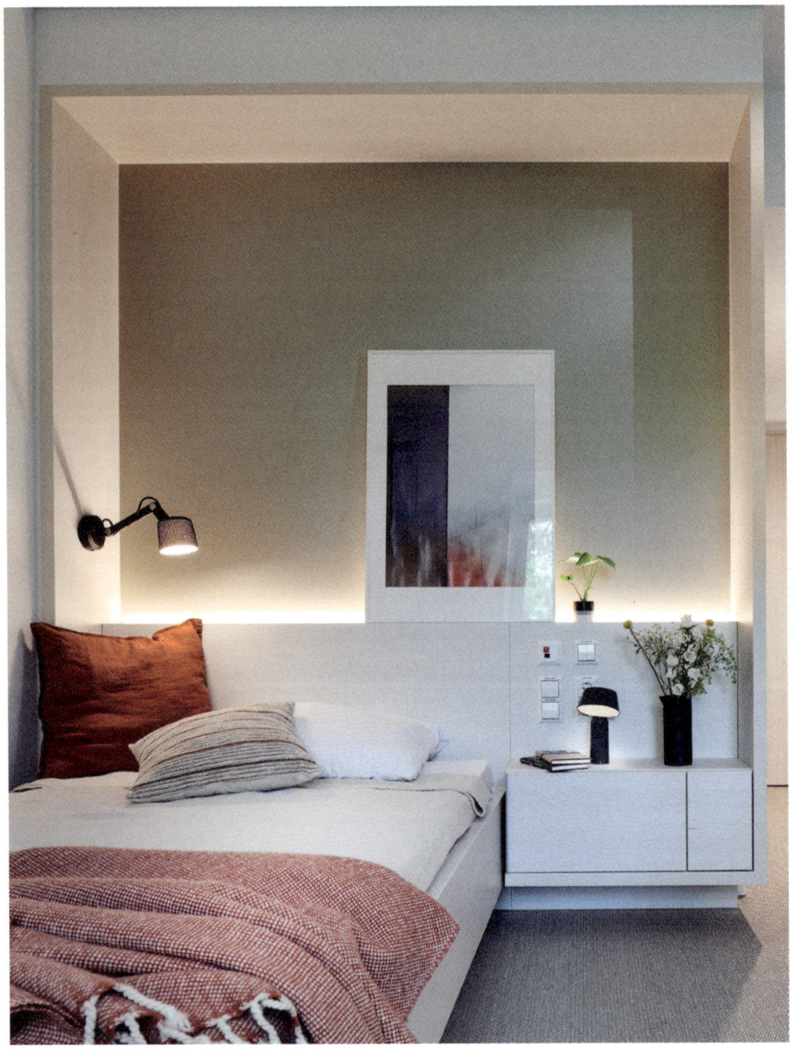

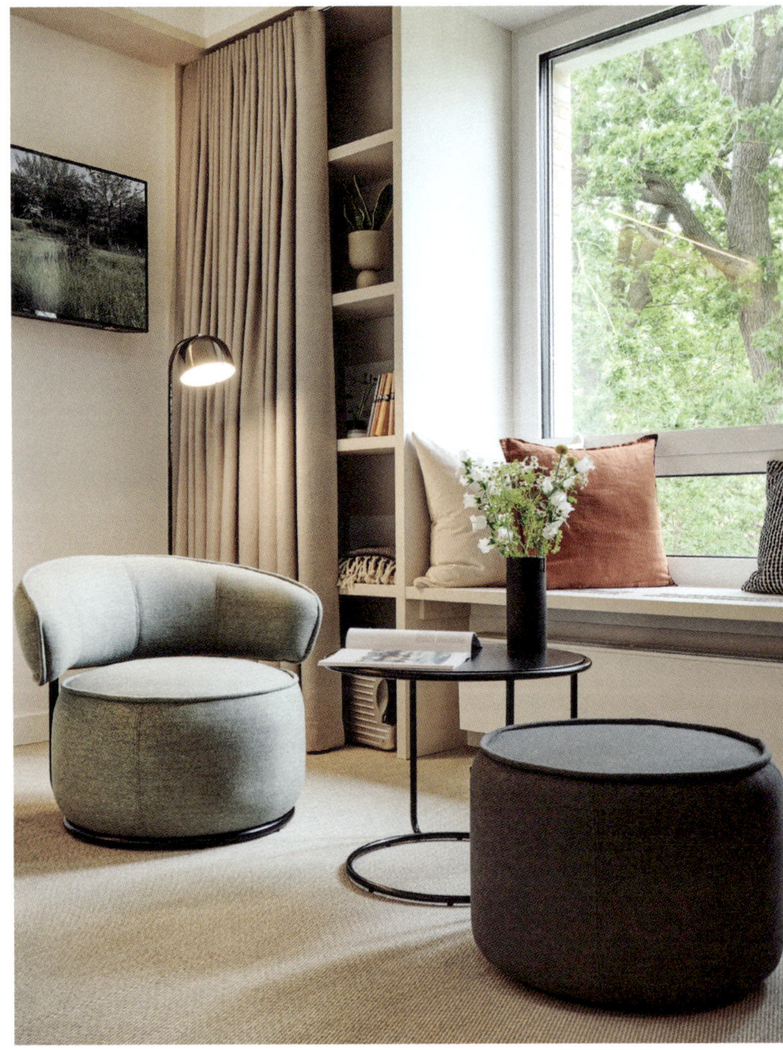

Color coordinated patient's room in green.

Thoughtful and sensitive interiors with generous windows, allowing expansive views of nature complete the rooms.

Floor plan of a two-bed and one-bed patient room.

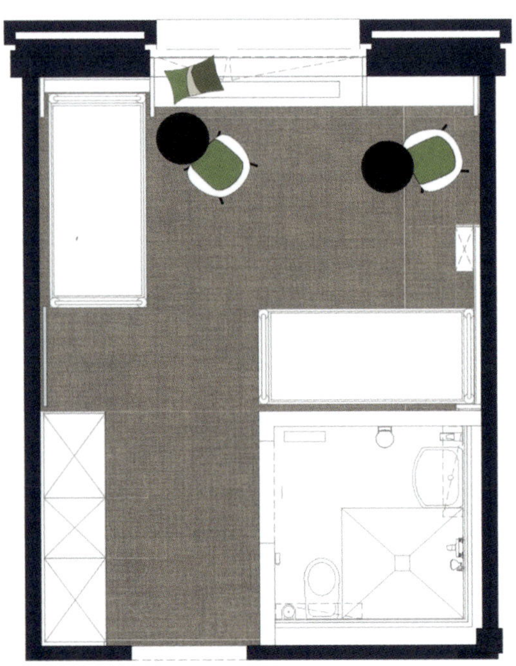

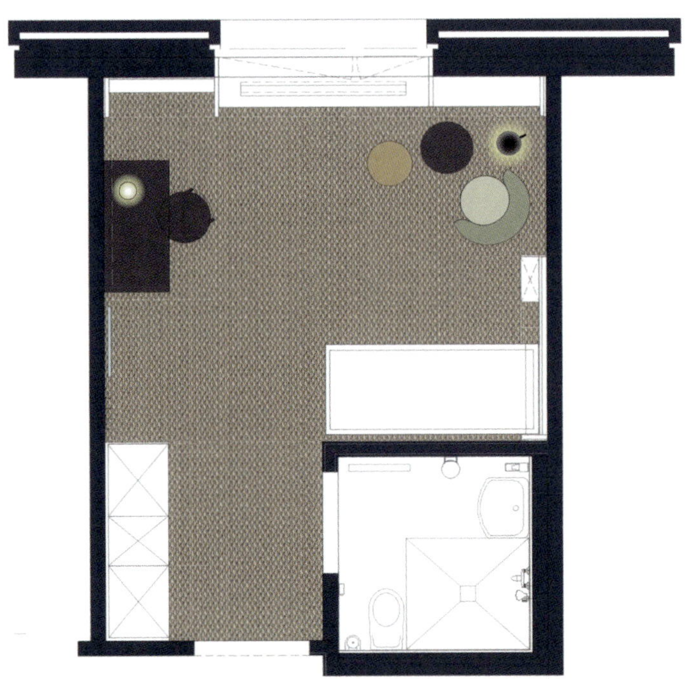

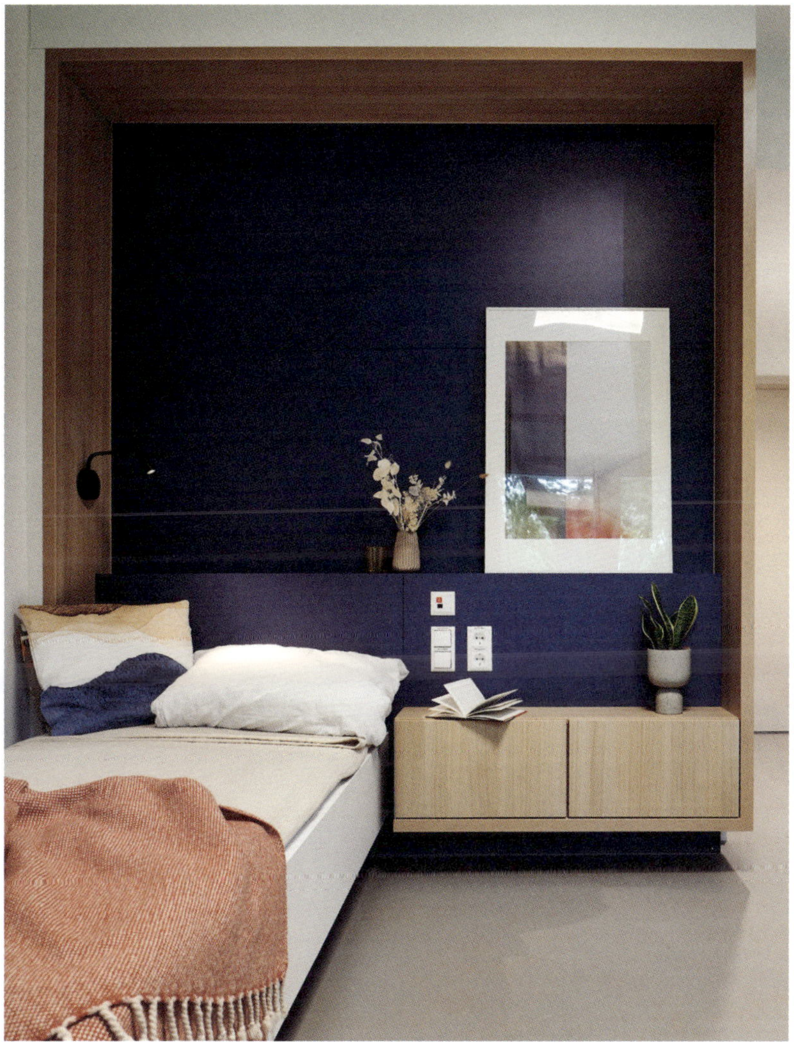

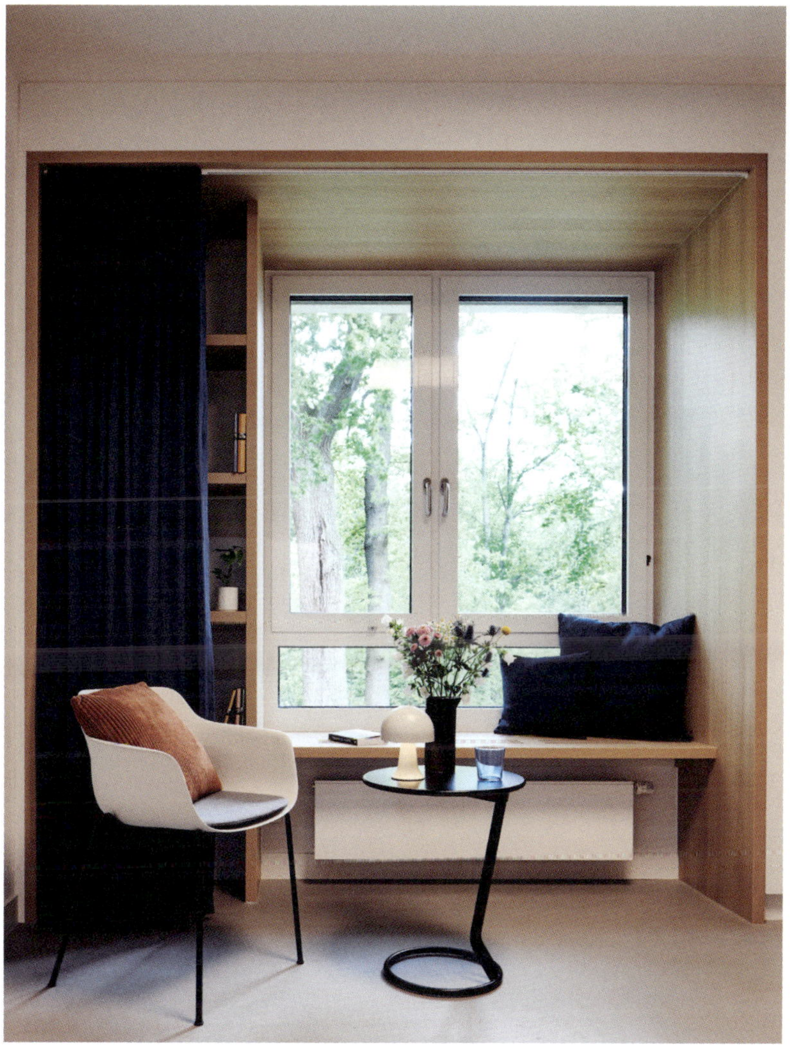

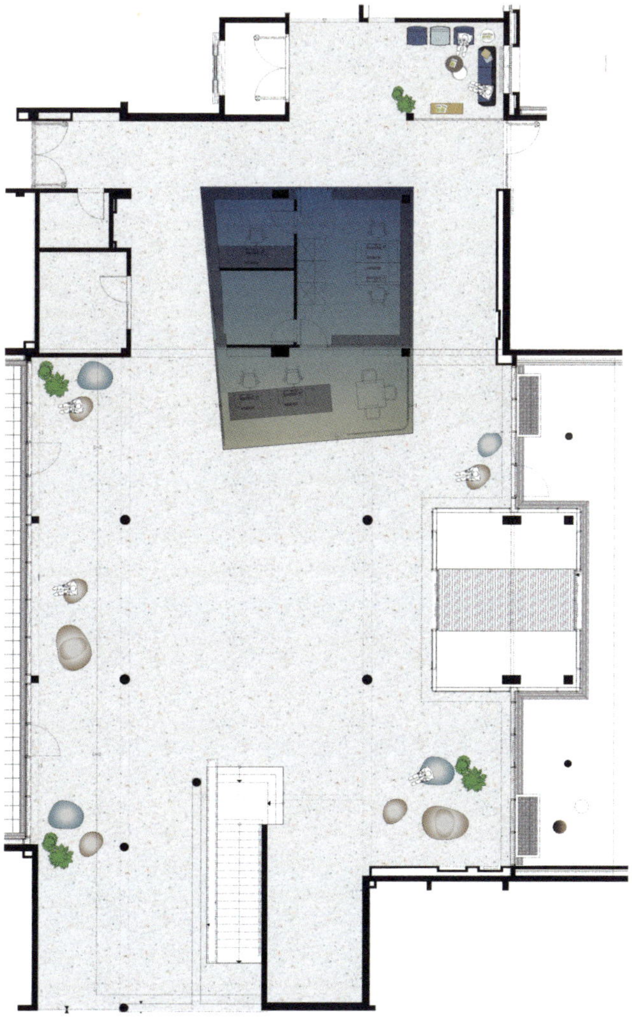

Color coordinated patient's room in blue.

The rooms use a color-coding system to aid identification, orientation, and create a homelike atmosphere.

Floor plan of the lobby.

Tiemann-Petri Koch
Freie Architekten

Bolzano
Italy

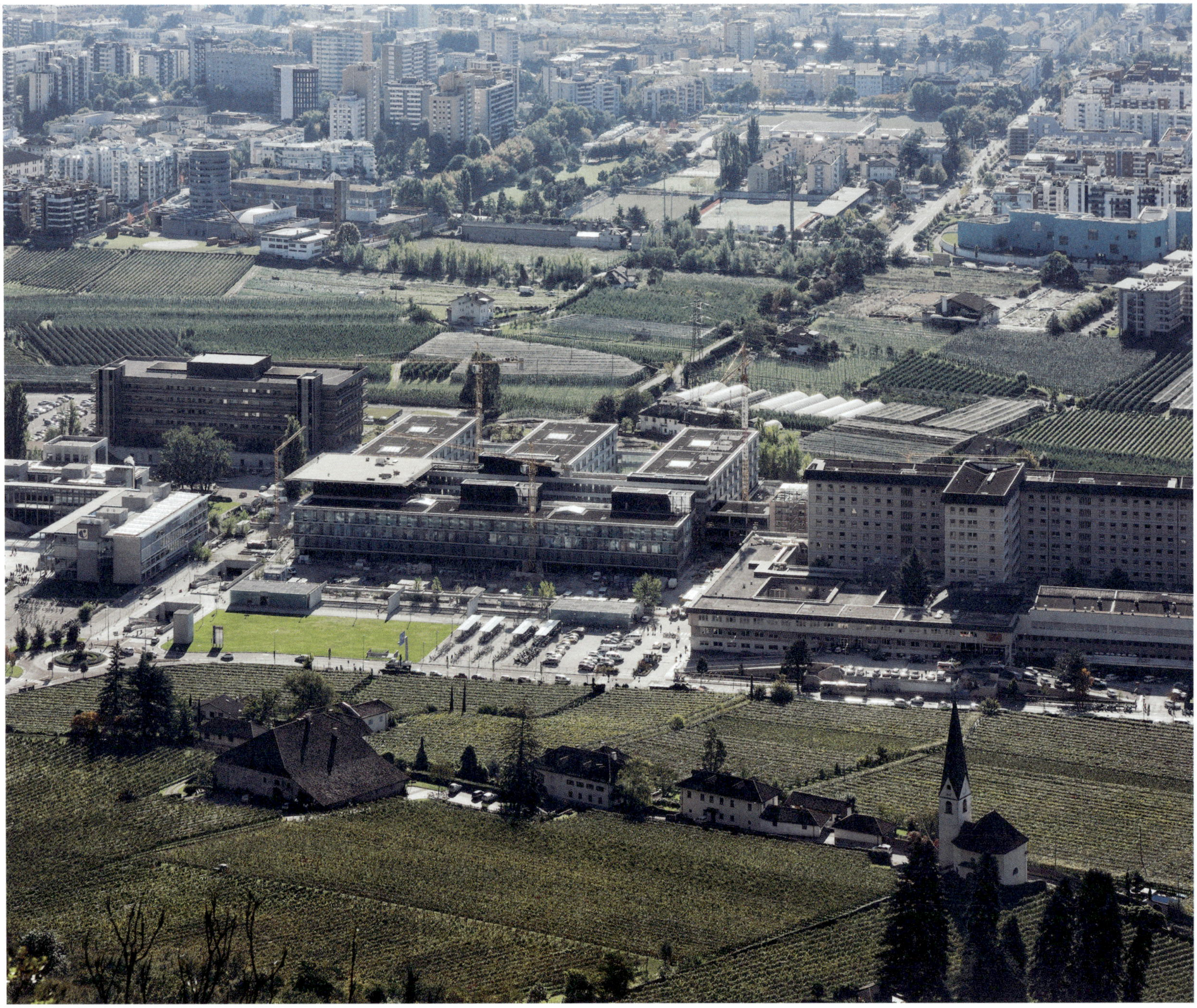

Aerial view of the hospital.

Garden courtyard for the patients.

Central piazza with water feature.

New Clinic Building Bolzano Central Hospital

The project reorganizes and extends Bolzano hospital into a structured and adaptable campus. The design establishes a clinic quarter that integrates the existing buildings with new medical functions and areas for future development within the surrounding landscape. A central glass-roofed passage connects new and existing constructions and serves as the main circulation axis, providing clear orientation from the central piazza to all functional areas. The extension is based on a modular system, enabling flexibility for changing requirements. The layout and moderate building heights create a well-lit and green ensemble, fostering a patient-friendly atmosphere. The program includes an interdisciplinary emergency department, outpatient clinics, an operating department, care units, public amenities along the main passage, and a rooftop helipad.

Address: Lorenz-Böhler-Straße 5, 39100 Bolzano, Italy | **Client:** Autonomous Province of Bolzano-South Tyrol | **Completion:** 2020 | **Size:** 58,920 m² | **Sector:** state | **Specialization:** tertiary care hospital | **Number of treatment rooms:** 140 | **Number of patient rooms:** 218 | **Open space design:** Entwicklung und Gestaltung von Landschaft, Erlangen

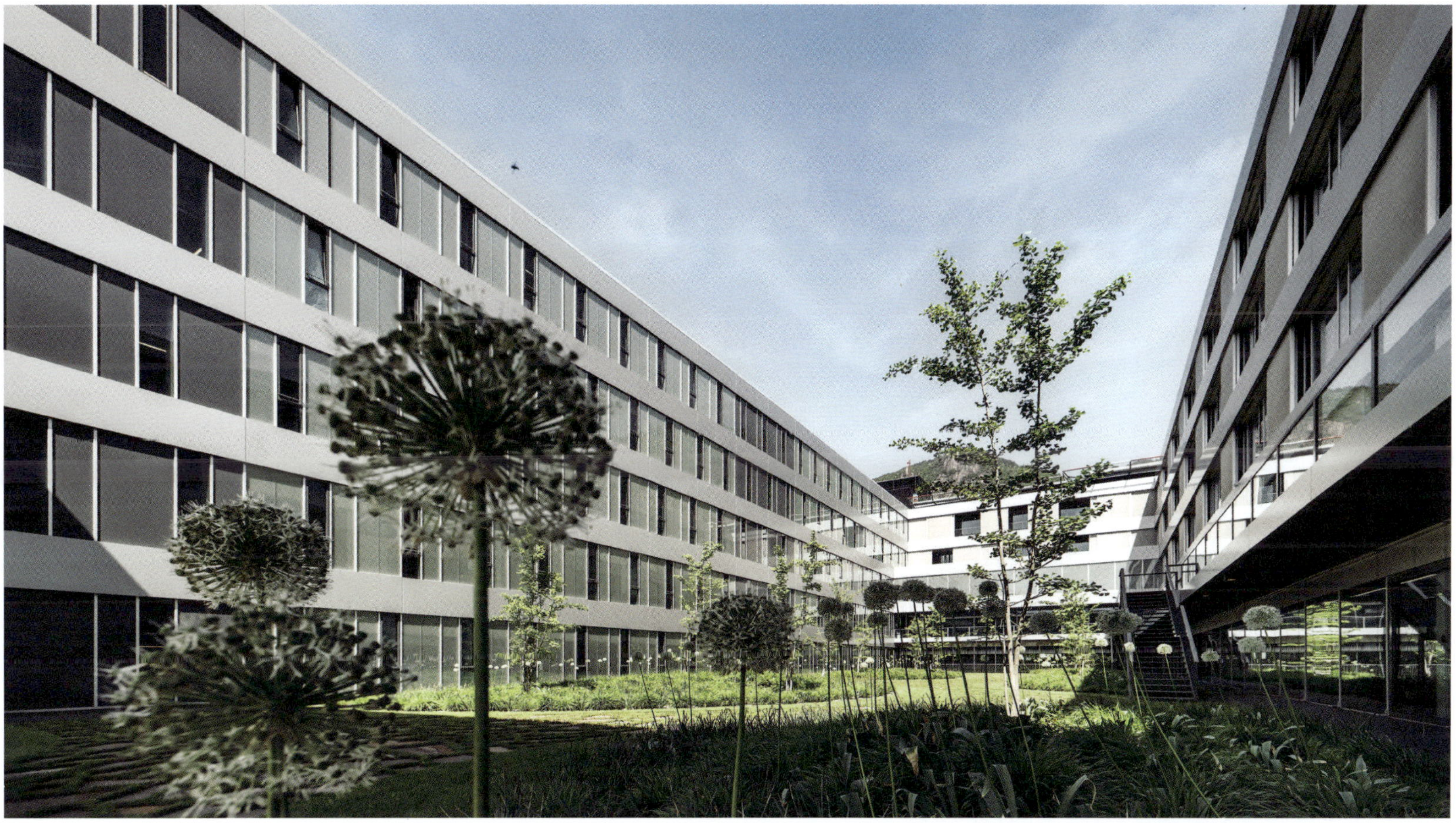

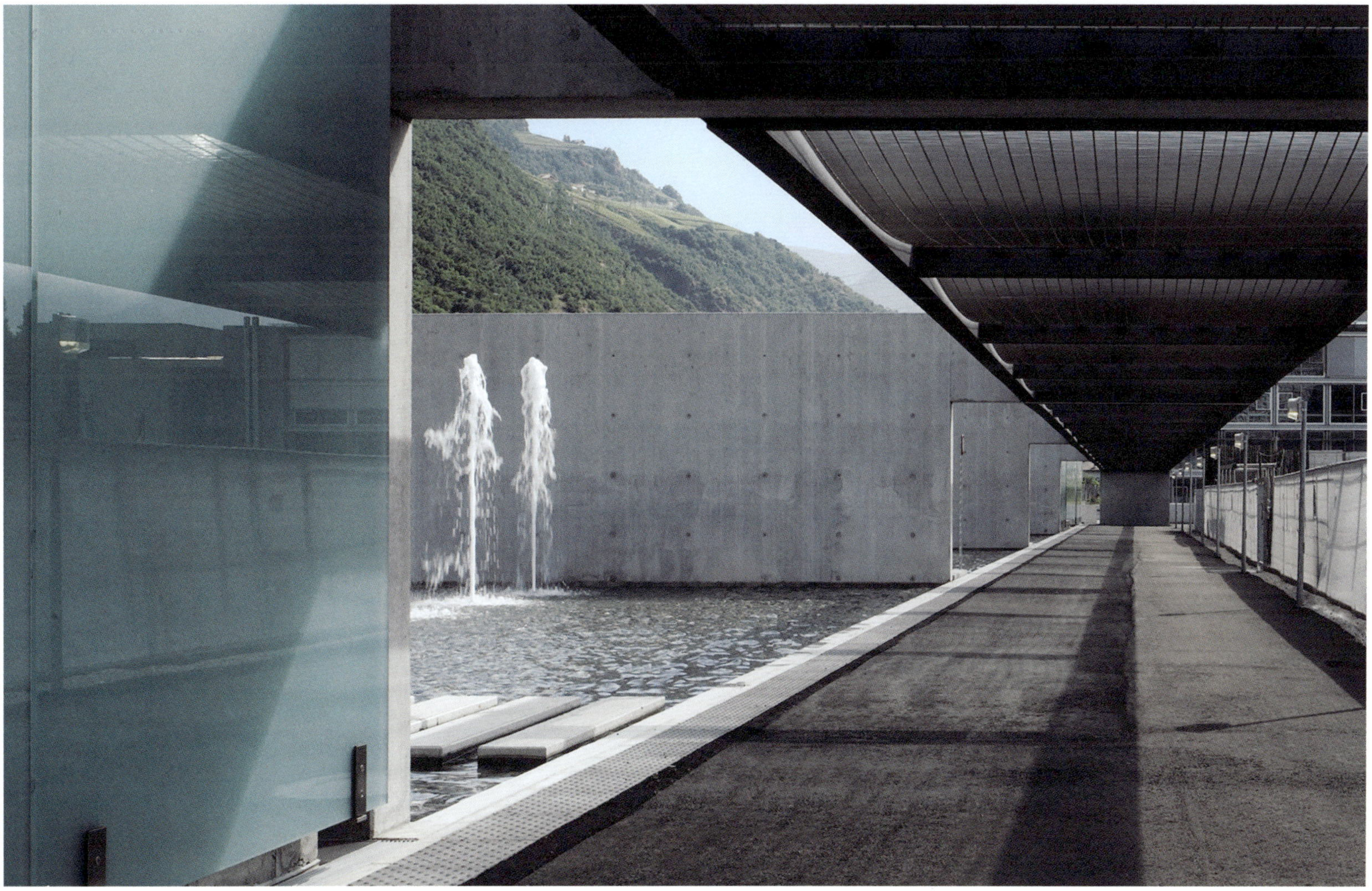

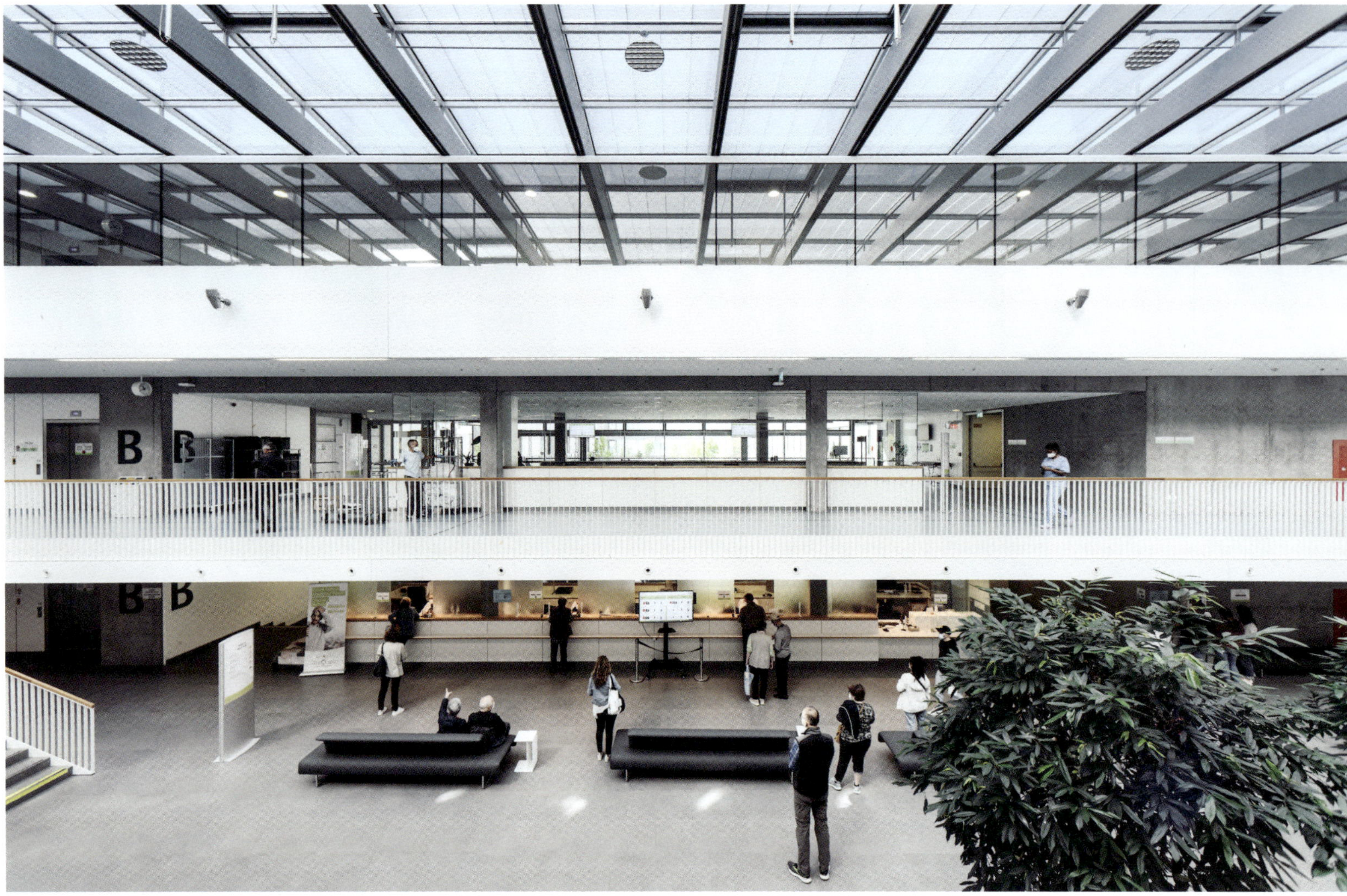

Central passage of the hospital with reception area.

Ground floor plan.

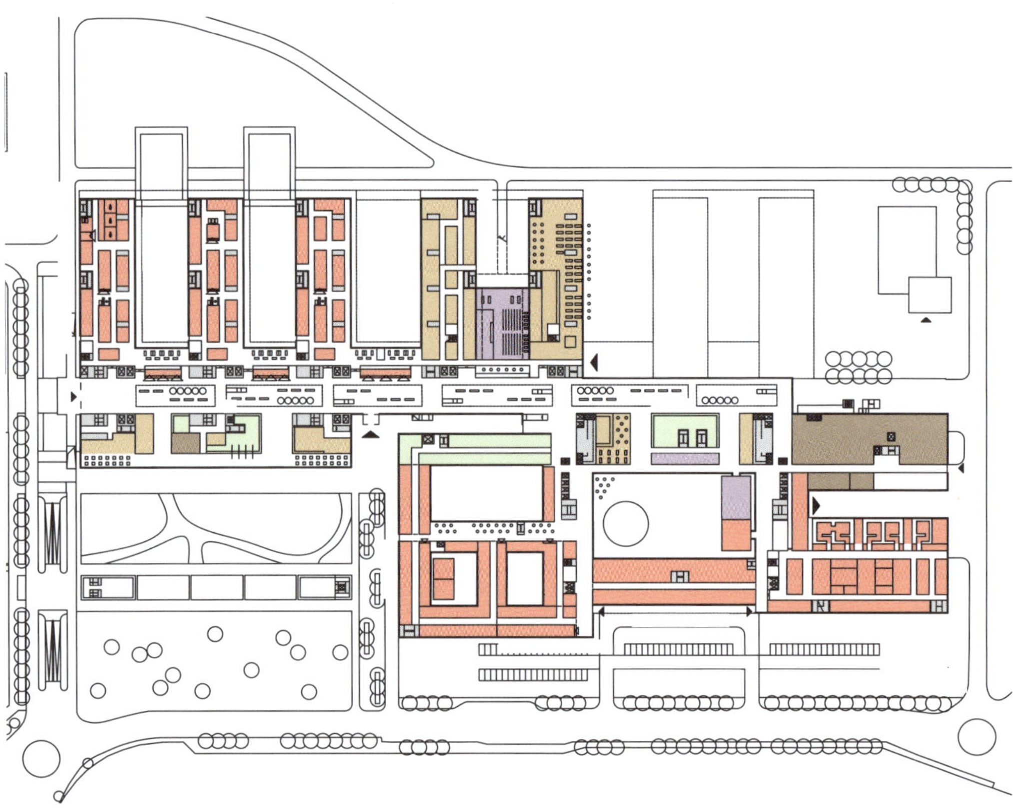

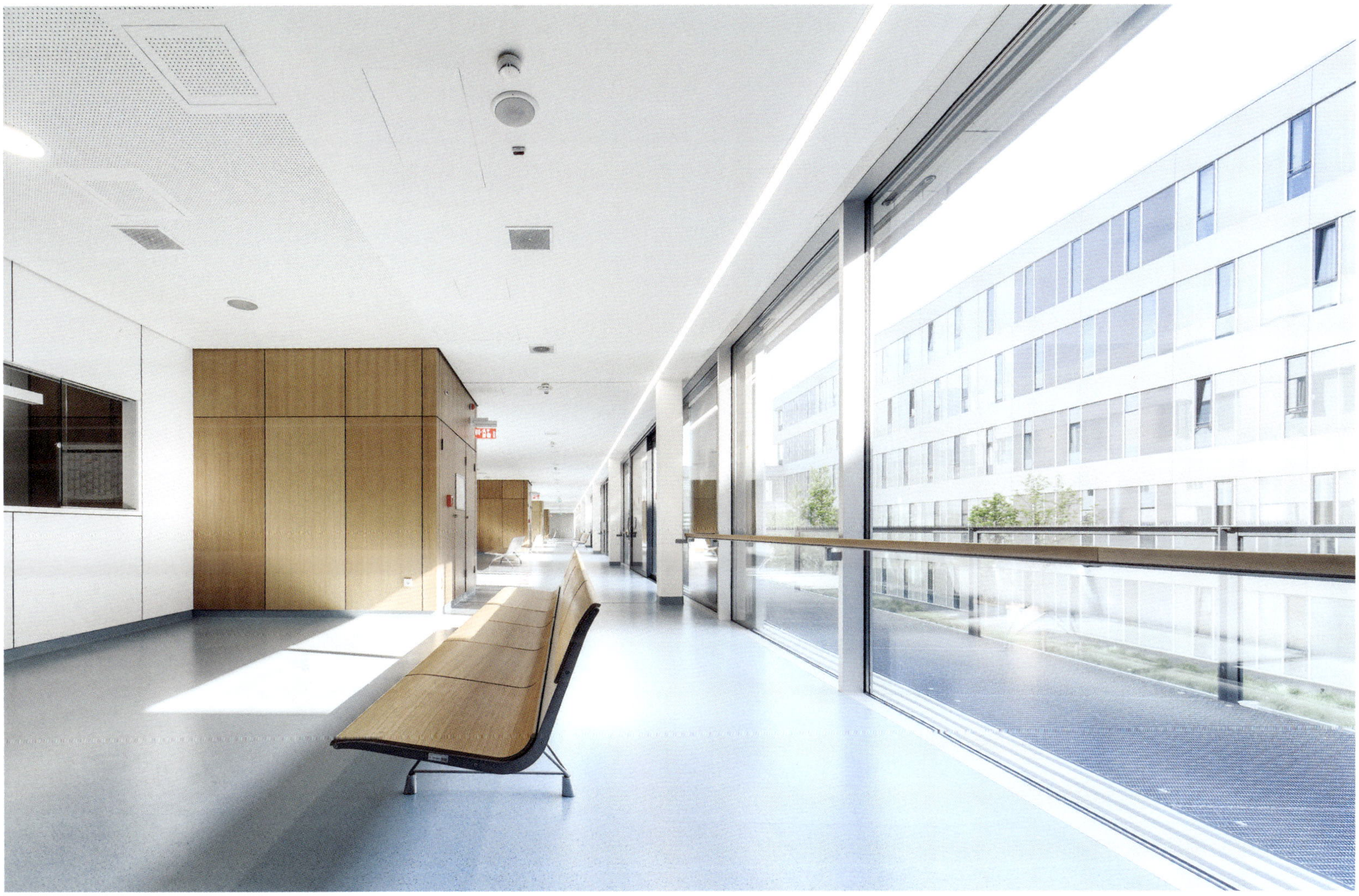

Outpatient waiting area.

Master plan.

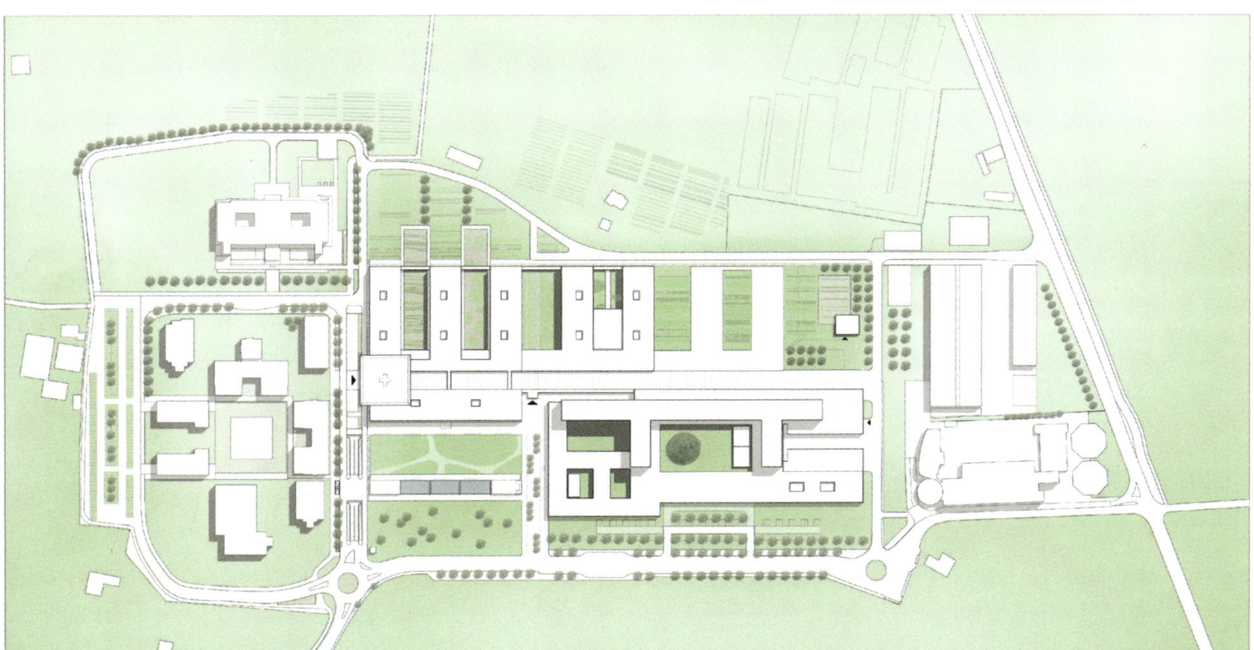

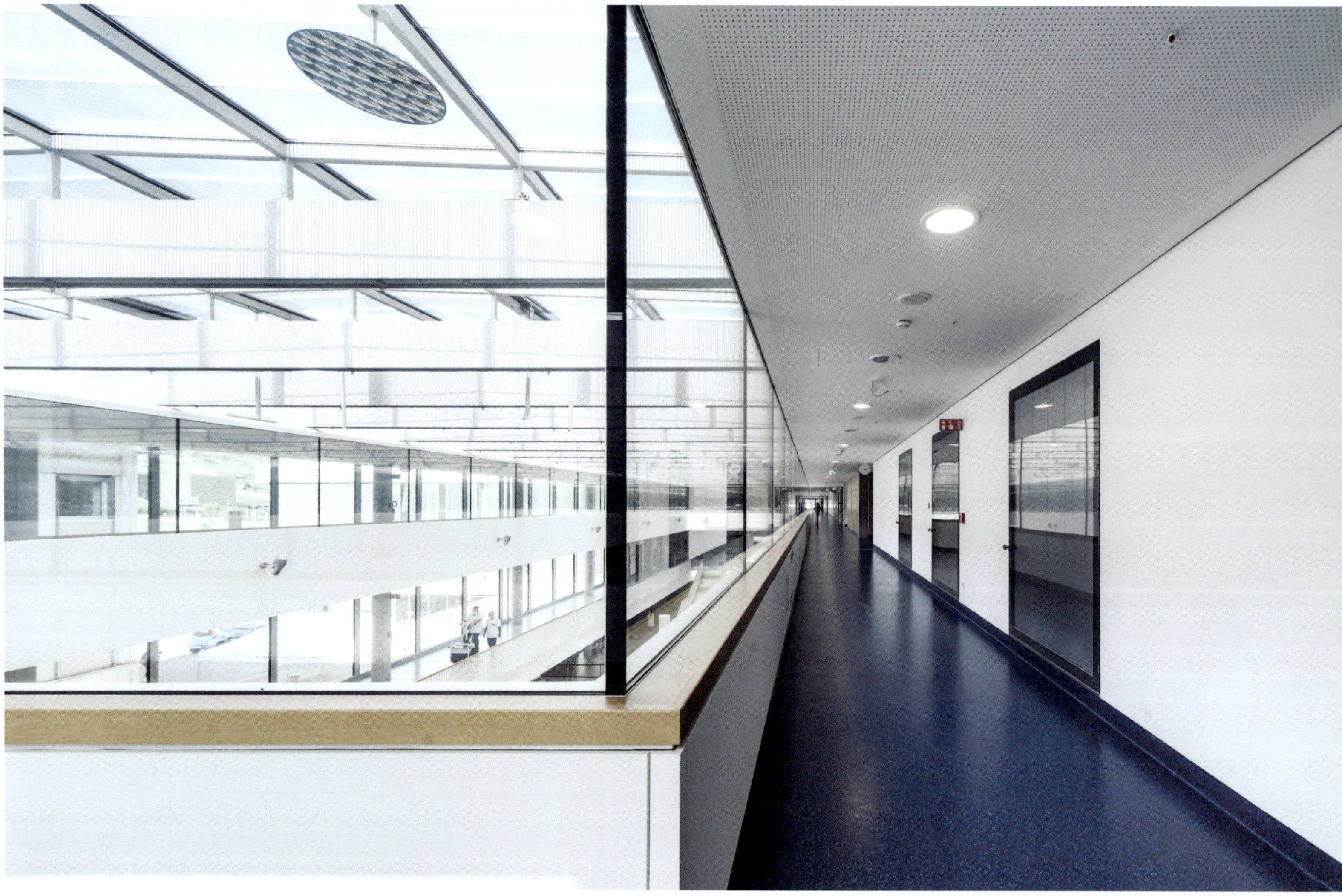

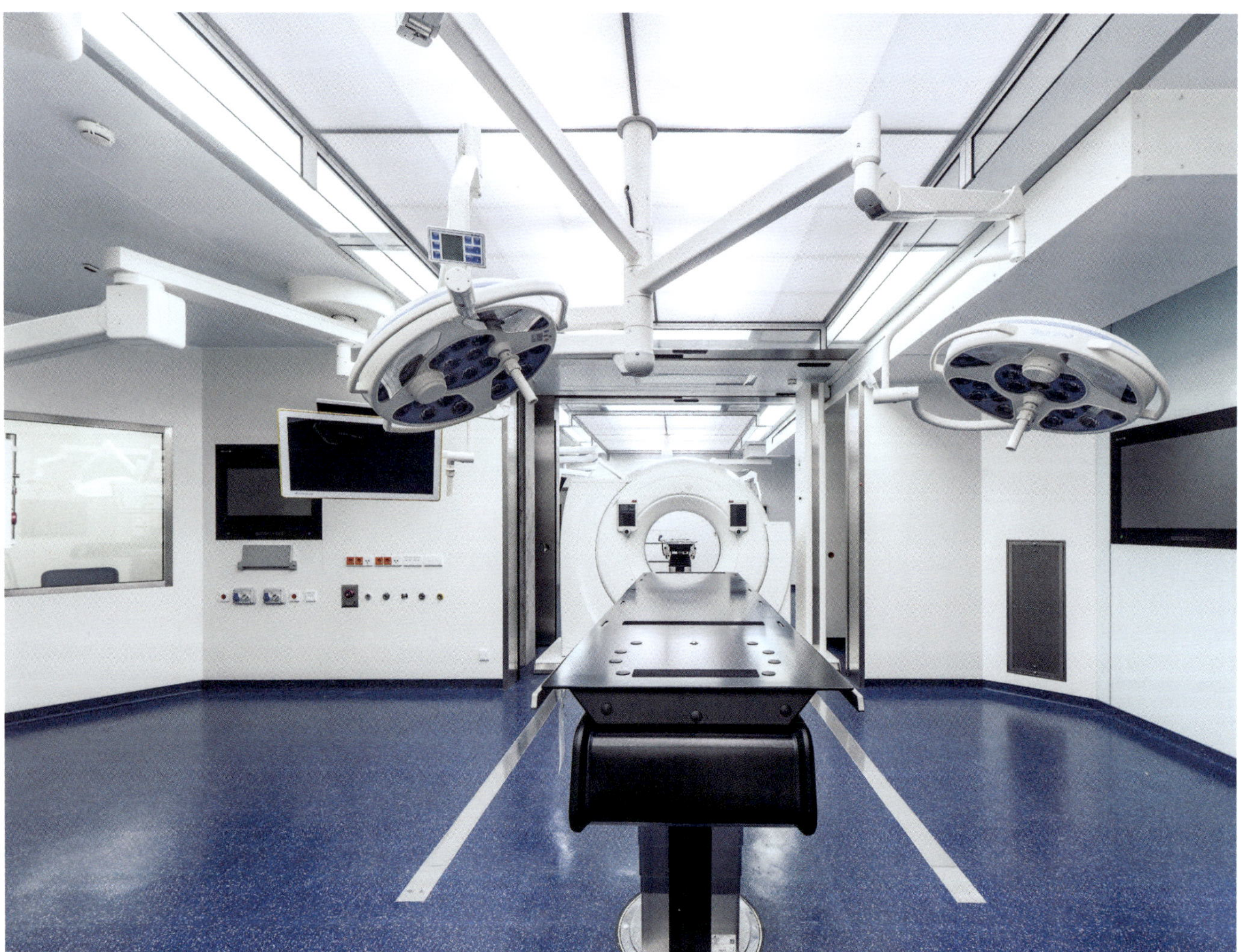

Connection ICU and operating department.

Operating room with CT scanner.

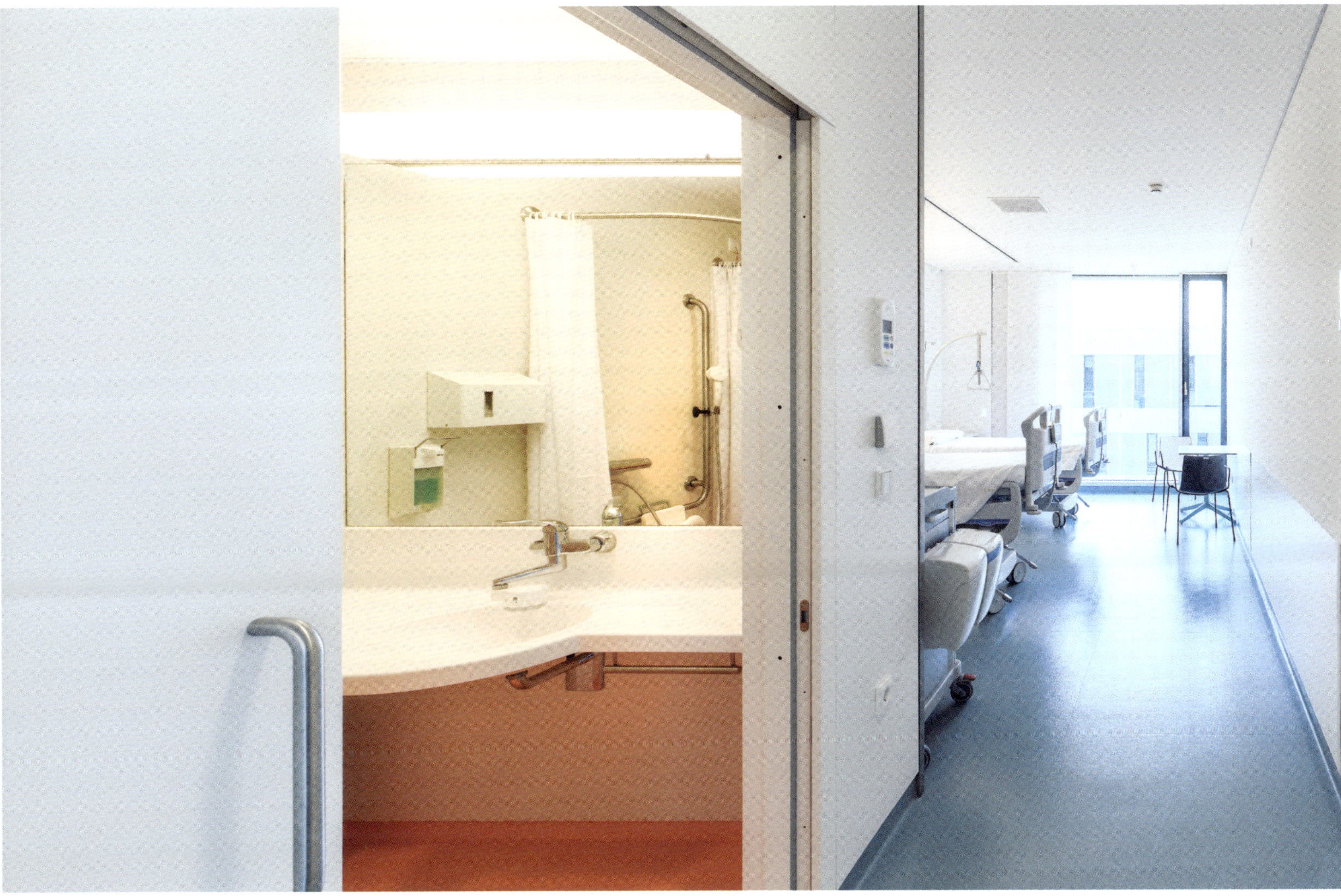

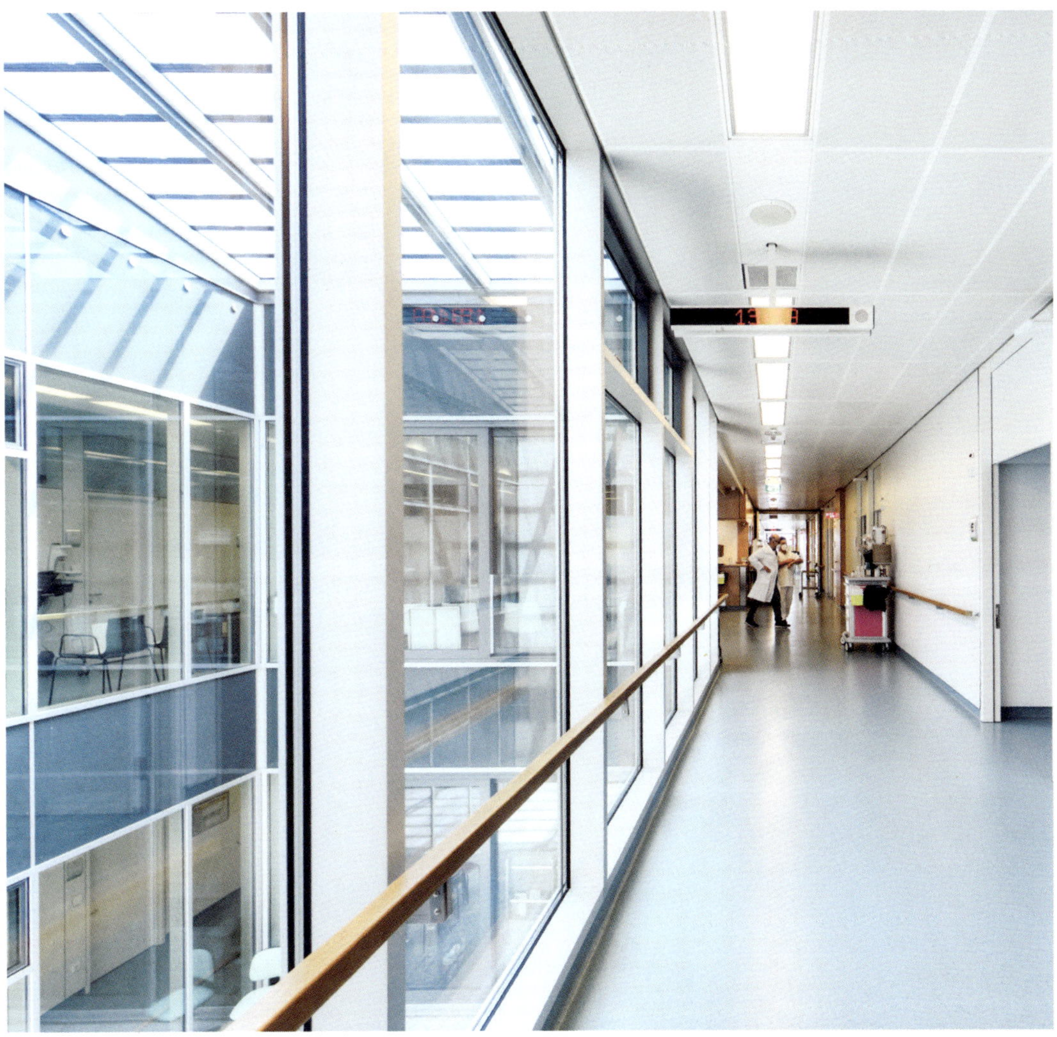

Patient room with en-suite bathroom.

Spacious and well lit corridor.

Studio Altieri

Kuwait City
Kuwait

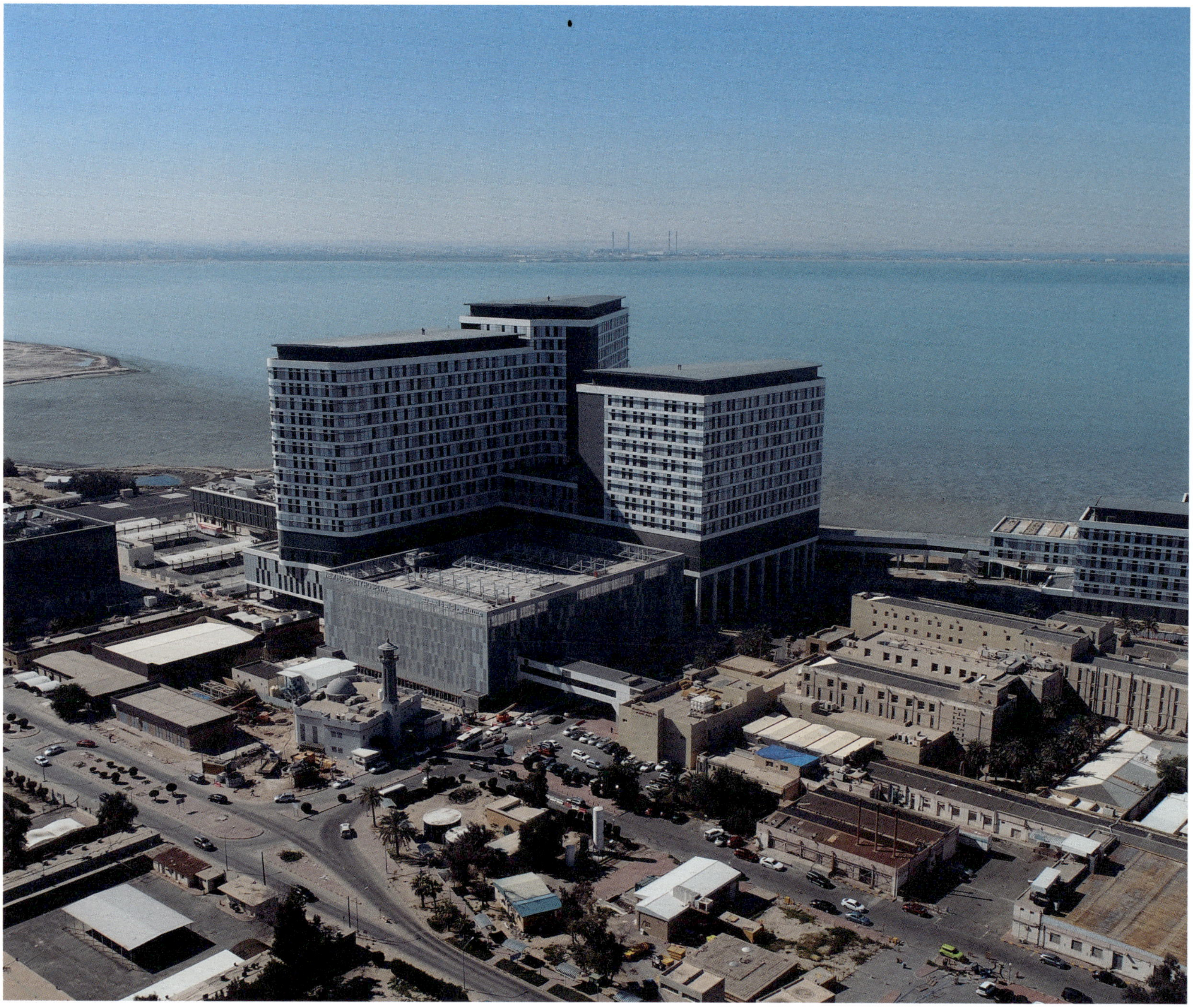

Landscape integration of the hospital.

Lateral aerial view.

Detail of the glass façade.

New Maternity Hospital – Kuwait

The New Maternity Hospital in Kuwait City is a cutting-edge facility for maternal and neonatal care, with 780 beds, 27 operating theaters, and 60 labor and delivery rooms. Soaring inpatient towers rise from a dense clinical podium, connecting seamlessly to outpatient clinics, parking, and a multi-level entry atrium. Situated on the coast of Kuwait Bay, the design maximizes sea views for 70 percent of rooms, while landscaped pedestrian paths and triangular flowerbeds draw visitors' gaze toward the water. The expansive outdoor areas are organized into thematic zones with gardens, seating, and refreshment spaces, creating a public environment that celebrates new life and welcomes the large family visitations that accompany births. In this harsh desert climate, the building envelope is carefully engineered to optimize insulation and solar control.

Address: Shuwaikh, Al Sabah Medical District, Kuwait City, Kuwait | **Client:** Ministry of Public Works of Kuwait | **Completion:** 2024 | **Size:** 351,300 m² | **Sector:** state | **Specialization:** obstetrics, gynecology, and neonatology | **Number of treatment rooms:** 27 | **Number of patient rooms:** 540

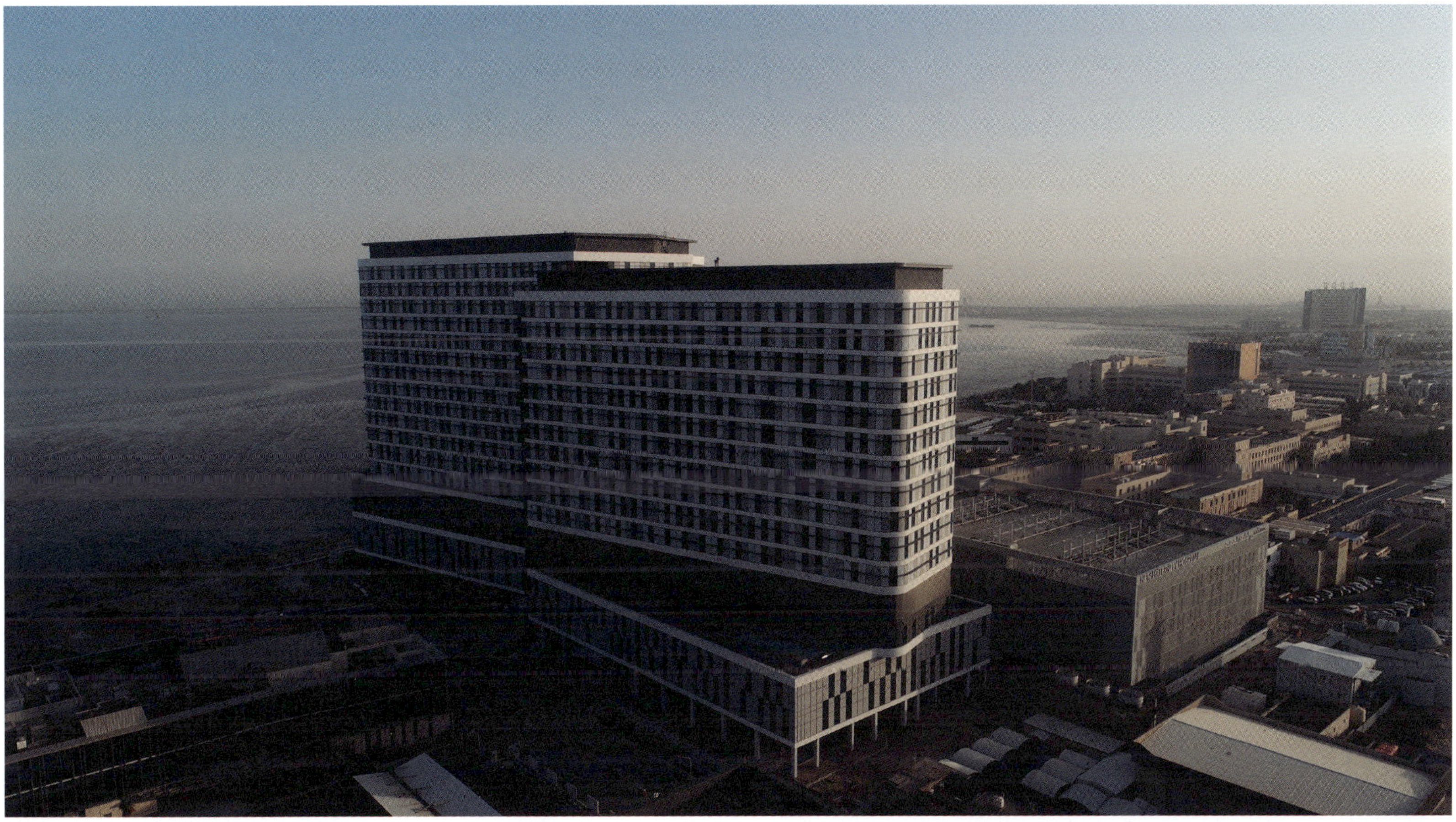

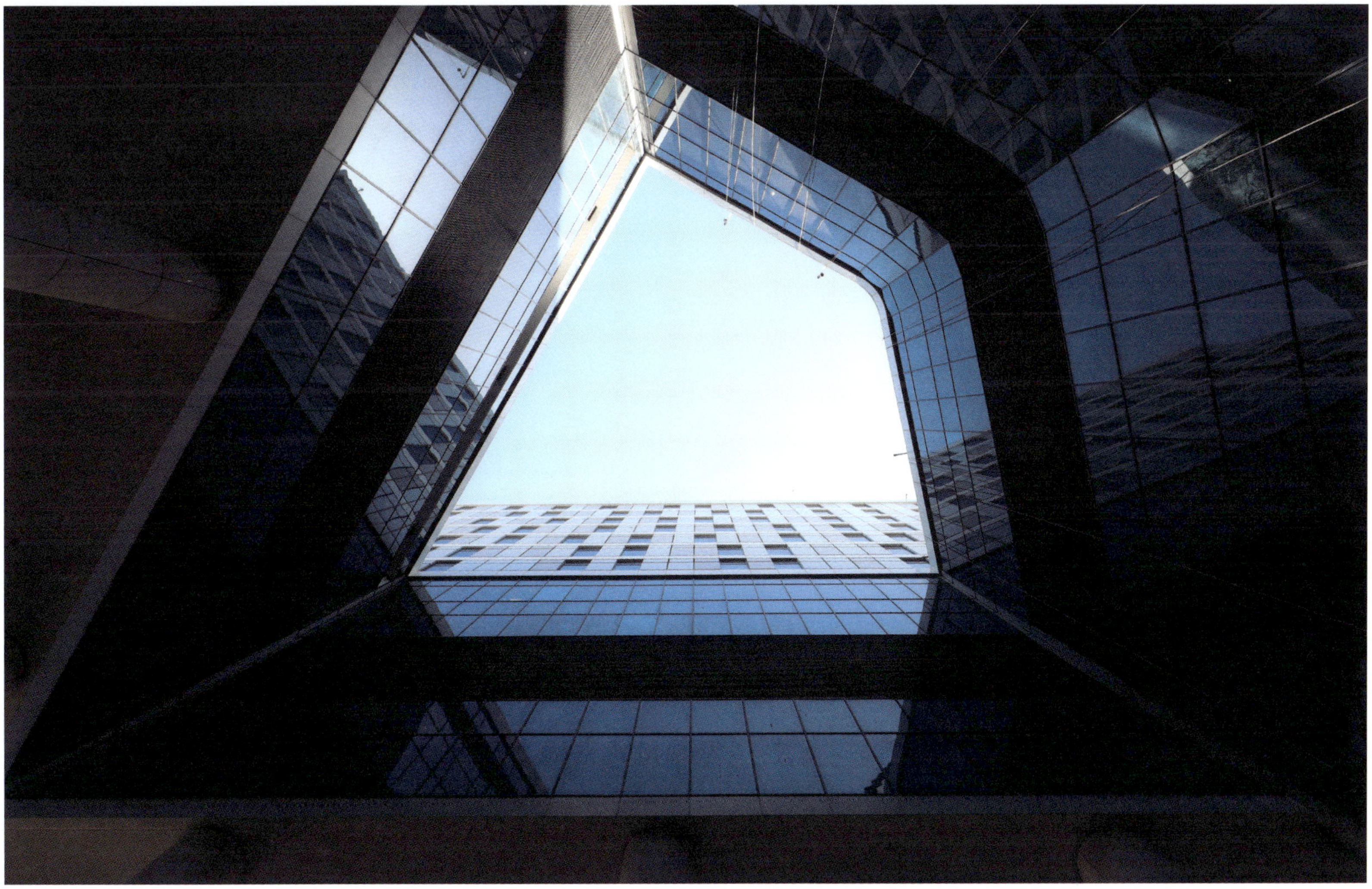

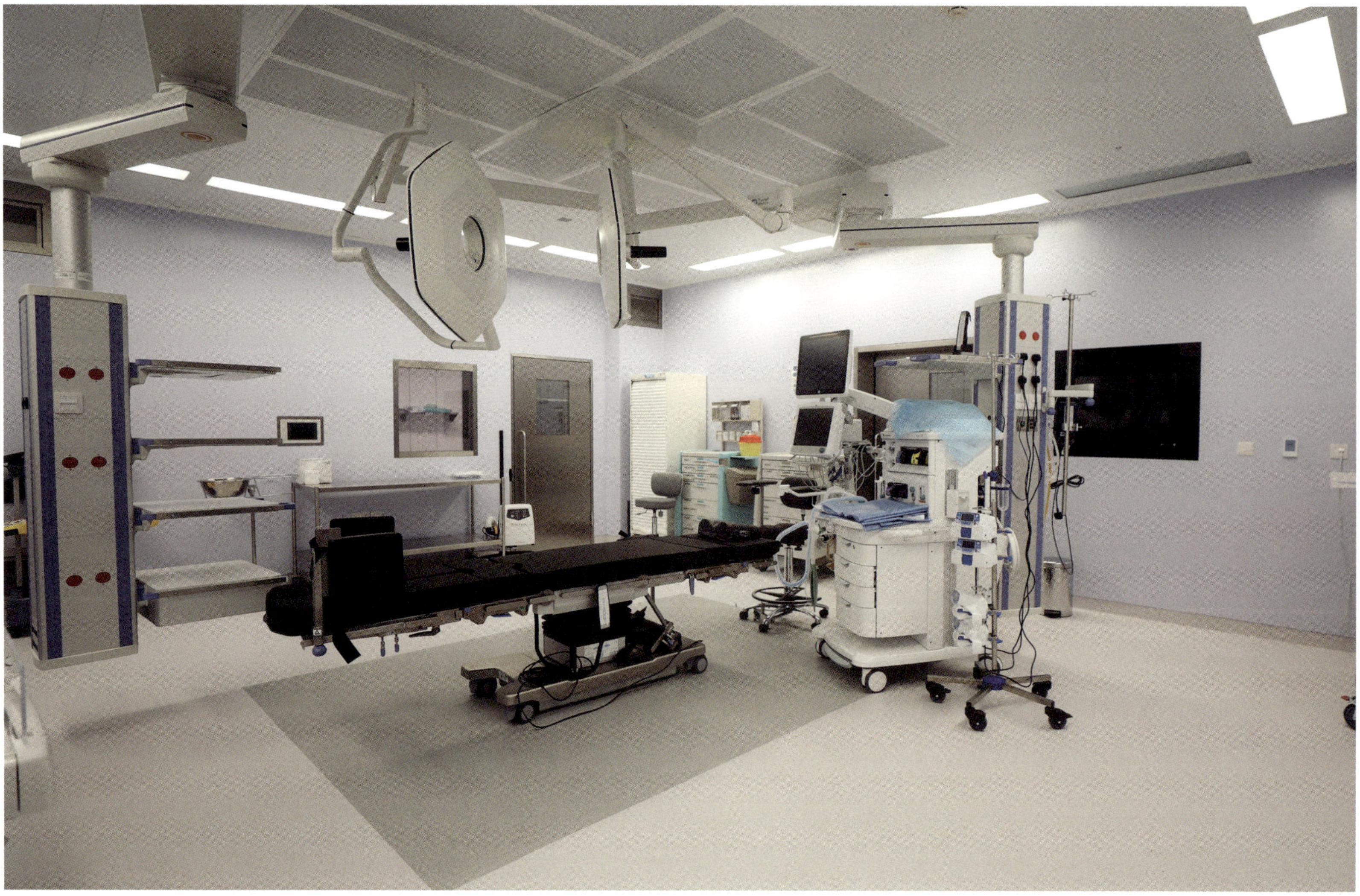

Hospital's fully-equipped operation theater.

Third floor plan – surgical block.

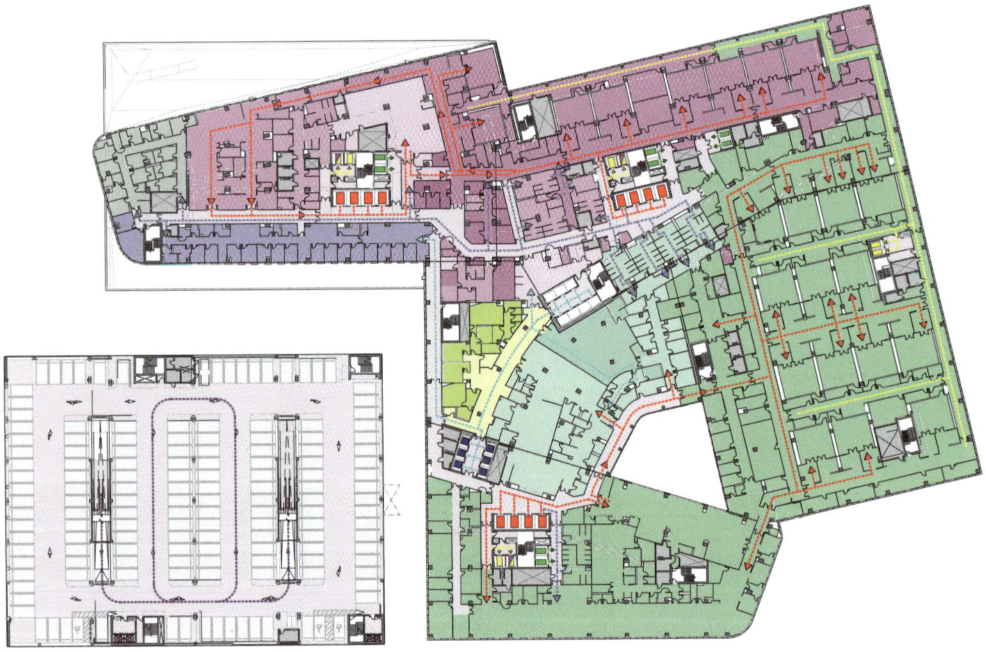

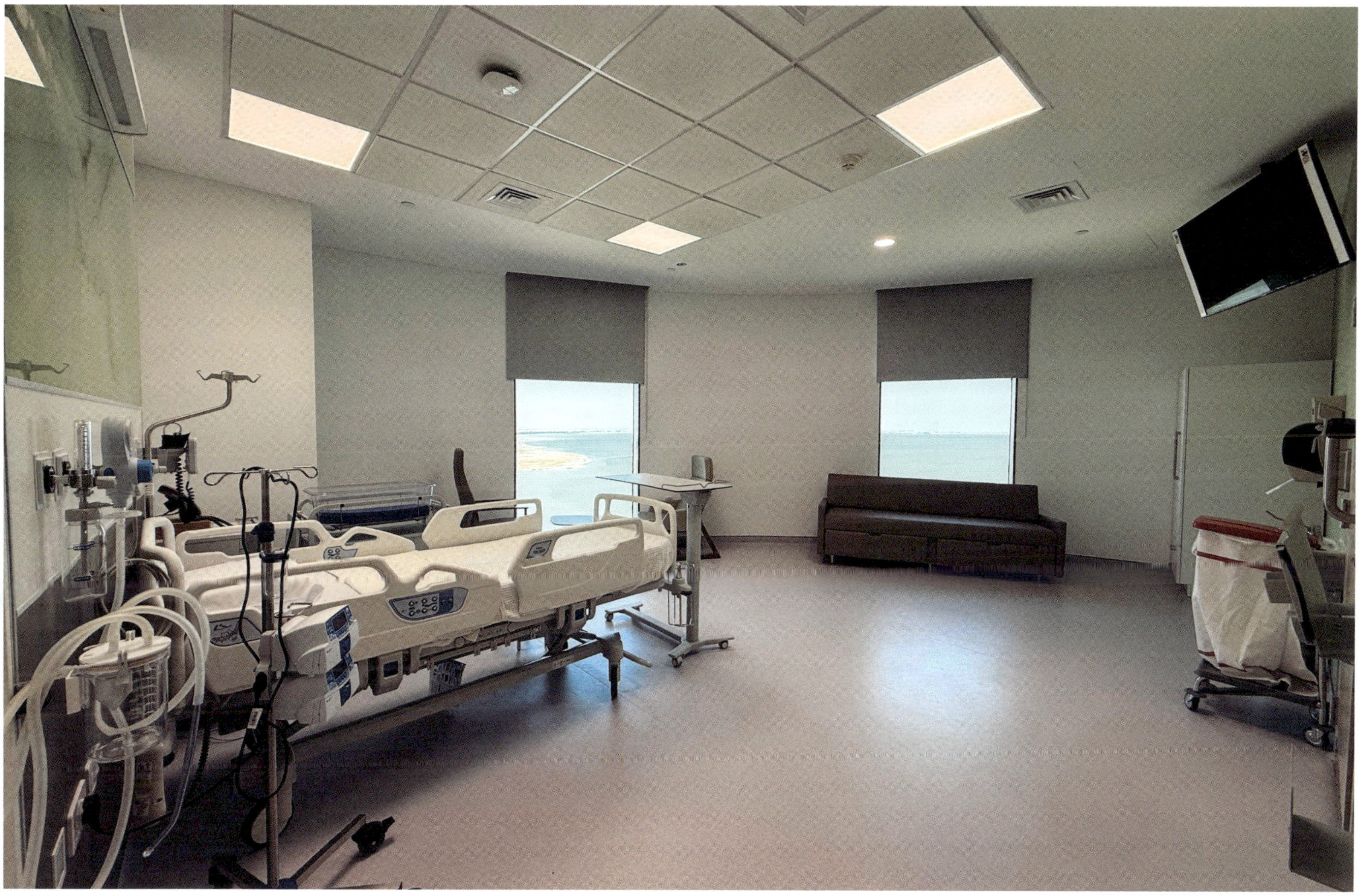

Postpartum room with full-height windows and sea view.

Typical ward plan.

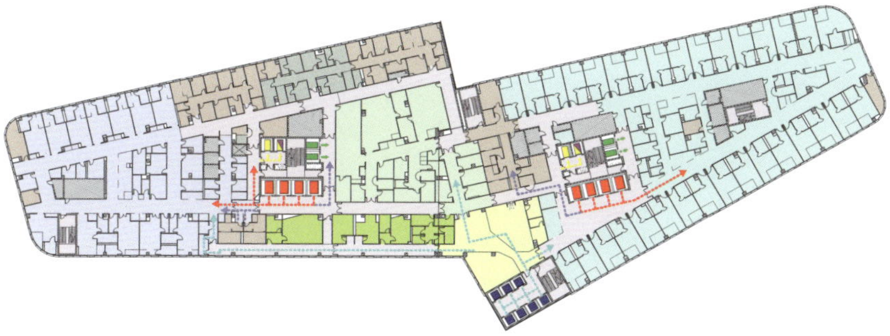

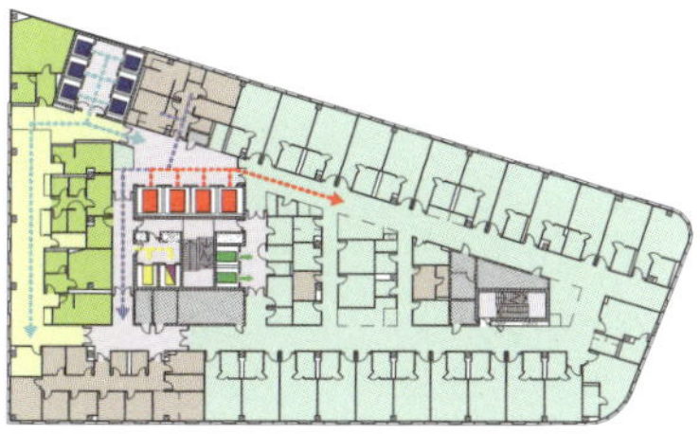

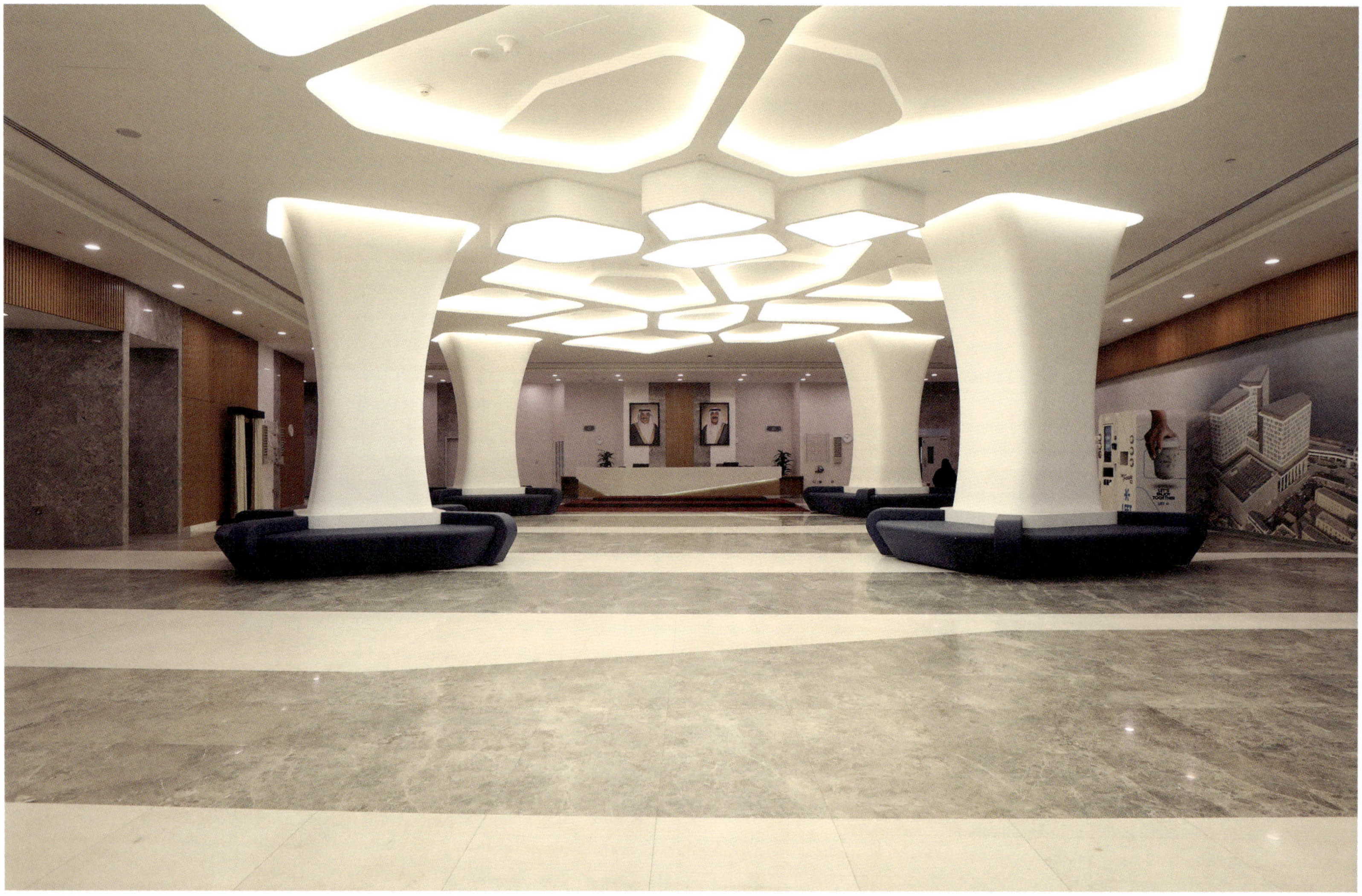

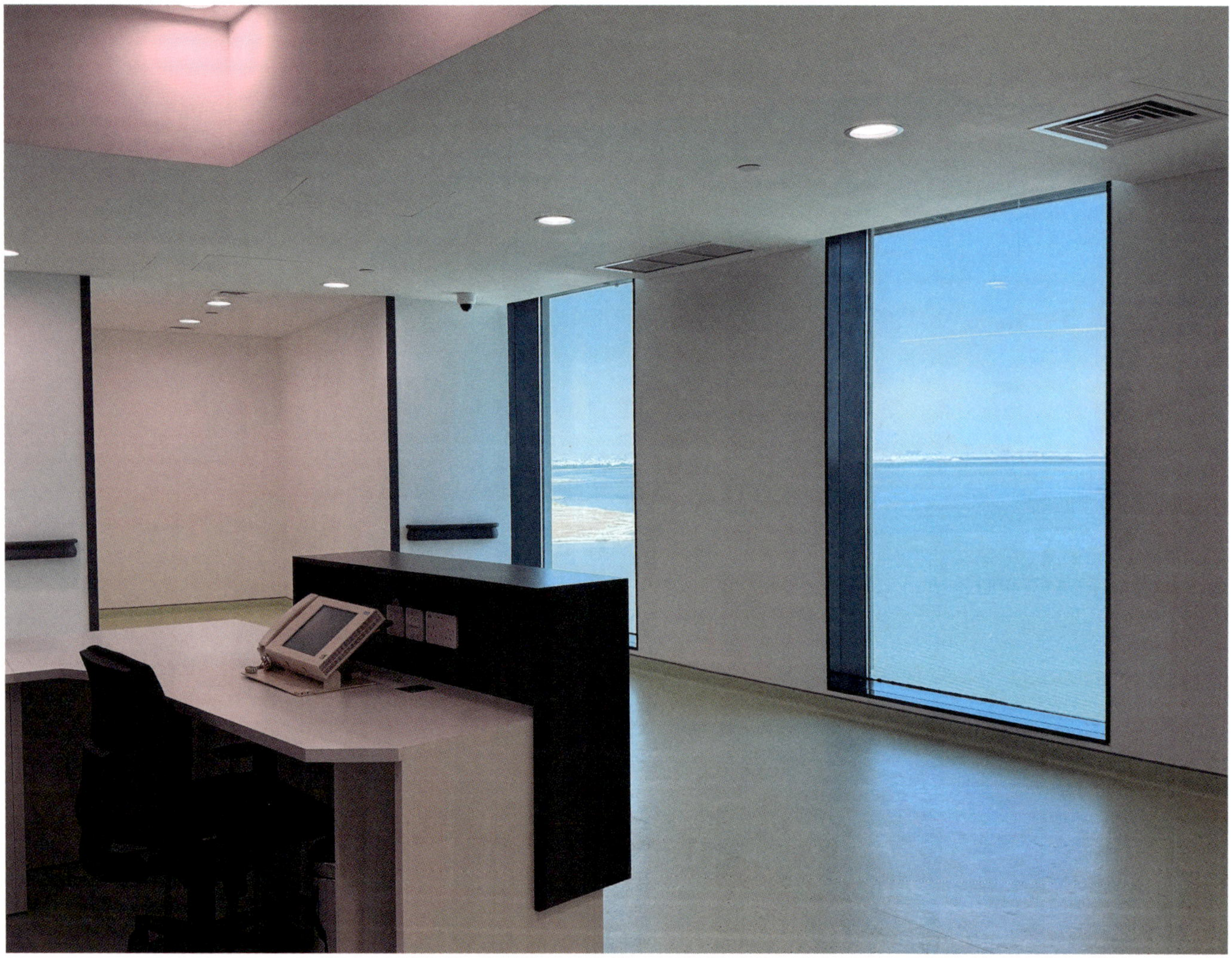

View from the main entrance court.

Nurse station with full-height windows and sea view.

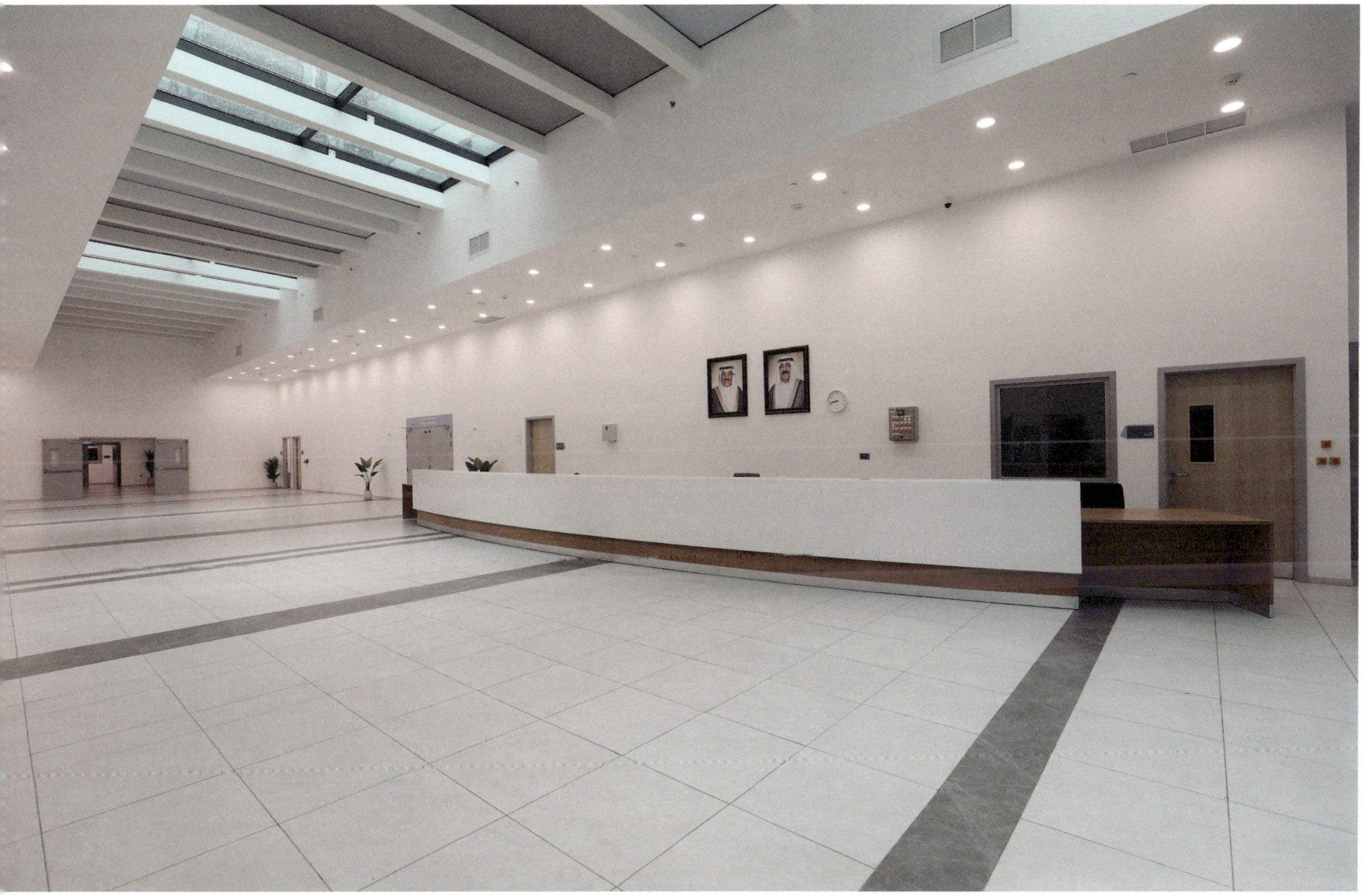

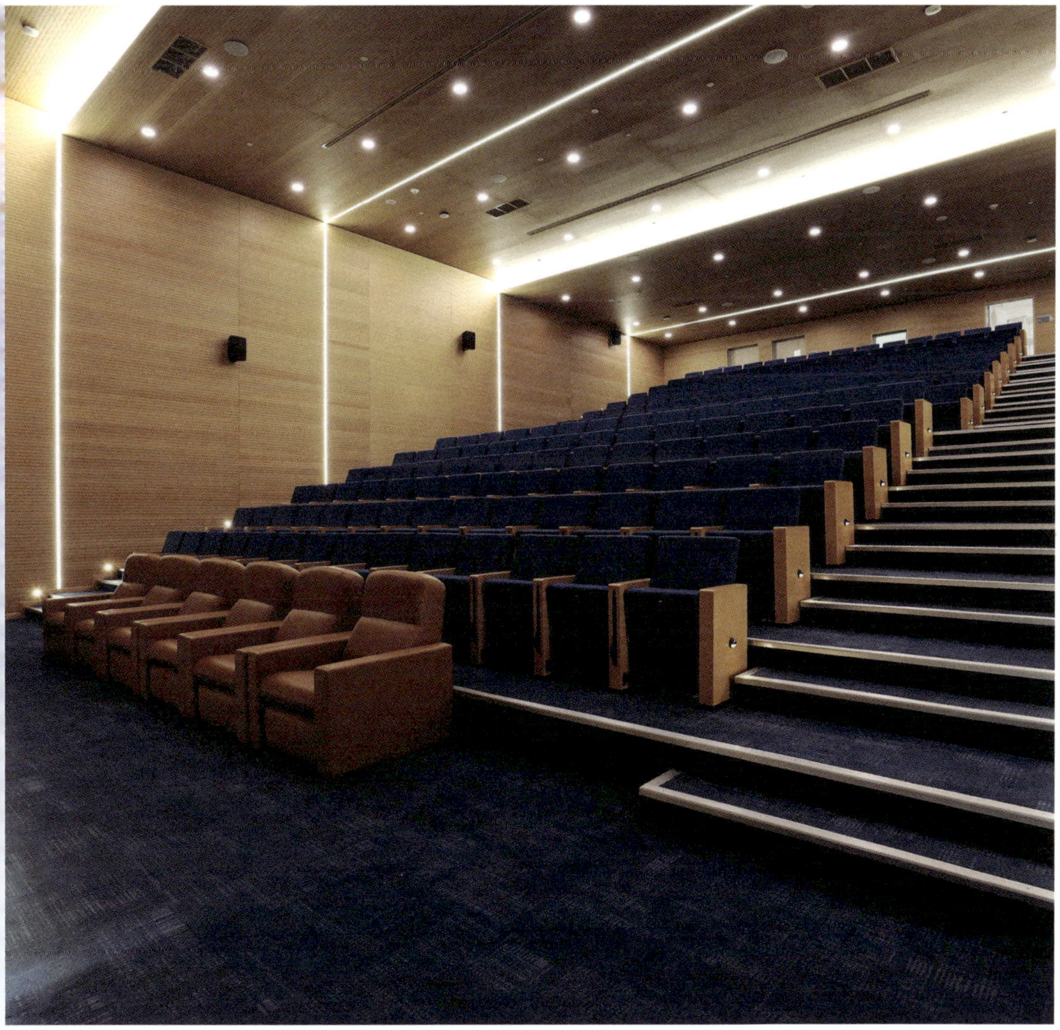

Outpatient clinic main entrance.

Hospital's auditorium.

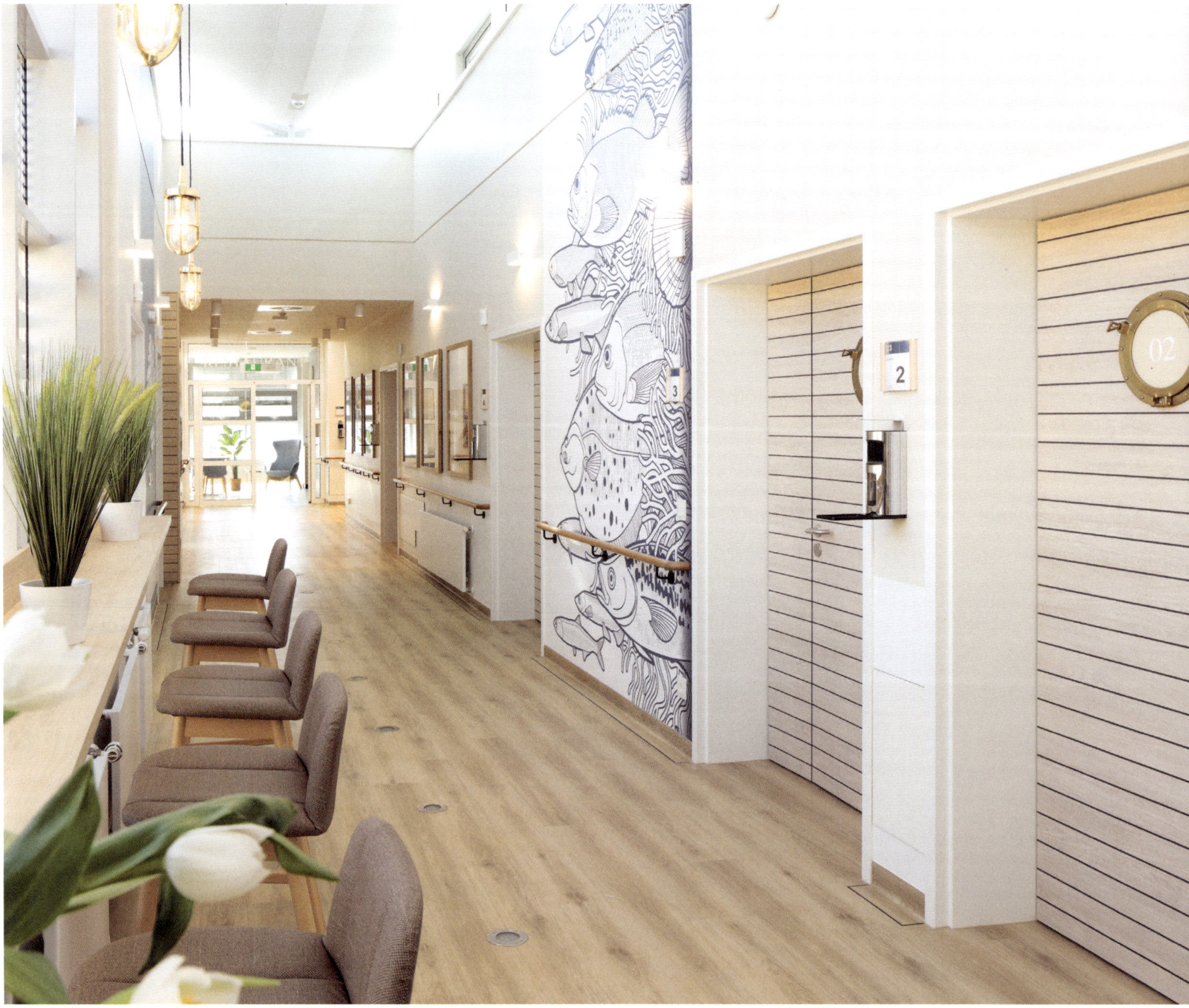

Spacious corridor with beautiful interiors.

Hospital's nursing station and common room.

Interdisciplinary Ward 11.2 B

The new Interdisciplinary Ward 11.2 B at Greifswald University Hospital was realized by space4life association, with ppm planung + projekt management GmbH as general contractor and in collaboration with partners KEUCO, Gira, and Häfele. This place combines medical excellence with emotional well-being – through architecture, design, and atmosphere. Even in the concept phase, it was clear that this ward should be more than just a functional space. A design concept inspired by maritime themes had been developed: sand and blue tones that radiate calm and depth; ship-style flooring, portholes, and brass details – elegant references to boat building – combined with sophisticated lighting and carefully selected materials that connect function with emotion. Bright, open spaces with clean lines, abundant daylight, and thoughtfully designed furnishings create an environment that offers both comfort and orientation.

Address: Fleischmannstraße 10, 17489 Greifswald, Germany | **Client:** Greifswald University Hospital | **Completion:** 2025 | **Size:** 750 m² | **Sector:** state | **Specialization:** interdisciplinary elective services ward | **Number of patient rooms:** 10

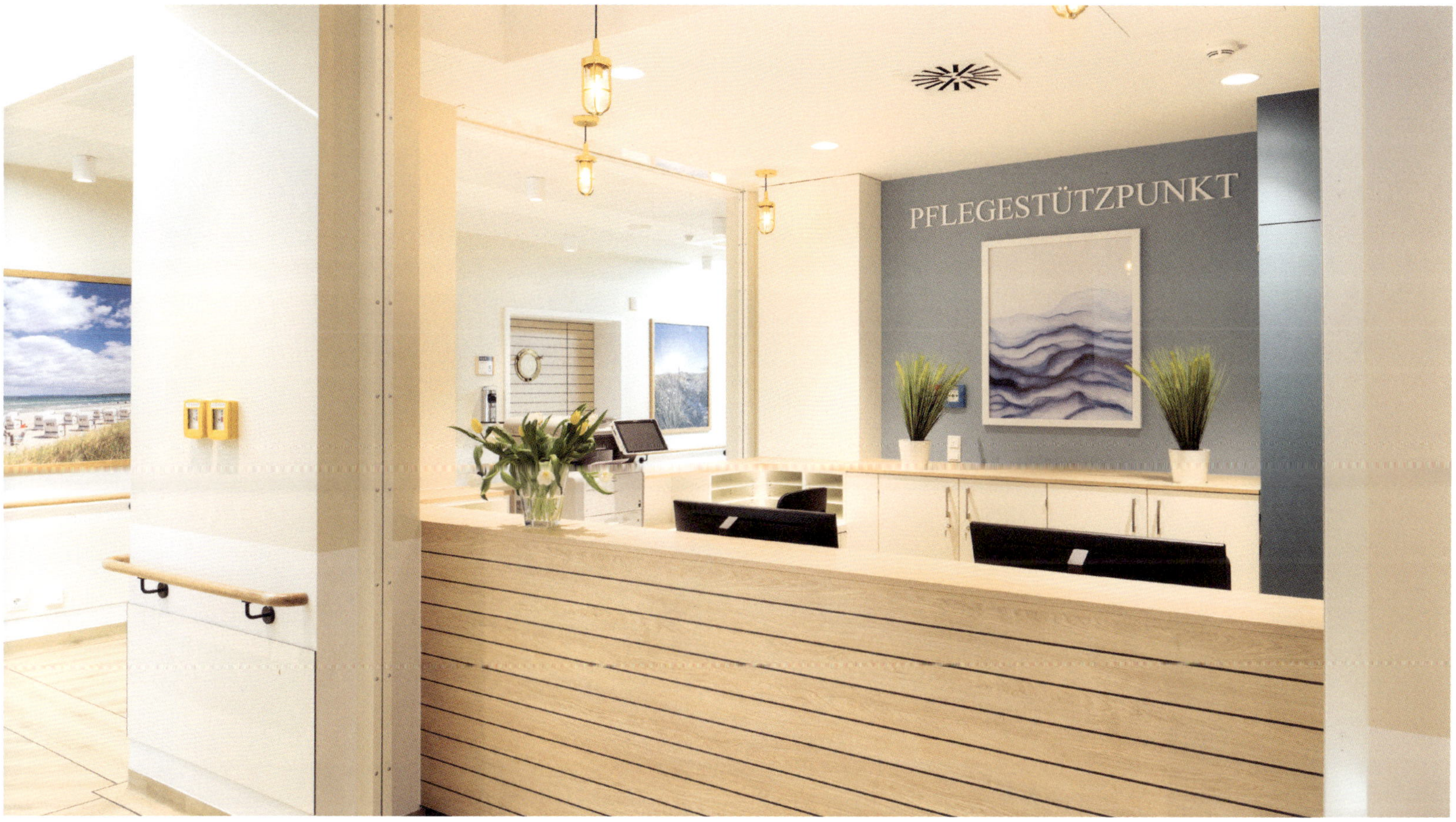

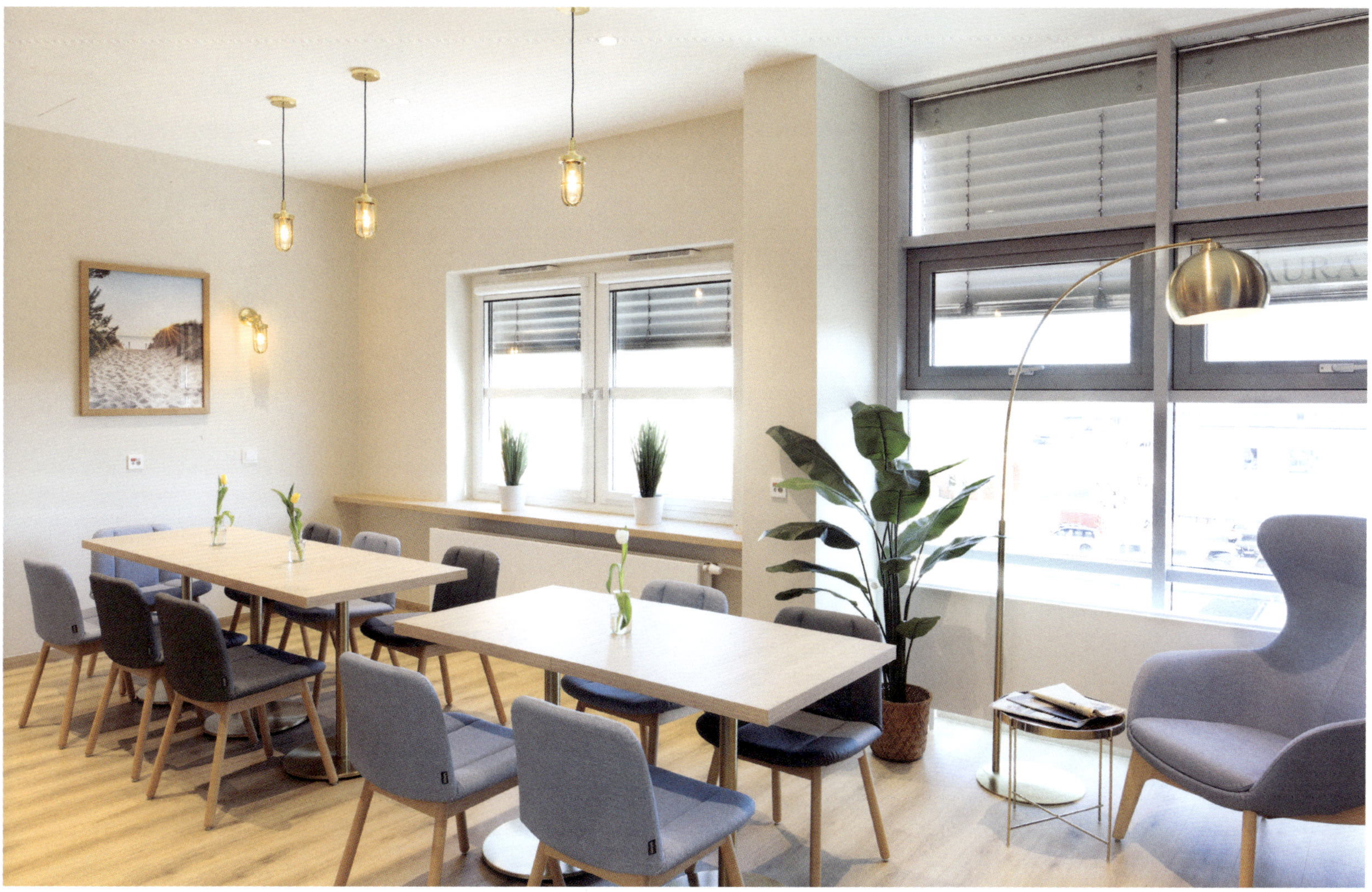

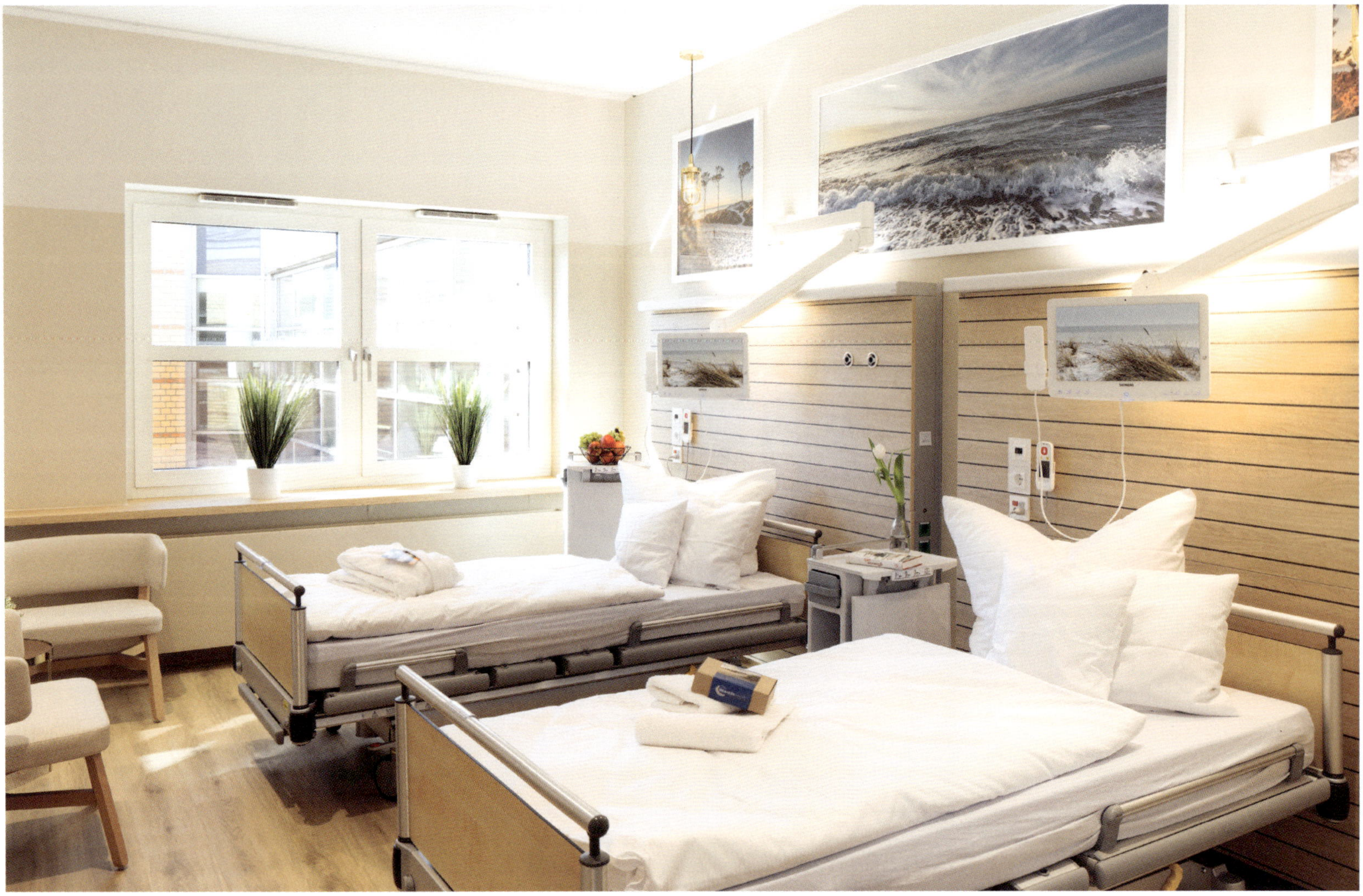

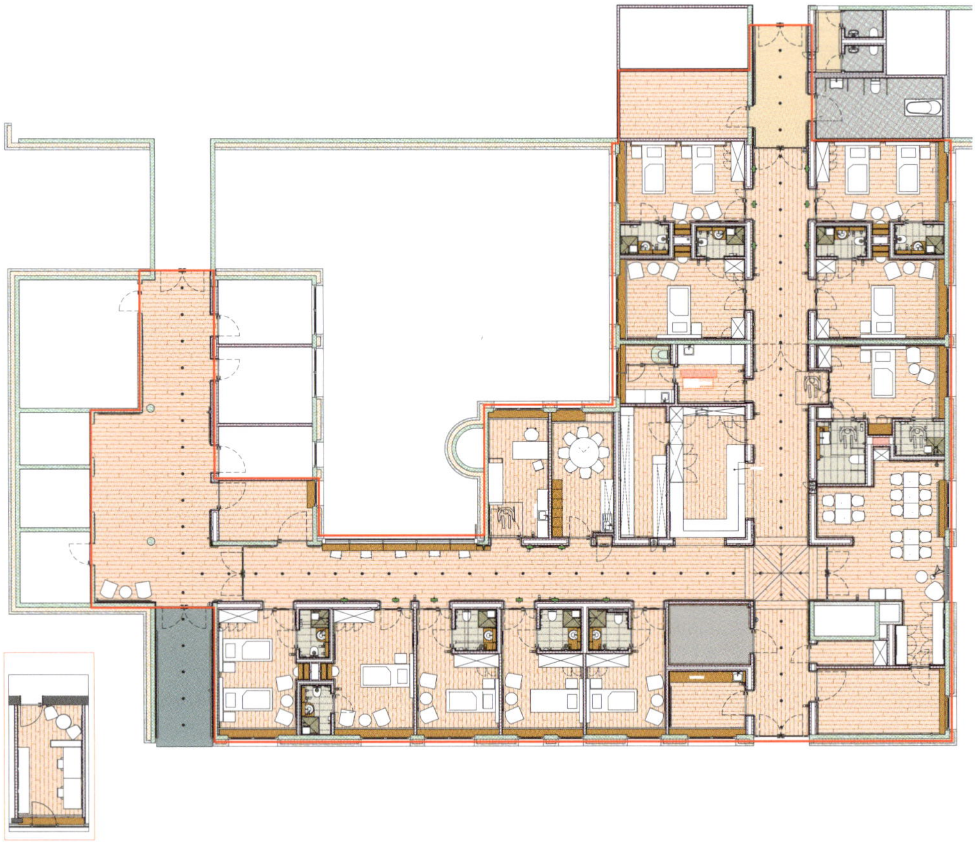

Tastefully designed twin patient's room.

Room layout plan after renovation.

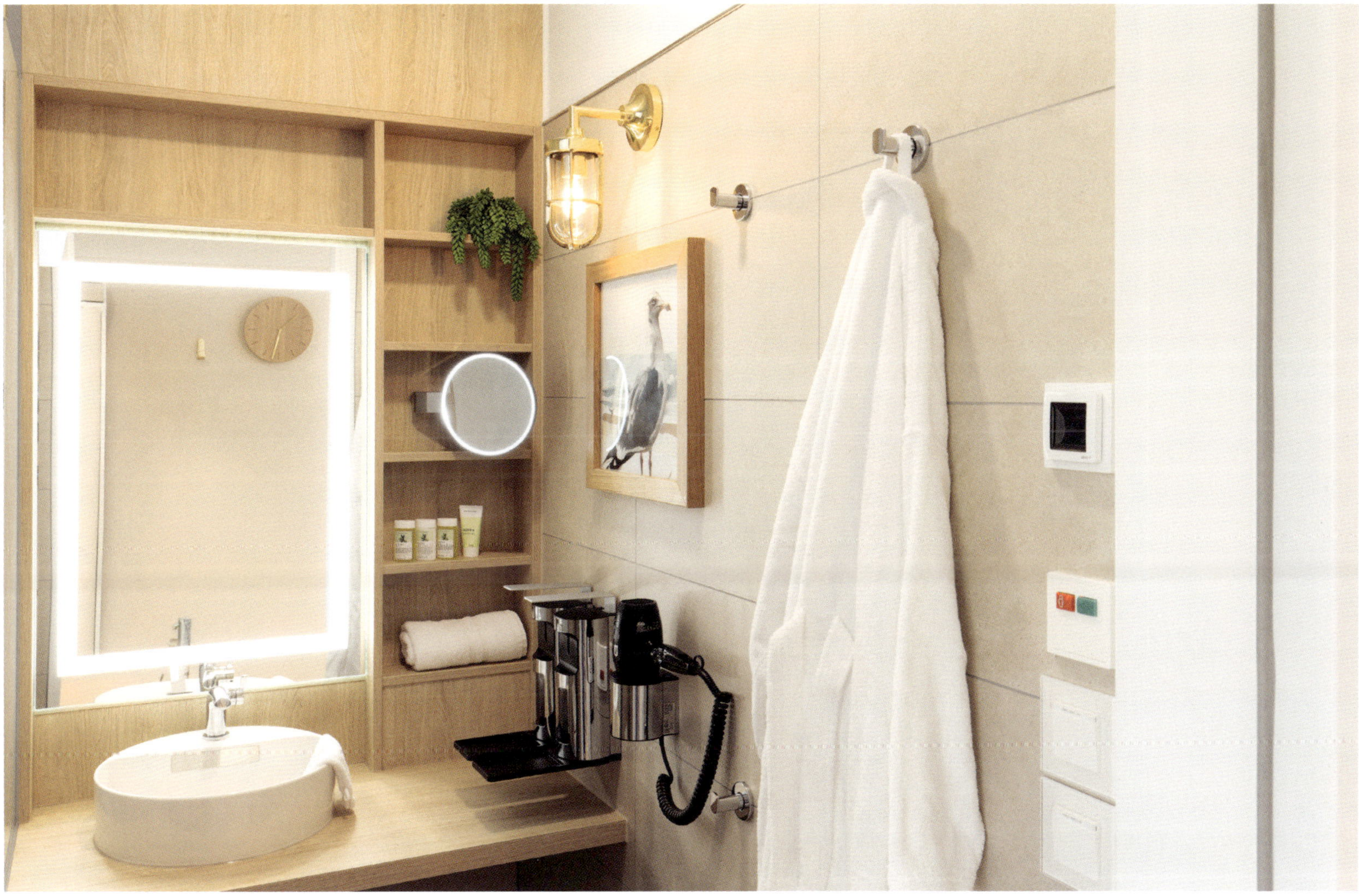

Fully renovated and modern bathroom.

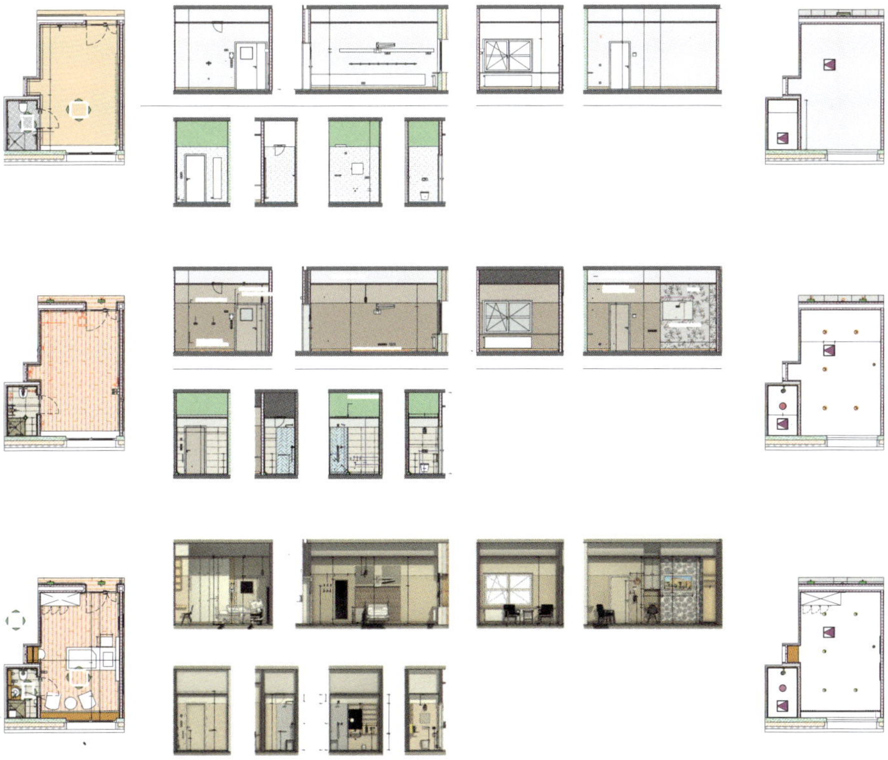

Patient's room floor plan.

EGM architects
JKMM Architects

Jyväskylä
Finland

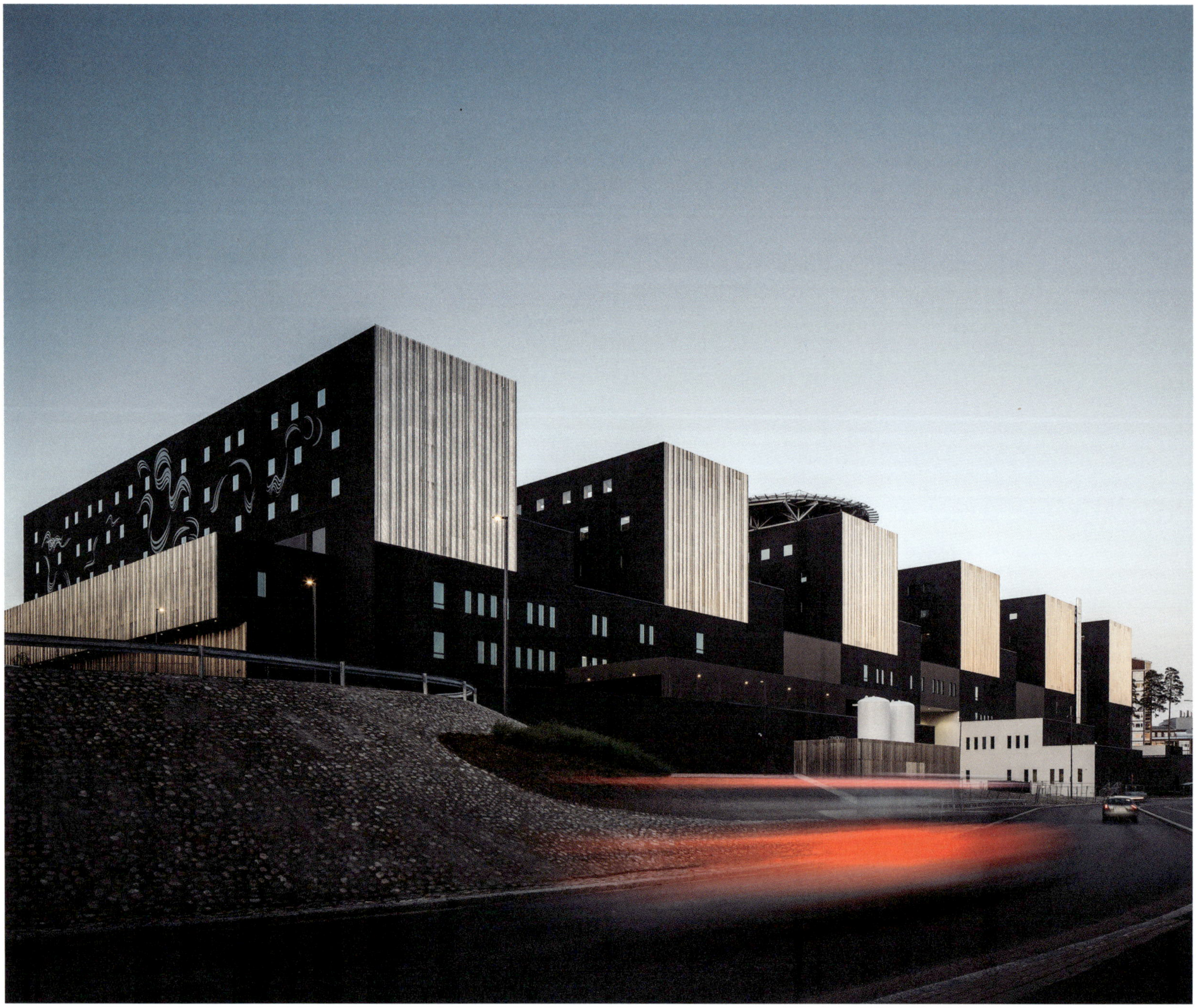

Exterior view of the building volumes.

Atrium hall with waiting area and light installation.

Hospital Nova

The KSSHP Hospital Nova is located in central Finland and is the first entirely new hospital to be built in Finland in the last 20 years. At the core of the project lies a patient-centered philosophy that translates into spatial clarity and experiential quality. It aims to actively involve patients in their care, providing a healing environment for rehabilitation. Its design speaks a clear yet touchingly soothing language. The 450-beds hospital offers nearly all medical specialities, education, research, and includes 24 operating theaters including a hybrid theater. Despite its scale, the design is compact with a clear layout and human scale, is highly sustainable, and integrates advanced technologies such as a fully automated waste-transport system and an automated trolley system for logistics. Hospital Nova is designed by JKMM Architects in collaboration with EGM architects.

Address: Hoitajantie 3, 40620 Jyväskylä, Finland | **Client:** Keski-Suomen sairaanhoitopiiri | **Completion:** 2020 | **Size:** 102,000 m² | **Sector:** public | **Number of patient rooms:** 383

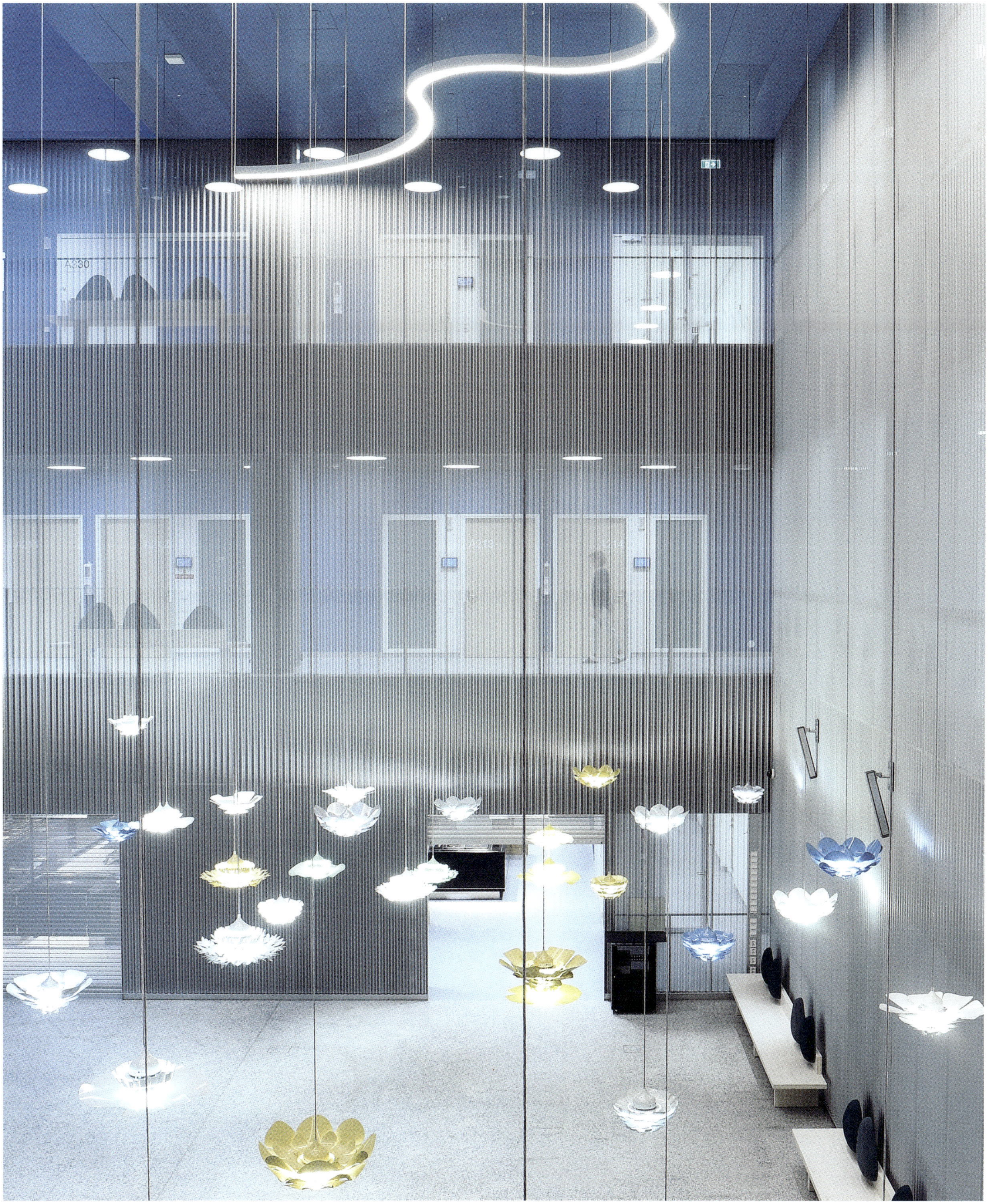

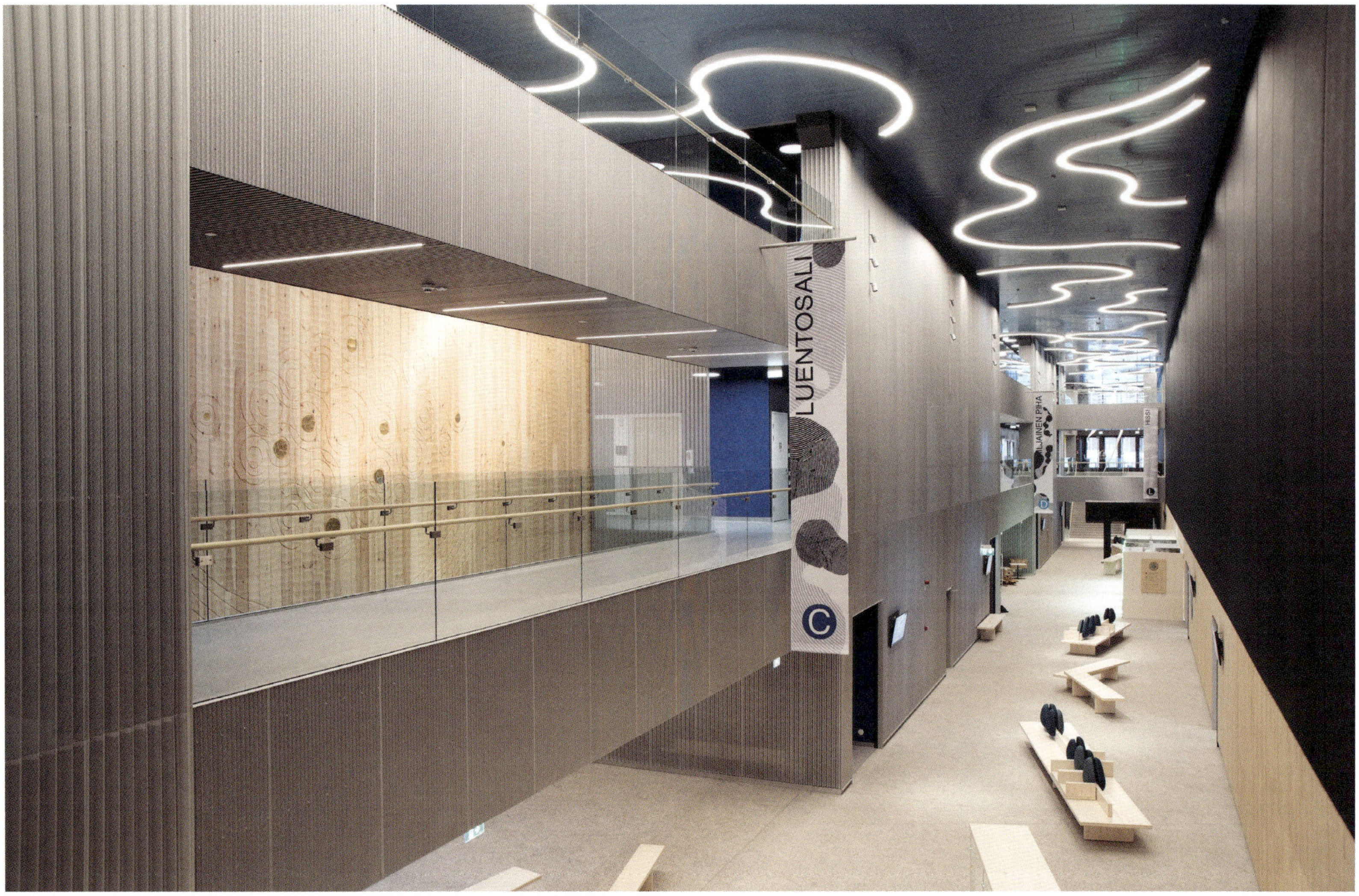

Main passage with gallery.

Ground floor plan.

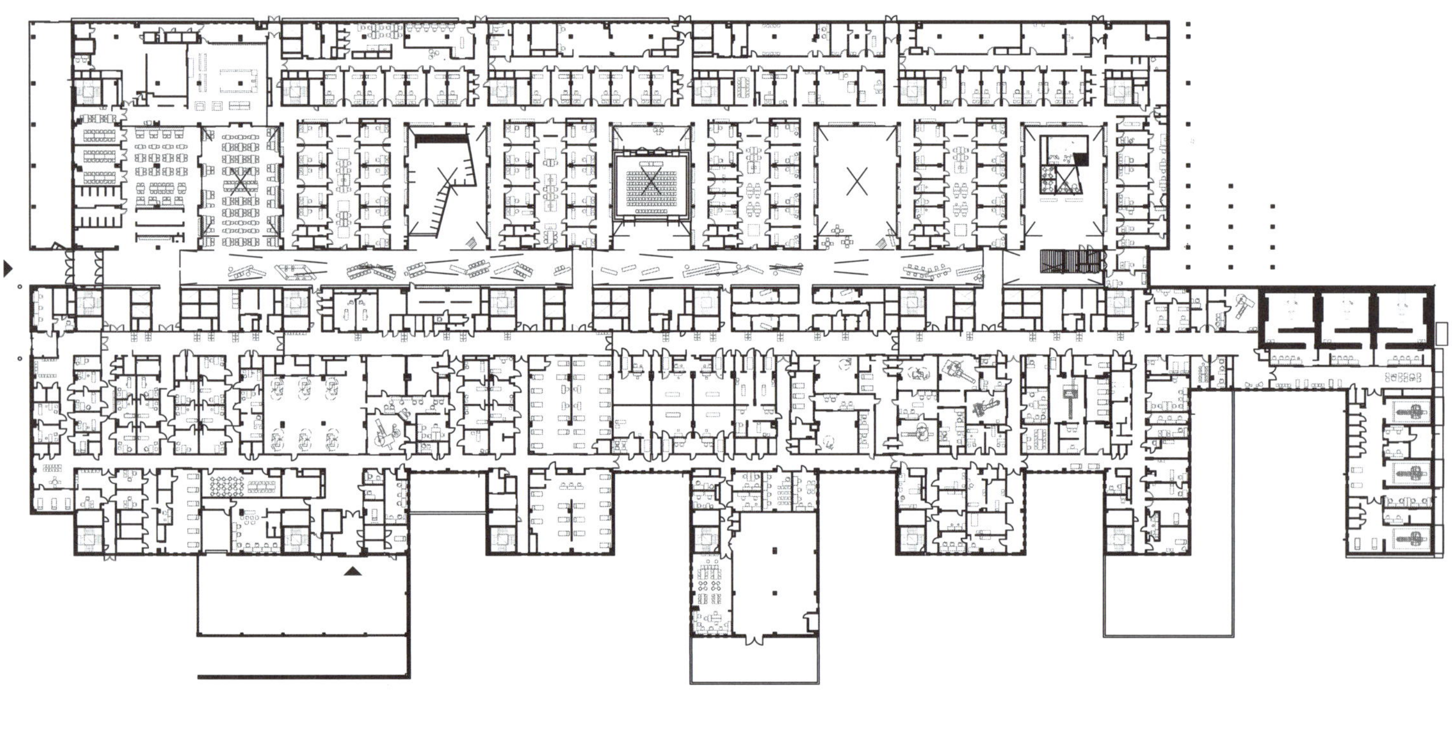

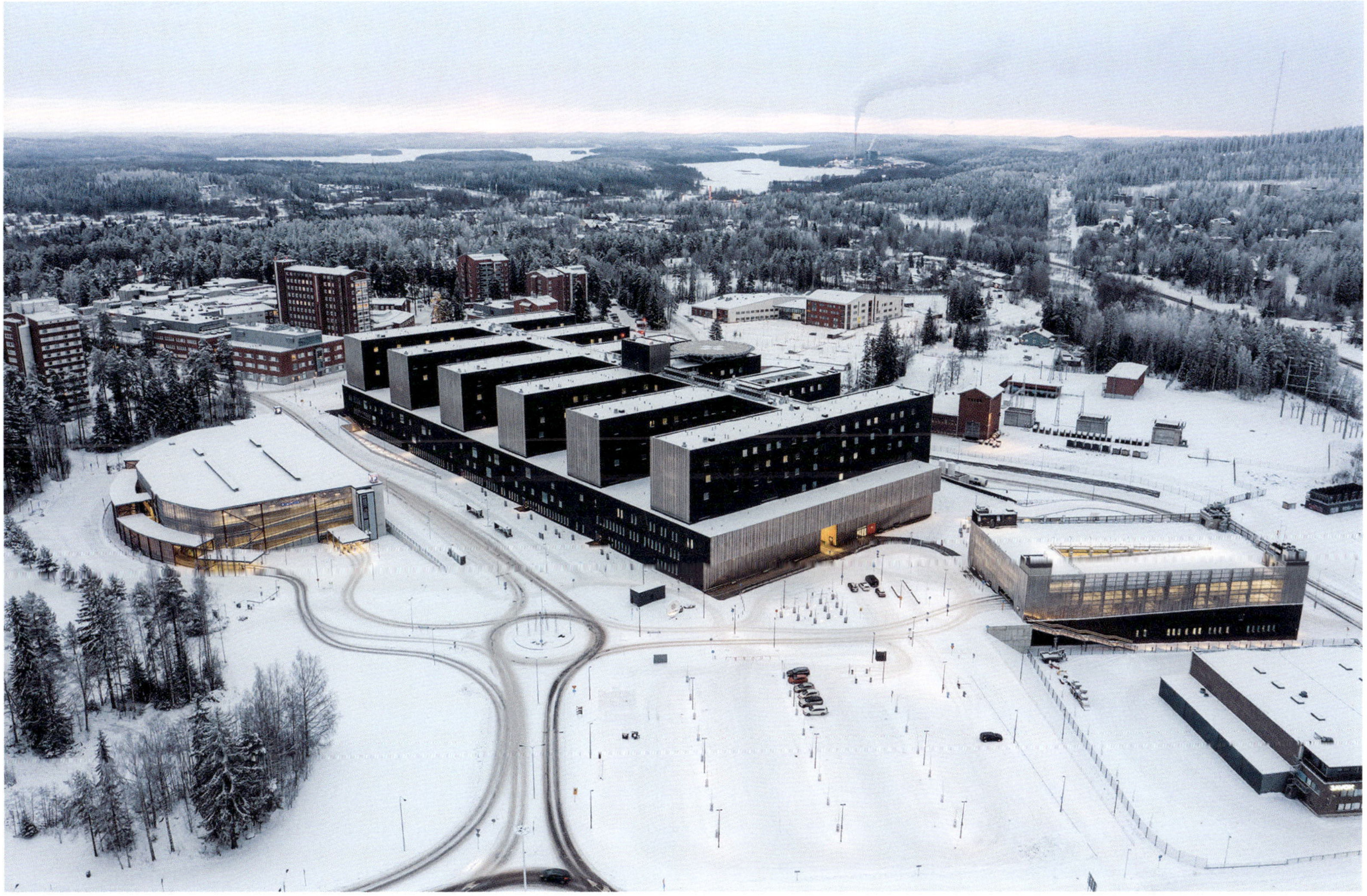

Bird's-eye view of the building.

Pictogram illustrating the composition of the building.

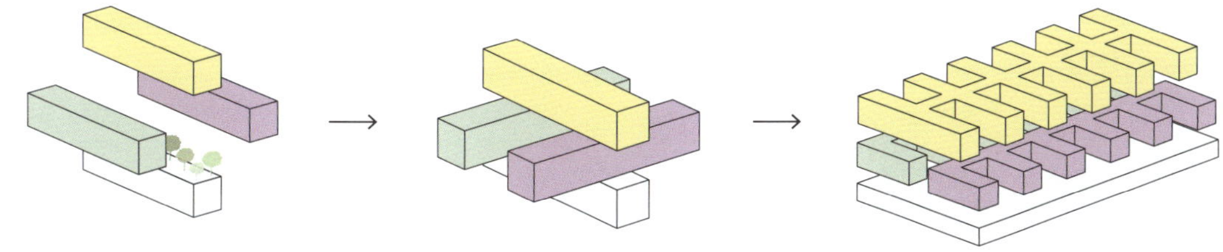

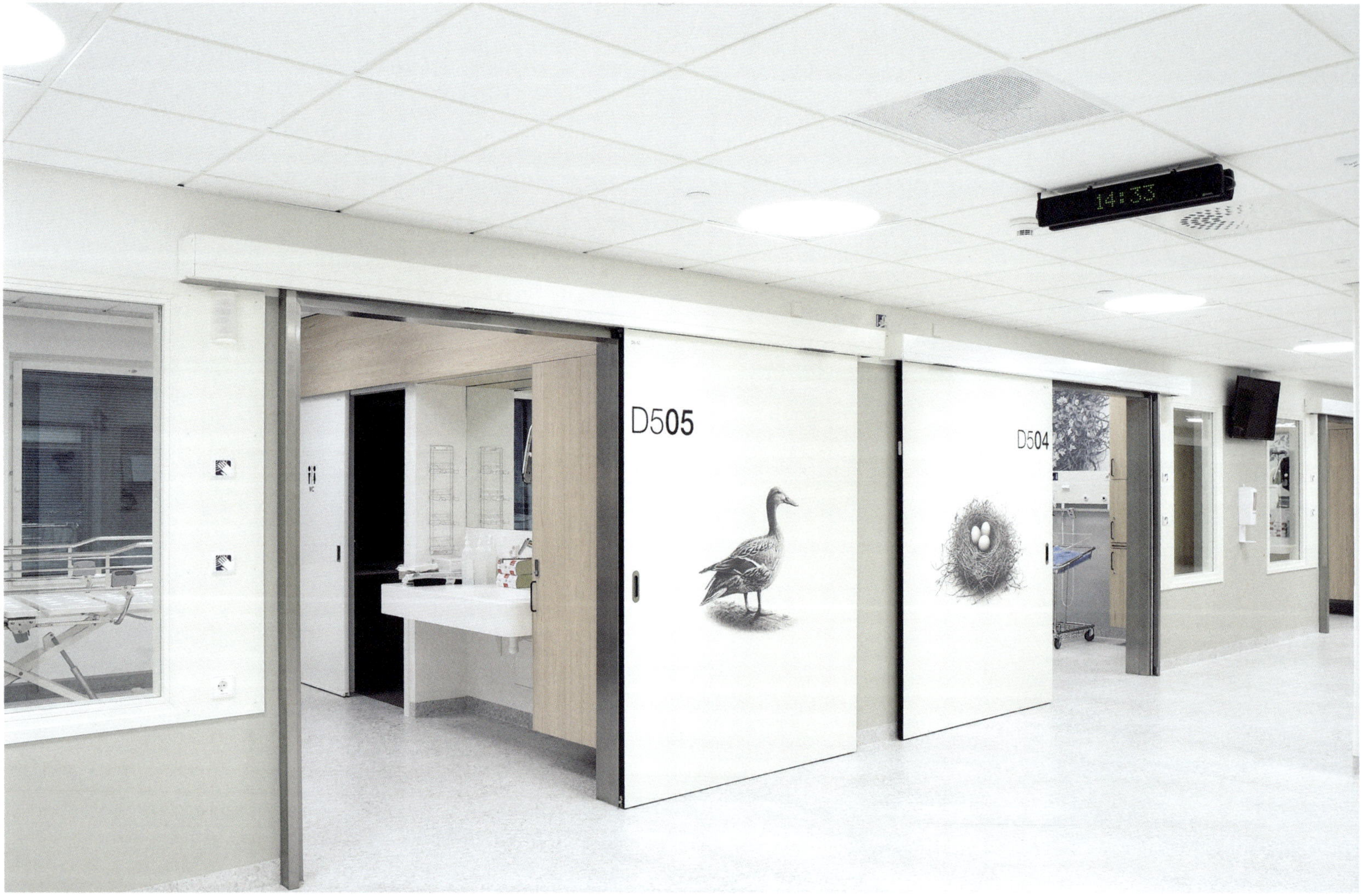

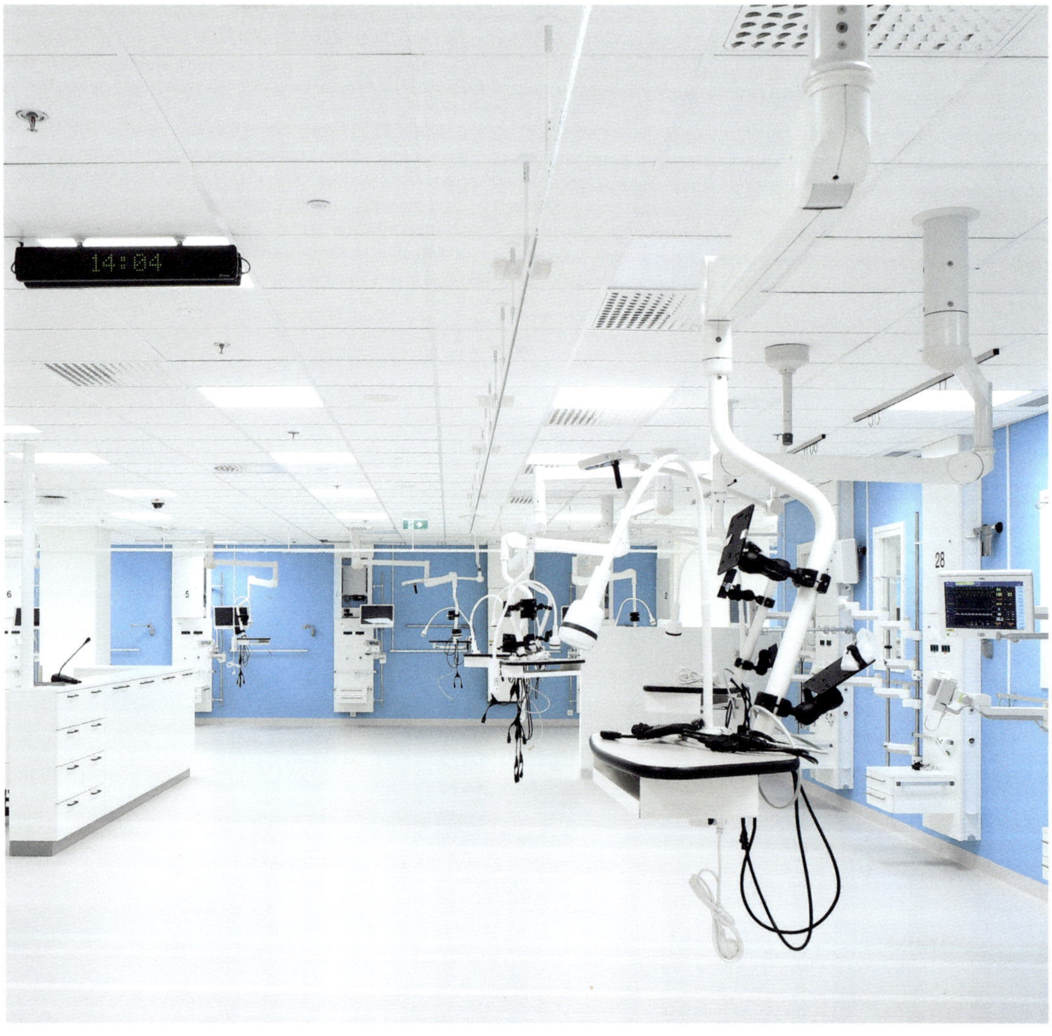

View of the wards.

Holding-recovery room.

Isometric drawing.

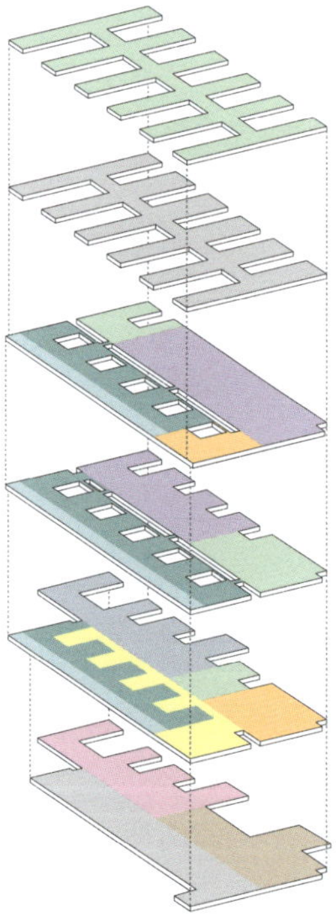

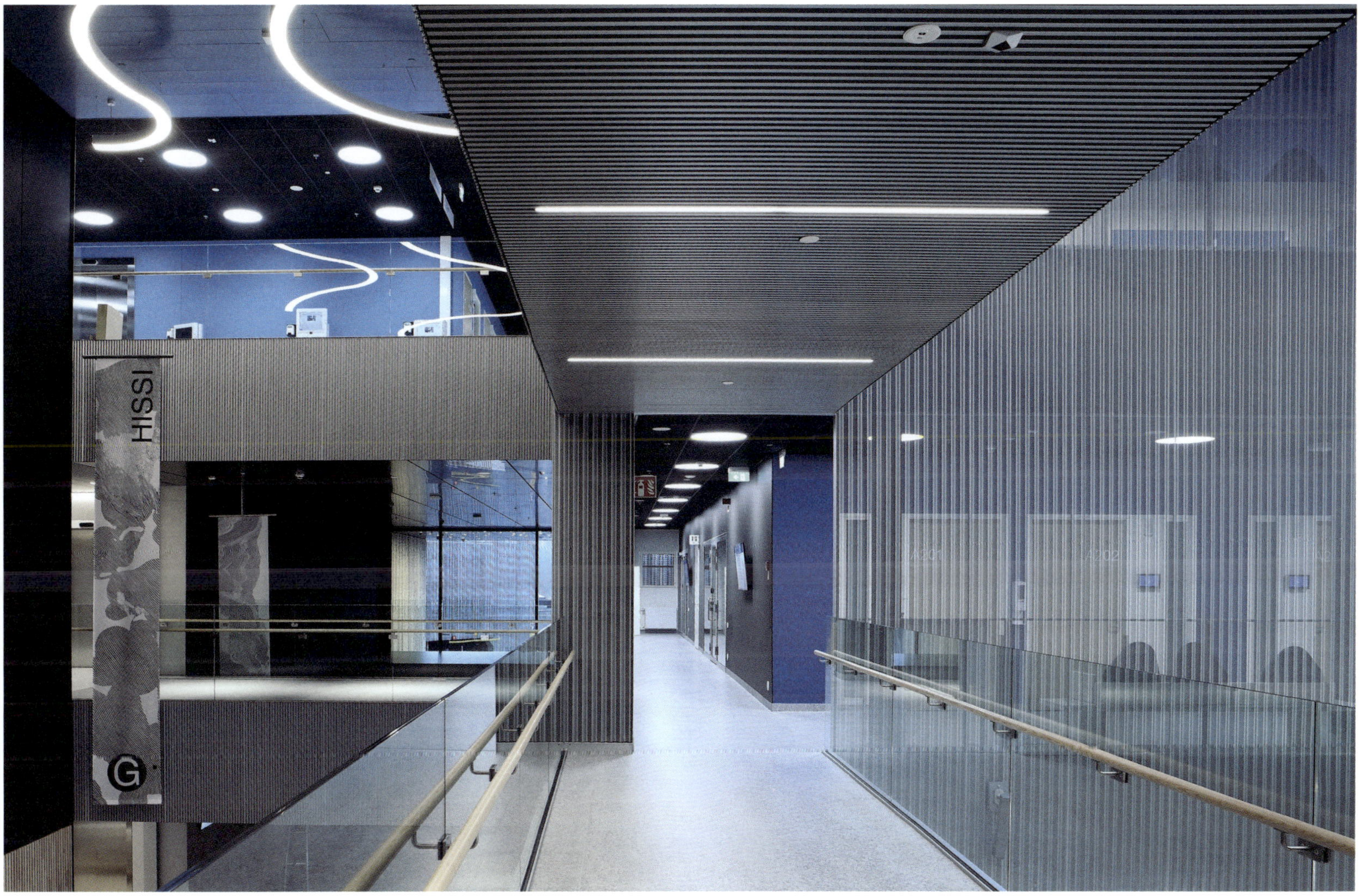

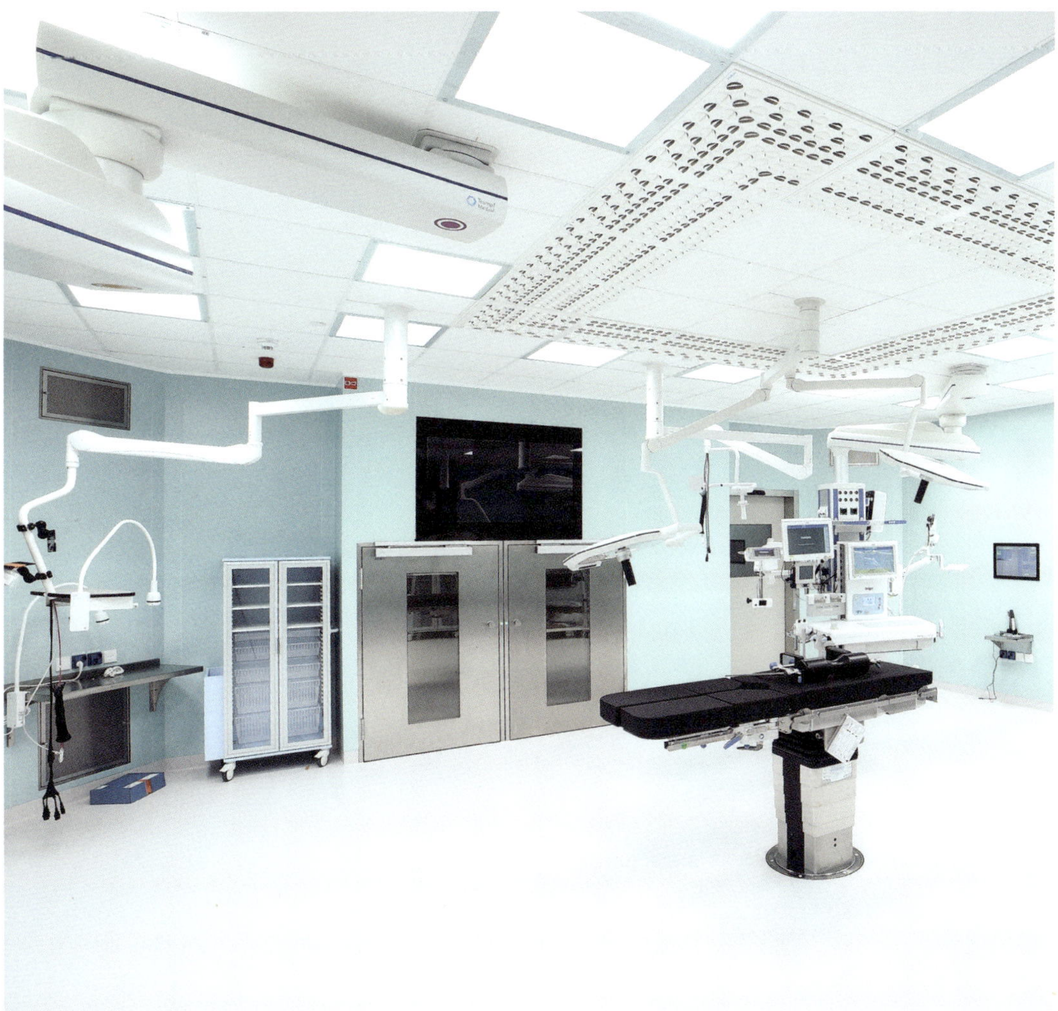

View from the gallery of the main passage.

Operating room.

APC Architectural
Pioneering Consultants

Burtinle
Somalia

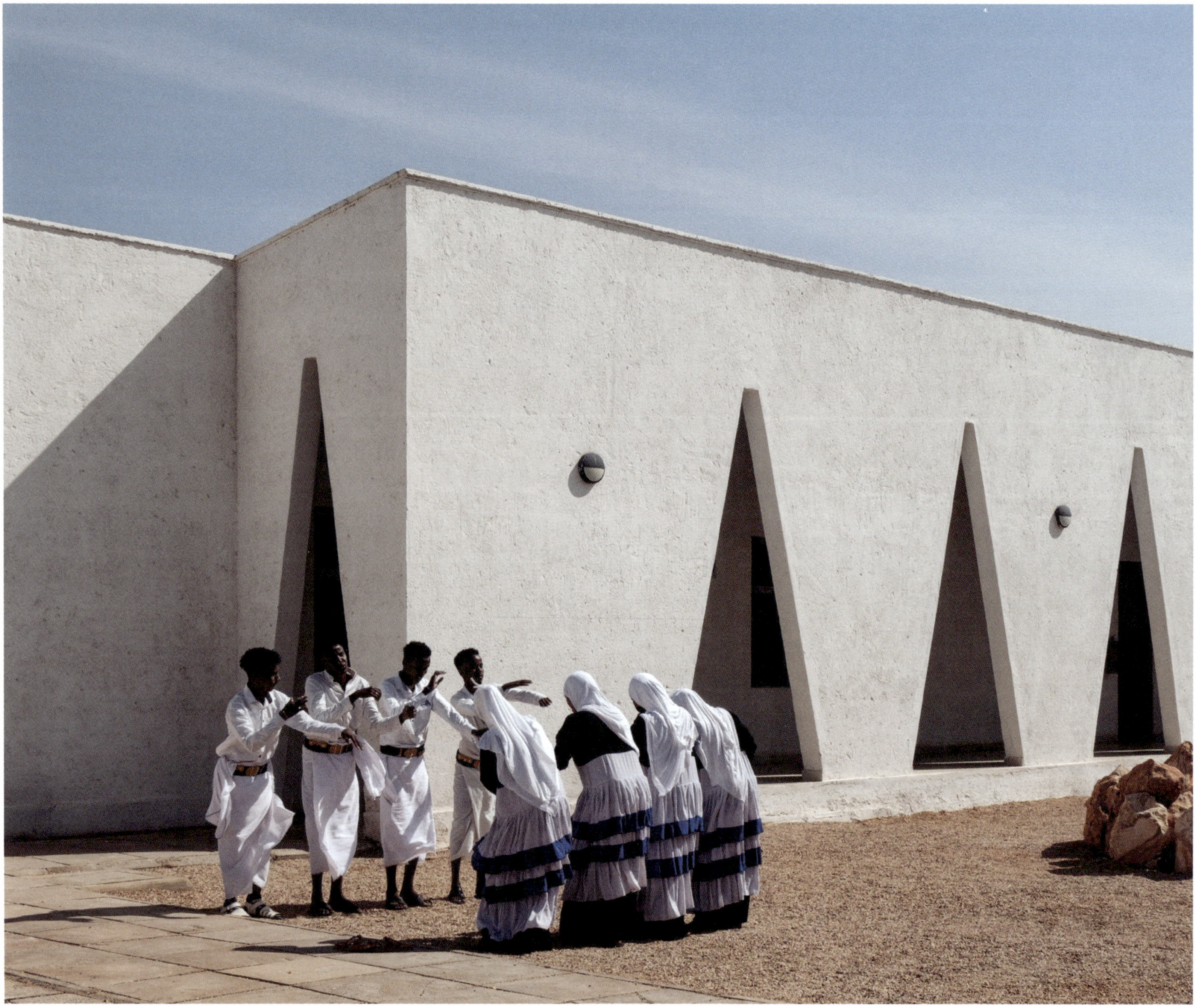

Triangular false arches define the visual identity of the hospital courtyard.

Wind towers act as visible landmarks within the town.

The clearly organized hospital corridors follow the arrangement of the wind tunnels underground.

Burtinle District Hospital – isbitaalka degmada burtinle

Responding to the urgent need for accessible healthcare in Burtinle, Puntland, Burtinle District Hospital – commissioned by UNICEF Somalia – transforms an abandoned site into a compact, courtyard-based medical compound. Three new buildings and an adapted existing structure define a central garden that functions as both organizational core and therapeutic landscape. Shaded verandas and planted areas create protected zones for waiting and gathering, while ensuring privacy in line with local social and religious practices. Environmental strategies such as wind towers, rainwater harvesting and solar-powered water treatment support passive cooling and self-sufficiency. Locally sourced materials further root the hospital in its arid context, establishing a restrained yet resilient model of healing architecture.

Address: Burtinle Town, MR3H+JWF, Burtinle, Somalia | **Client:** UNICEF Somalia | **Completion:** 2023 | **Size:** 1,257 m² | **Sector:** state | **Number of treatment rooms:** 7 | **Number of patient rooms:** 12

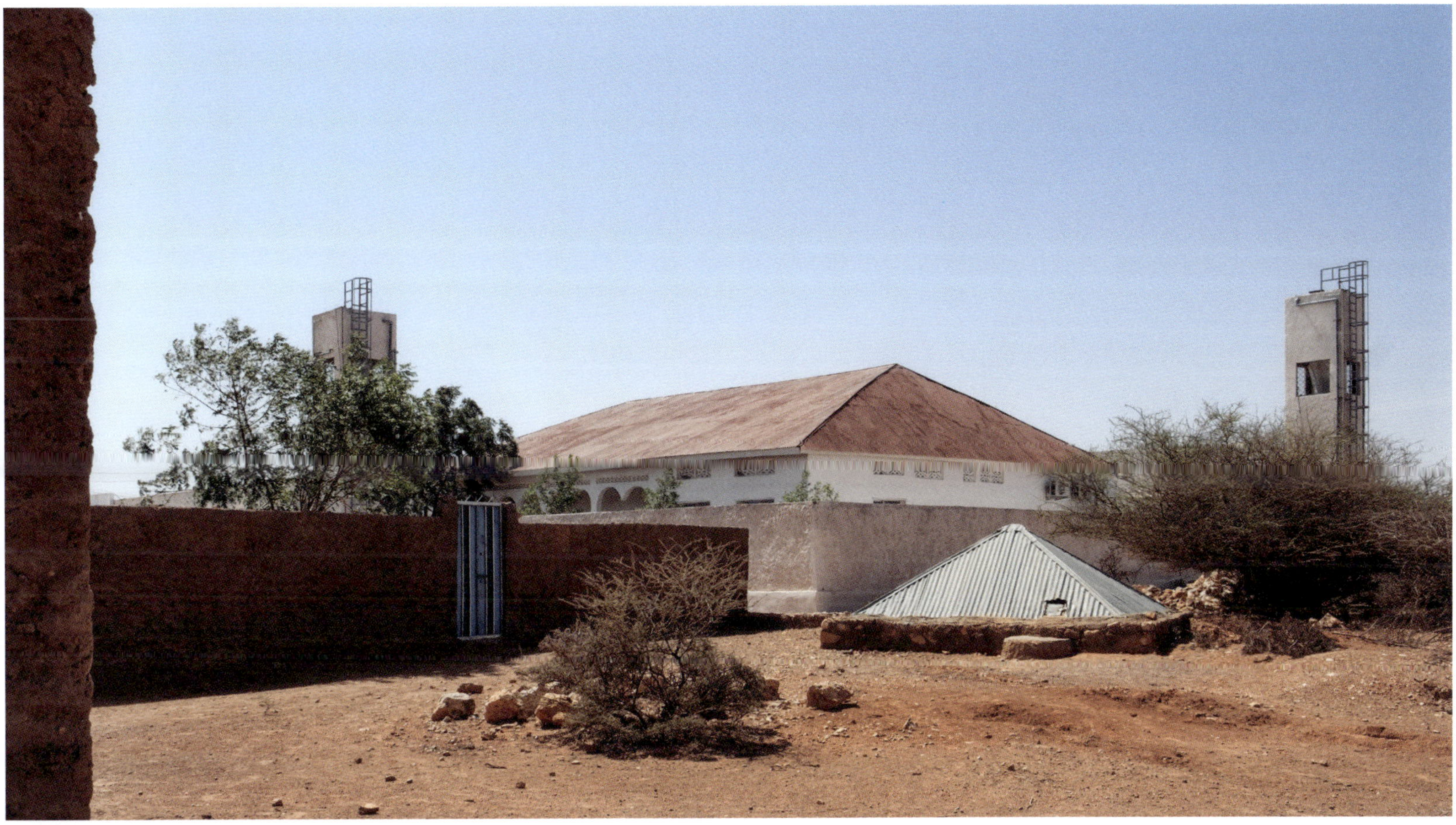

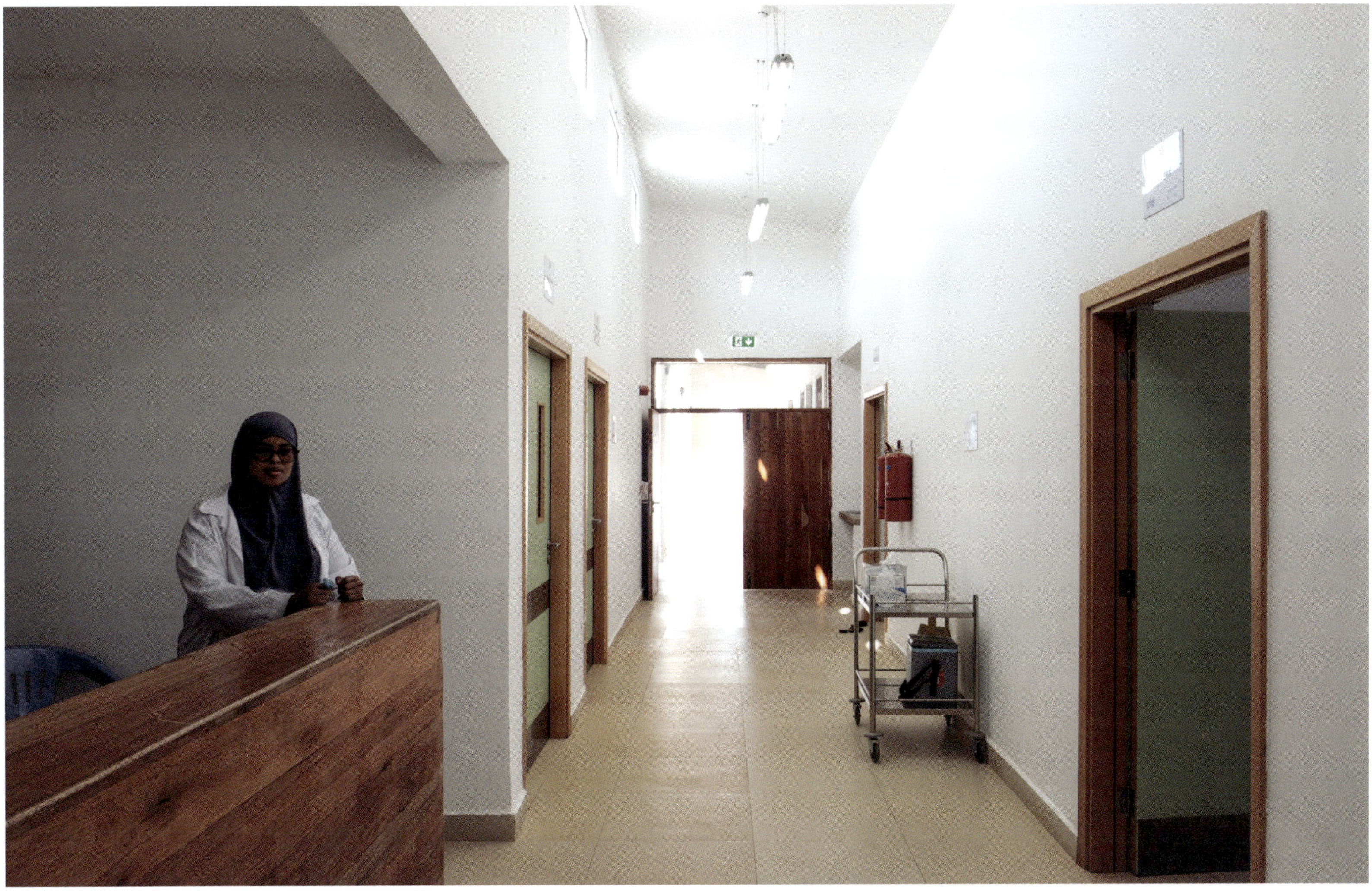

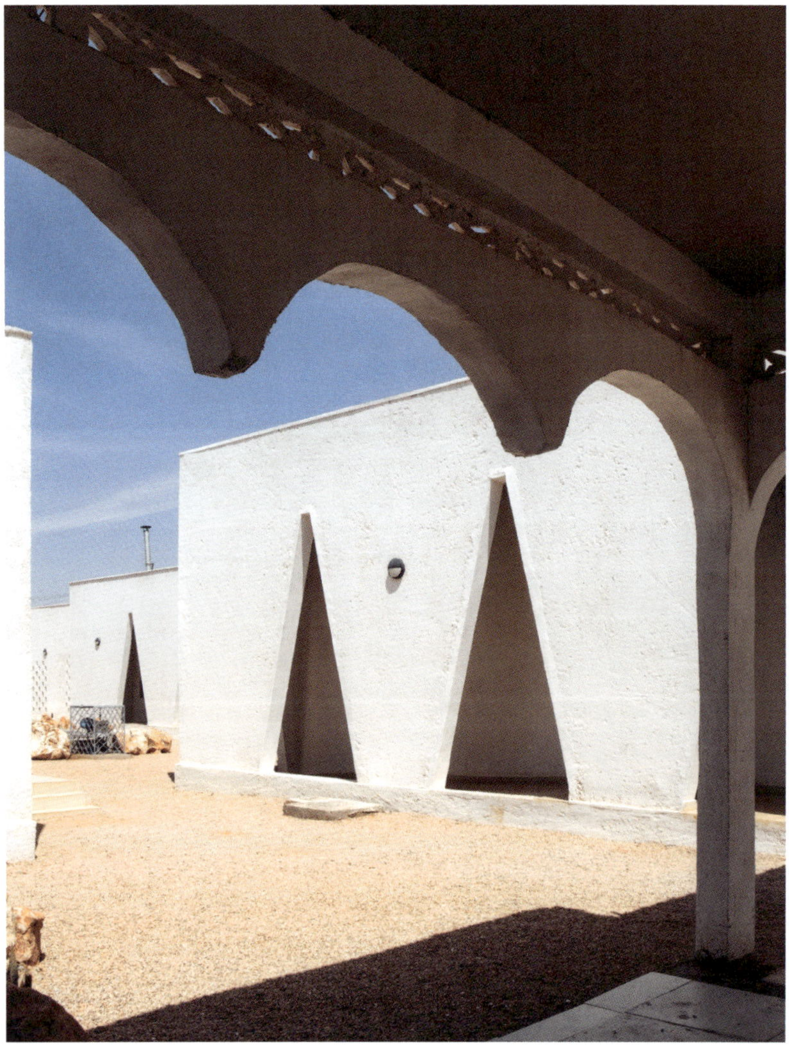

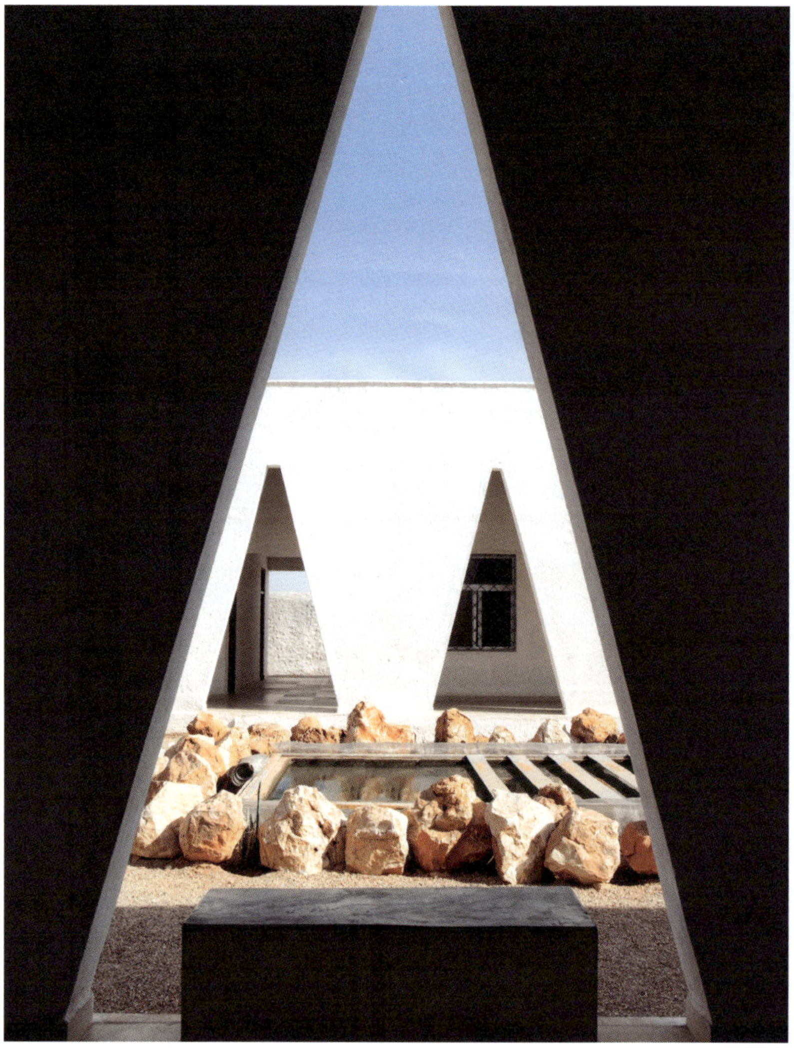

Verandas are a continuous feature of both existing and new structures.

A water body frames the courtyard.

Floor plan.

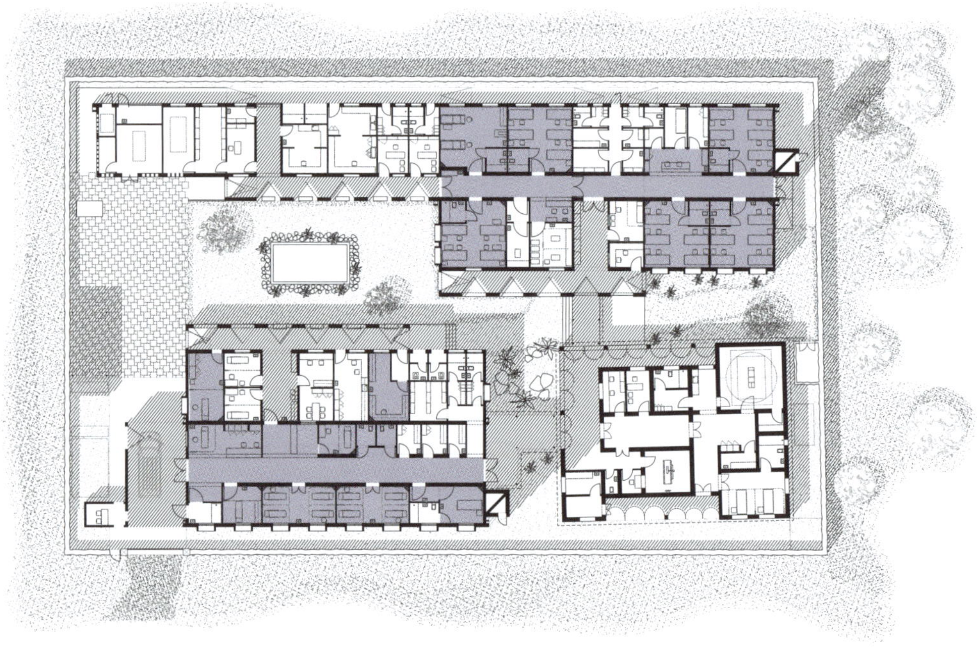

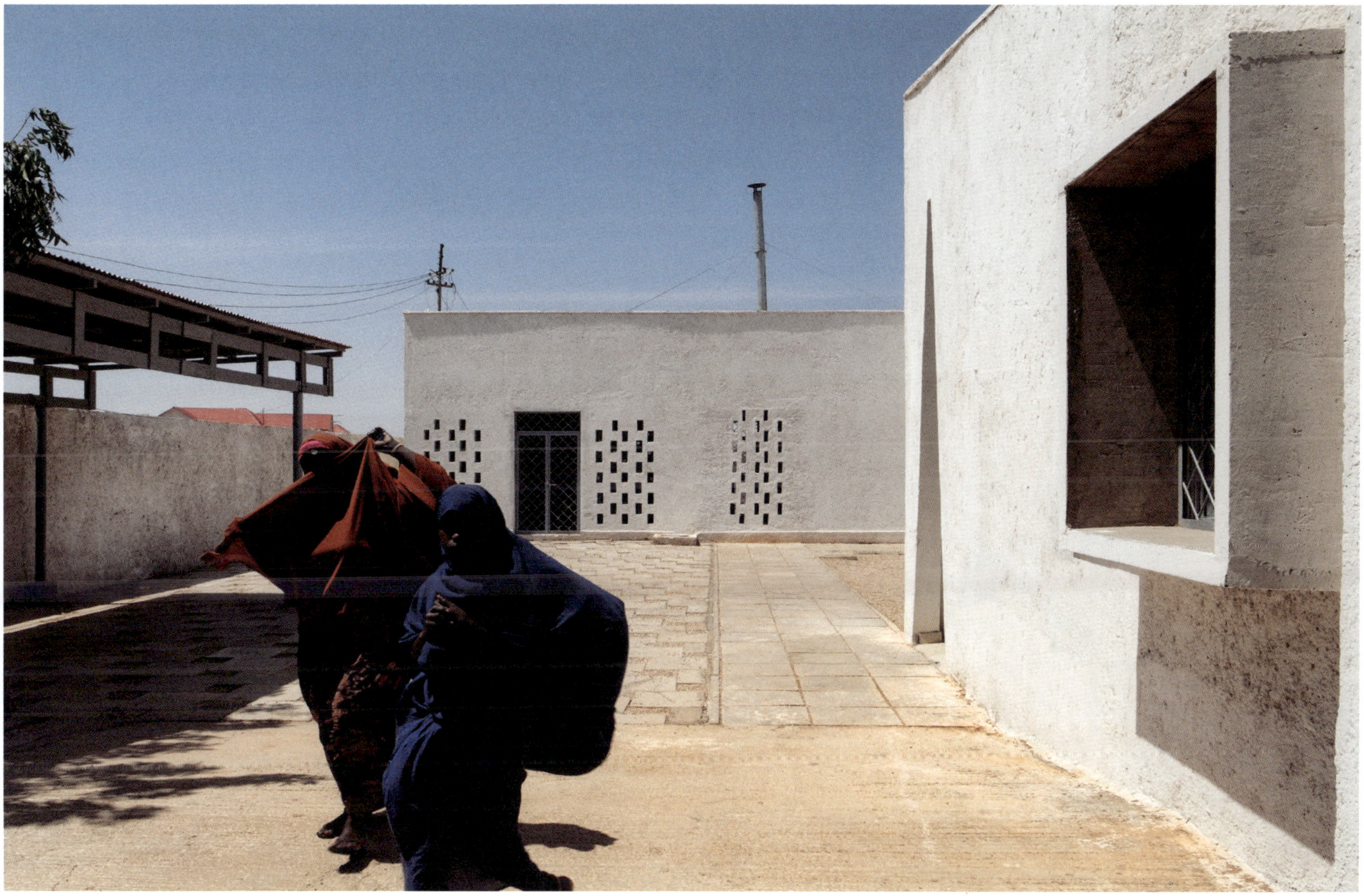

Entrance area articulated through clean geometry and subtle material transitions.

Cross section.

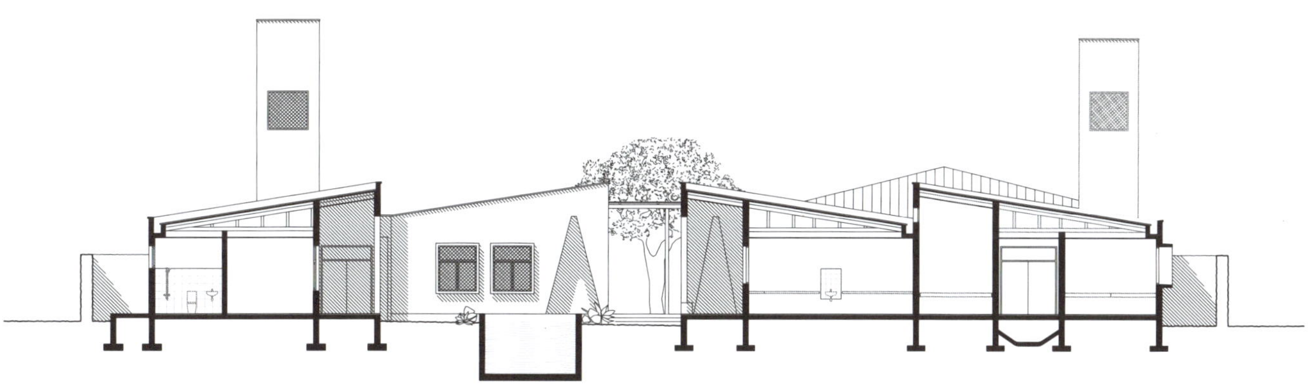

H2M Architekten
a|sh sander.hofrichter architekten

Munich
Germany

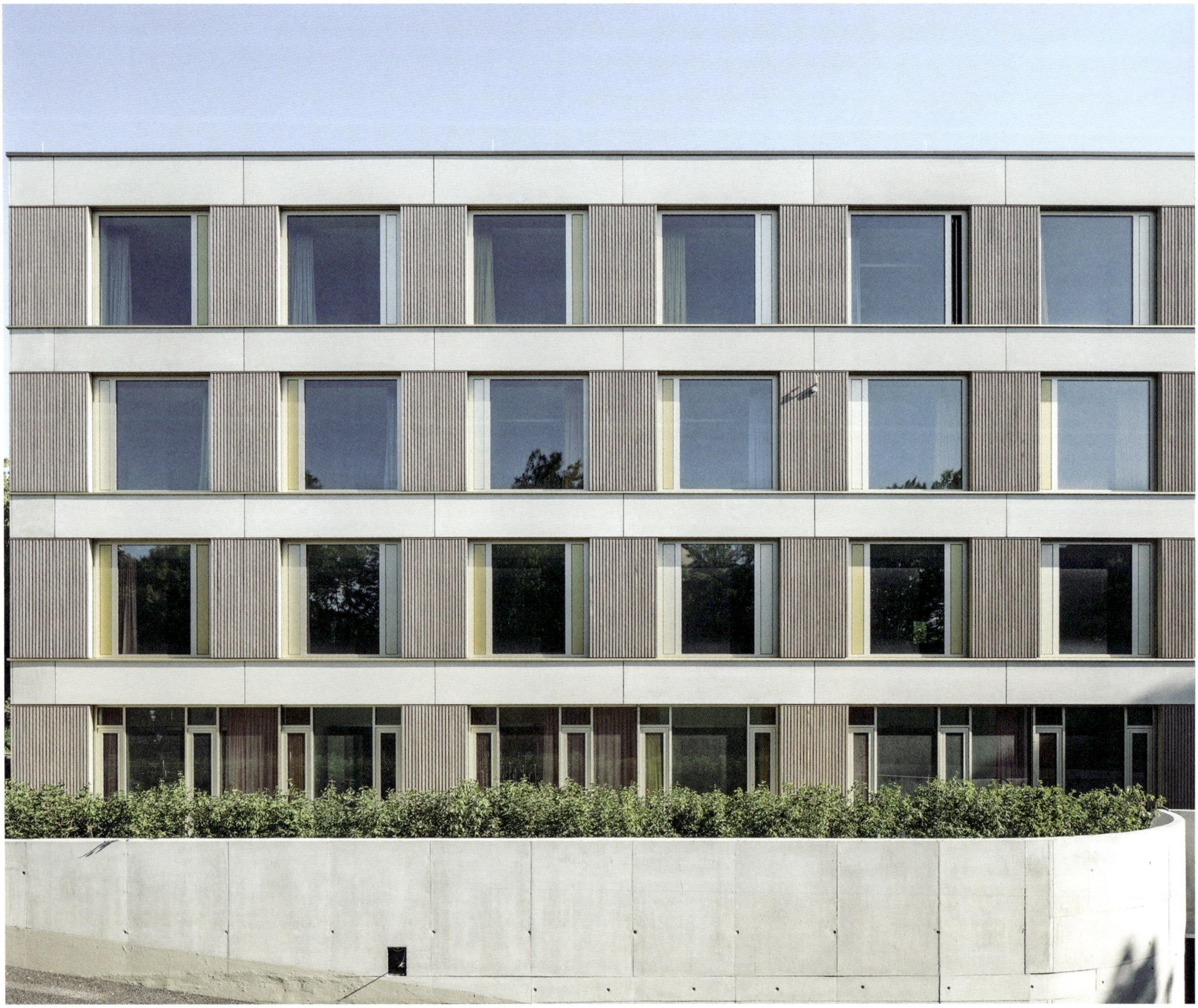

Hospital's façade with large glass windows.

Inner courtyard and glass façade.

kbo Children's Center, Munich

A home for children, parents, and staff – the new kbo Children's Center in Munich is a place that fosters a sense of community. The design complements the existing development in a way that makes urban planning sense – creating a cohesive whole guided by the principles of Montessori education. Arrive, orient, feel at home: visitors enter through a newly landscaped forecourt into a light-filled entrance hall, from which a colorful wayfinding system intuitively guides them to all central areas. Short distances and a welcoming atmosphere – all outpatient, day clinic, and shared therapy facilities are located near the entrance on the ground floor. Bavaria's first Childhood House is also located here. The wards on the first and second floors are designed to provide privacy and a sense of security. A circular movement system shortens distances and supports operationally optimized 'floating.'

Address: Heiglhofstraße 69, 81377 Munich, Germany | **Client:** kbo-Kinderzentrum München gGmbH | **Completion:** 2023 | **Size:** 14,700 m² | **Sector:** state | **Specialization:** social pediatric center and specialized clinic for social pediatrics and developmental rehabilitation | **Number of treatment rooms:** 113 | **Number of patient rooms:** 56 | **Landscape design:** Rainer Schmidt Landschaftsarchitekten | **Signage and Wayfinding system:** designgruppe koop

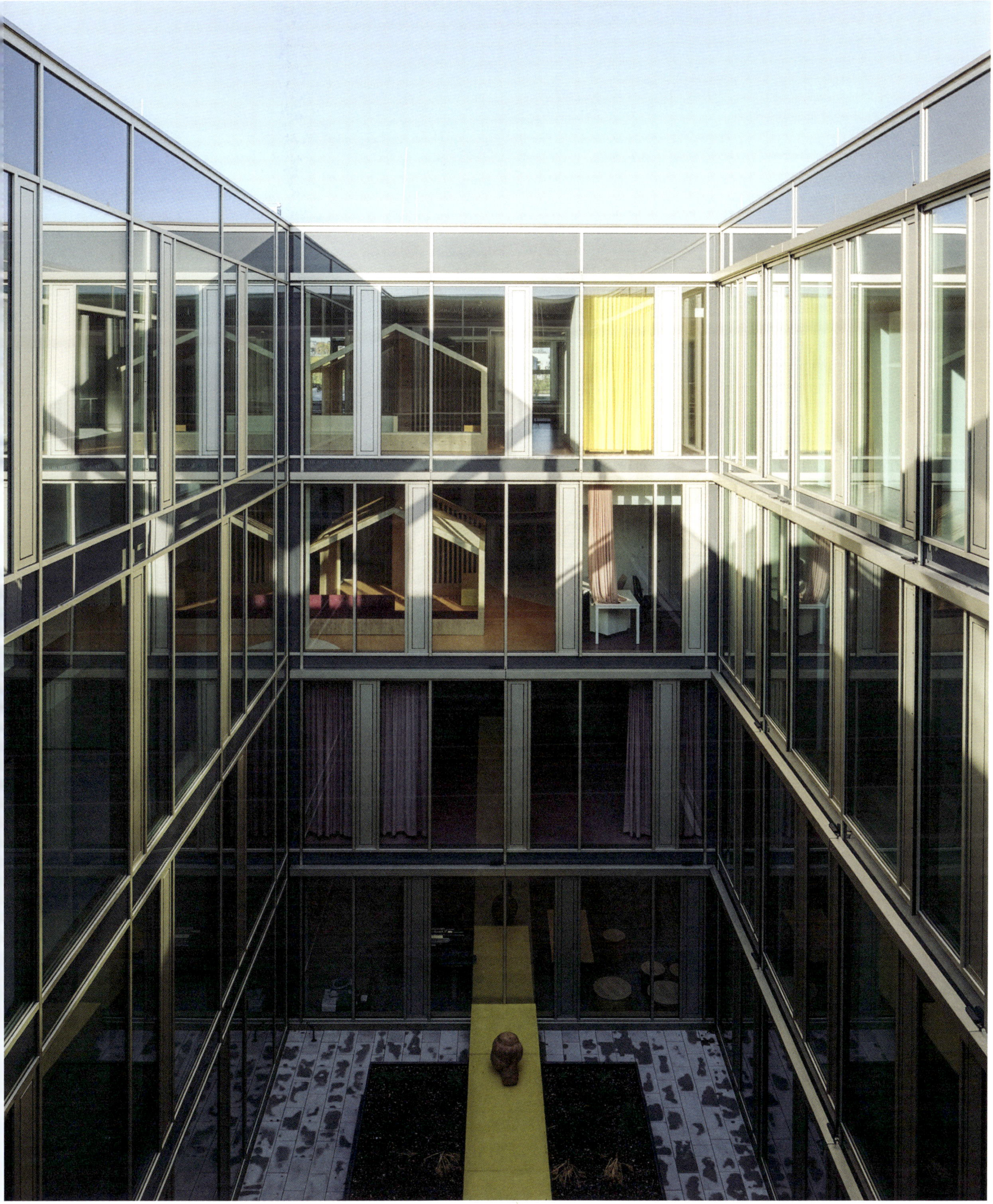

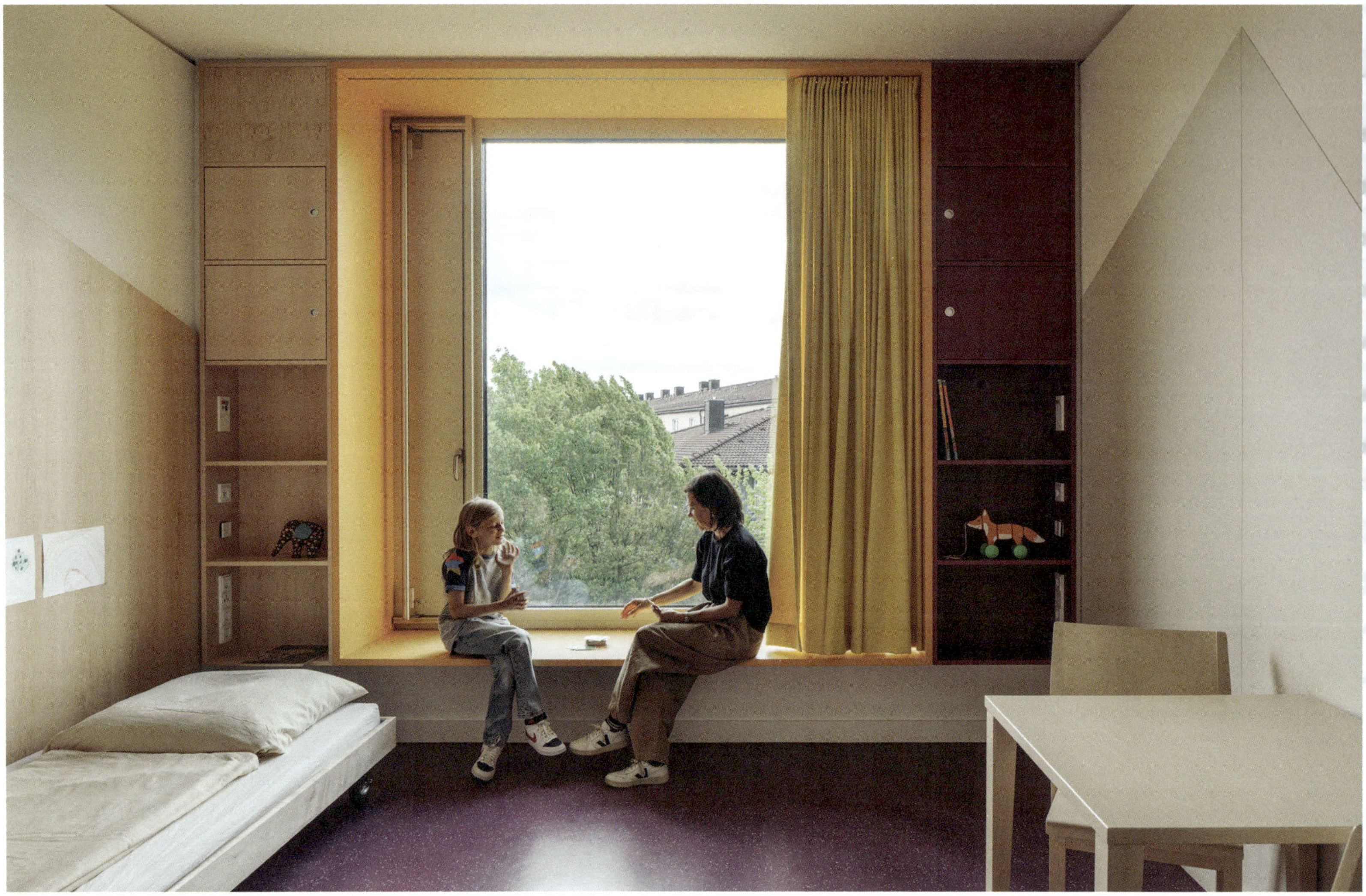

Playful and colorful patient's room.

Ground floor plan.

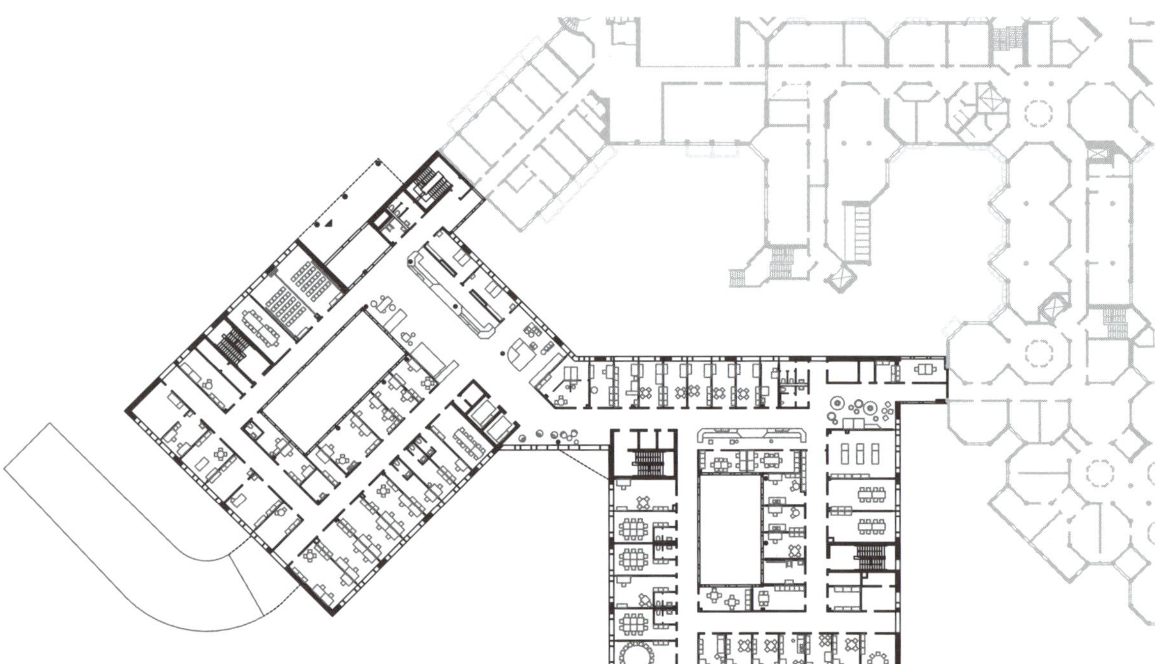

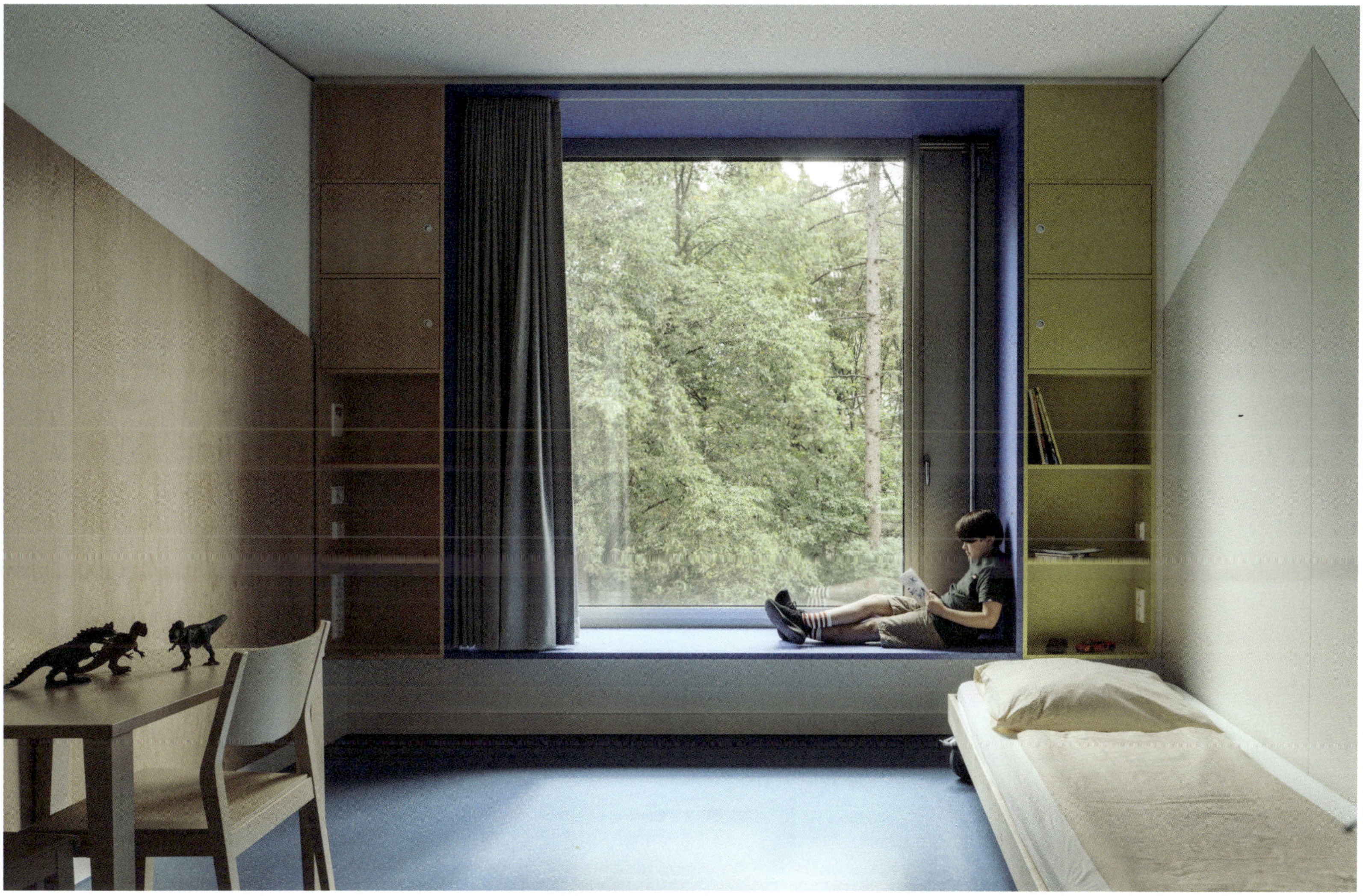

Passepartout windows frame the green trees.

Site plan showing tree locations.

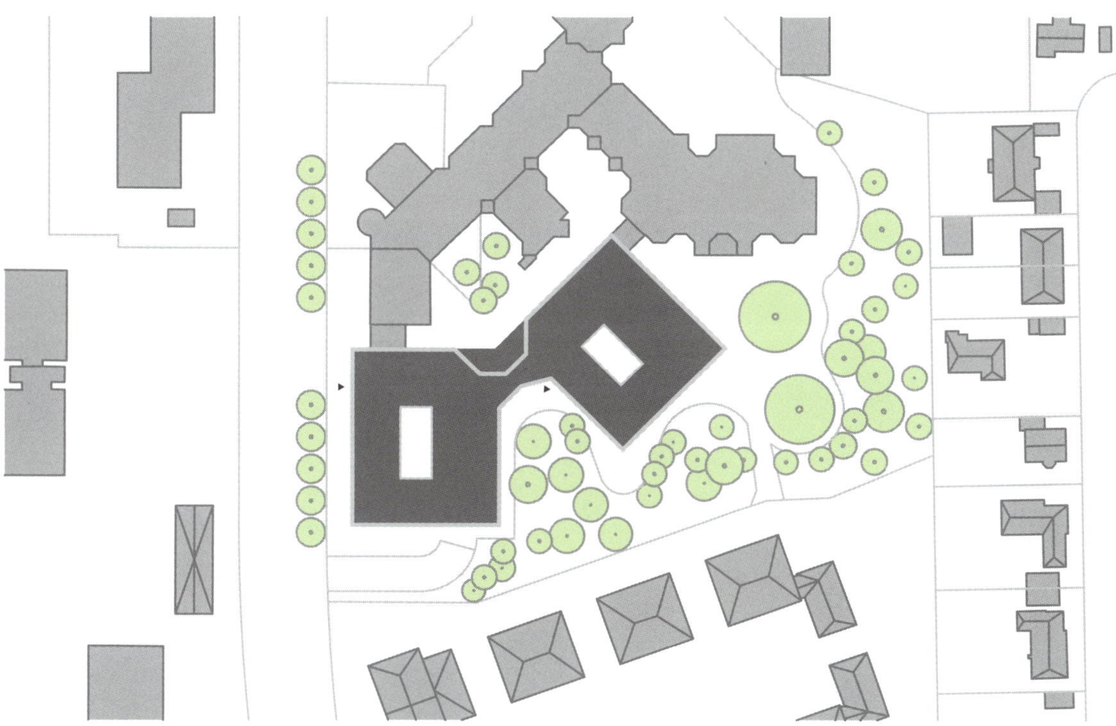

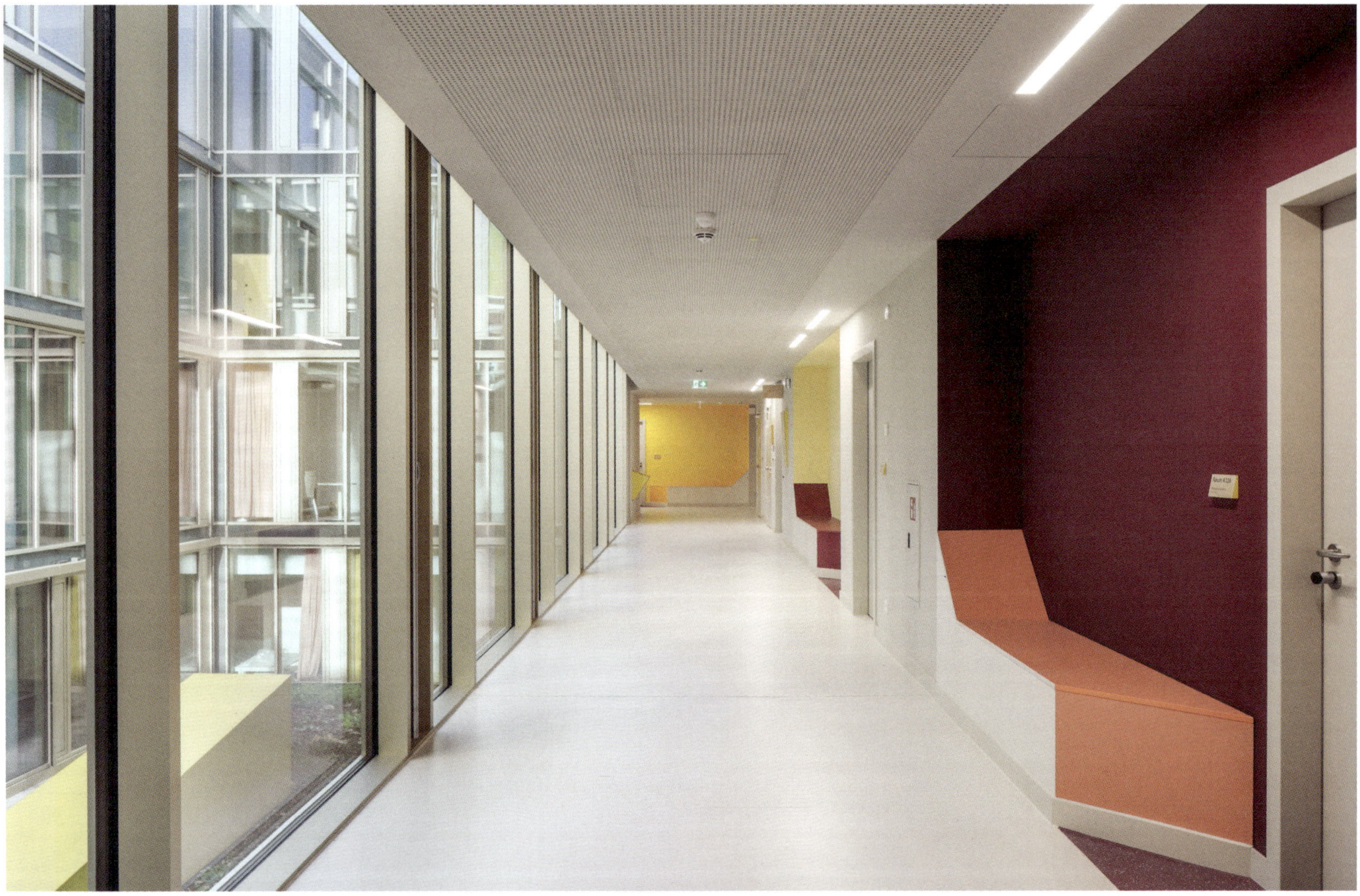

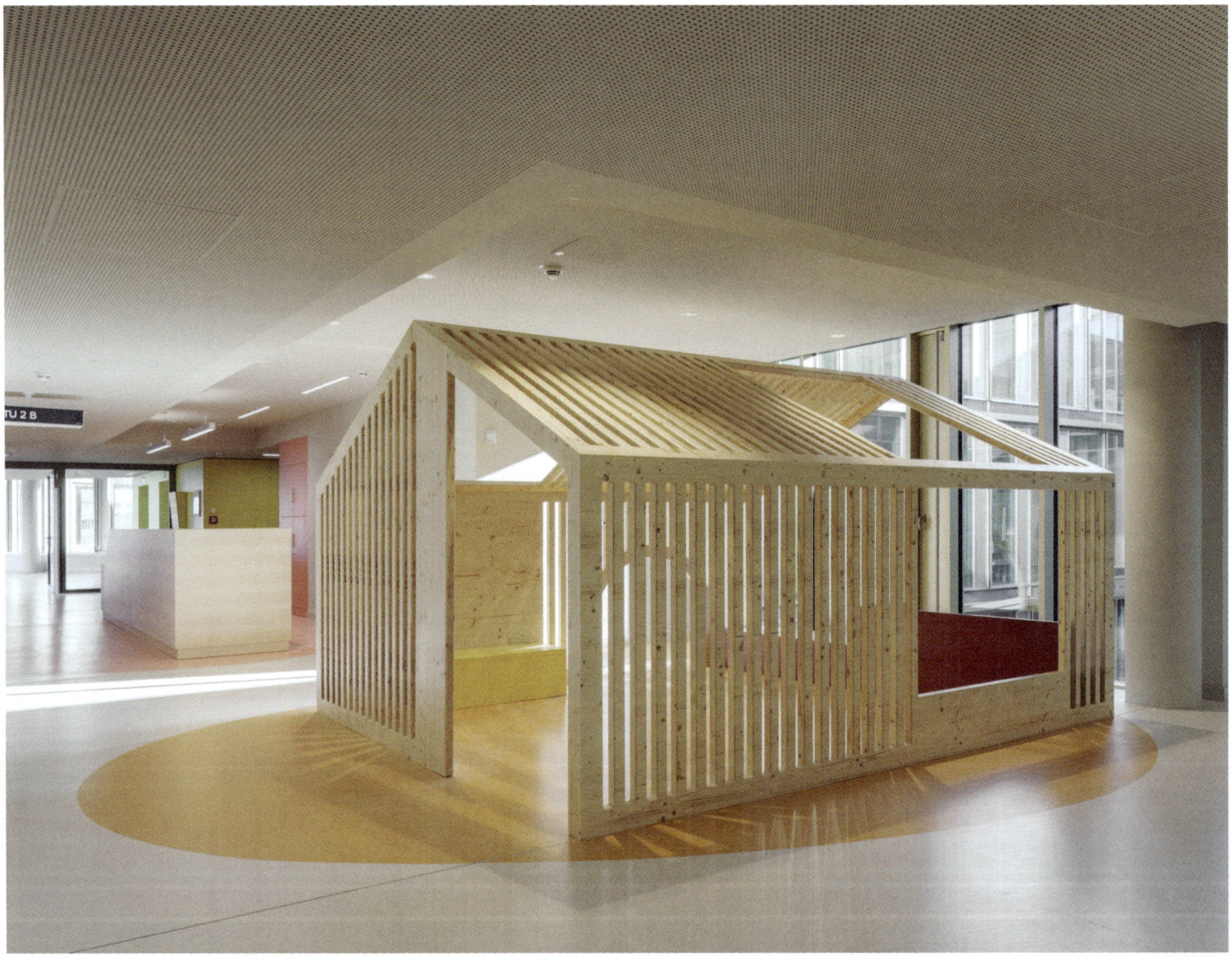

Hallway with seating niches and a view into the courtyard.

Play street with floor markings and Children's House.

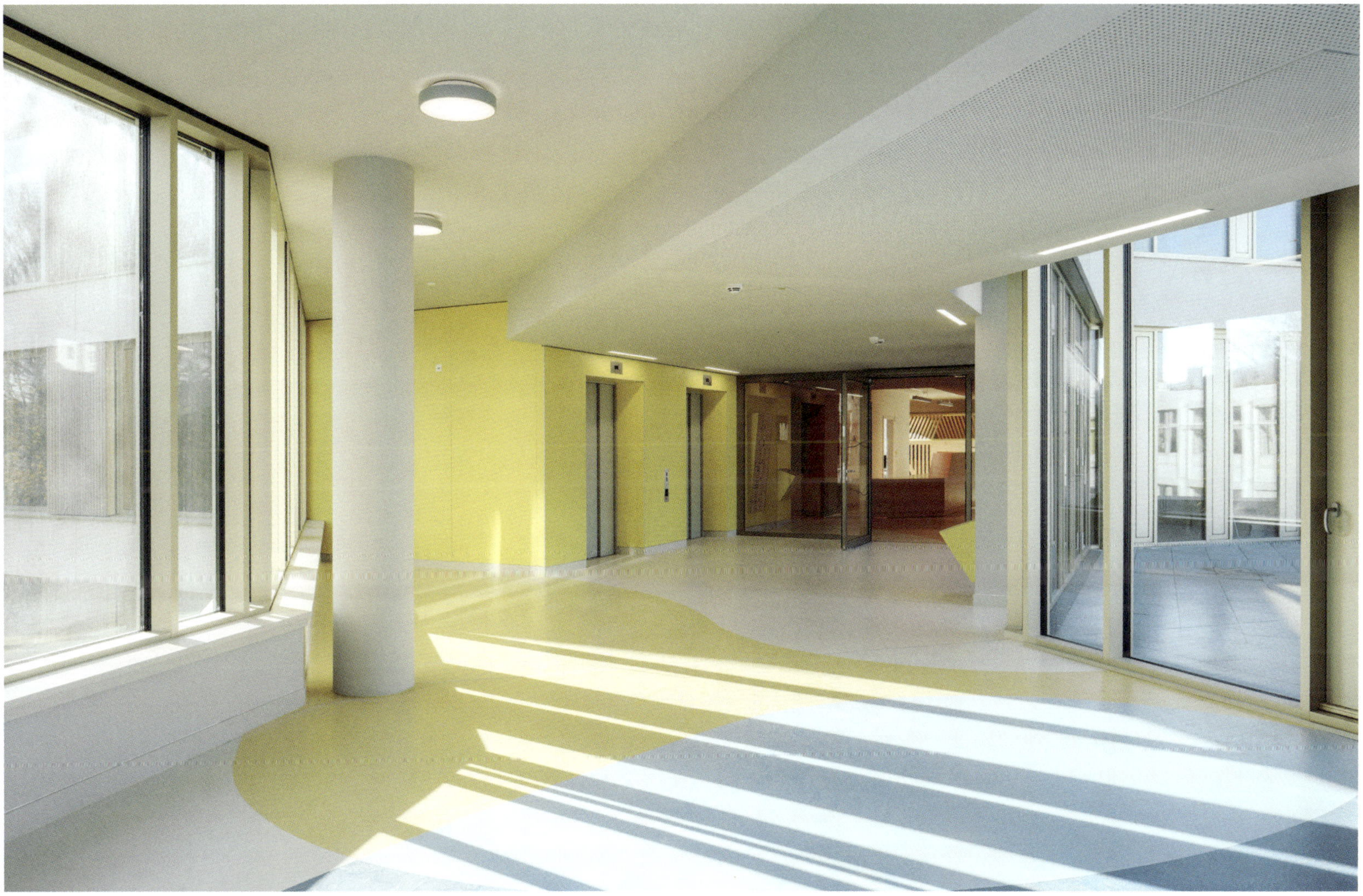

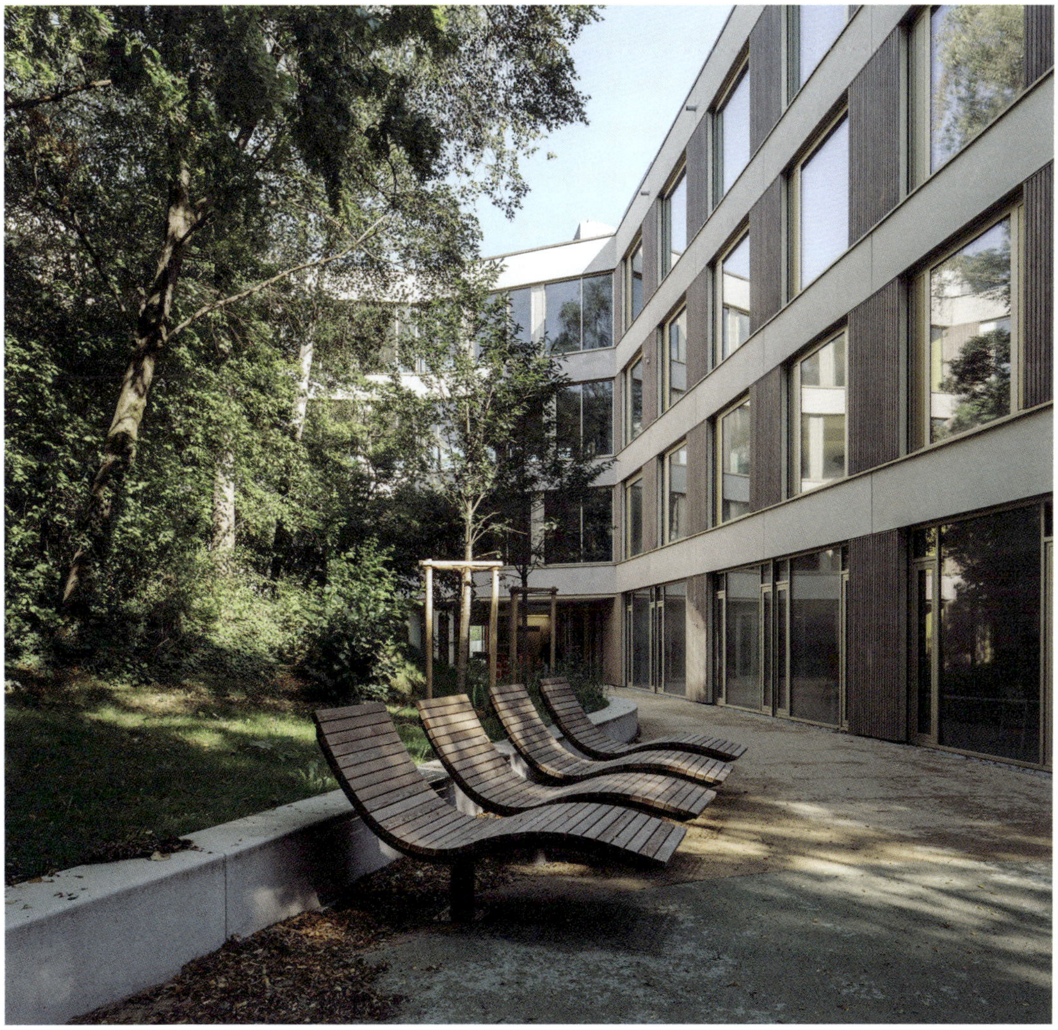

Bright colorful an well lit connecting corridor.

A green retreat for patients and visitors.

skyline architekten

St. Veit im Pongau
Austria

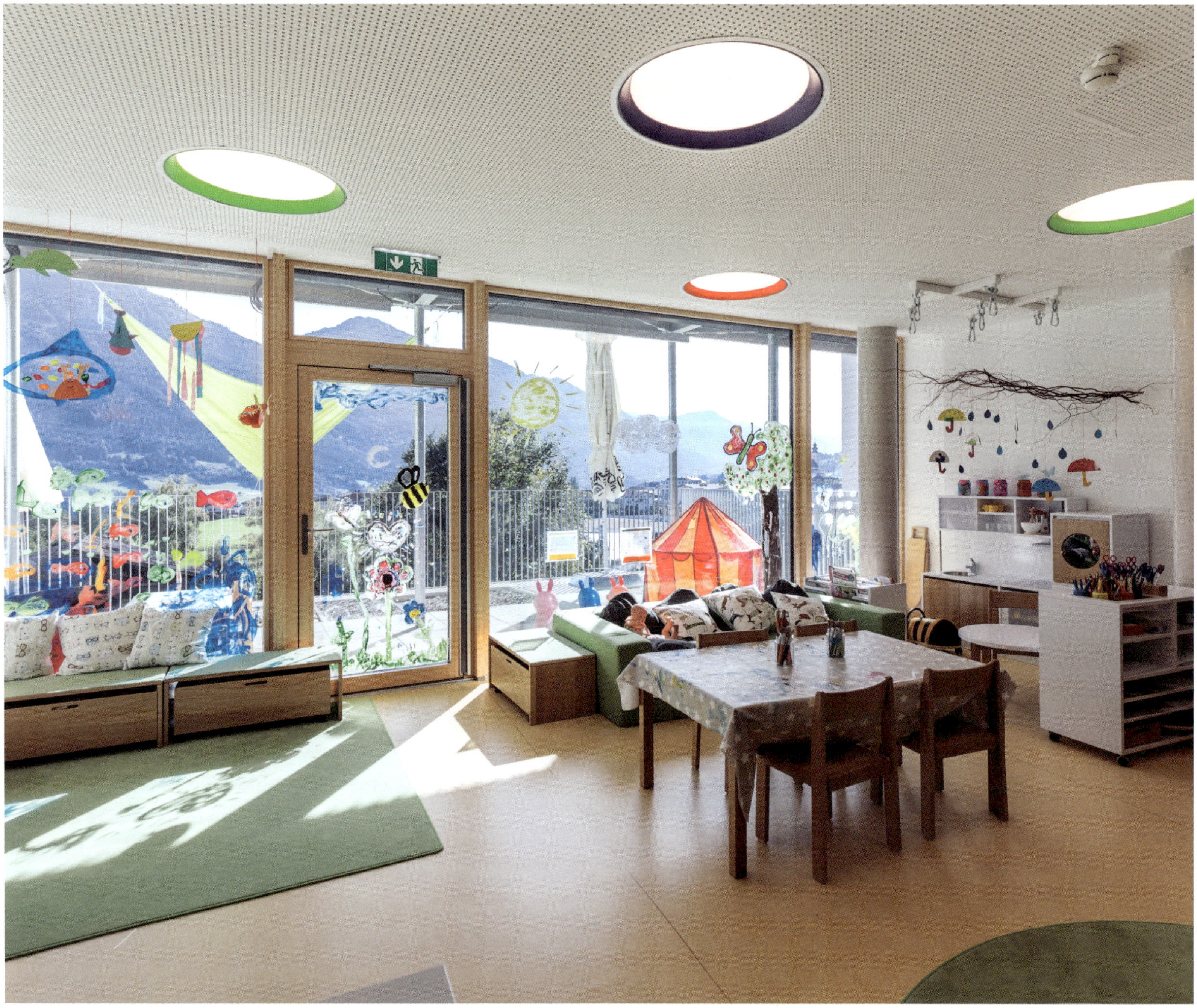

Hospital's kindergarten area.

Valley side view of the hospital.

Main entrance area.

Leuwaldhof Rehabilitation Center for Children and Adolescents

The Leuwaldhof is Austria's first rehabilitation center for children and adolescents with cancer and metabolic disorders. It takes a holistic, family-oriented approach that also involves the young patients' immediate family members. The extension to the existing adult oncology rehabilitation facility offers extensive therapy options, including a swimming pool, school, and kindergarten groups, as well as dining and common areas and a thoughtfully designed outdoor space concept featuring a therapy garden and playgrounds. Exposed wooden ceilings and walls in areas permitted by health regulations, combined with wood-aluminum windows and soothing color tones and appropriate daylighting make an important contribution to the concept of healing as well as to physical and mental well-being. The concrete, wood, and hybrid construction method allowed for a construction period of only 12 months.

Address: St. Veiter-Straße 48a, 5621 St. Veit im Pongau, Austria | **Client:** VAMED Standortentwicklung und Engineering GmbH | **Completion:** 2018 | **Size:** 6,830 m² | **Original building:** Architekt Robert Soyka, 2013 | **Sector:** private | **Specialization:** rehabilitation center for children and adolescents with cancer and metabolic disorders | **Number of treatment rooms:** 20 | **Number of patient rooms:** 116

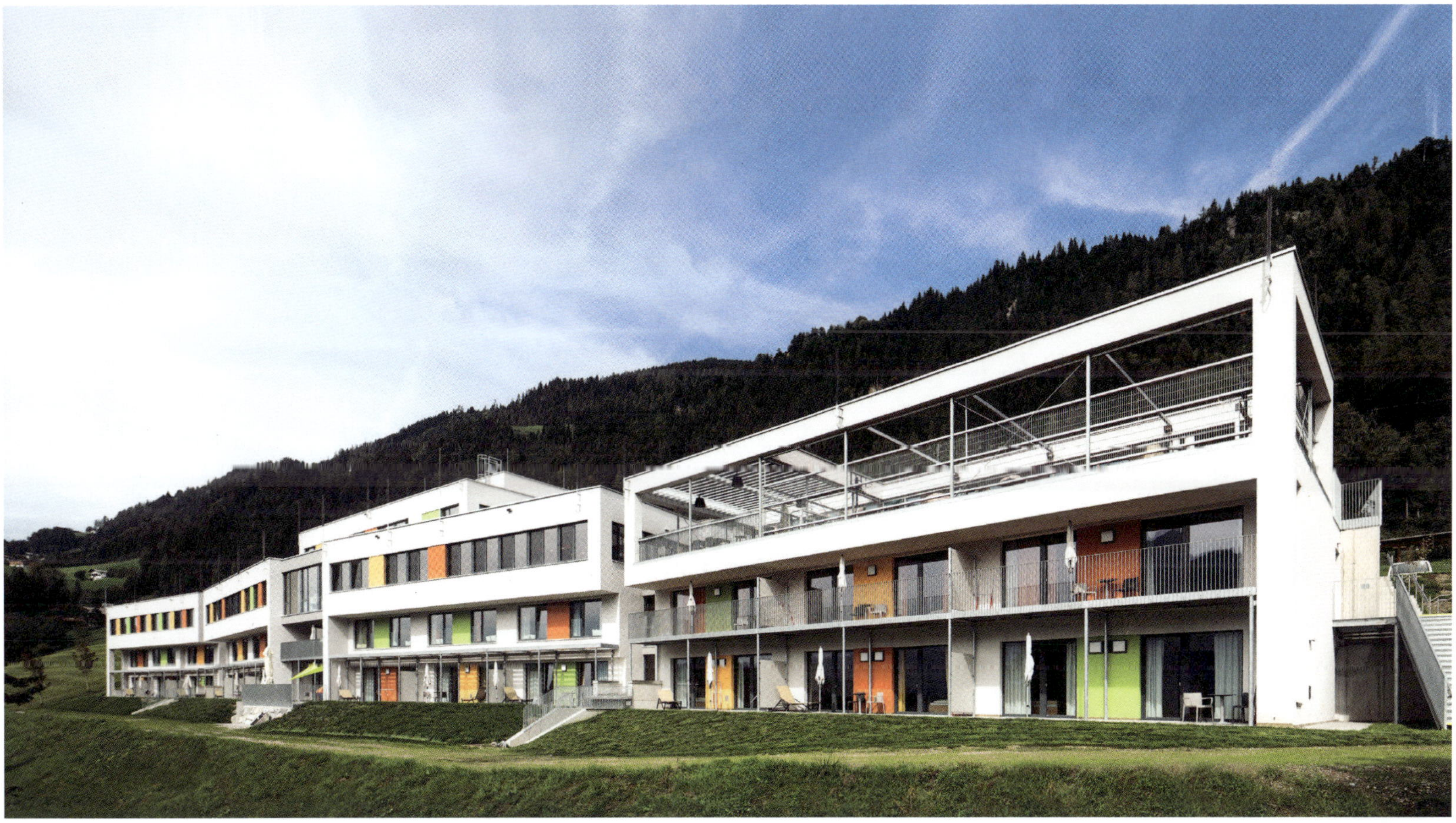

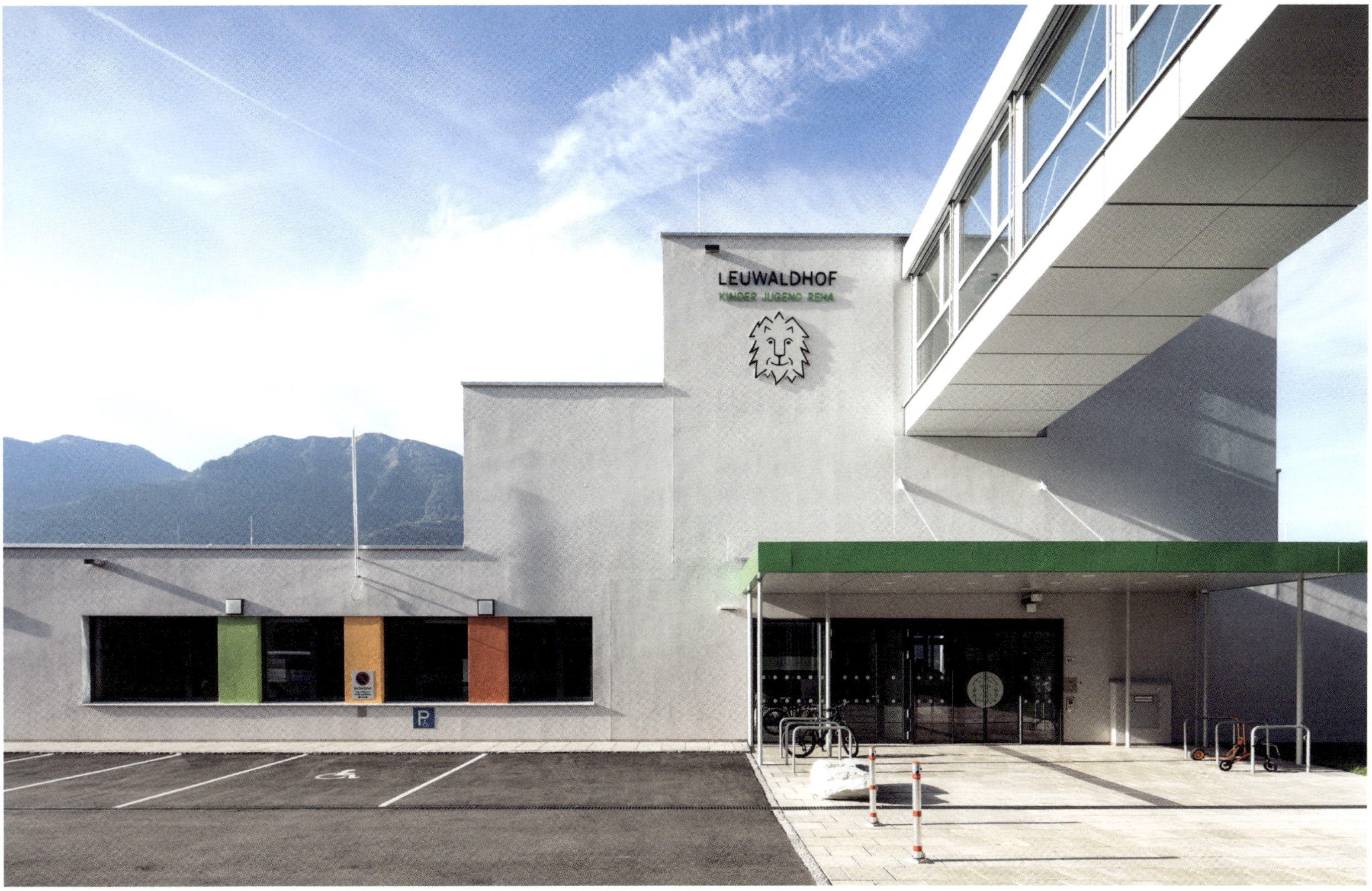

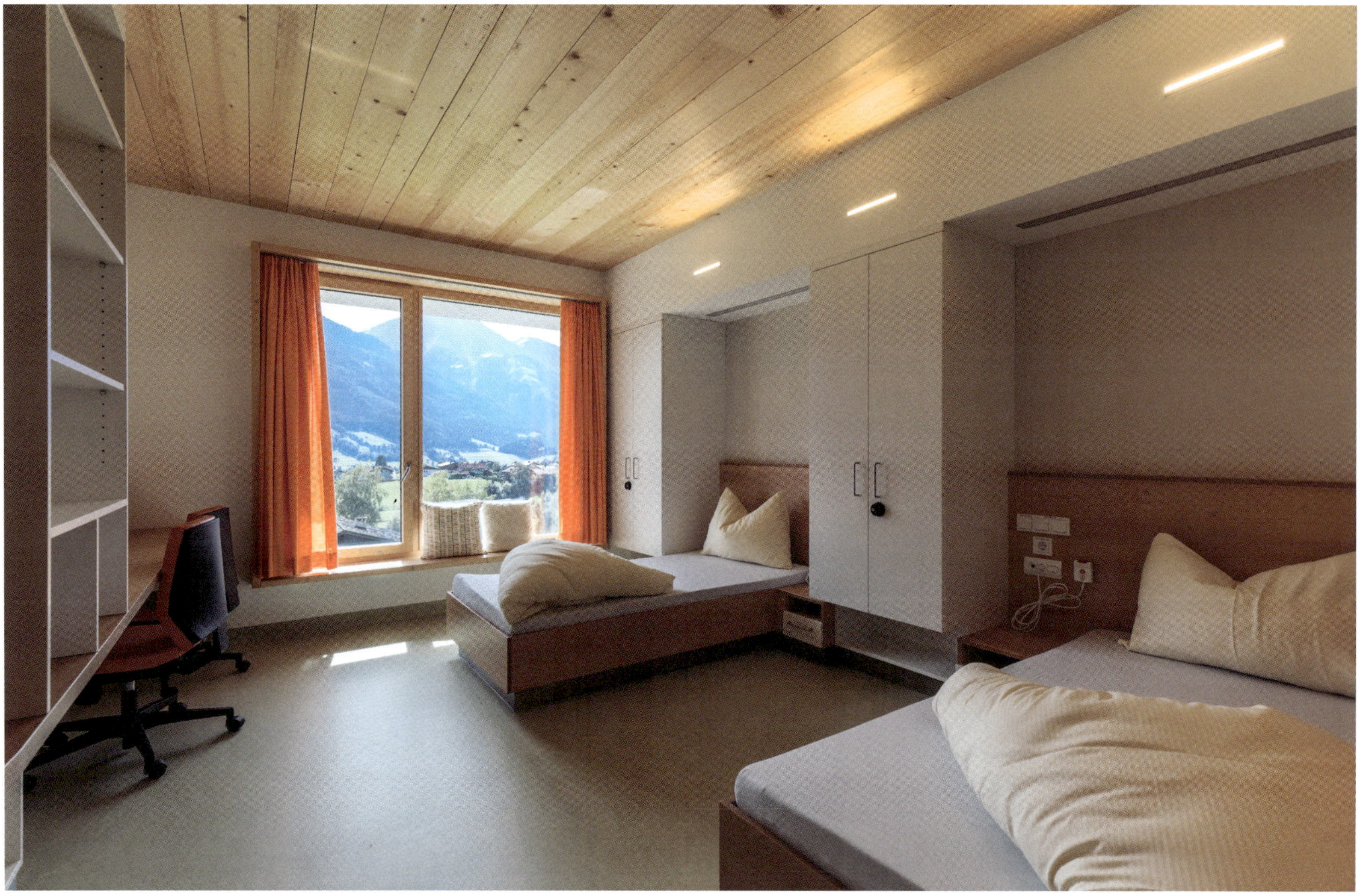

Spacious and well-designed twin room.

Site plan.

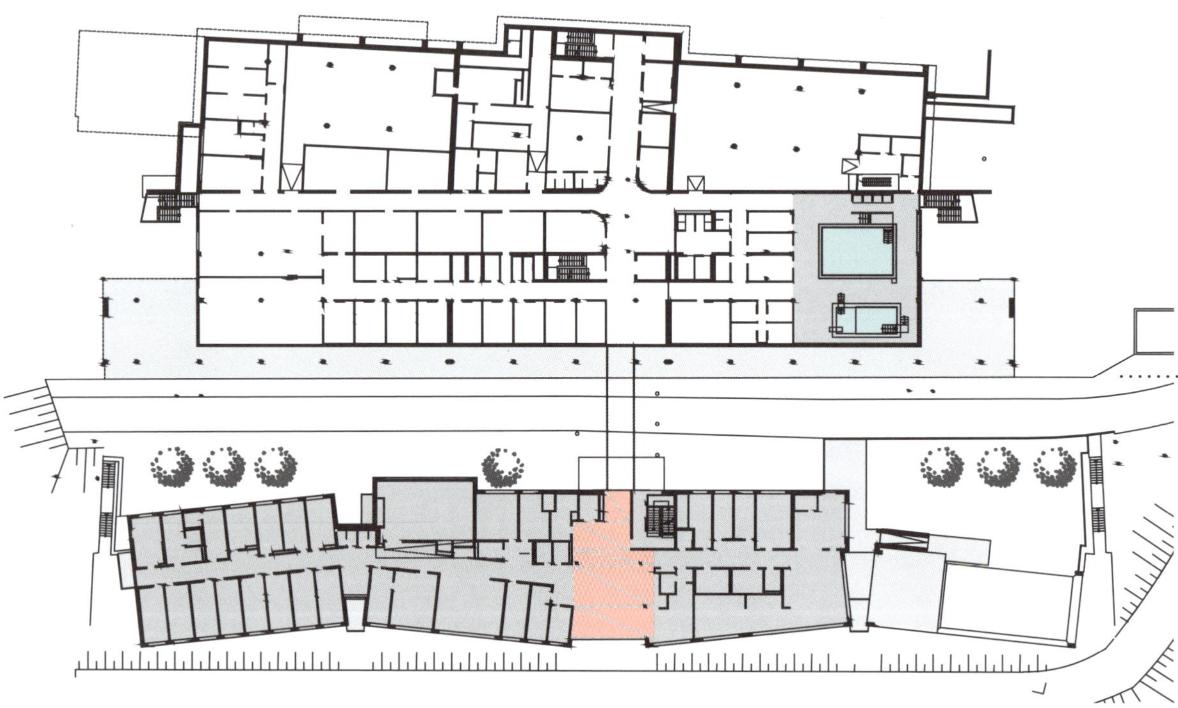

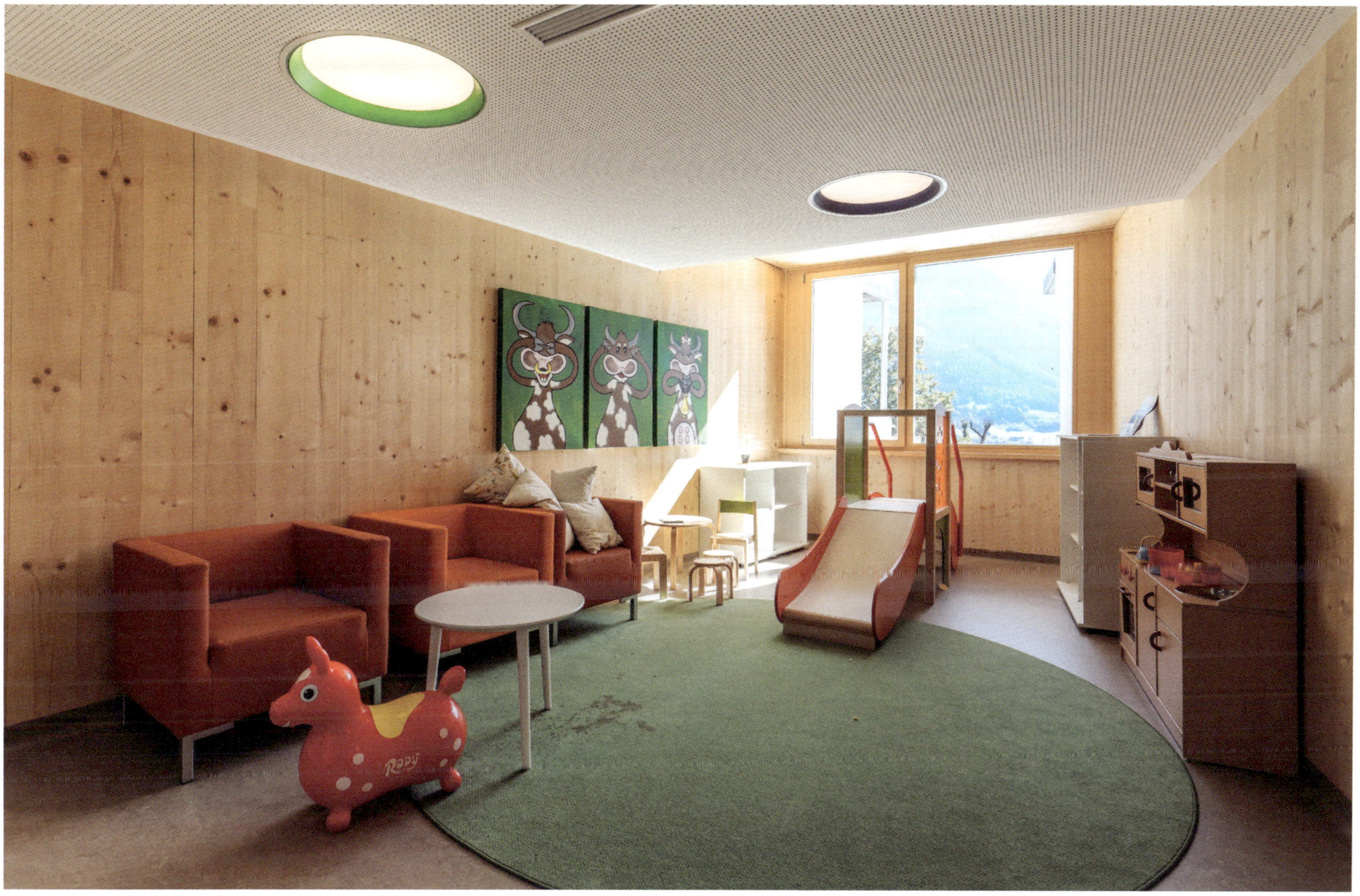

Colorful and playful waiting room.

Section and typical floor plan.

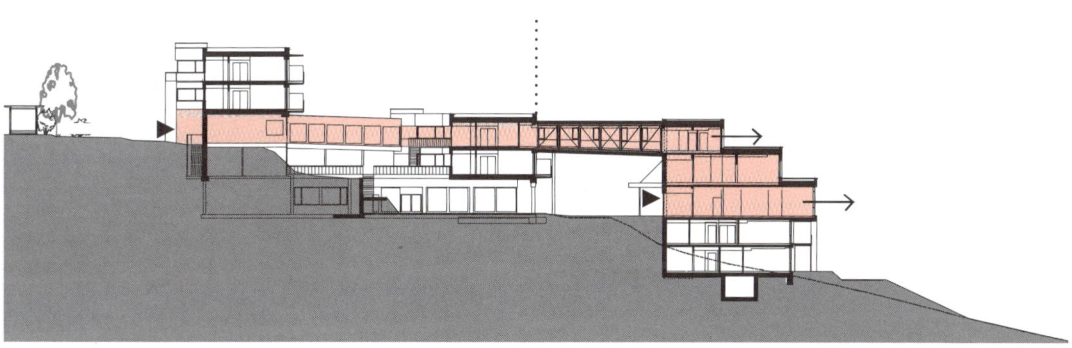

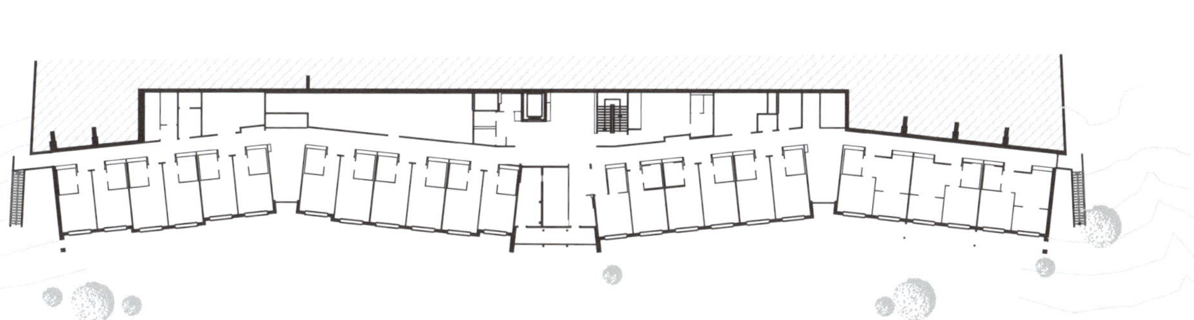

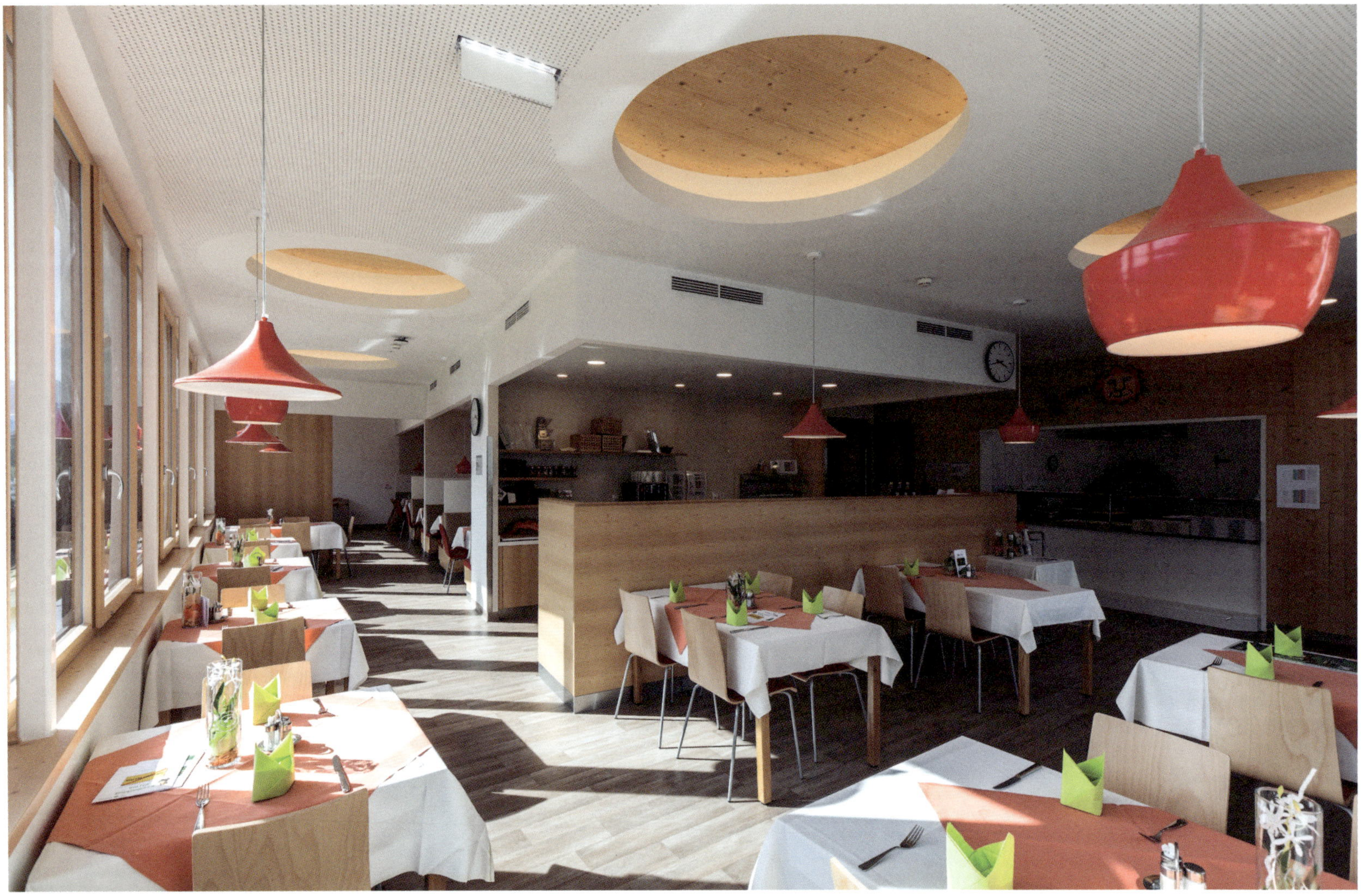

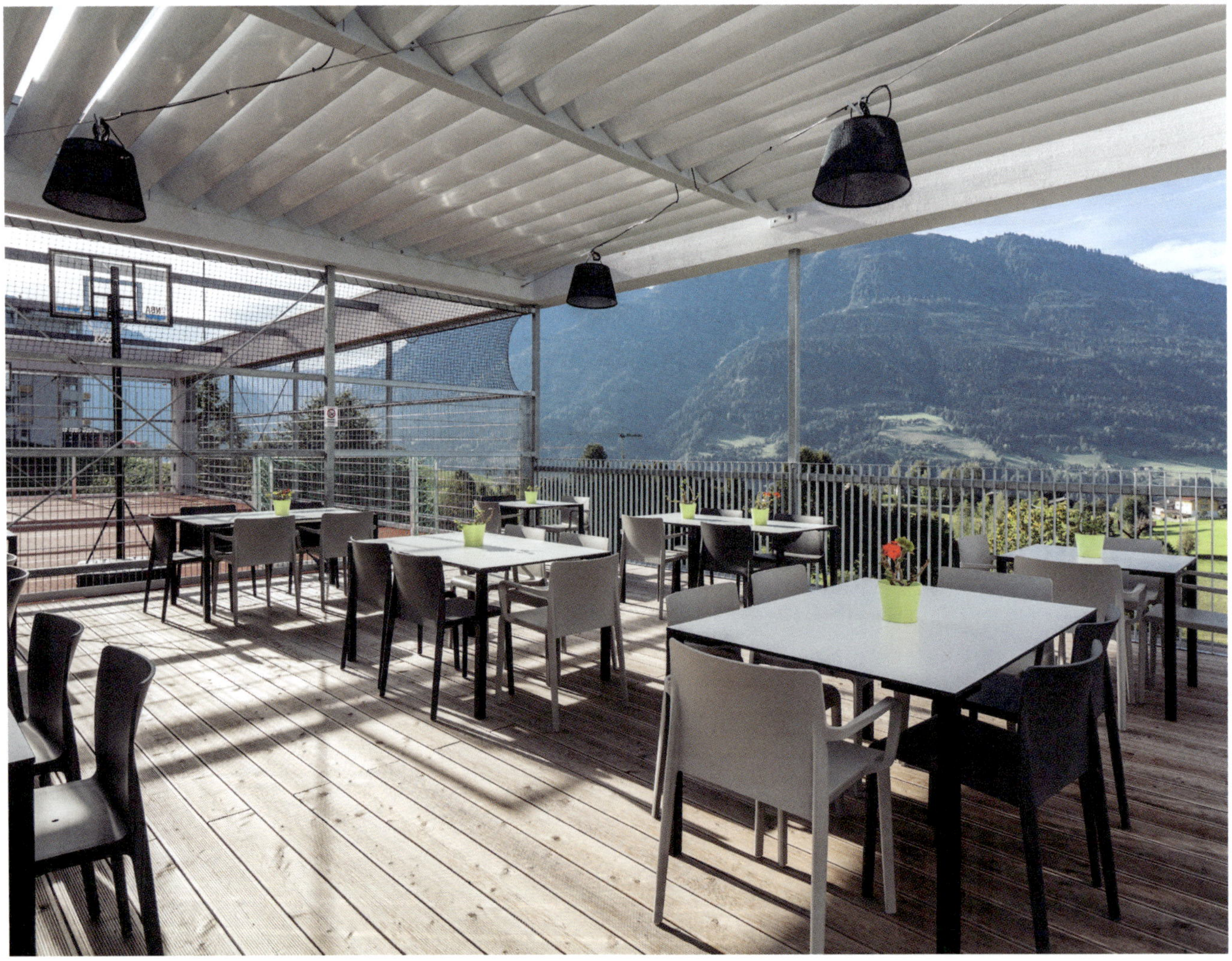

Hospital's dining room for children and families alike.

Roof terrace dining room with a beautiful view.

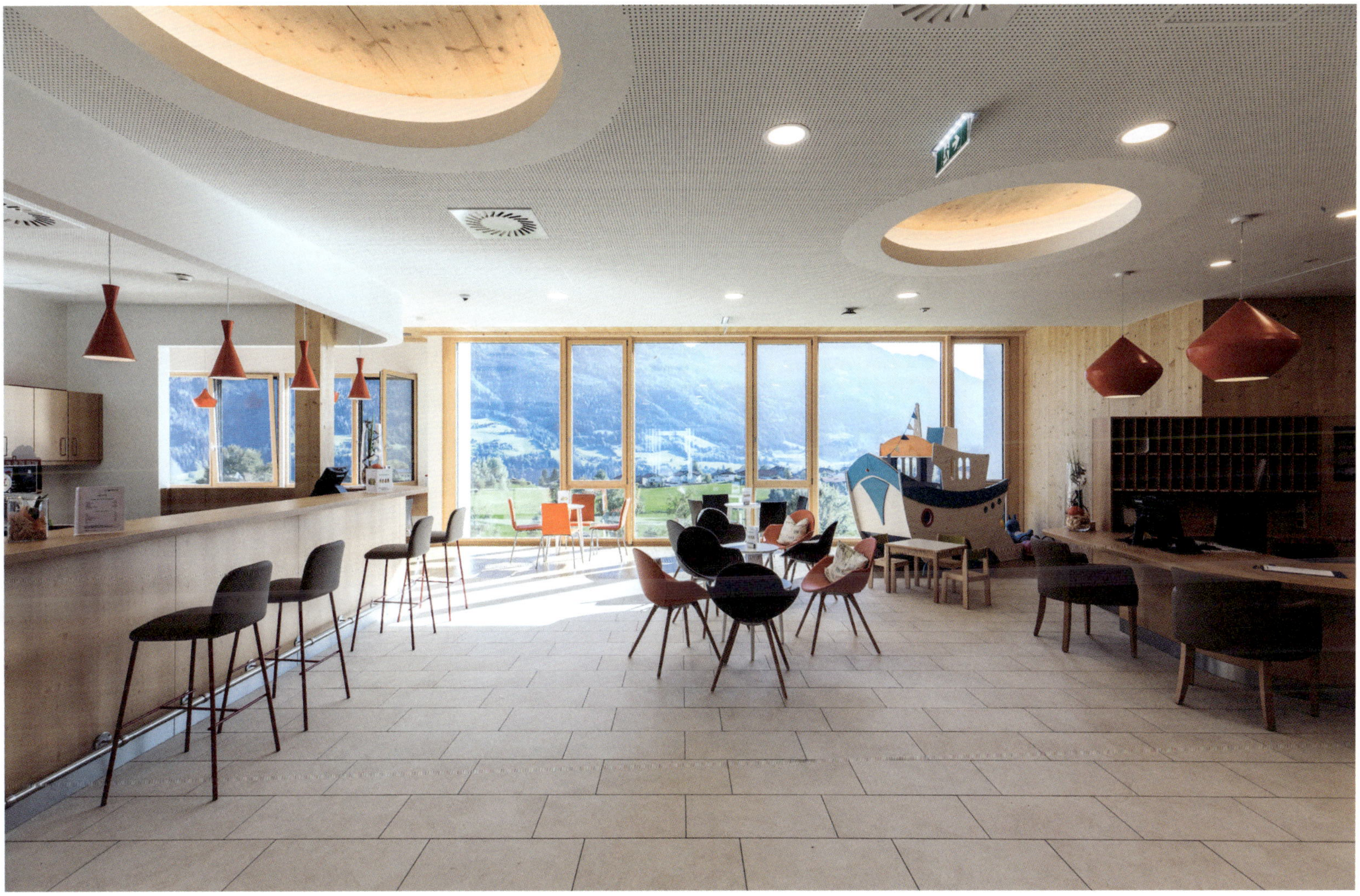

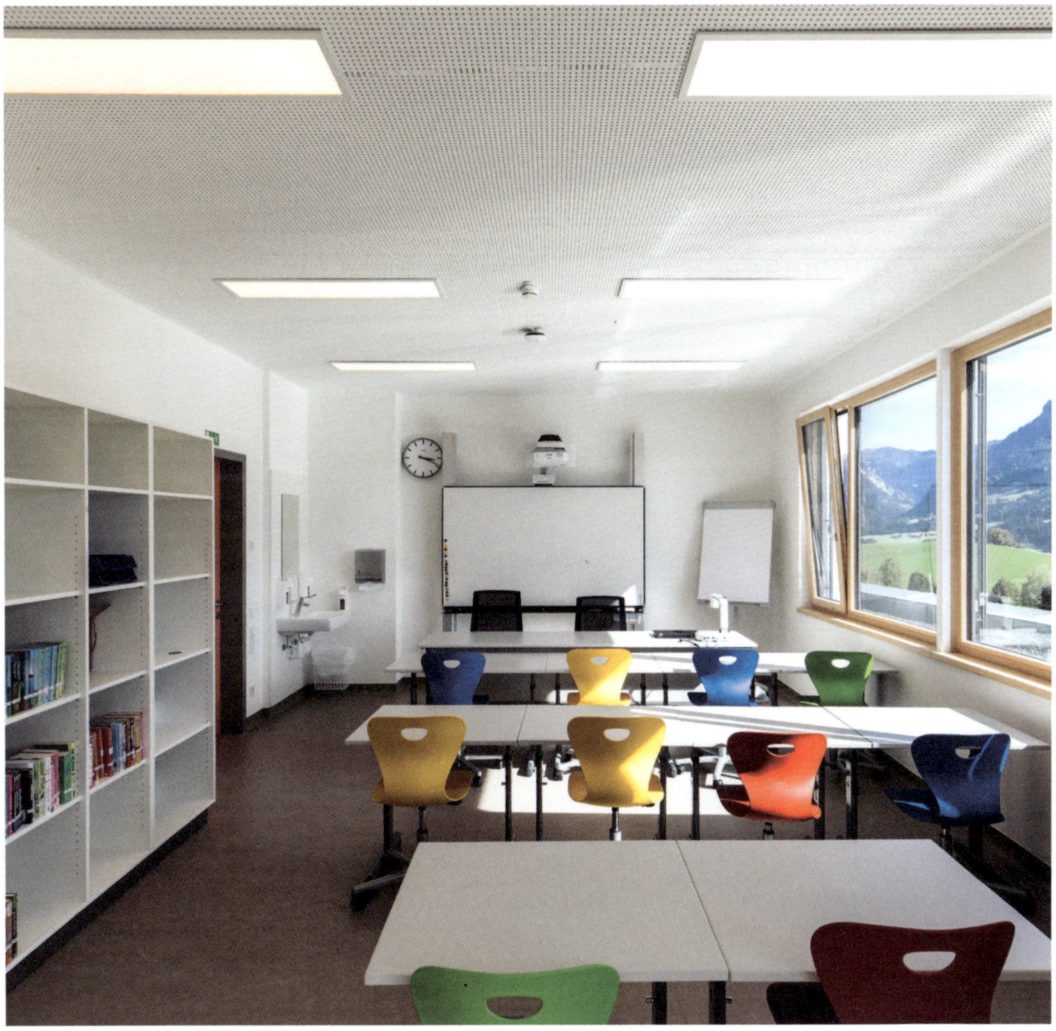

Main entrance hall of the hospital.

Sanatorium school inside the hospital.

Architecturestudio

Guadeloupe
French West Indies
France

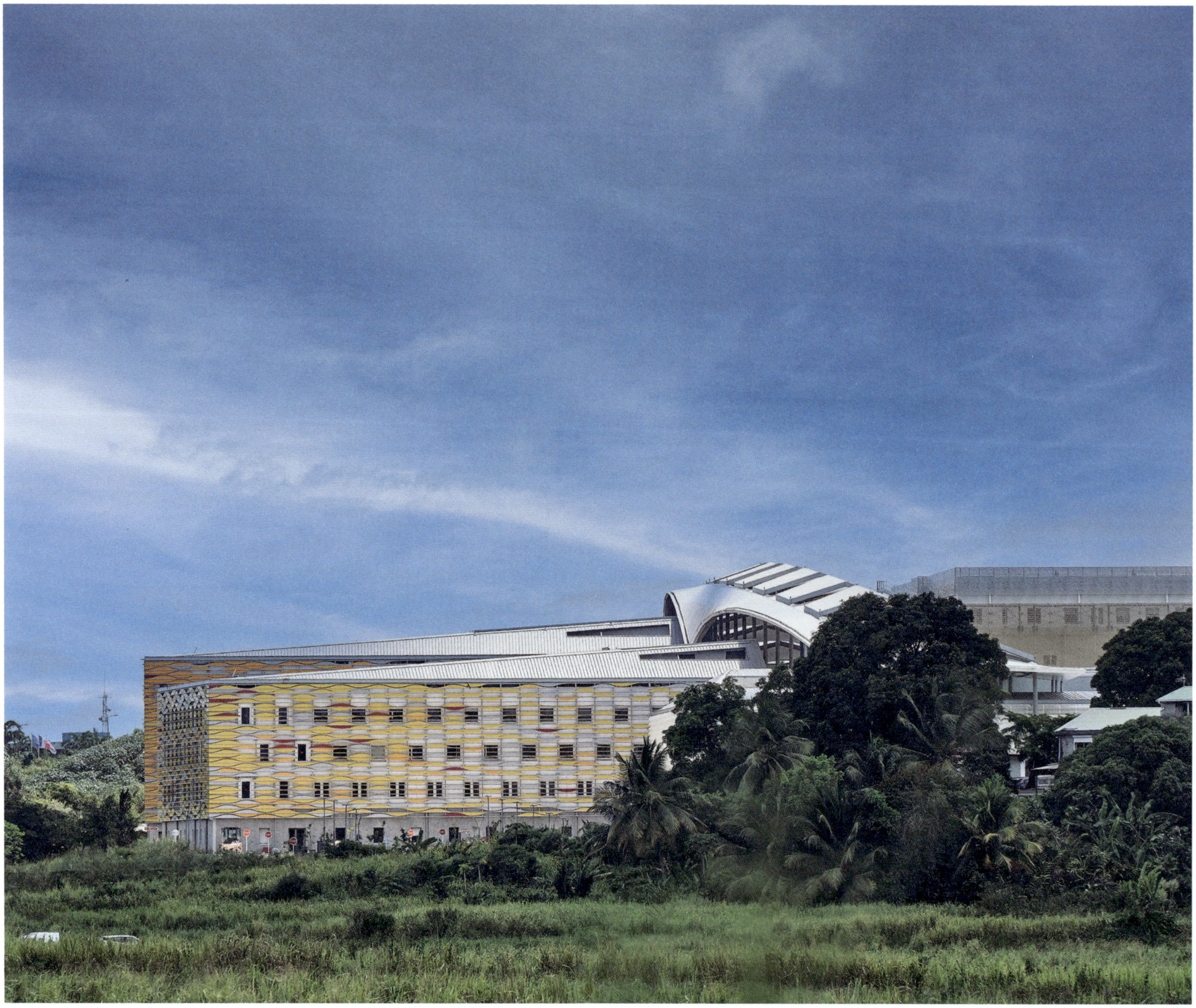

Hospital's inpatient building in the midst of nature.

Public access for patients and visitors.

Hospital's colorful roof detailing.

Guadeloupe University Hospital

The new Guadeloupe University Hospital is an innovative facility designed to combine modularity, resilience, and cultural integration while balancing medical excellence with environmental sustainability. Resilient to major seismic and hurricane risks, the hospital is designed to adapt in the event of a health crisis. Conceived on a 19-hectare site, it is a complex of interconnected buildings organized around a shared technical platform. The medical program comprises a comprehensive medical, surgical, and obstetric university hospital with a technical platform, mounted on seismic isolators, housing emergency services, imaging, operating rooms, neonatology, nuclear medicine, radiation therapy, critical care, laboratories, and more. Its architecture, structured around a central Caribbean street, optimizes patient flow, orientation, and reception. Agility and sustainability are at the heart of the project.

Address: 97139 D106, Les Abymes 97142, Guadeloupe, French West Indies, France | **Client:** Guadeloupe University Hospital | **Completion:** 2026 | **Size:** 85,000 m² | **Sector:** state | **Number of beds:** 700

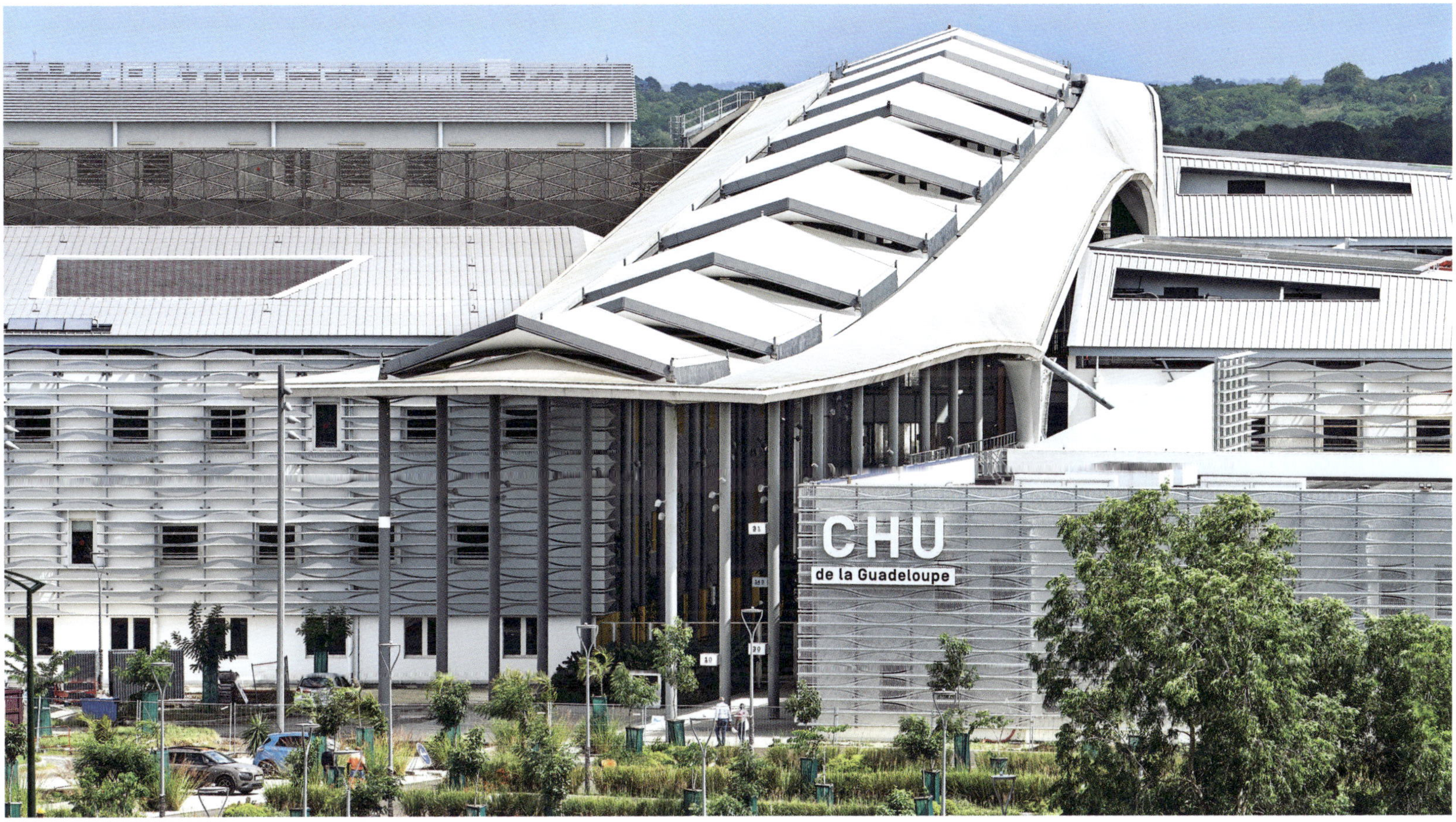

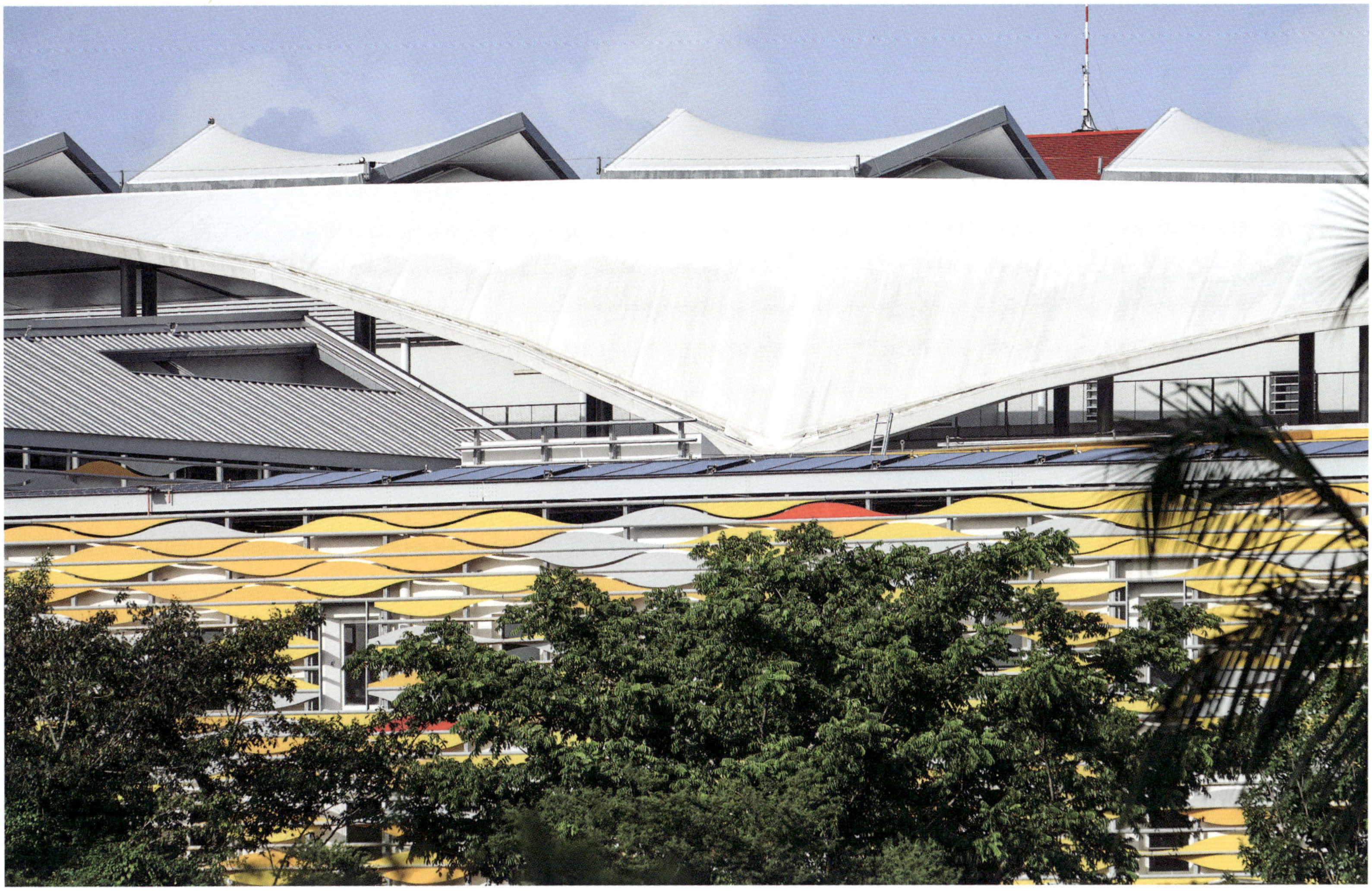

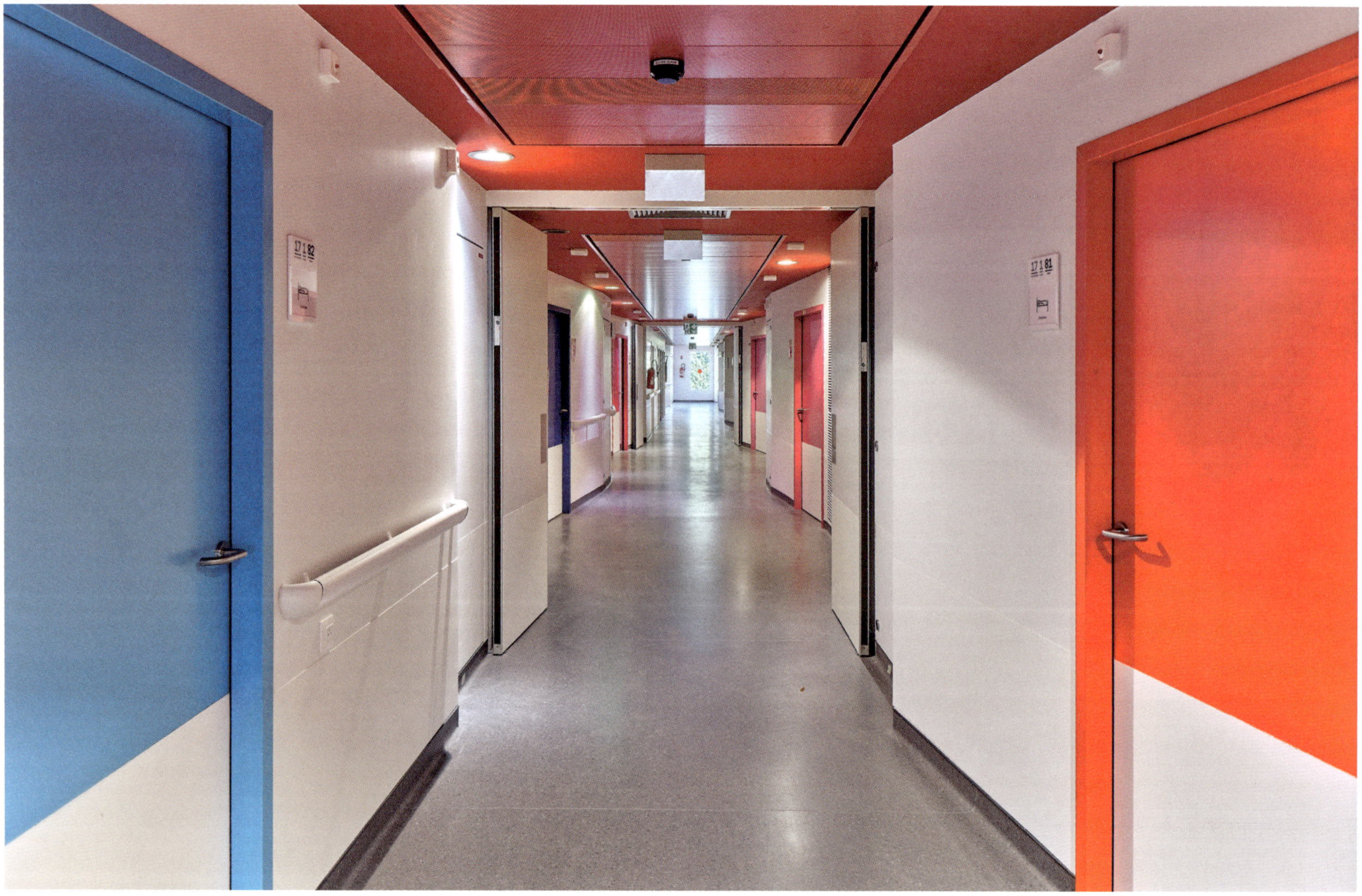

Bright and colorful corridor in an inpatient unit.

Ground floor plan.

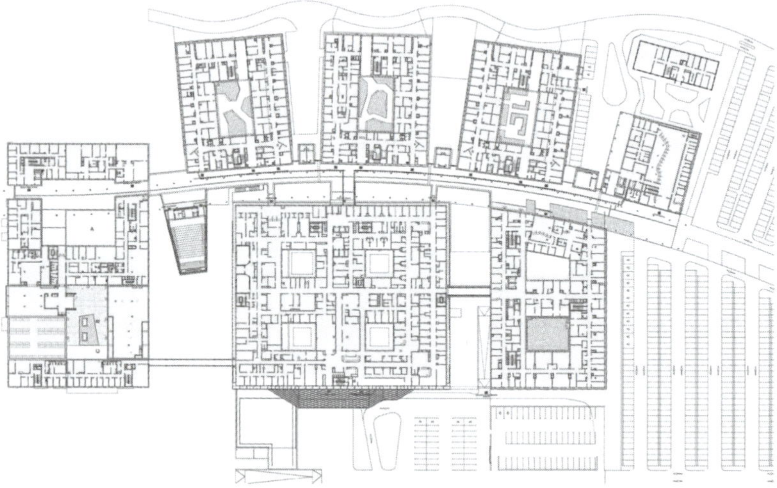

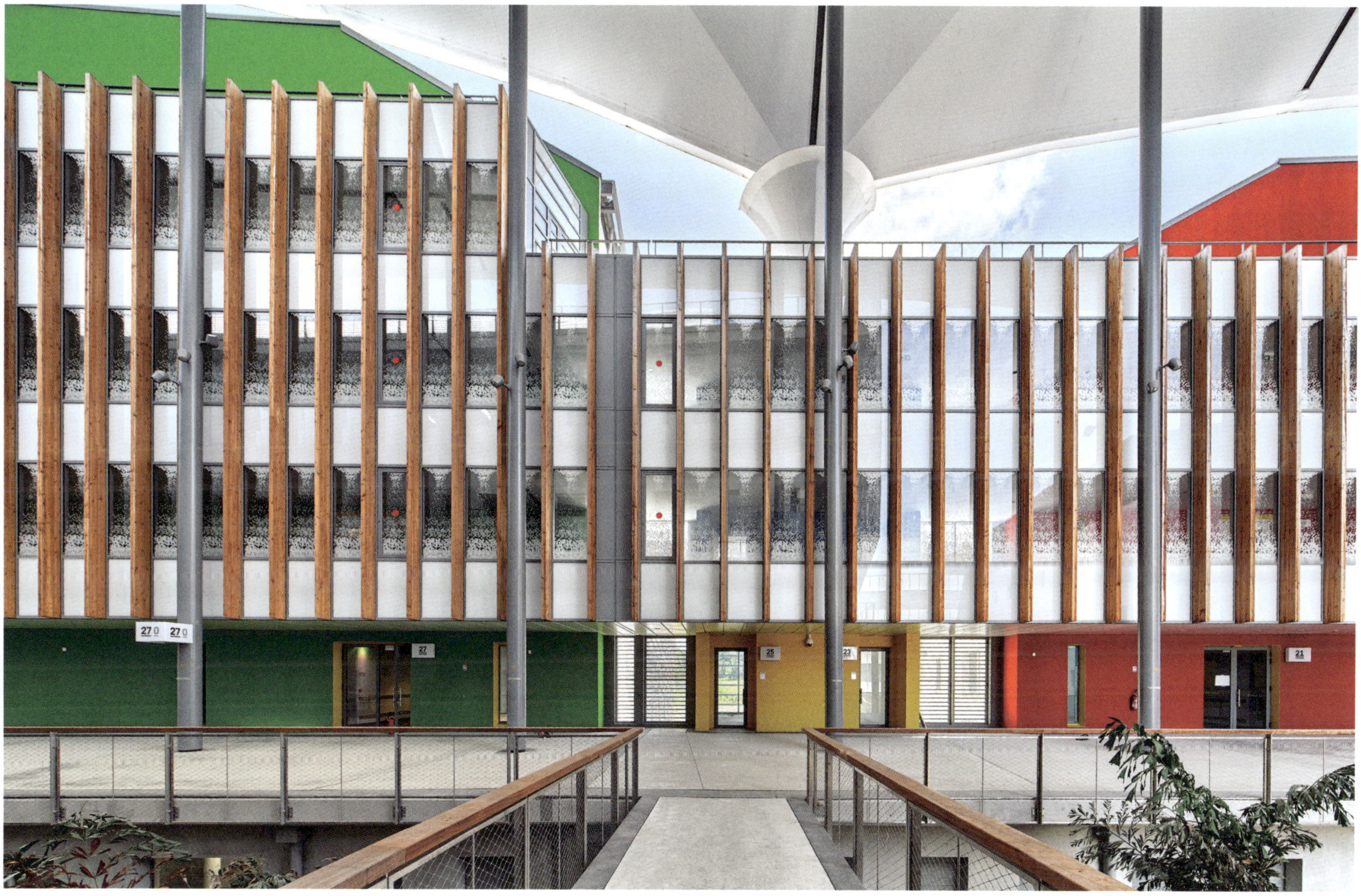

Medical corridors on the first floor.

Section.

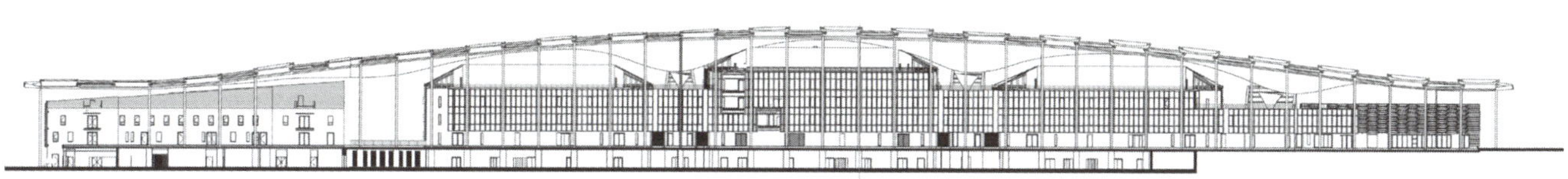

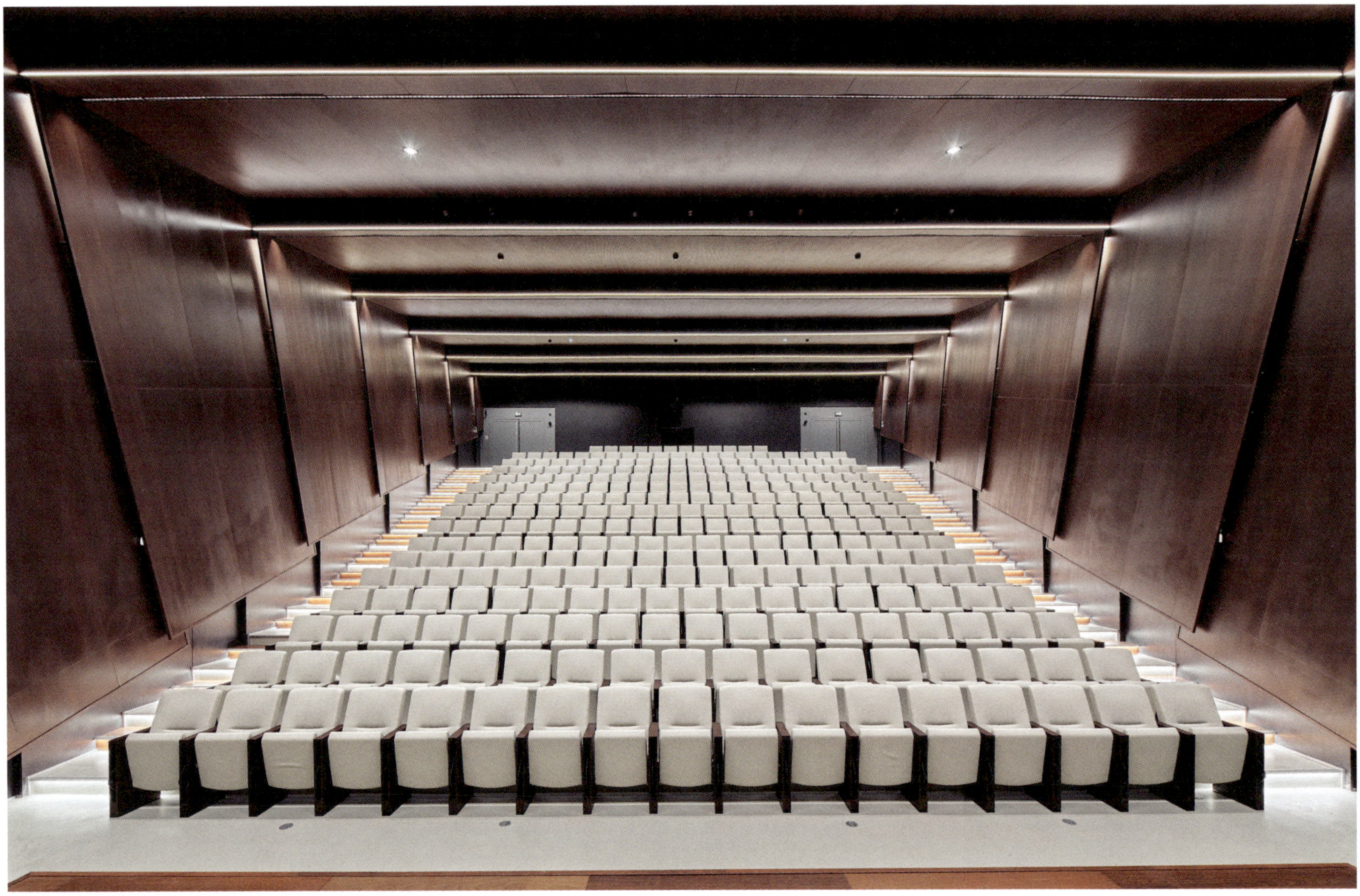

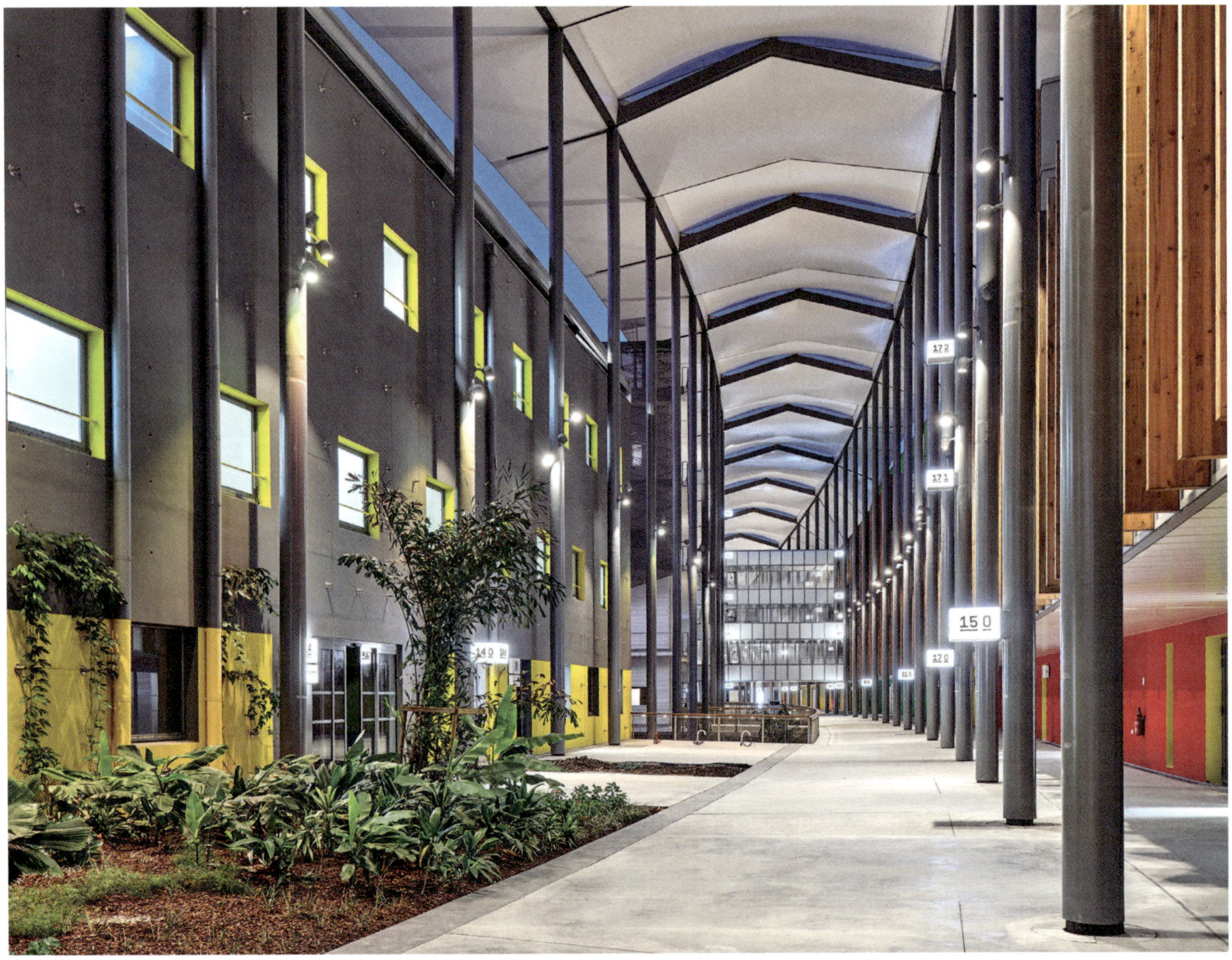

Hospital's amphitheater.

Well lit and color-coordinated indoor circulation.

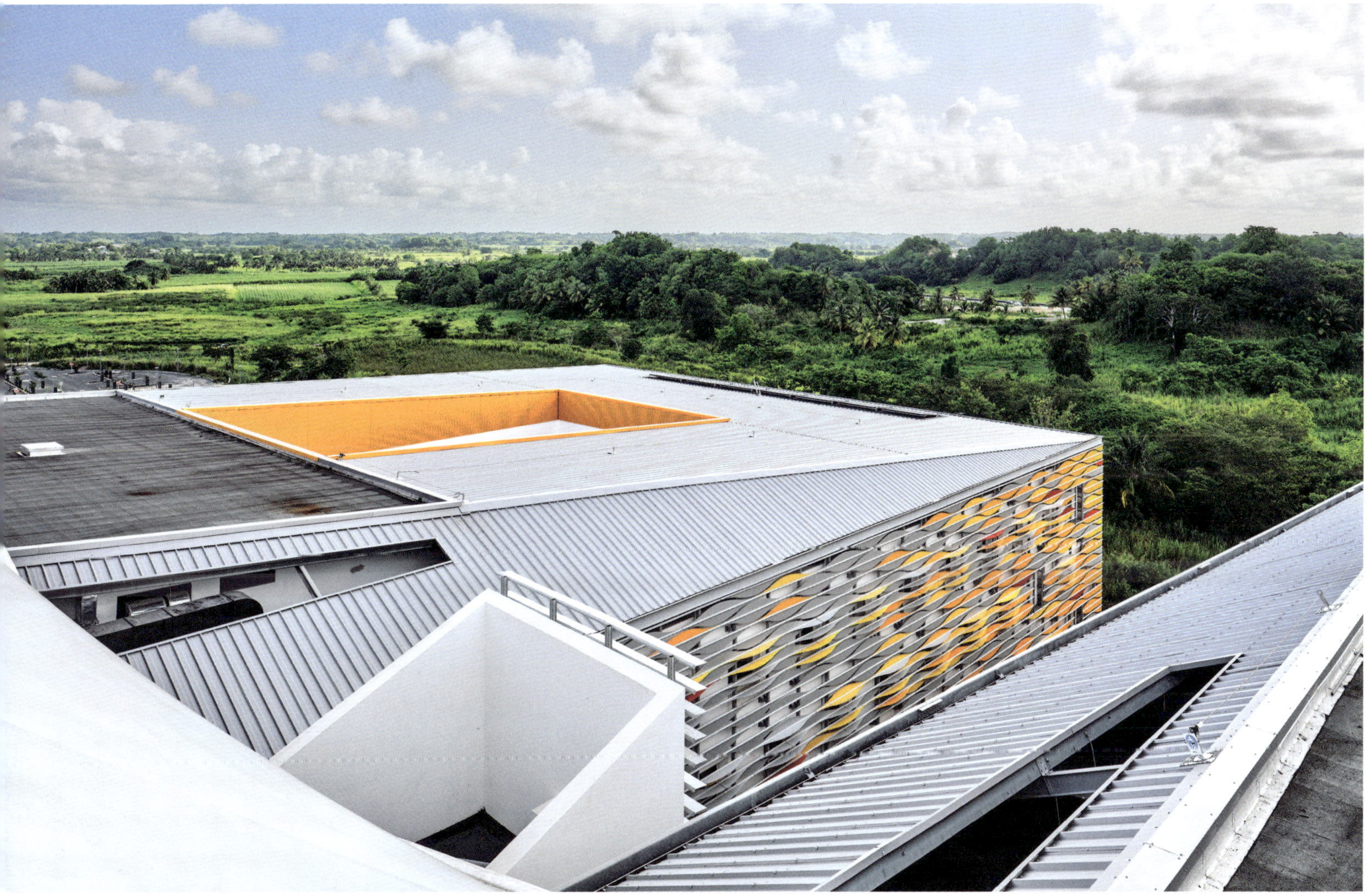

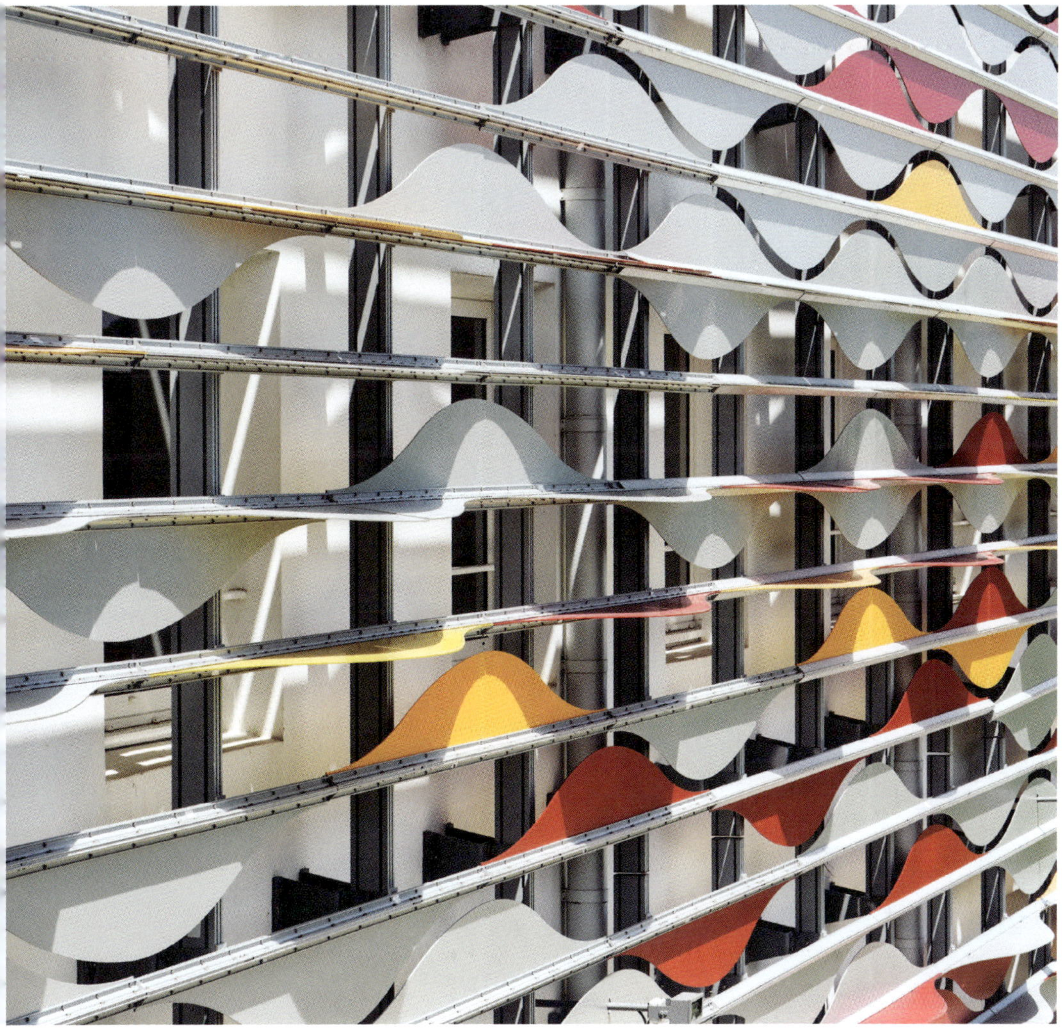

View of the inpatient building from above.

Detailing of the hospital's sunshades.

kerstin gierse architekten

Düsseldorf Germany

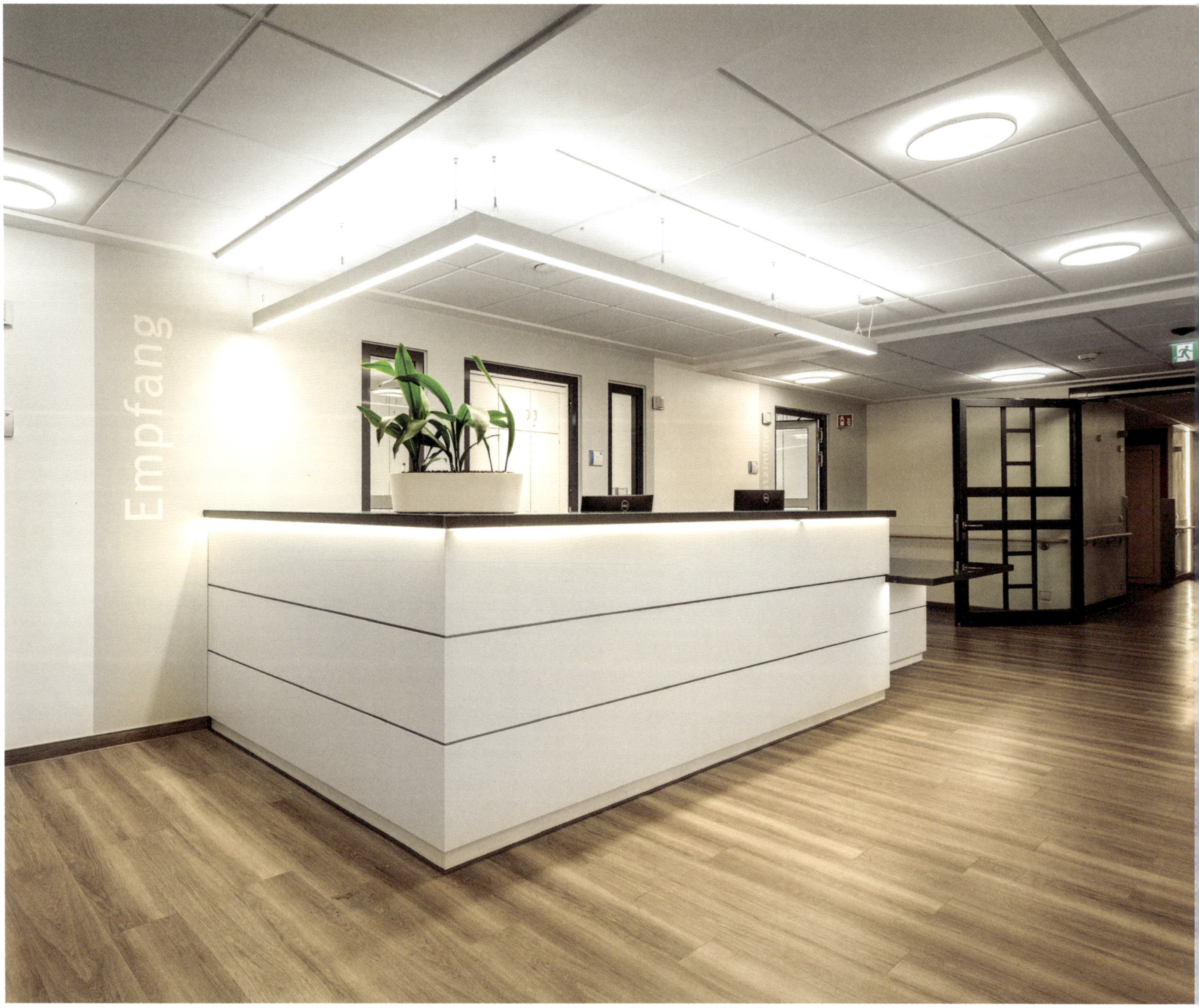

The spacious, newly redesigned reception area for two state-of-the-art wards.

Gray and natural tones, comfortable seating, and soft lighting create a cozy atmosphere in the common areas.

The functional floor plan and the overall interior design concept were developed in hand-in-hand.

Oncology Center and Palliative Care Unit at Florence Nightingale Hospital

In 2021, a modern Oncology Center and a new Palliative Care Unit were established at the Florence Nightingale Hospital in Düsseldorf. To achieve this, the entire first floor was gutted and completely rebuilt. The goal was to improve patients' quality of life and comfort. The former intensive care unit was removed, adjacent rooms were restructured, and the reception area was functionally redesigned. The result is bright single and double rooms with barrier-free bathrooms, pleasant lighting, and home-like furnishings. A large balcony with a view of the greenery and a new day room encourage social interaction and relaxation. The architecture emphasizes modern standards, short distances, and a calm atmosphere. Large-scale backlit images and wood-look flooring further create a warm, friendly environment and support optimal palliative care. In this way, functionality was combined with well-being.

Address: Kreuzbergstraße 79, 40489 Düsseldorf, Germany | **Client:** Kaiserswerther Diakonie | **Completion:** 2021 | **Size:** 850 m^2 | **Sector:** nonprofit | **Specialization:** oncology and palliative care | **Number of treatment rooms:** 2 | **Number of patient rooms:** 12

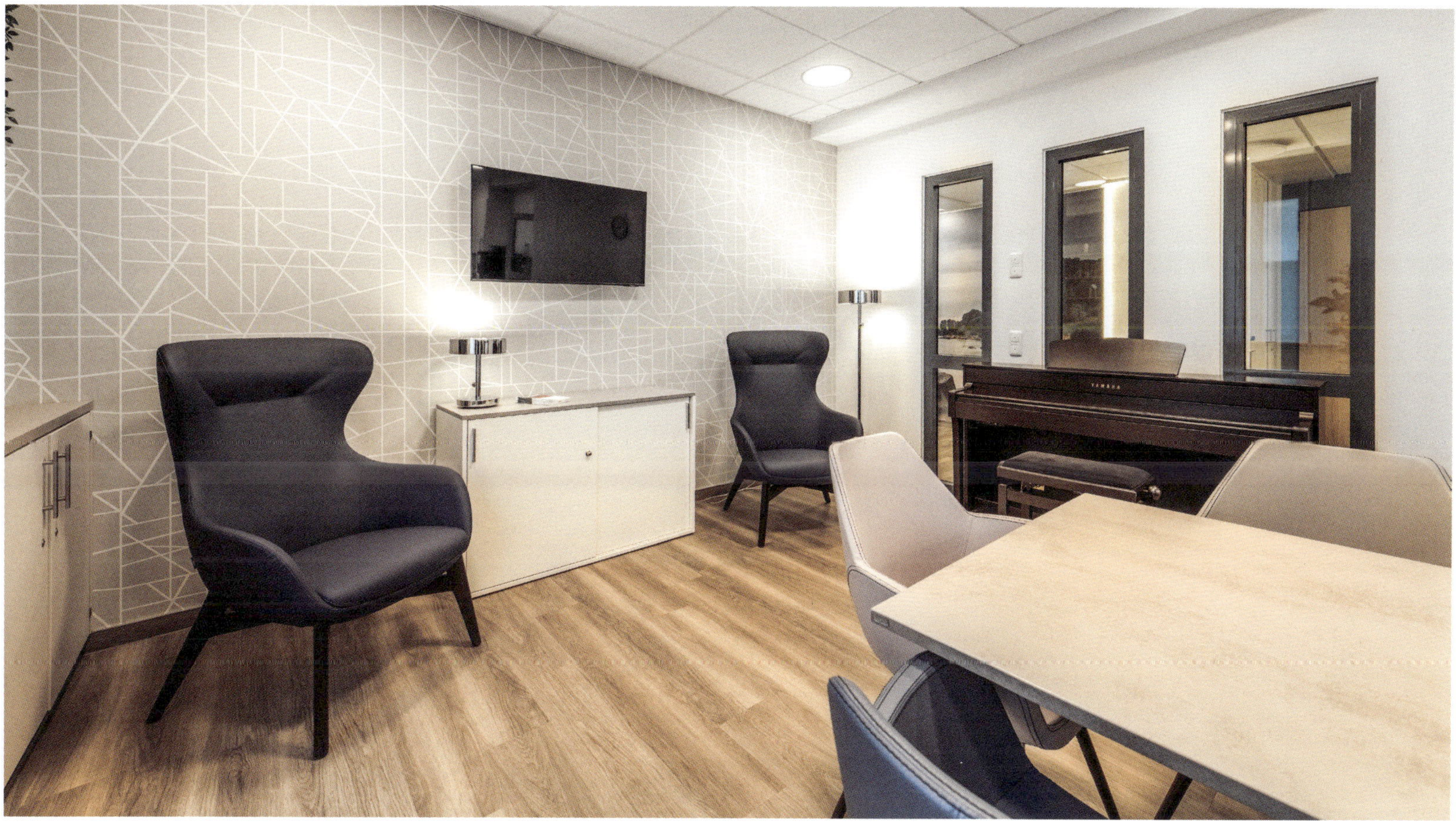

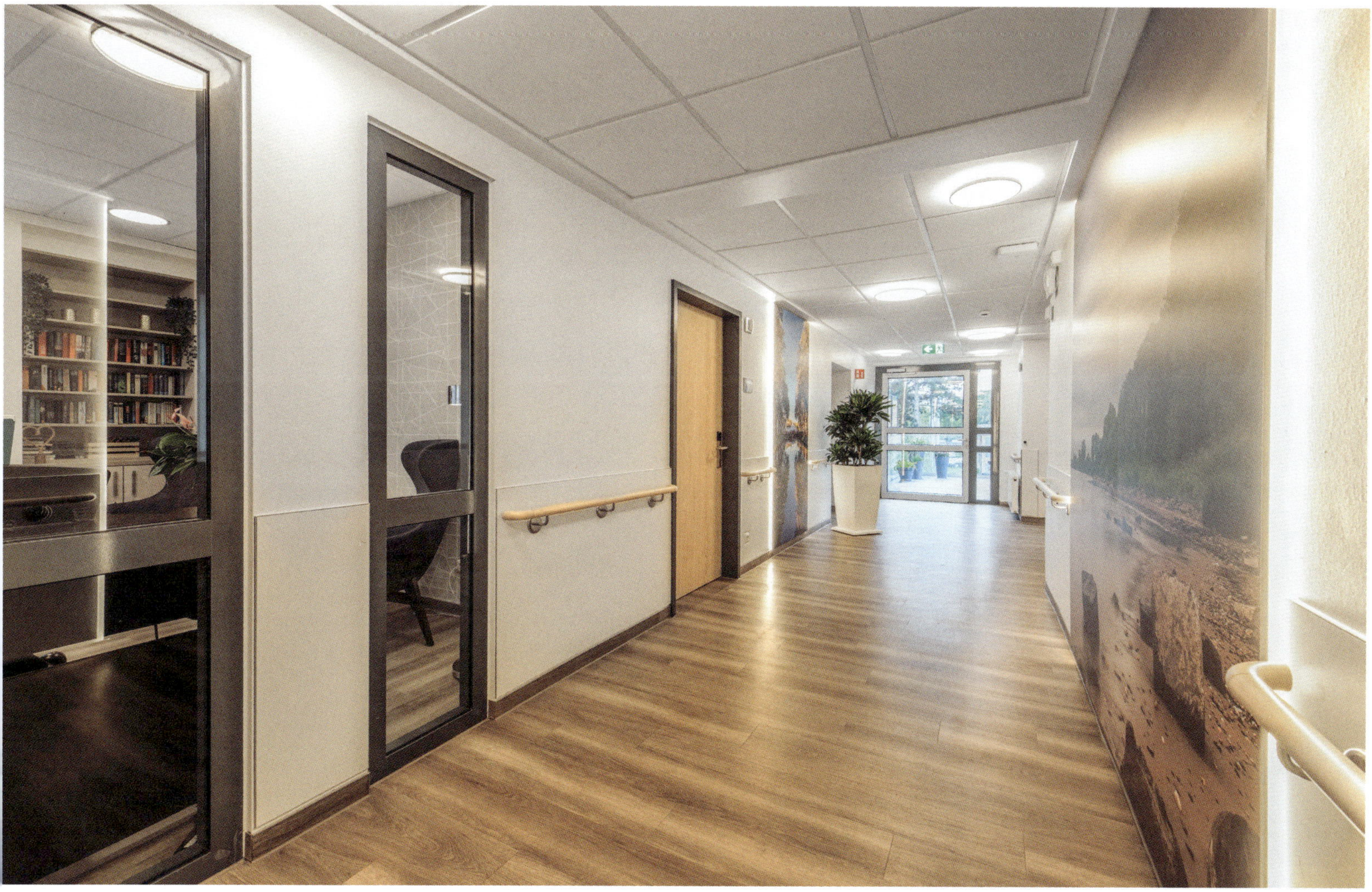

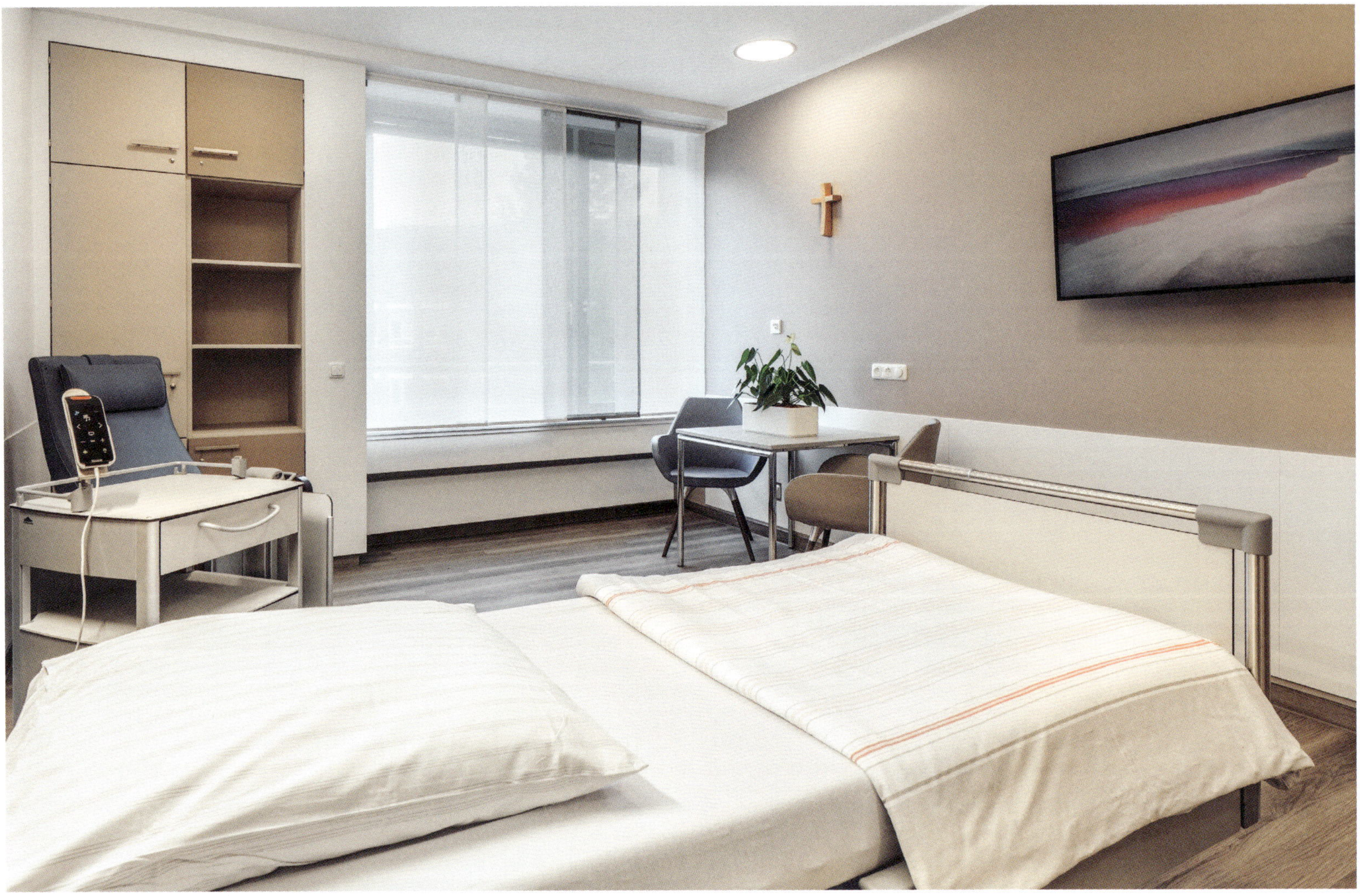

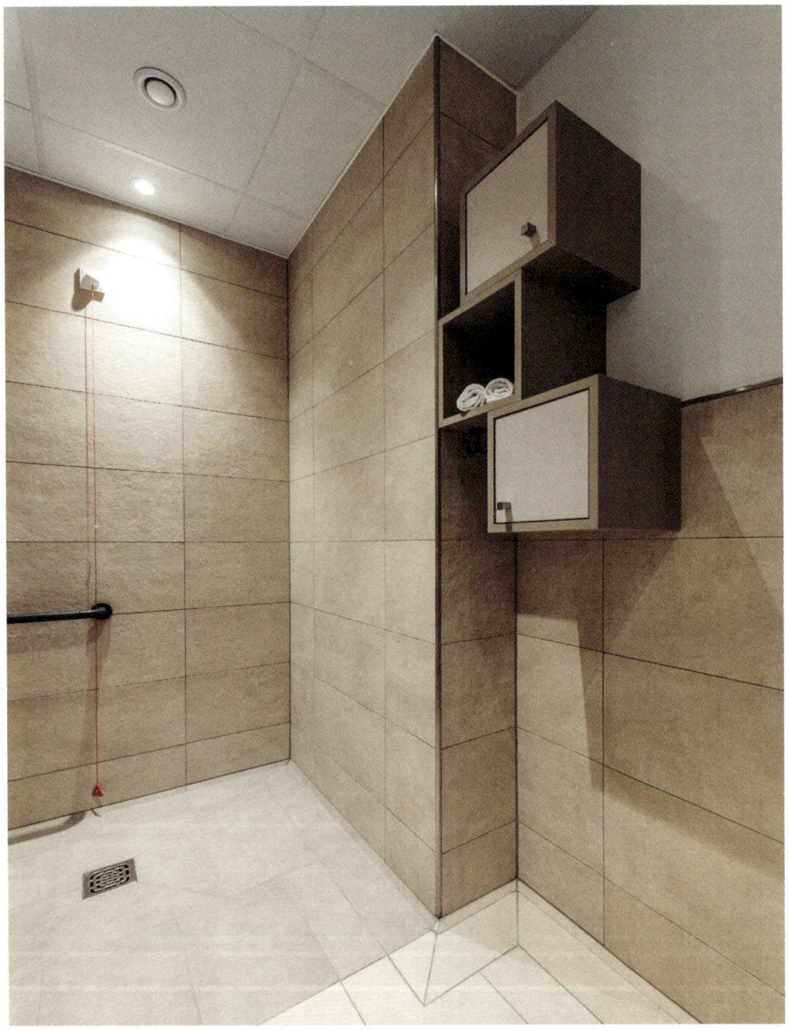

The entire first floor was completely gutted and renovated from the ground up while the clinic remained open.

An accessible, modern bathroom with porcelain tiles and high-quality fixtures.

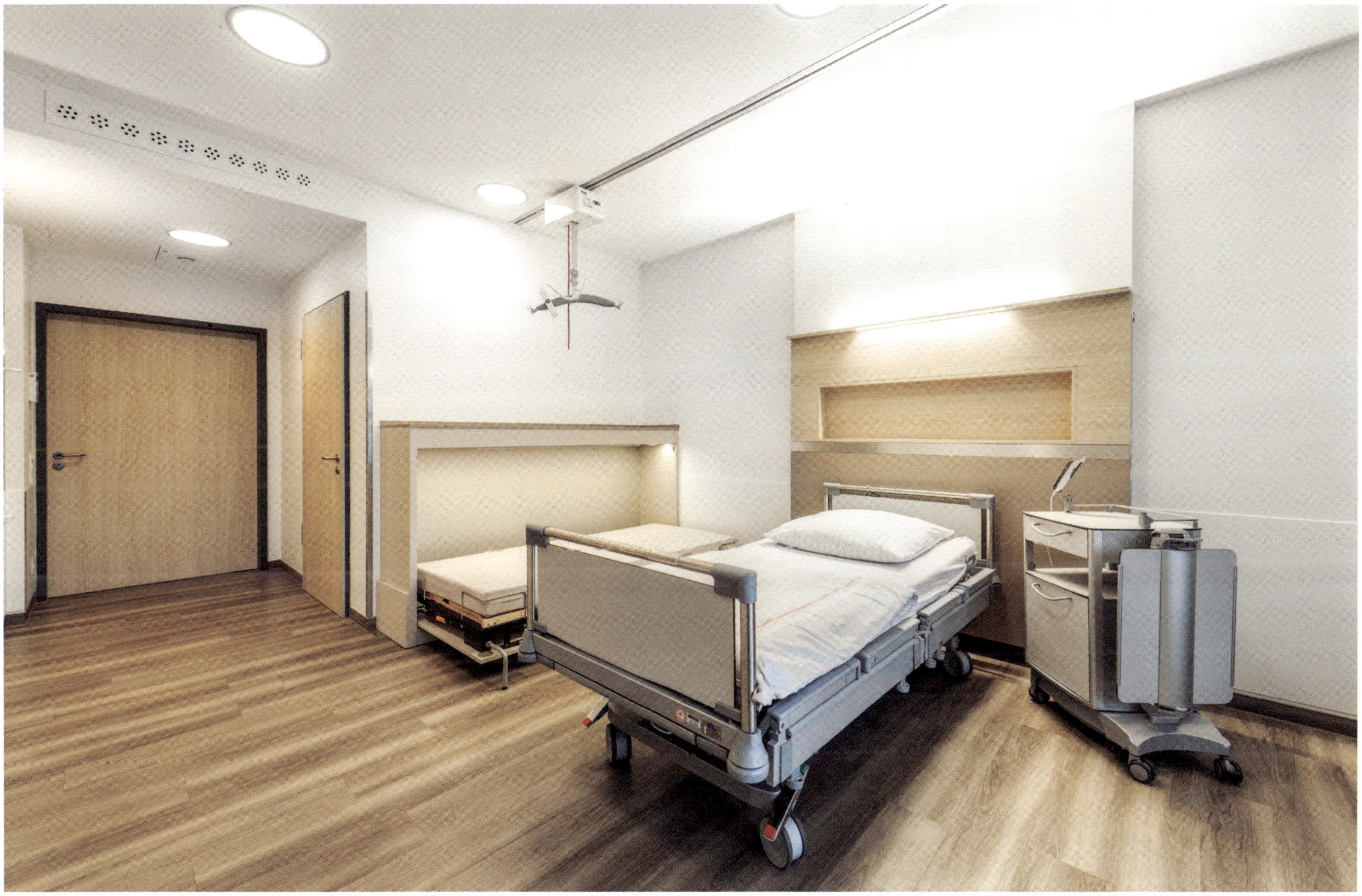

In the palliative care unit, family members can use built-in fold-out beds.

Floor plan.

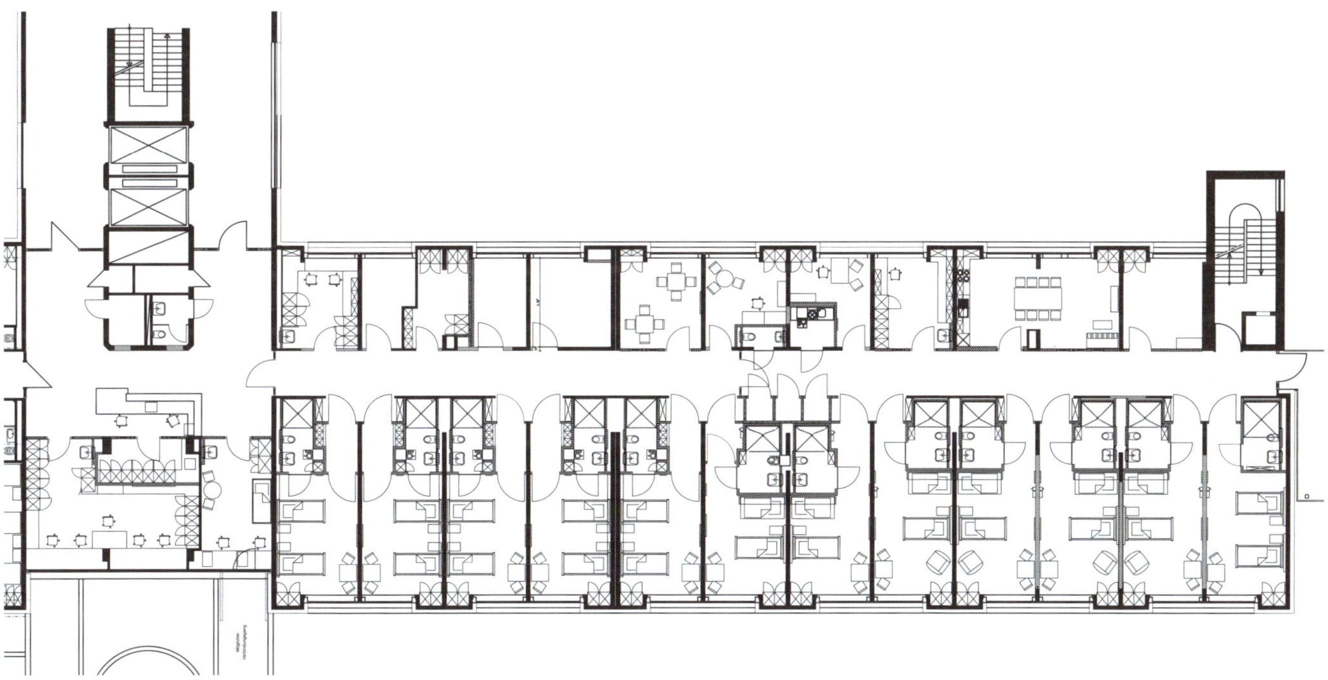

gmp · von Gerkan, Marg und Partner Architects
Ferrari Architectes

Lausanne
Switzerland

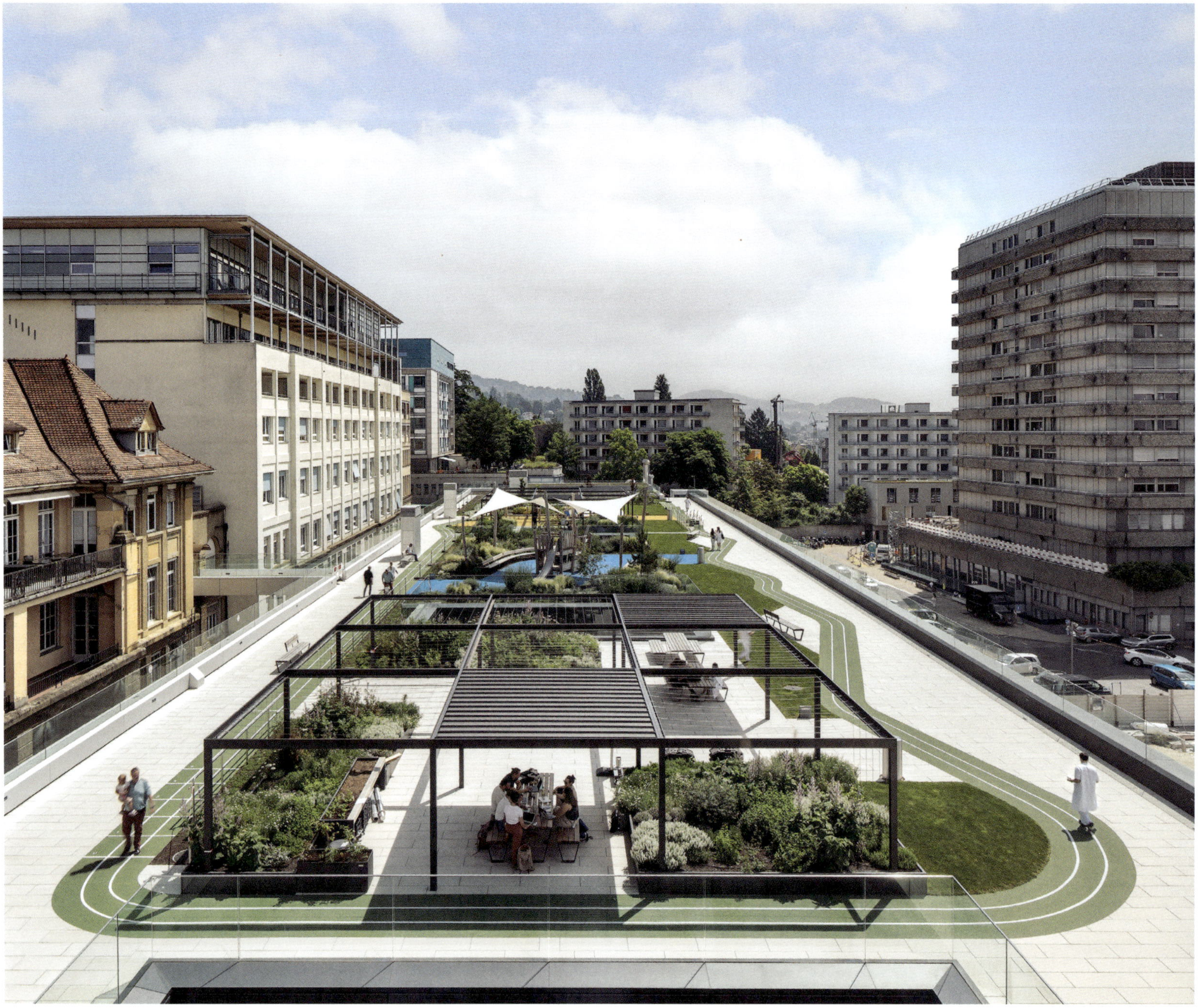

Roof top garden with gathering spaces and green track.

Façade view from the garden.

Children's Hospital at the Lausanne University Hospital

The children's hospital in the center of the campus of the Lausanne University Hospital (CHUV) appears in a dialogue with its urban surroundings drawing attention to a clear entrance situation and a disctinct façade design. It also integrates a subway station in its building volume and proves capable of adapting to evolving future needs. An important element of the concept are the gardens that are placed on the roof and the lower part of the building serving as a therapy and rehabilitation space as well as providing an outdoor area for the adjacent cafeteria. Special attention was paid to creating a family-friendly design. Ample natural light creates an atmosphere that is both soothing and stimulating, a harmonious color and material concept ensures a warm and inviting ambience. A unique interior design feature is a multifunctional bench along the window, which can be converted into an extra bed.

Address: Rue du Bugnon 50, 1011 Lausanne, Switzerland | **Client:** Etat de Vaud, DSAS, CHUV | **Completion:** 2025 | **Size:** 39,232 m² | **Sector:** public | **Specialization:** children's hospital | **Number of treatment rooms:** 14 | **Number of patient rooms:** 71 | **Landscape design:** Verzone Woods Architectes

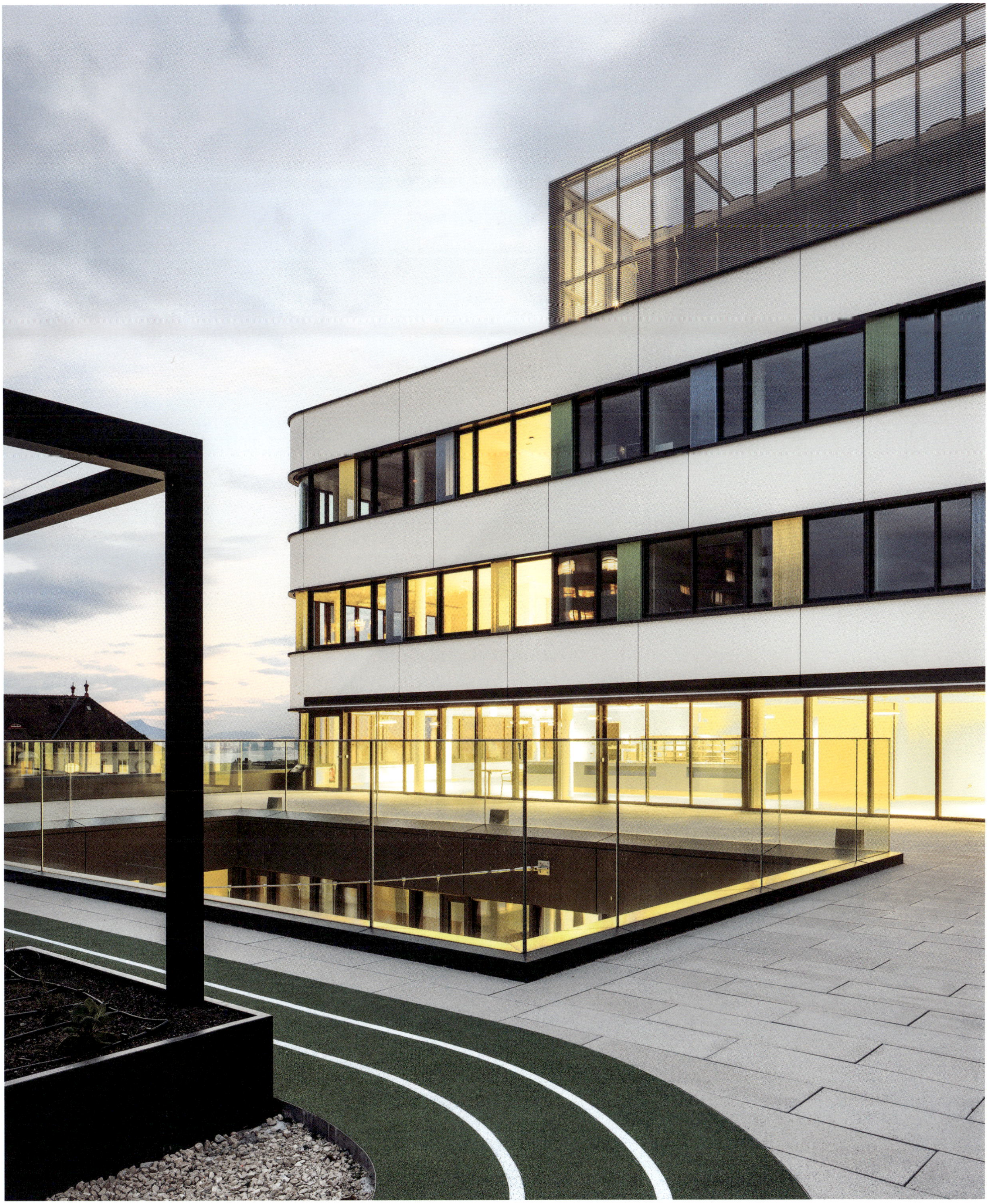

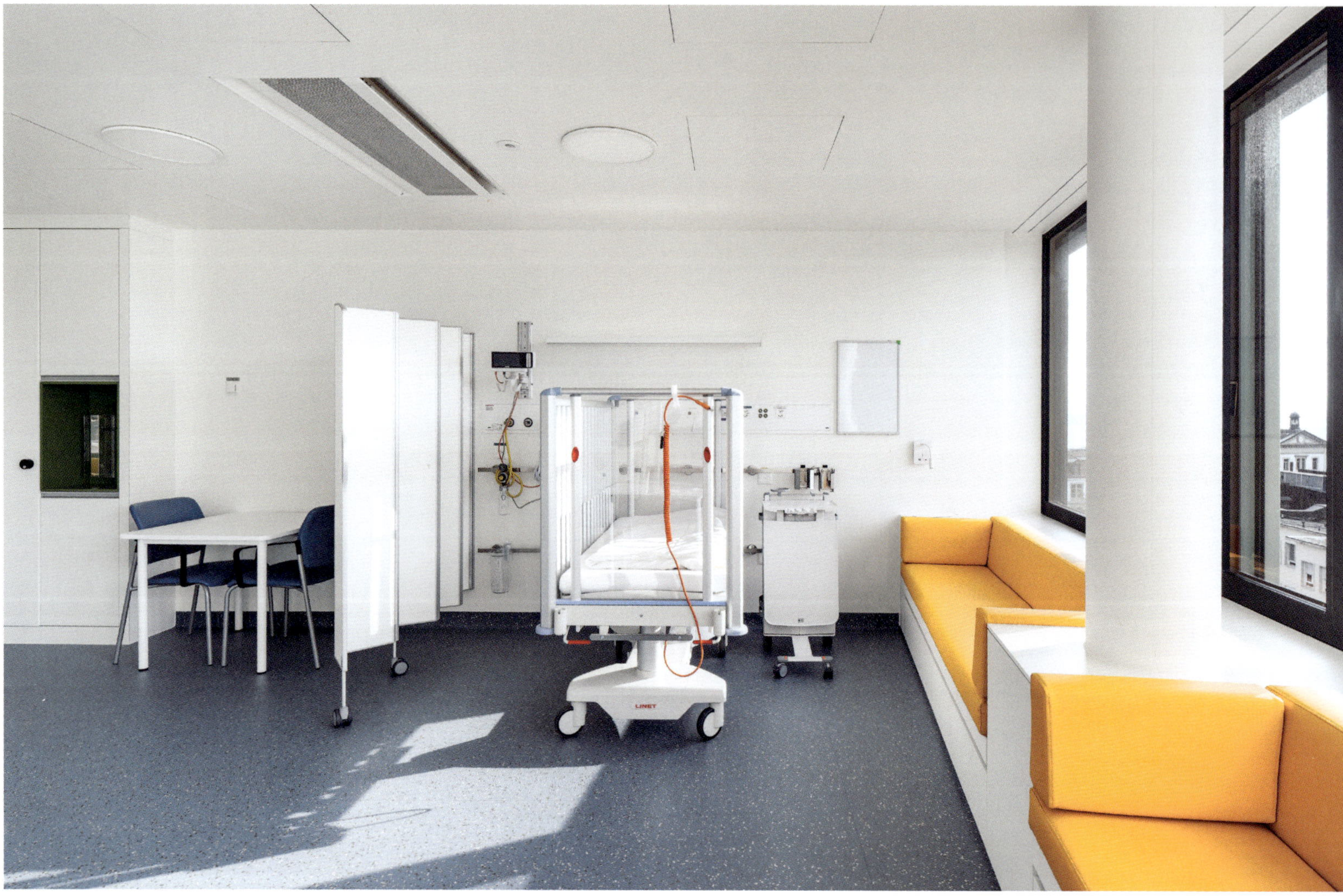

Room with convertible benches.

Ground floor plan.

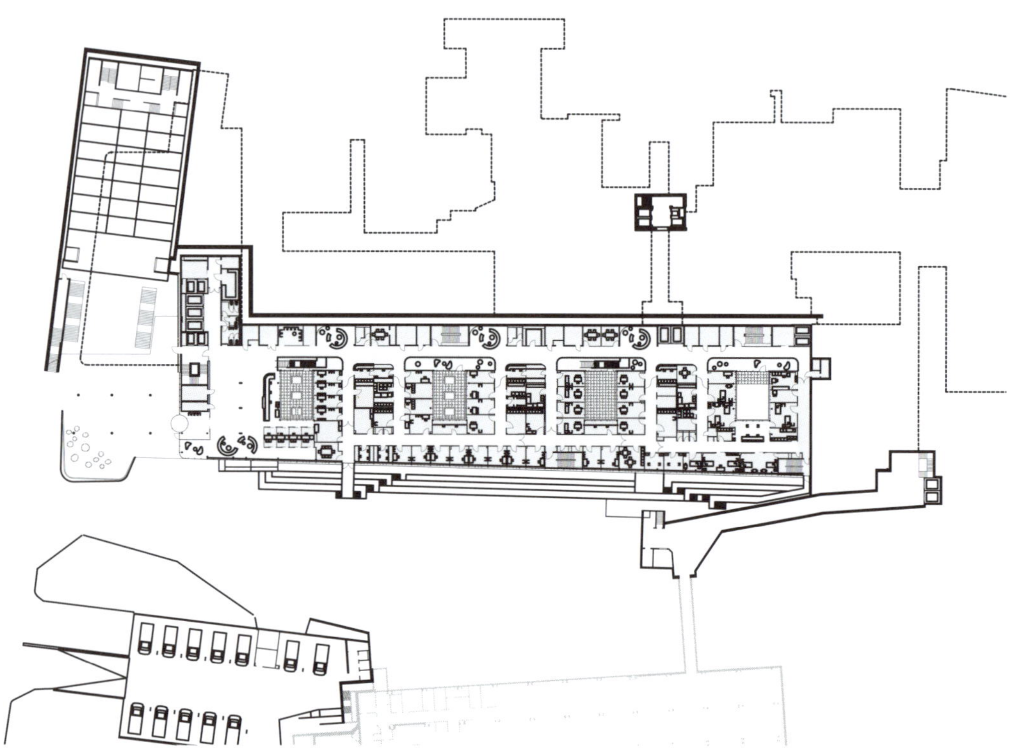

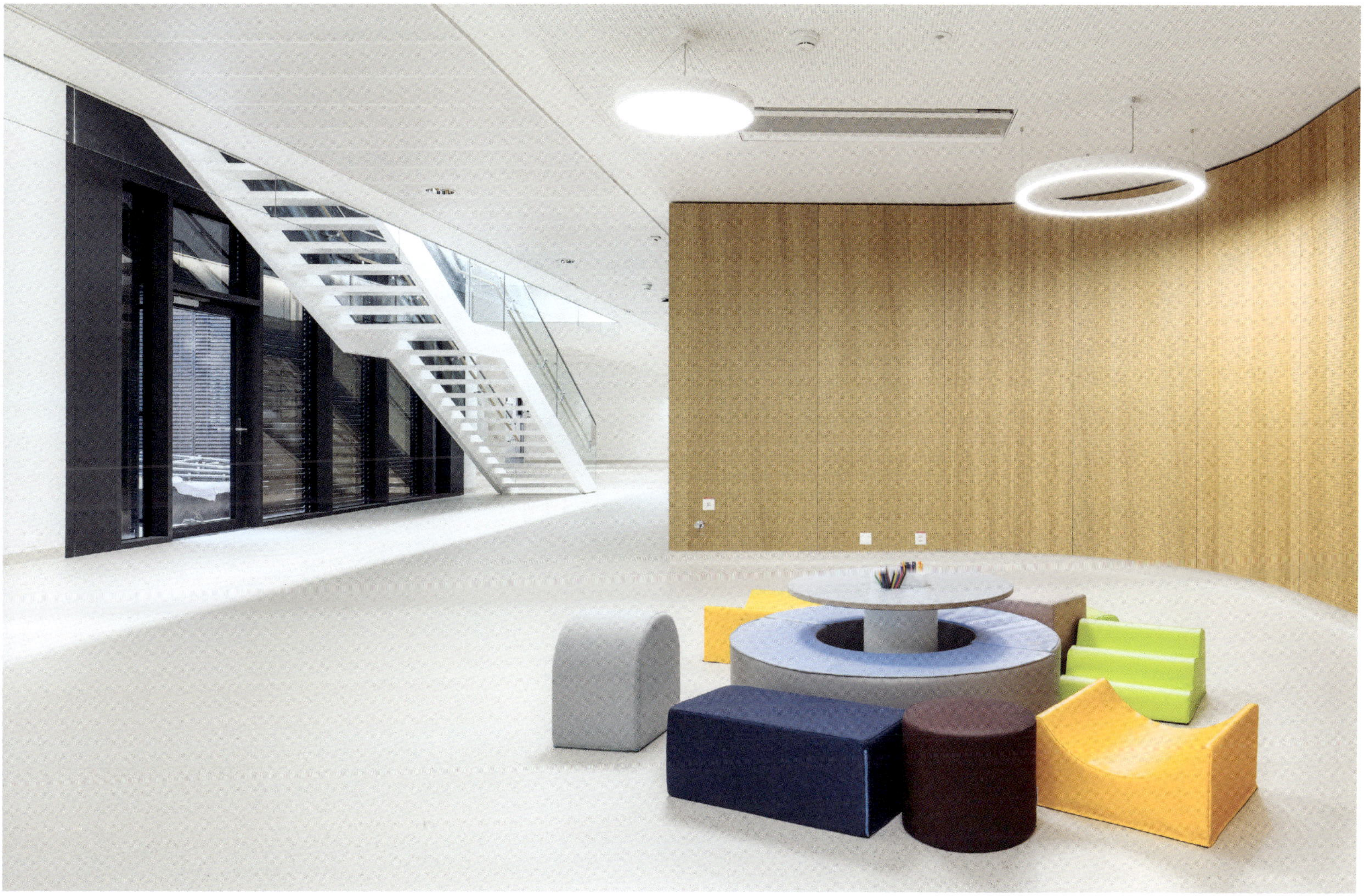

Entrance hall with colorful furniture.

Sections.

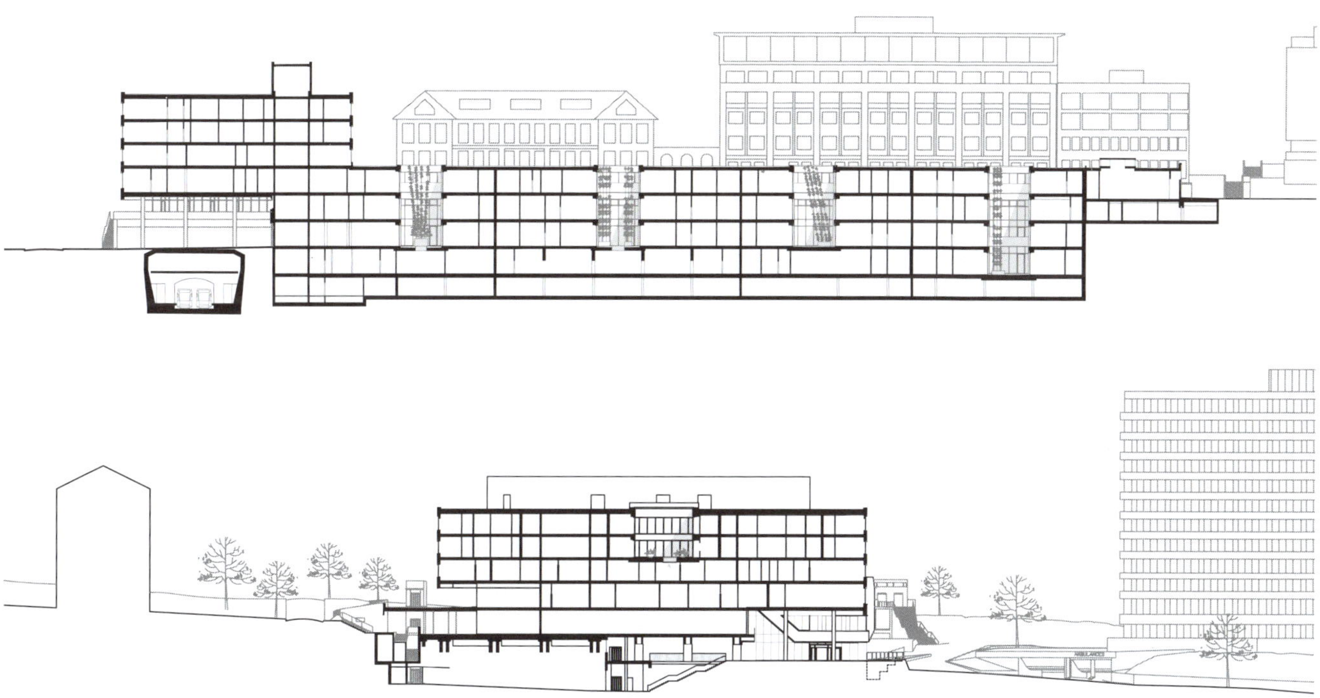

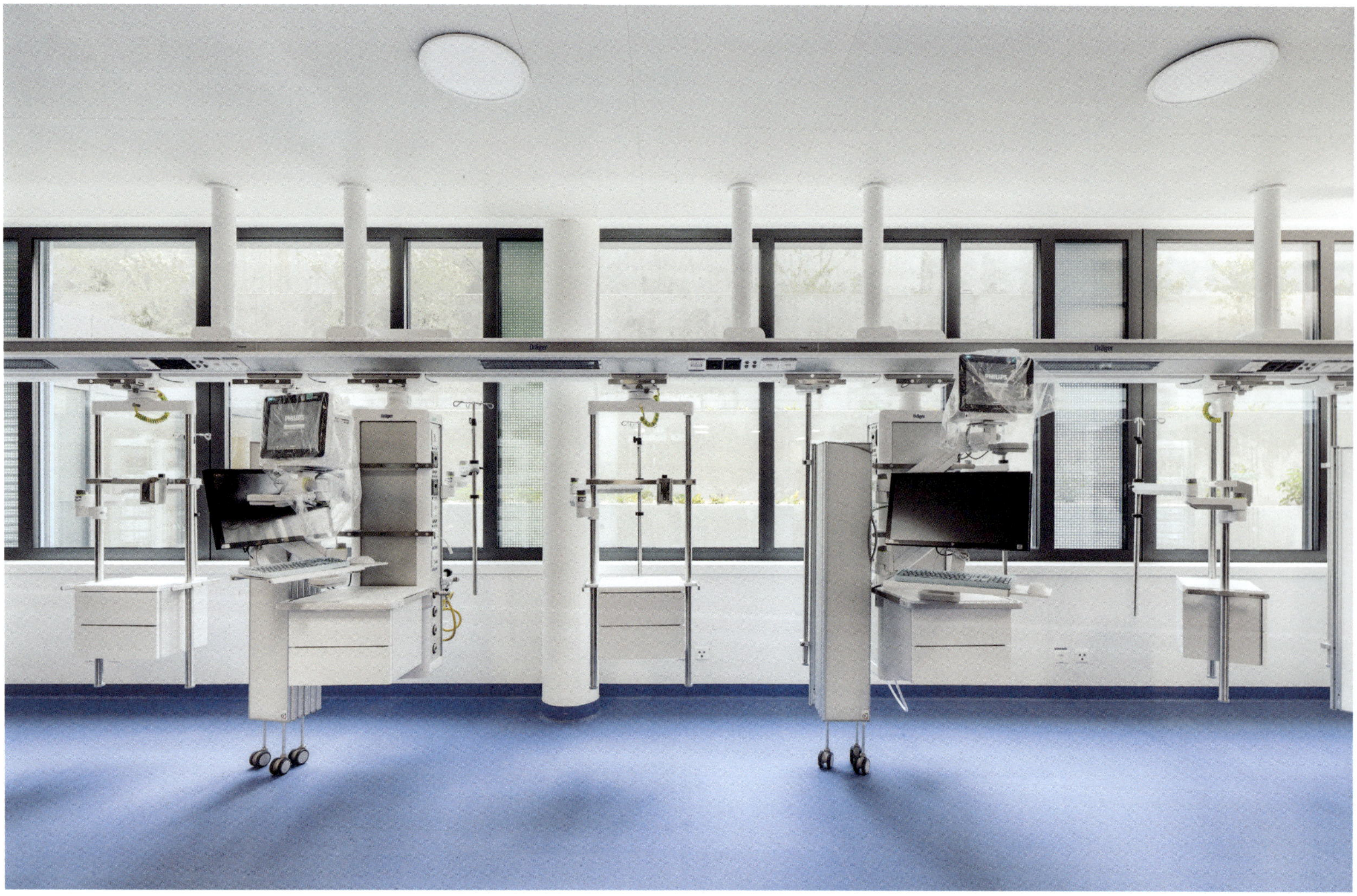

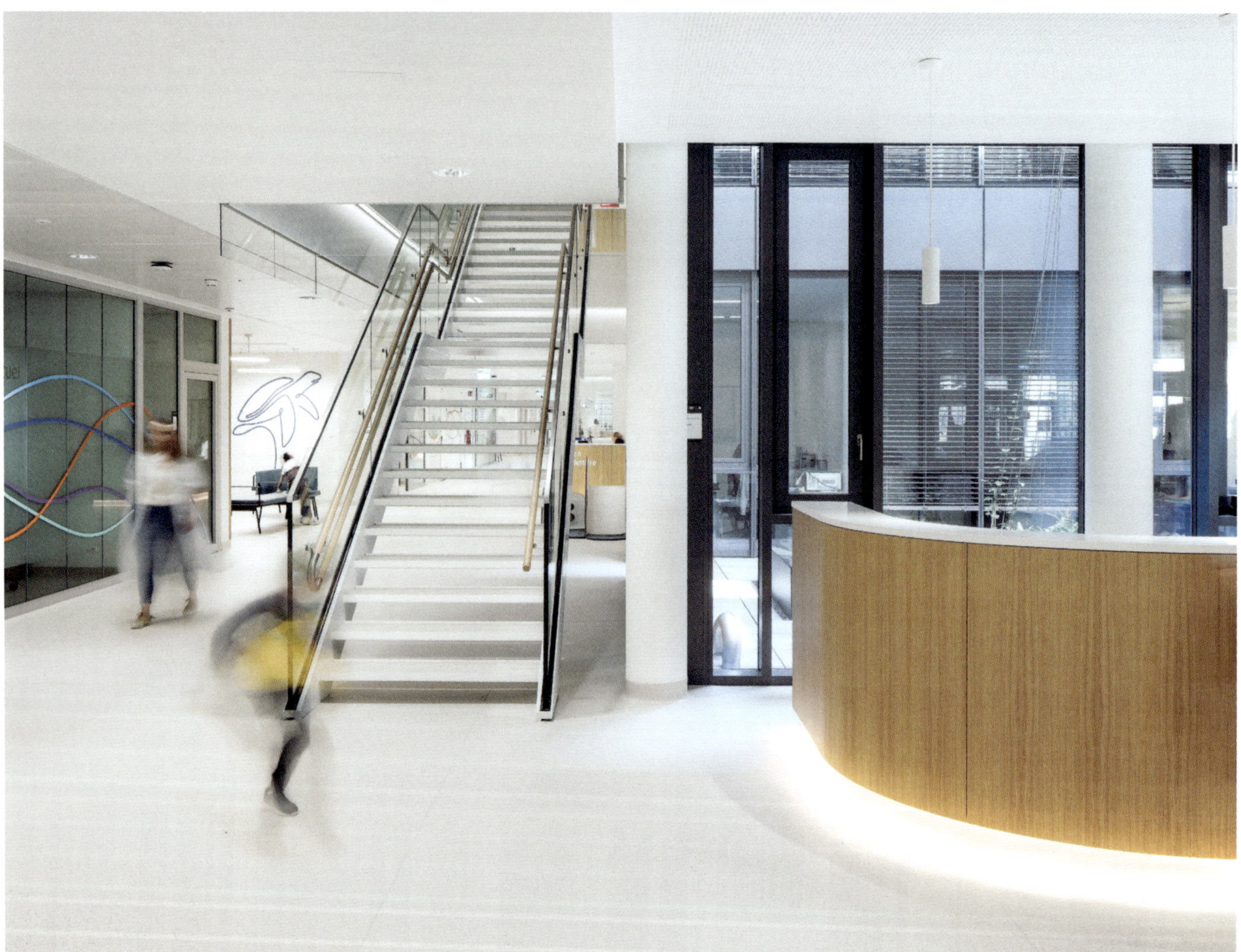

Examination room.

Main hall with abundant light.

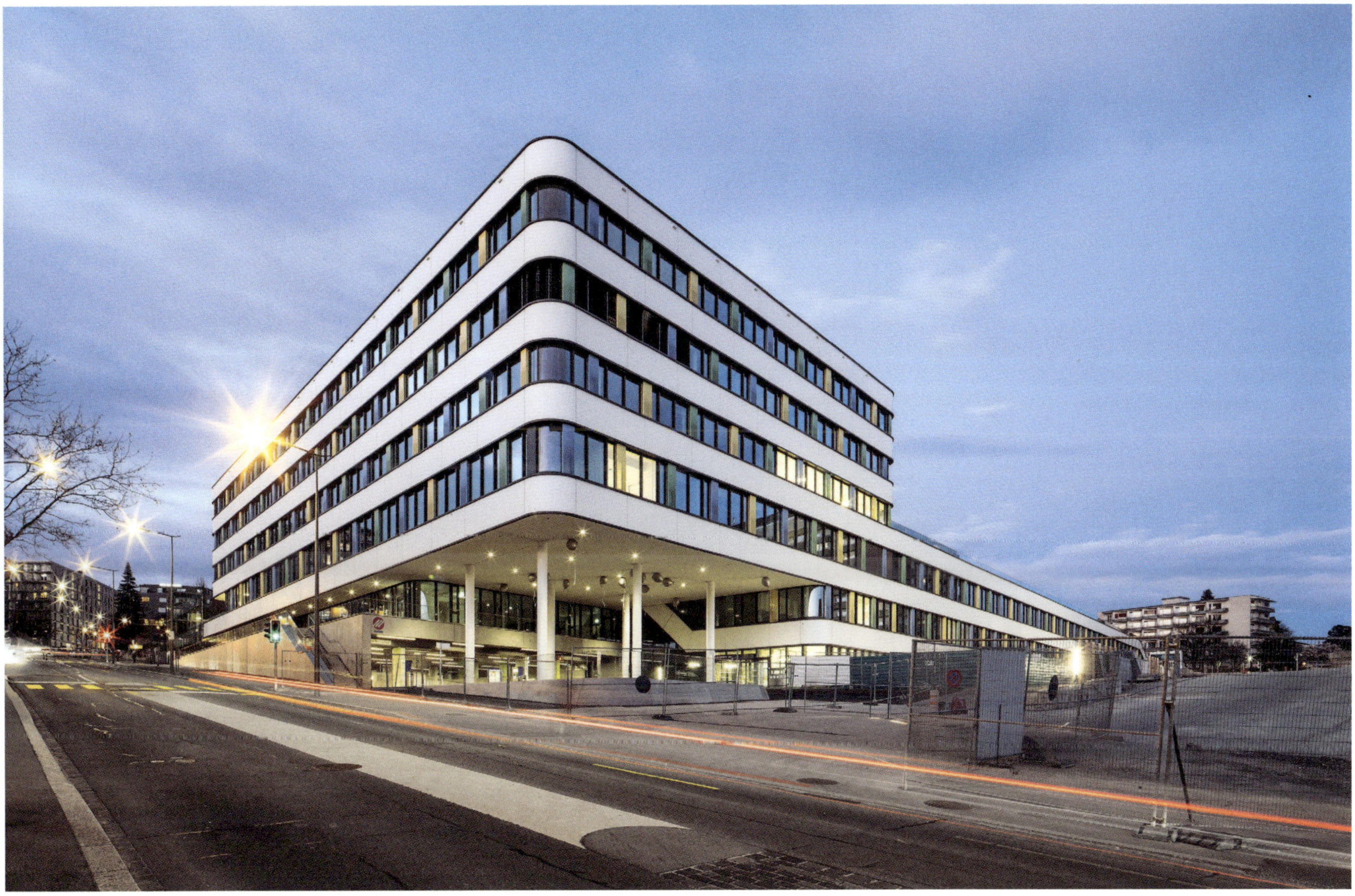

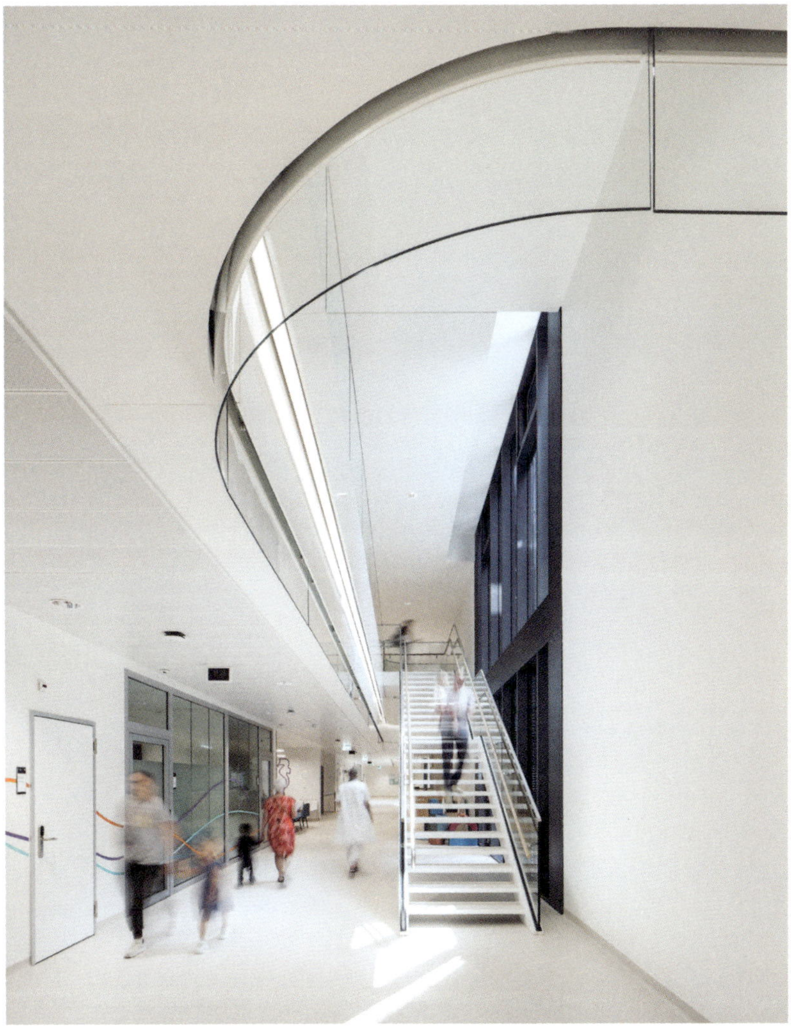

Building in its urban context.

Elegant staircase by the window.

Figure-ground plan.

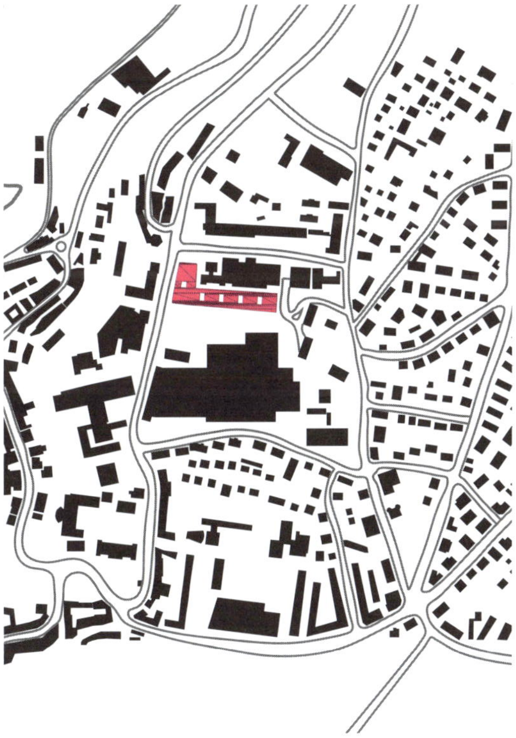

Felix+Jonas Architekten

Altötting
Germany

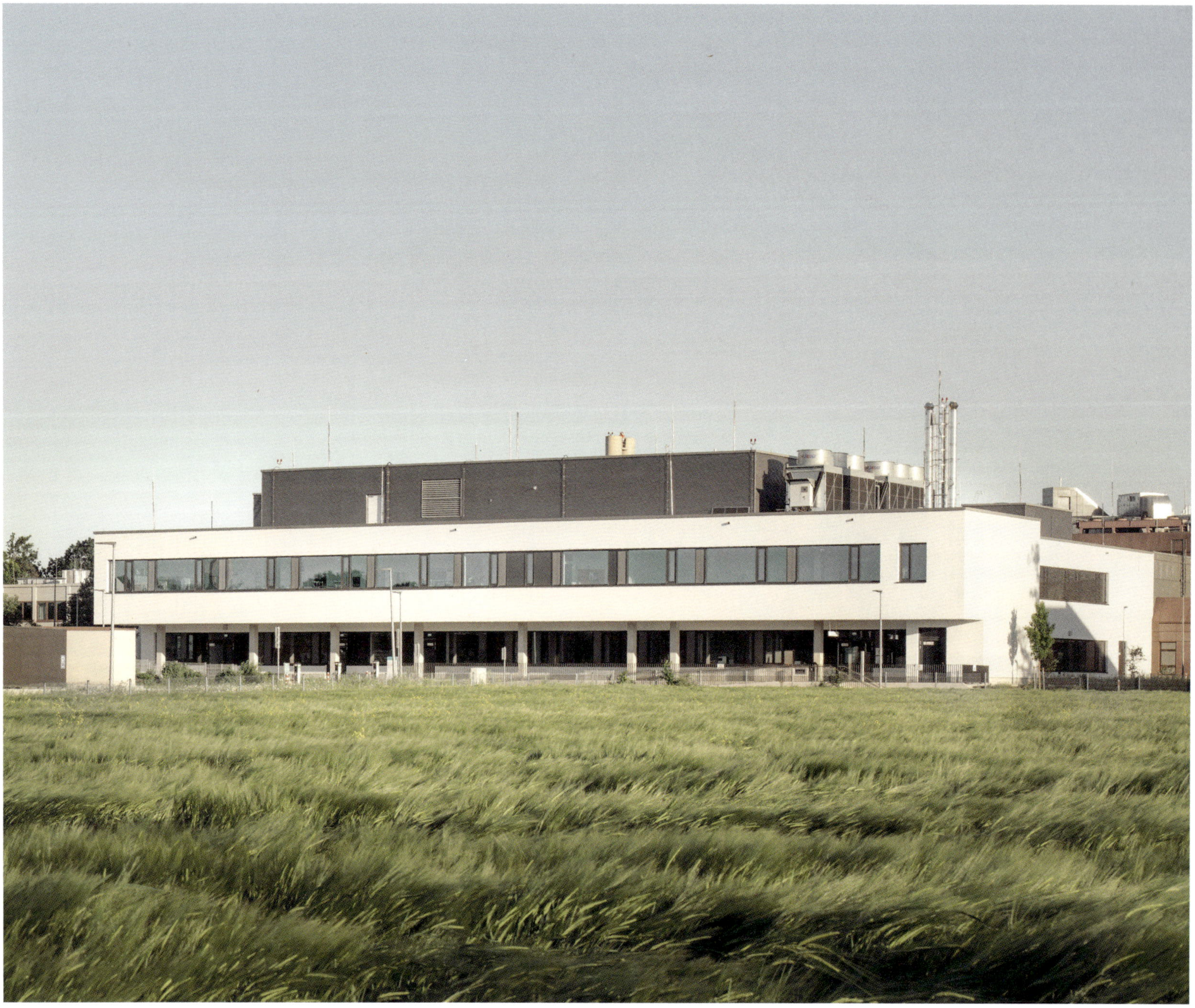

Altötting District Hospital Expansion and Addition

Exterior view of the new building and expansion, construction phase 1.

Modern operating room with a landscape photo, construction phase 1.

Hallway and hygiene area, construction phase 2.

The Innklinikum Altötting, constructed in a single phase beginning in 1982, underwent extensive modernization after approximately 30 years. Initial measures included the addition of a functional wing and the expansion of general care facilities on the third floor. This first phase was finished in 2021. Two years later the new building opened as well. It houses central medical departments such as the operating room, laboratory diagnostics, and the medical device reprocessing unit. To expand capacity by 120 beds, the existing ward buildings were raised by one story using lightweight construction methods to minimize the load on the existing structural framework. The rear-ventilated façades with color-coordinated metal cladding blend harmoniously into the existing structure. Inside, spacious single and double rooms with barrier-free bathrooms offer modern comfort and a high quality of stay.

Address: Vinzenz-von-Paul-Straße 10, 84503 Altötting, Germany | **Client:** Kreiskliniken Altötting-Burghausen | **Completion:** 2021 / 2023 | **Size:** BA1: 13,660 m² | **Original building:** Gerhard Lukas, 1984 | **Sector:** state | **Specialization:** surgery and care | **Number of treatment rooms:** 8 | **Number of patient rooms:** 120

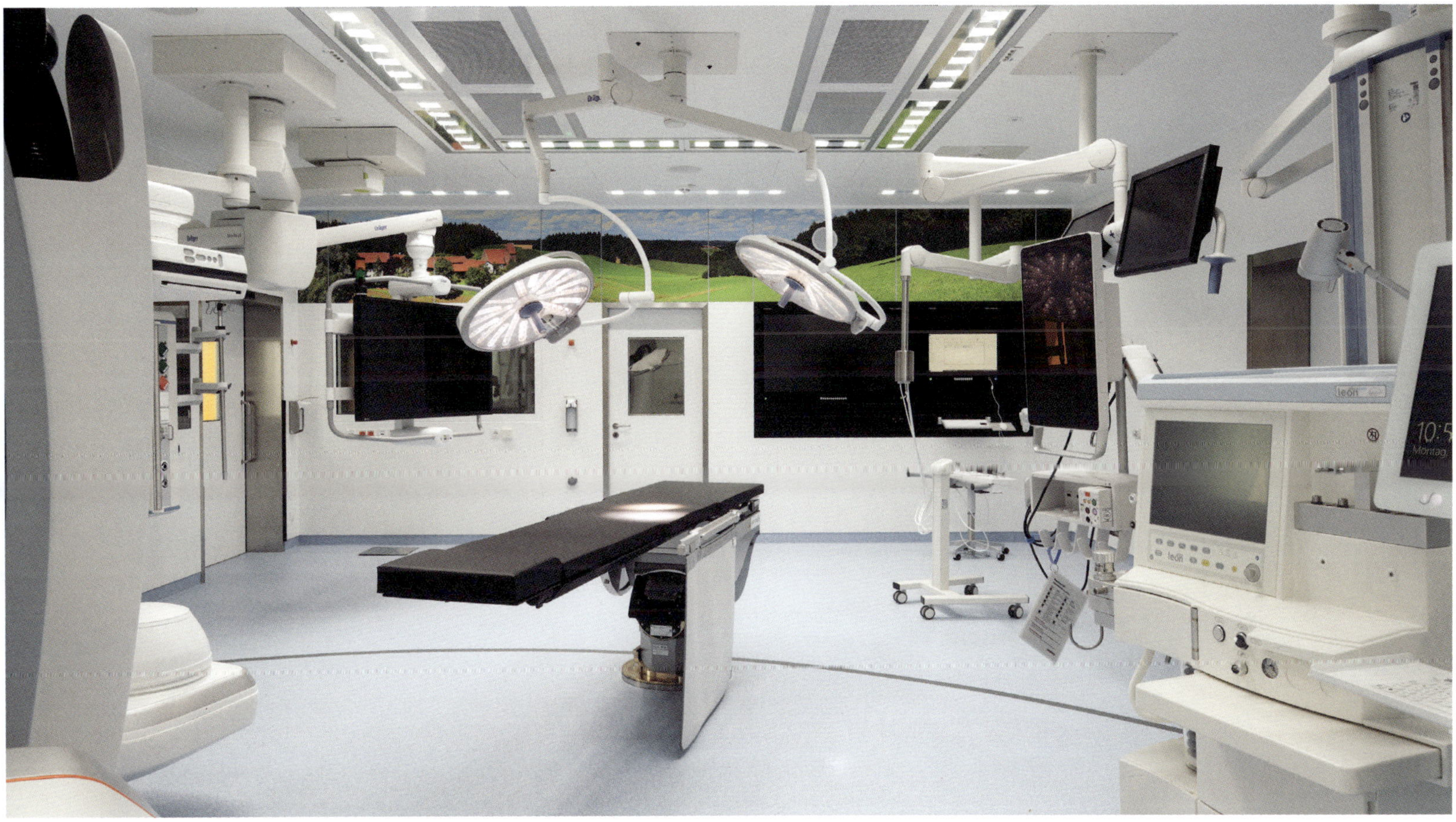

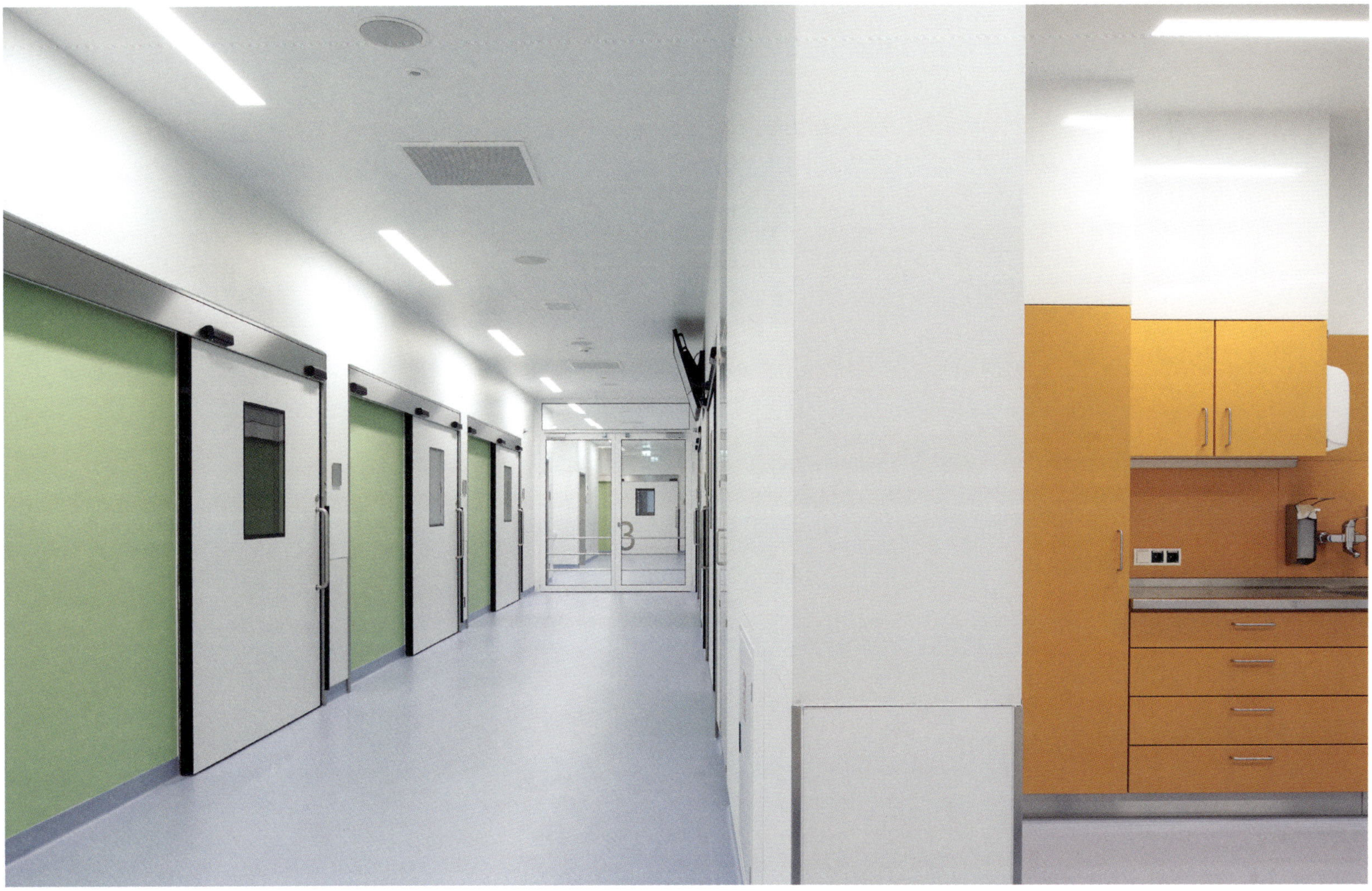

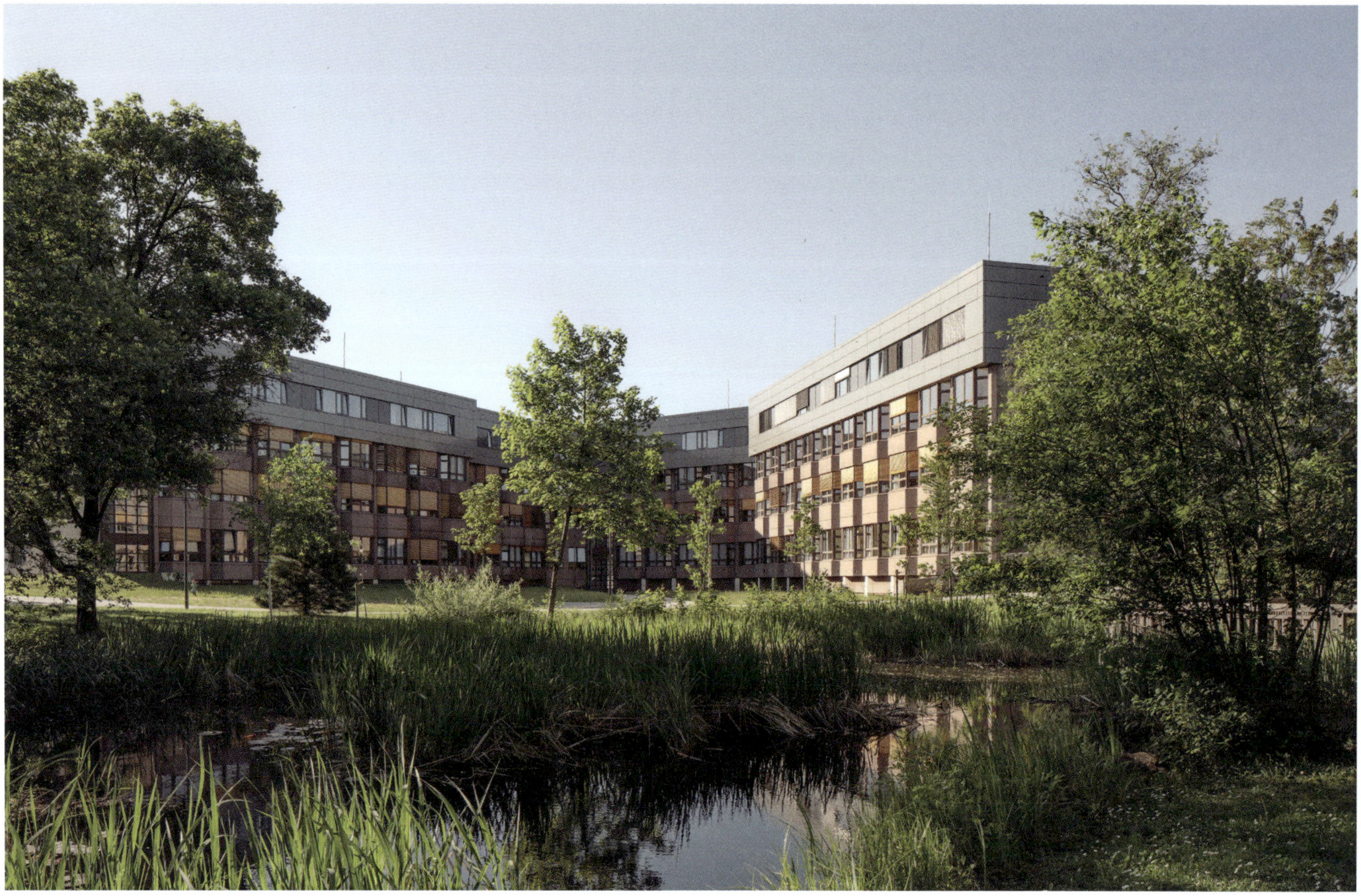

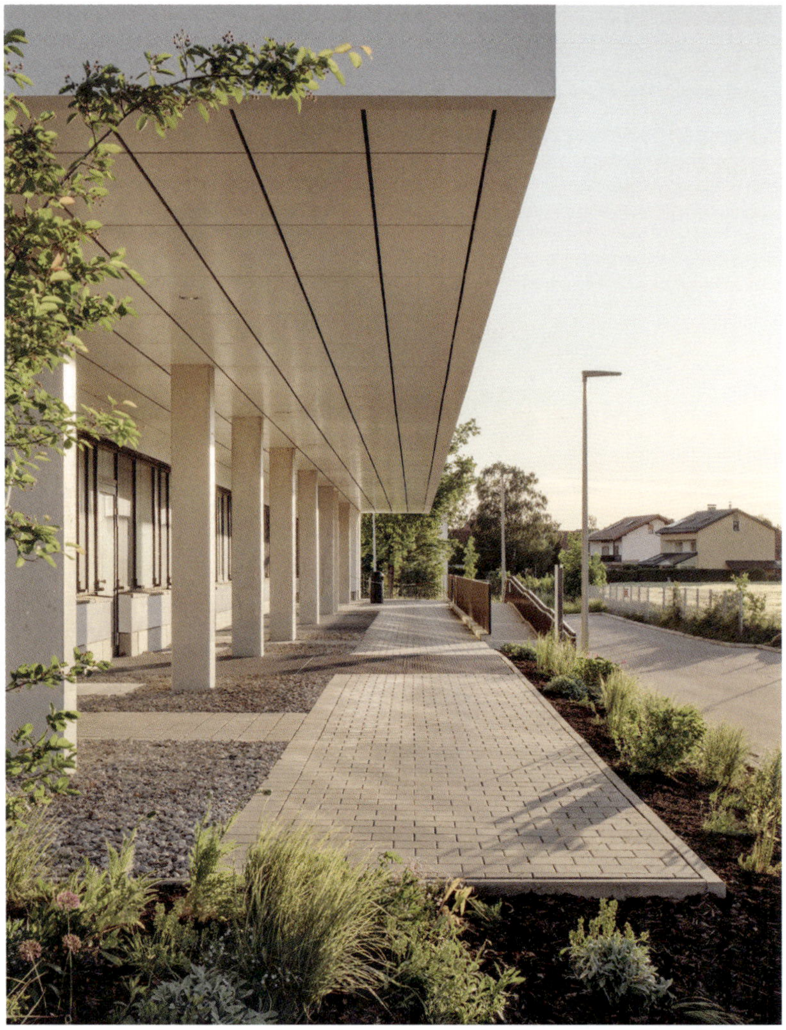

Exterior view of the added floor, construction phase 2.

Side entrance to the new building, construction phase 1.

Figure-ground plan with both construction phases.

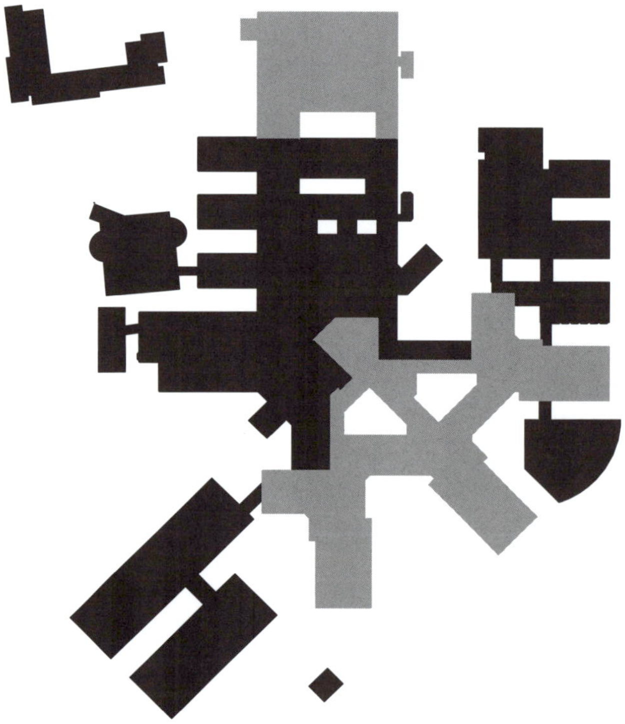

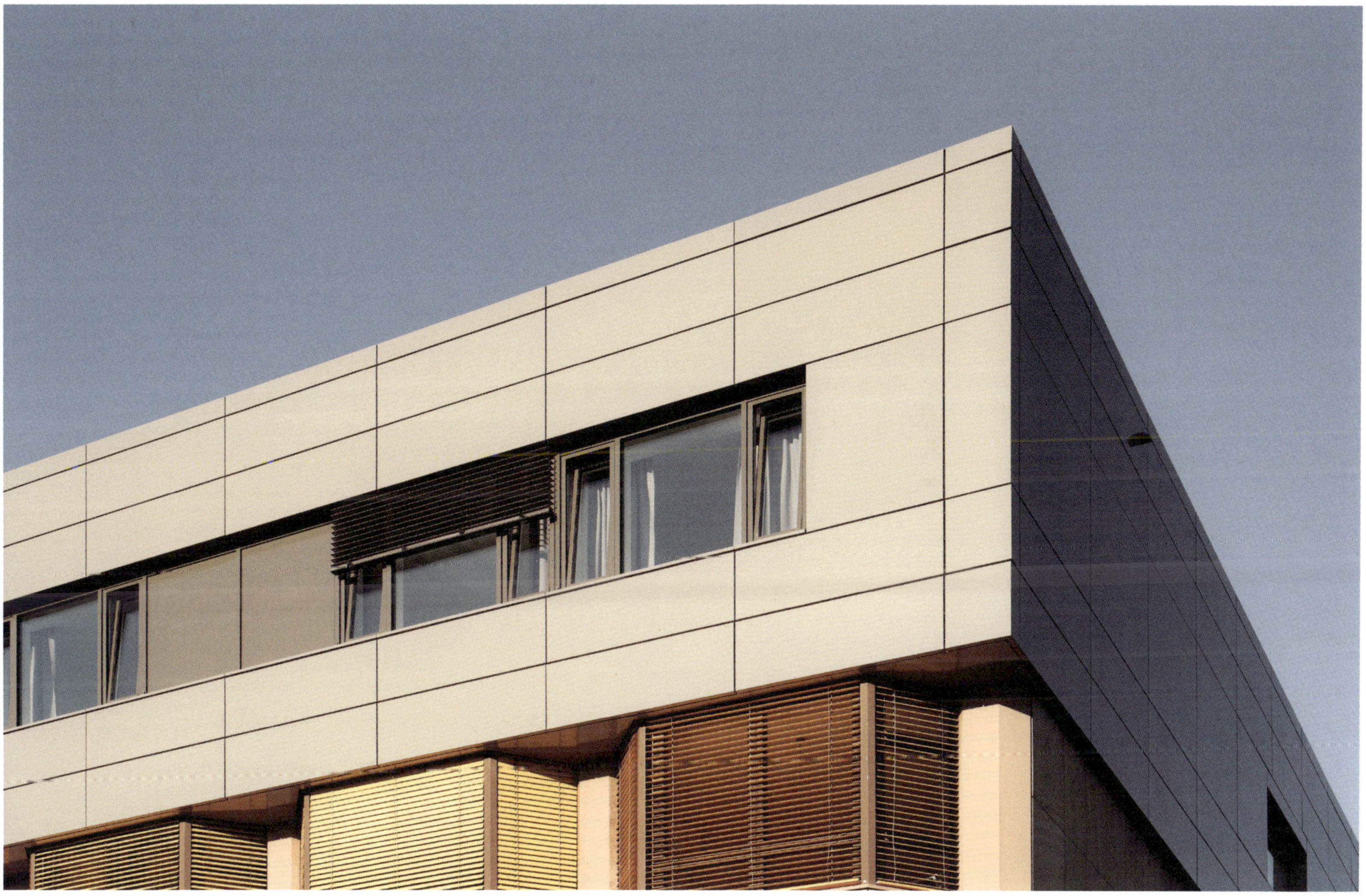

Detail of the added floor, construction phase 2.

Floor plan additional floor, construction phase 2.

Floor plan new build extension, construction phase 1.

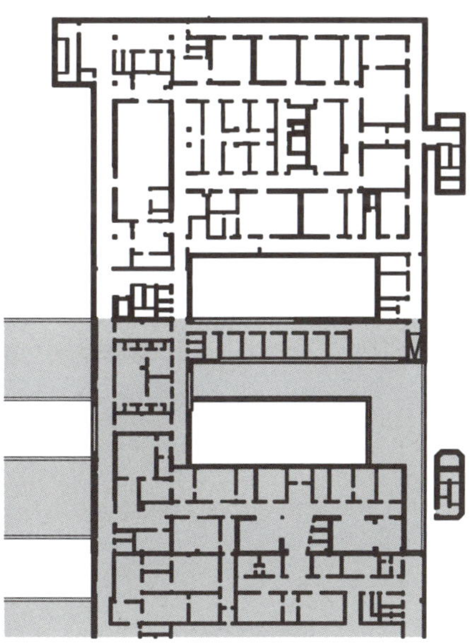

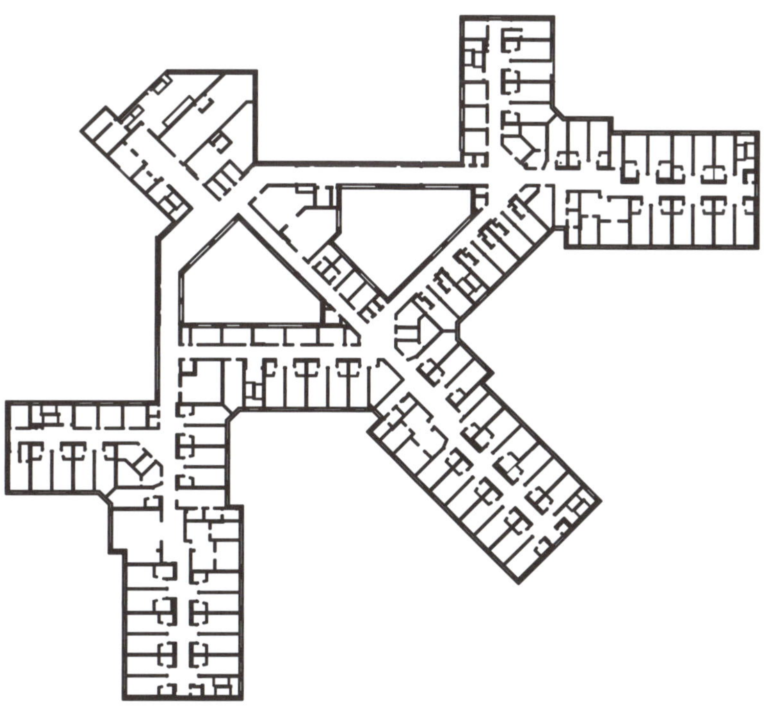

Architecturestudio

Tangier
Morocco

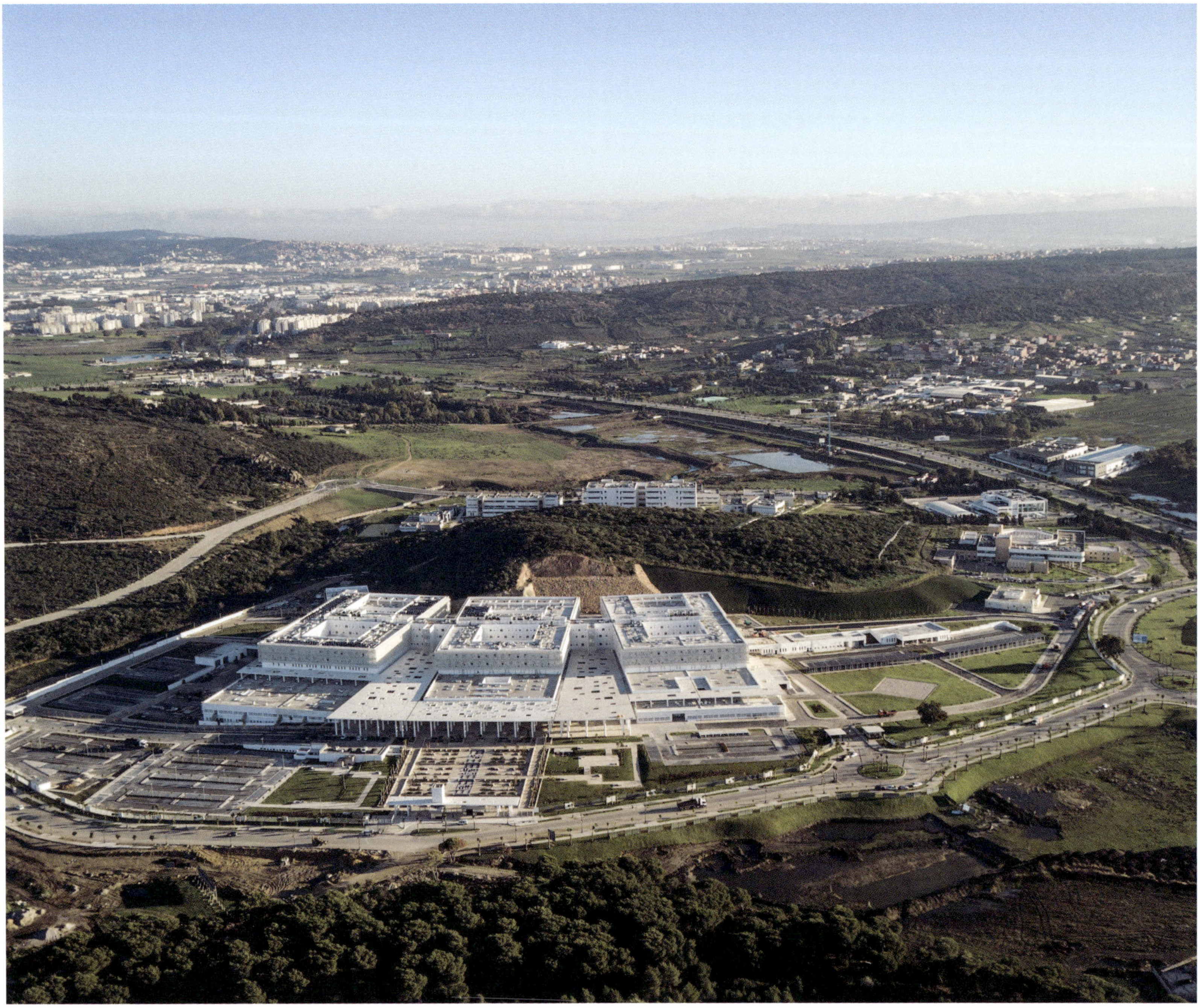

Ariel view of the hospital.

Hospital's main entrance with water fountains.

Expansive entrance with trees, water elements, and canopy.

Tangier University Hospital

Designed to accommodate 800 beds, the university hospital is organized into three building blocks set atop a base. The entrance plaza serves as the focal point for patient reception and connects the various sections of the site. Opening onto the city, the large canopy extends the mashrabiya that covers the entrance hall where visitors are welcomed. The base houses all logistical and reception activities, as well as a pavilion dedicated exclusively to the emergency department. The first level accommodates the operating rooms and a technical platform. The second level houses the laboratory and the hospital's administrative offices, and the upper levels bring together the three general inpatient units: medicine, surgery, and maternal-child health. This project places great emphasis on environmental considerations: the building is integrated into a landscaped park, blending seamlessly with the Mediterranean landscape.

Address: Route de Rabat, Km 17, P.O. Box 398, Gzinaya, Tangier, Morocco | **Client:** Ministry of Health – Kingdom of Morocco | **Completion:** 2022 | **Size:** 81,000 m² | **Sector:** state | **Number of beds:** 800 | **Technical Design Office:** NOVEC

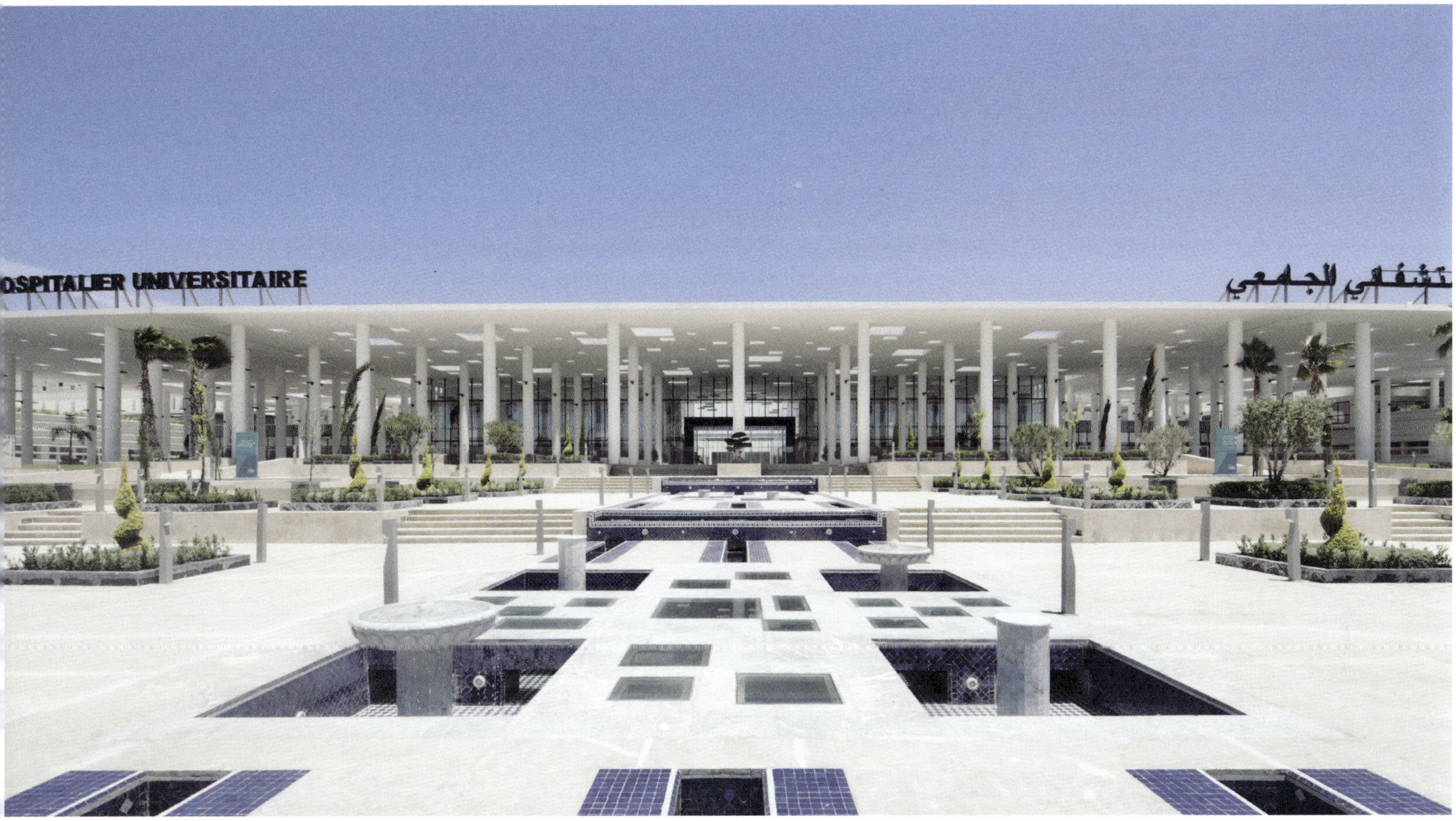

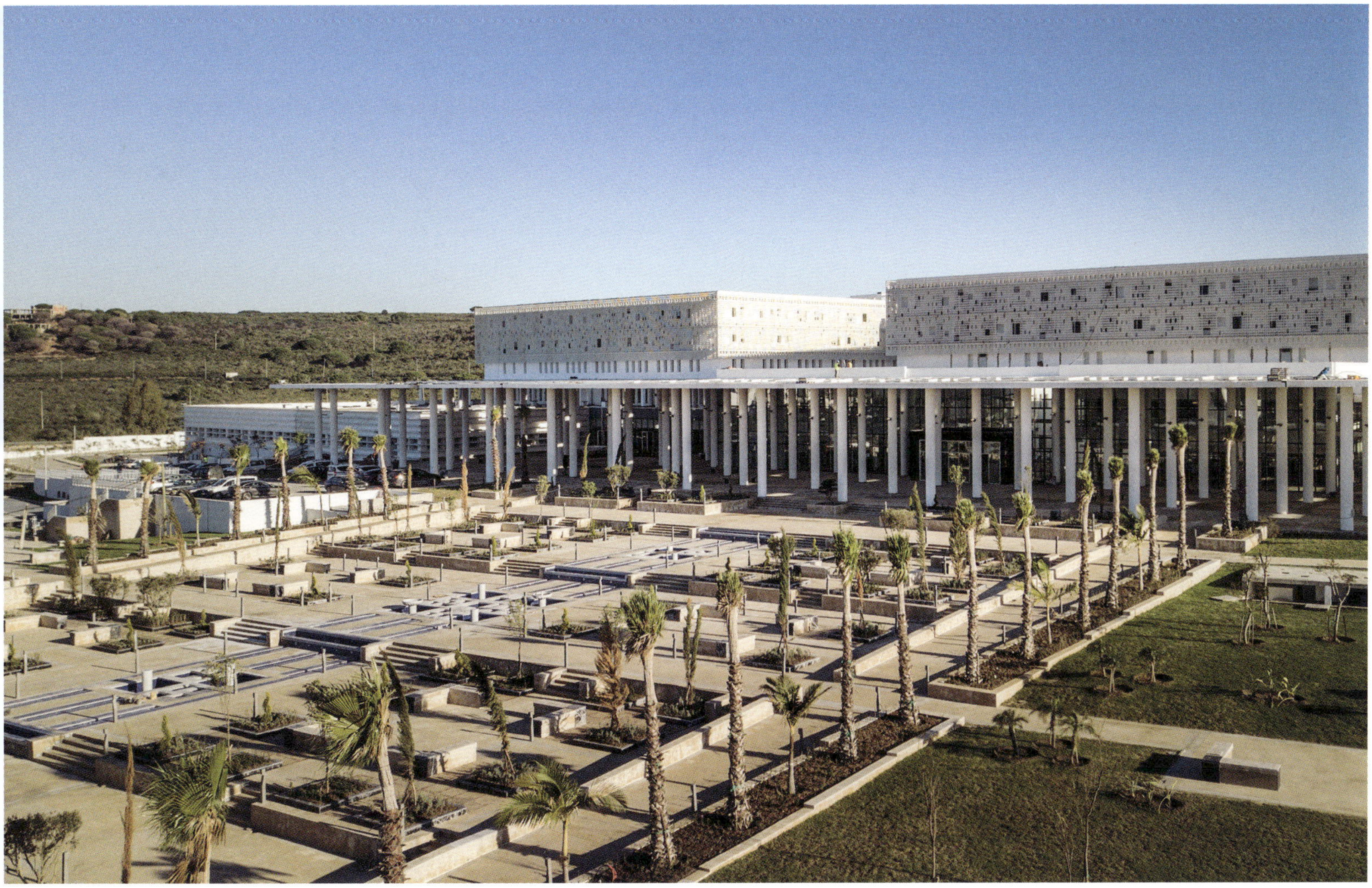

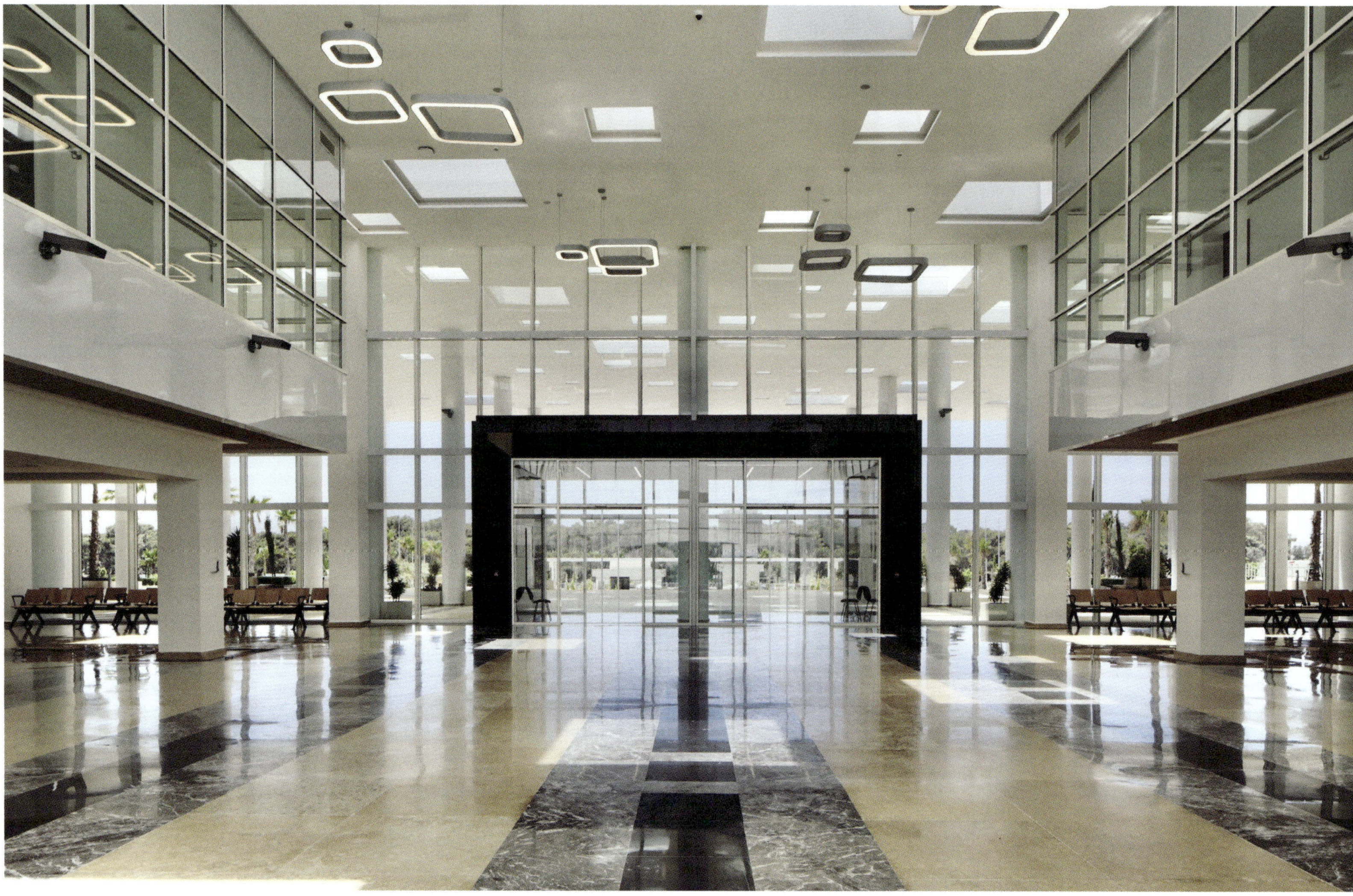

The entrance hall with large glass windows and ample natural light.

Ground floor plan.

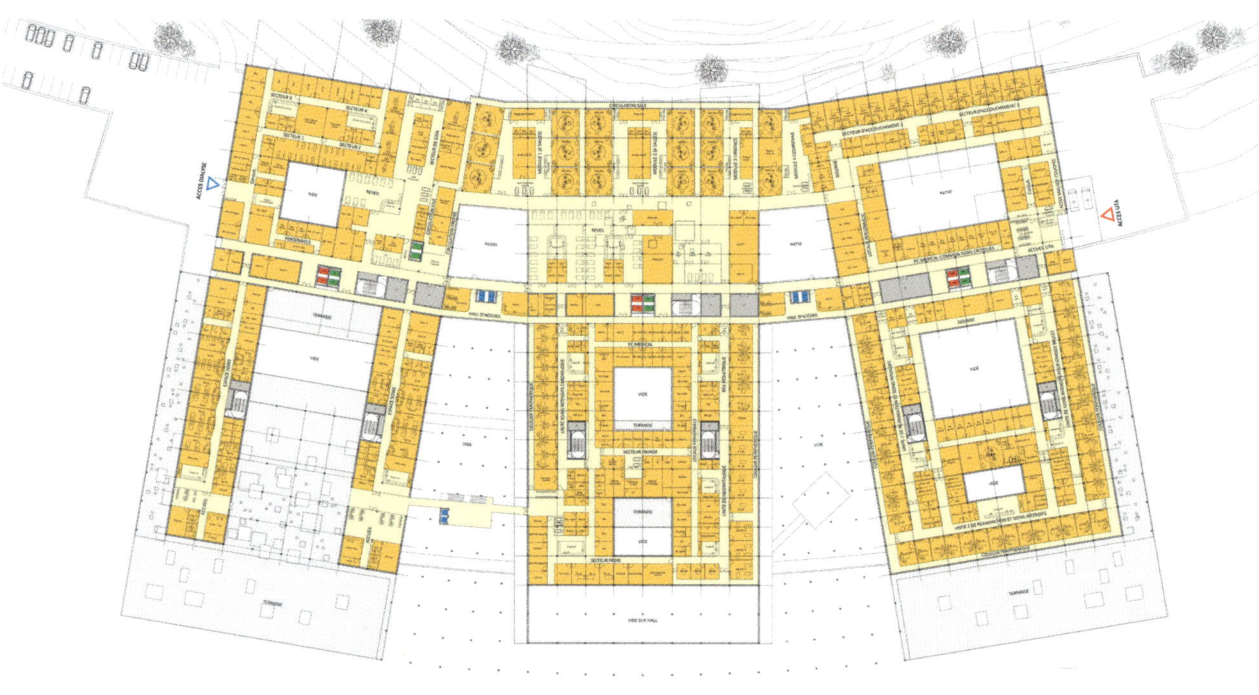

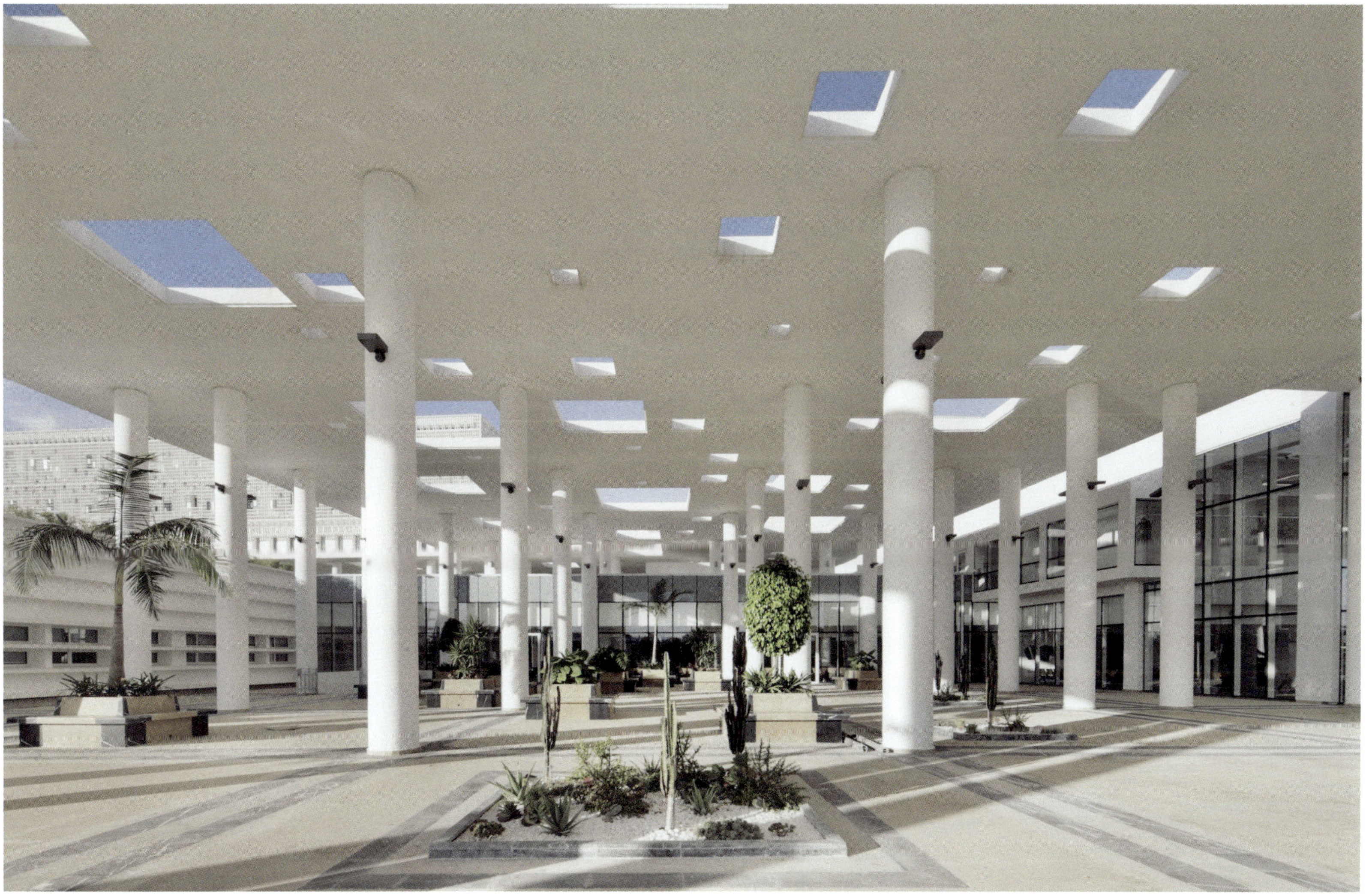

Canopy at the main foyer.

Third floor plan.

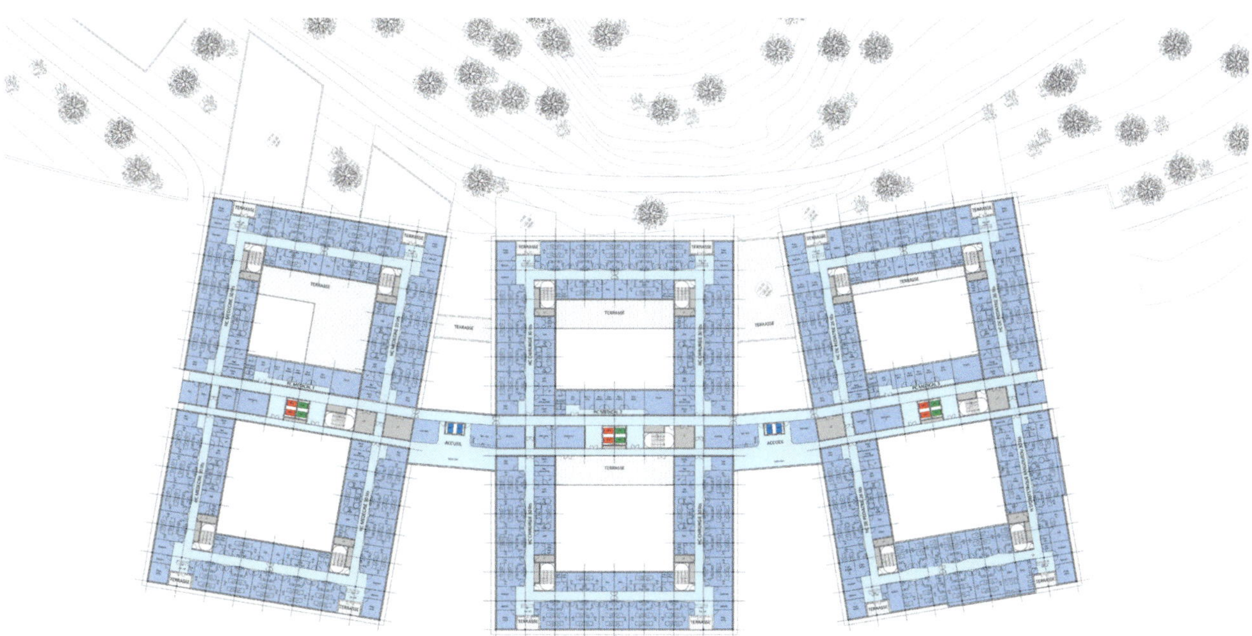

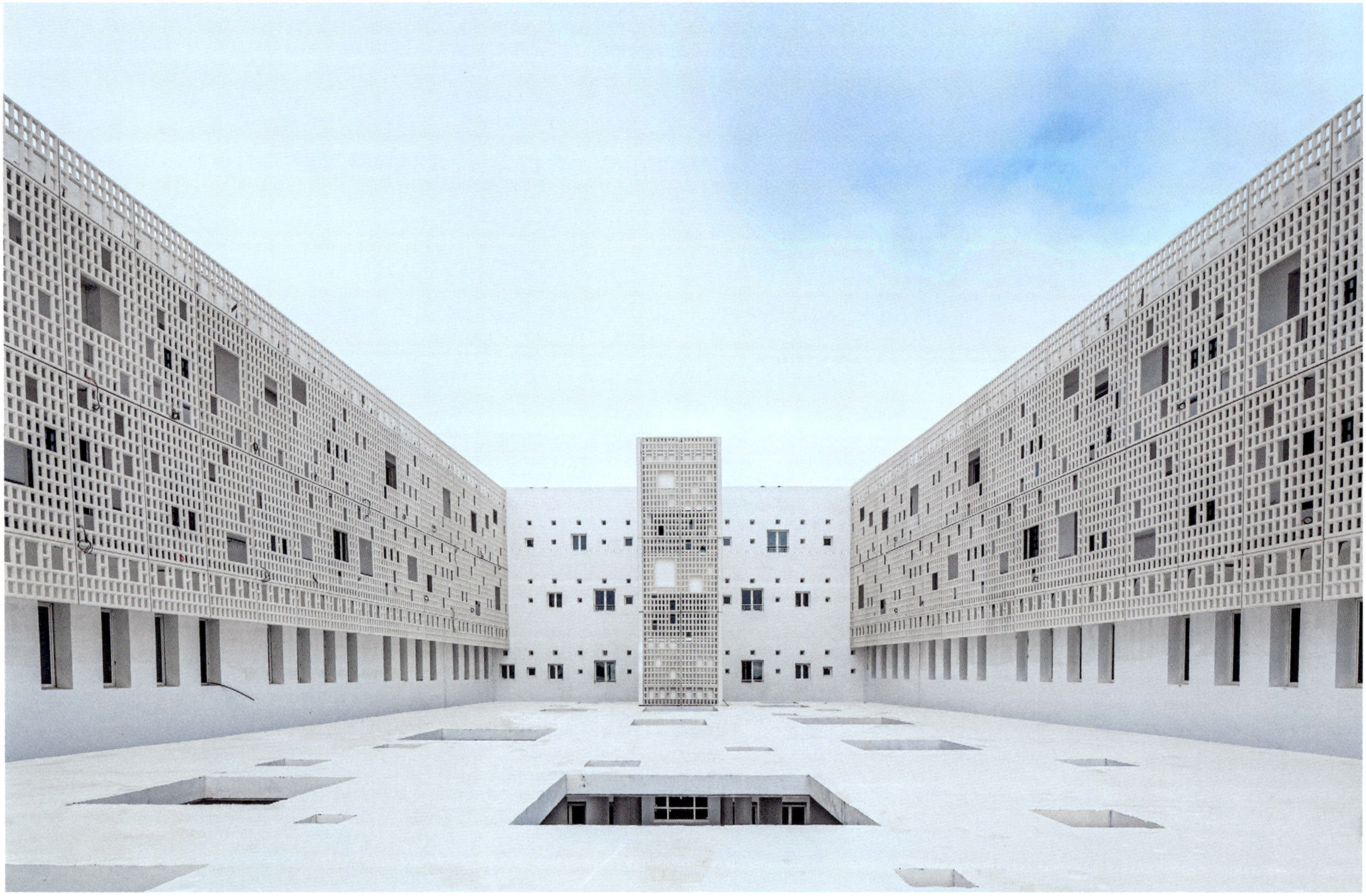

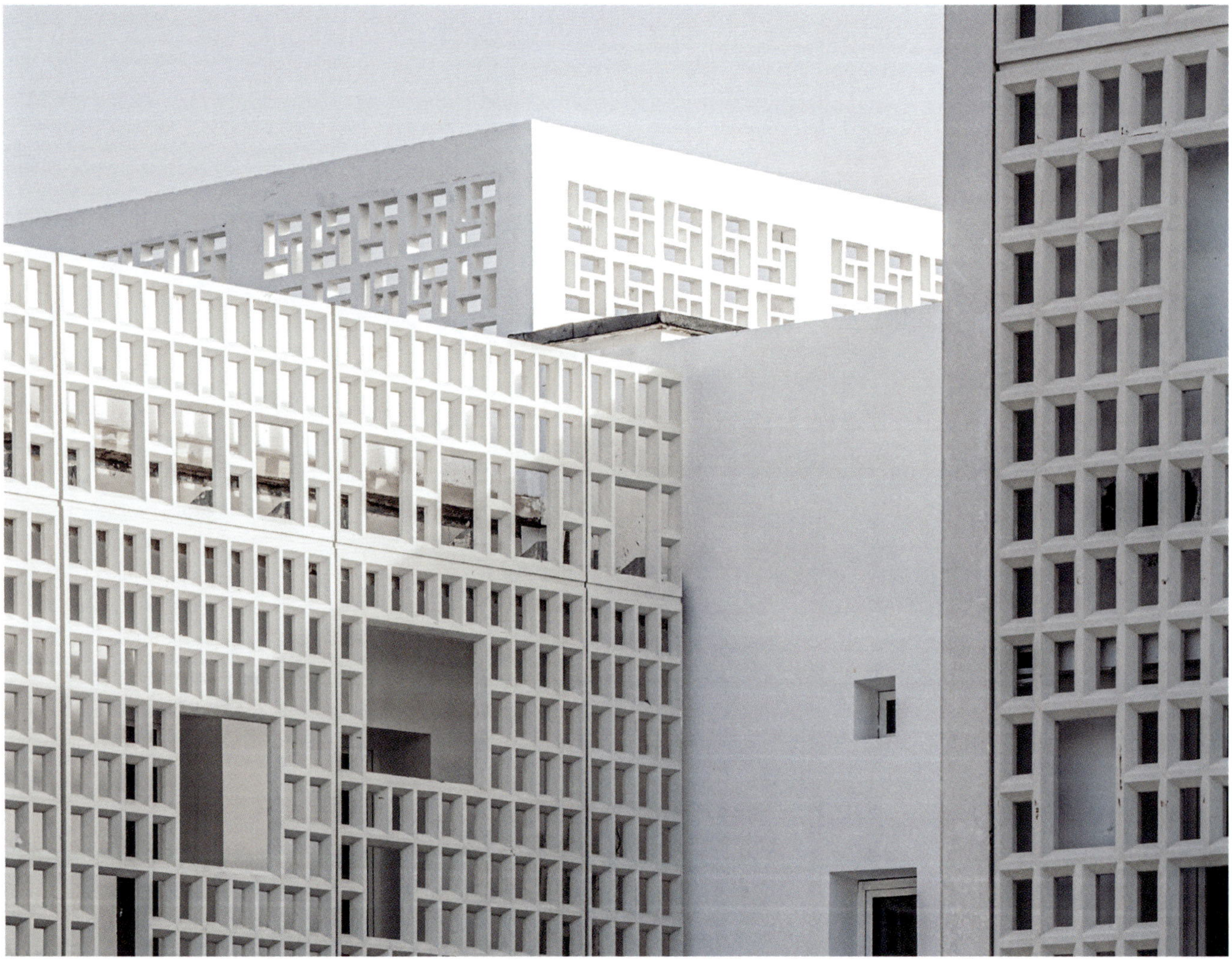

Hospital's all-white façade, a close-up of the mashrabiya.

Hospital's façade.

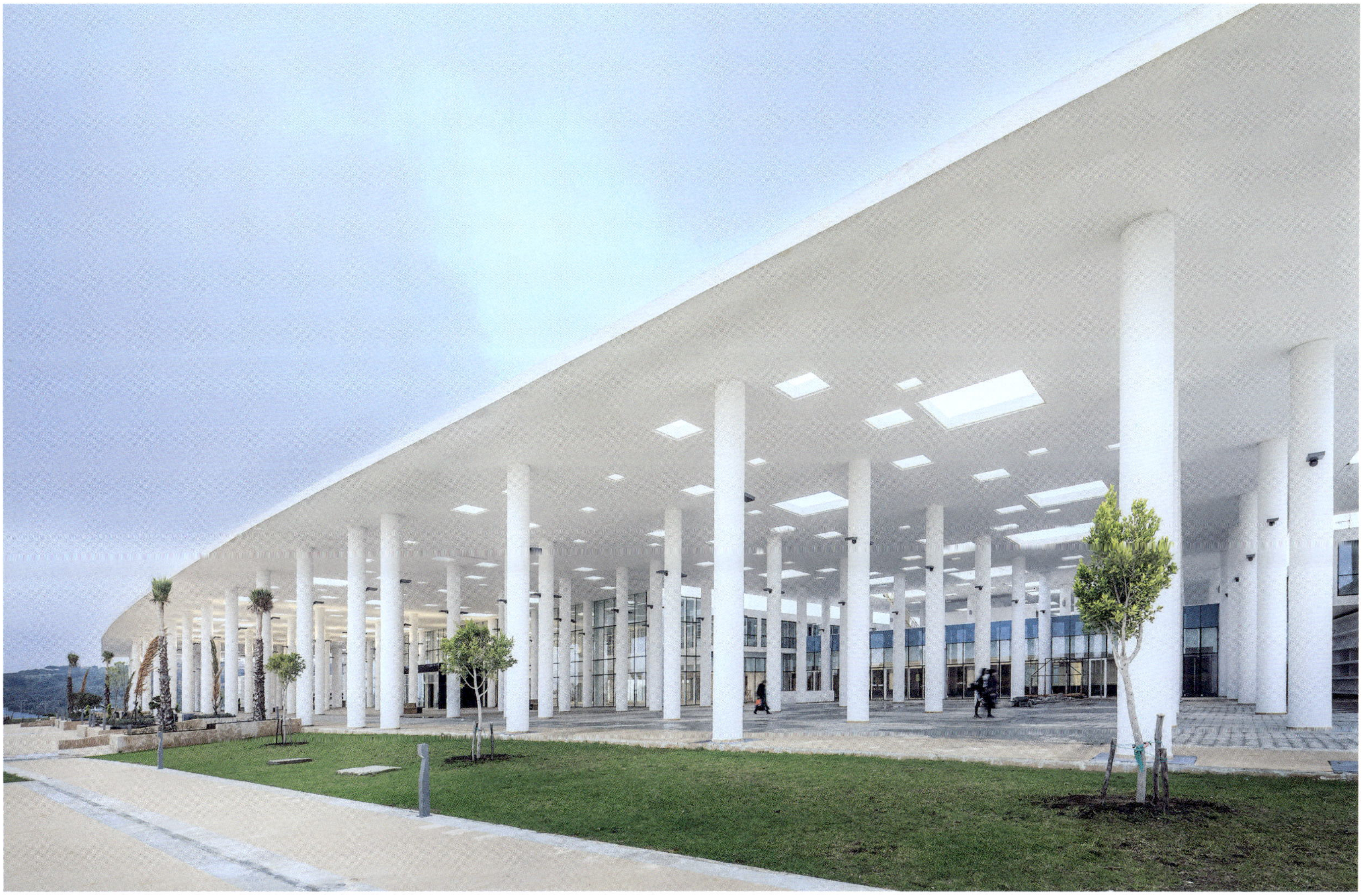

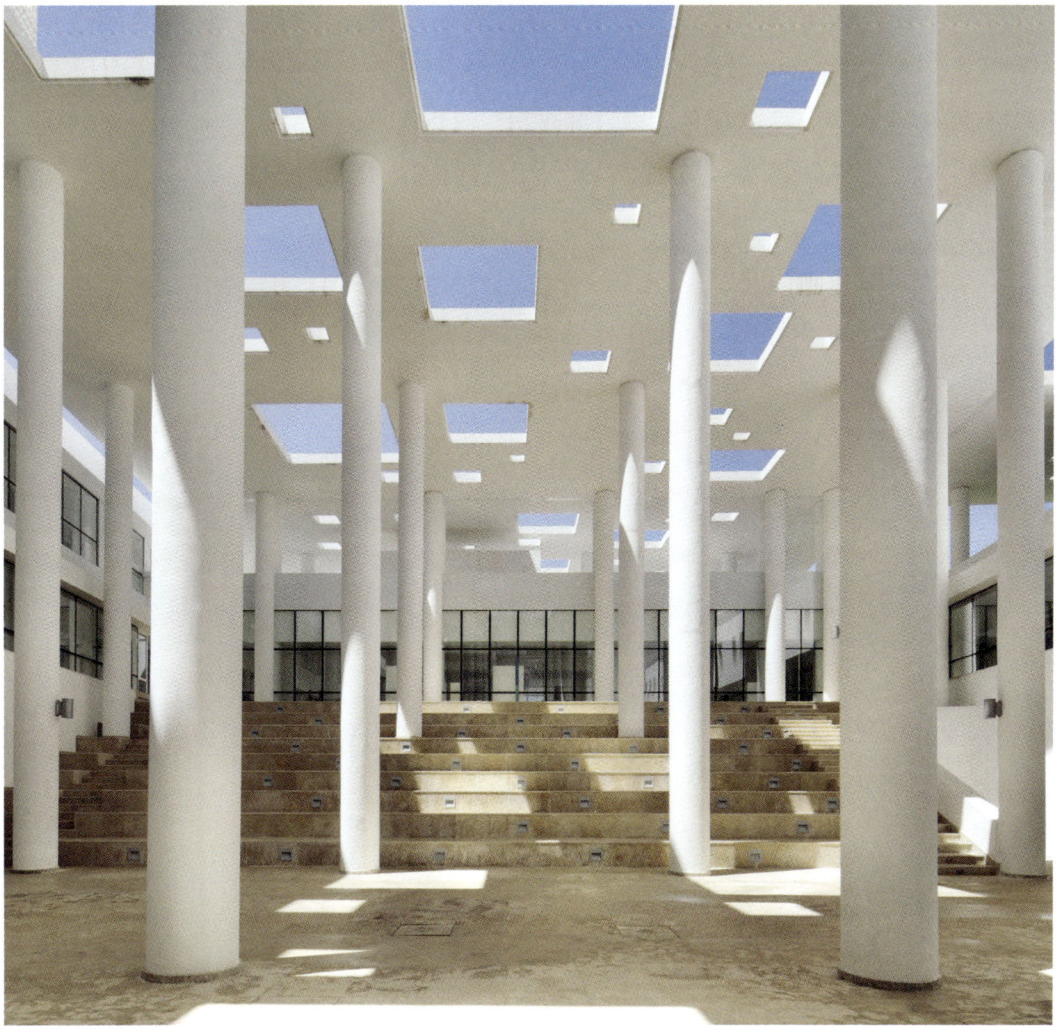

Canopy with several large pillars and cut-outs in the ceiling to allow more natural light in.

Large pillars add to the design element.

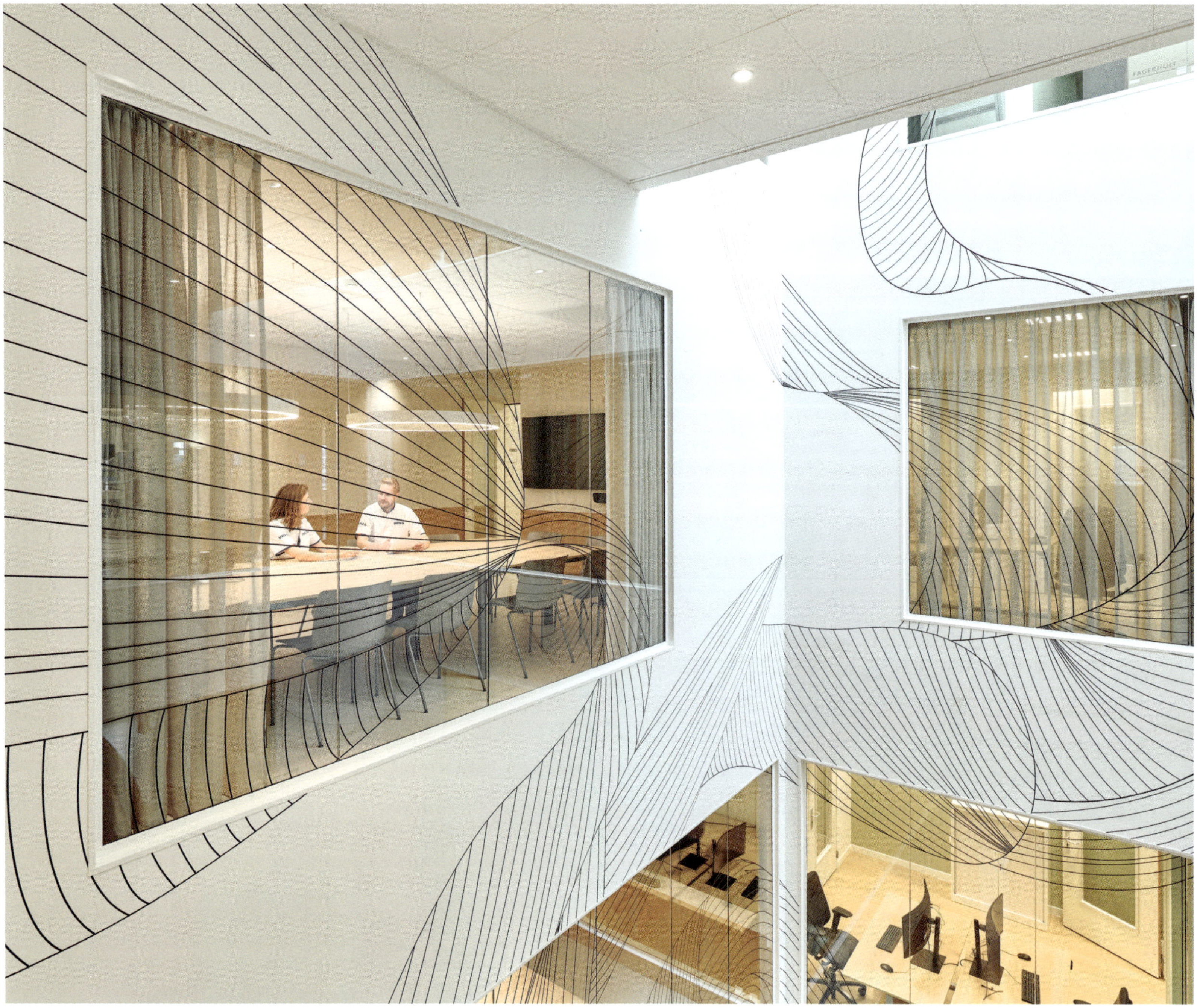

View onto the office spaces from the atrium.

The wooden spiral staircase in the atrium.

UMC Groningen A Tower

The A Tower houses a separate ENT clinic on the ground floor, then three floors intended for the ICU, and a new nursing ward on the fourth floor. The ICU is divided into three identical units, situated one above the other. On each of the three floors, the IC rooms are located on the façade side where there is plenty of daylight and are situated around identical facility spaces. On the other side of the building, adjacent to the internal street between the hospital wings, are the support spaces: the reception and accommodation areas for family (first floor), the break and changing rooms for staff (second floor), and the work and consultation areas for doctors, nurses, researchers, and residents (third floor). A three-story atrium with an attractive spiral staircase forms the light, bright heart of the ICU. The atrium serves as the connecting link between the IC rooms on one side and the support spaces on the other.

Address: Hanzeplein 1, 9713 GZ Groningen, The Netherlands | **Client:** UMC Groningen | **Completion:** 2025 | **Size:** 8,900 m² | **Sector:** universitairy | **Number of treatment rooms:** 26 | **Number of patient rooms:** 60 | **Interior design:** Wiegerinck

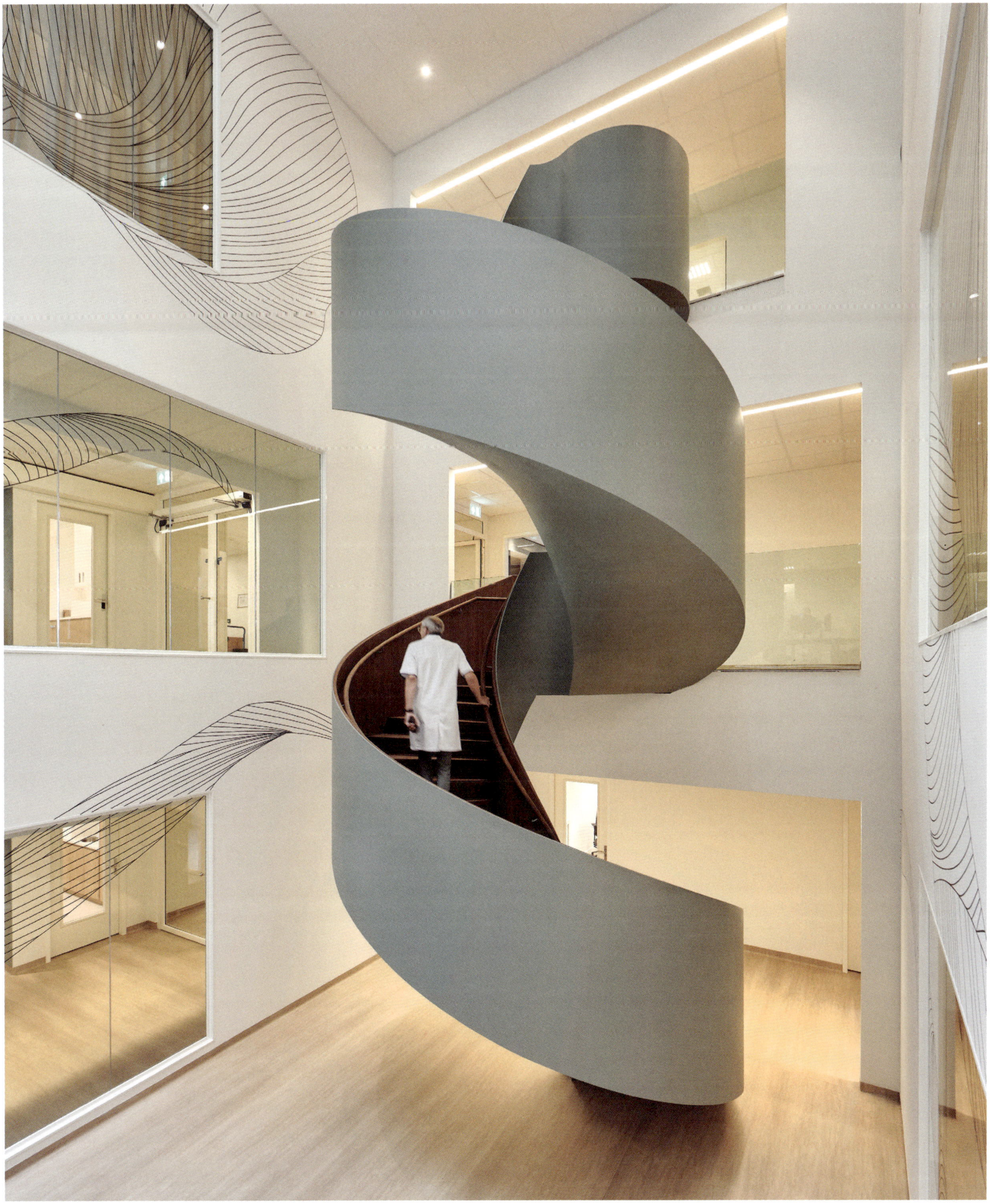

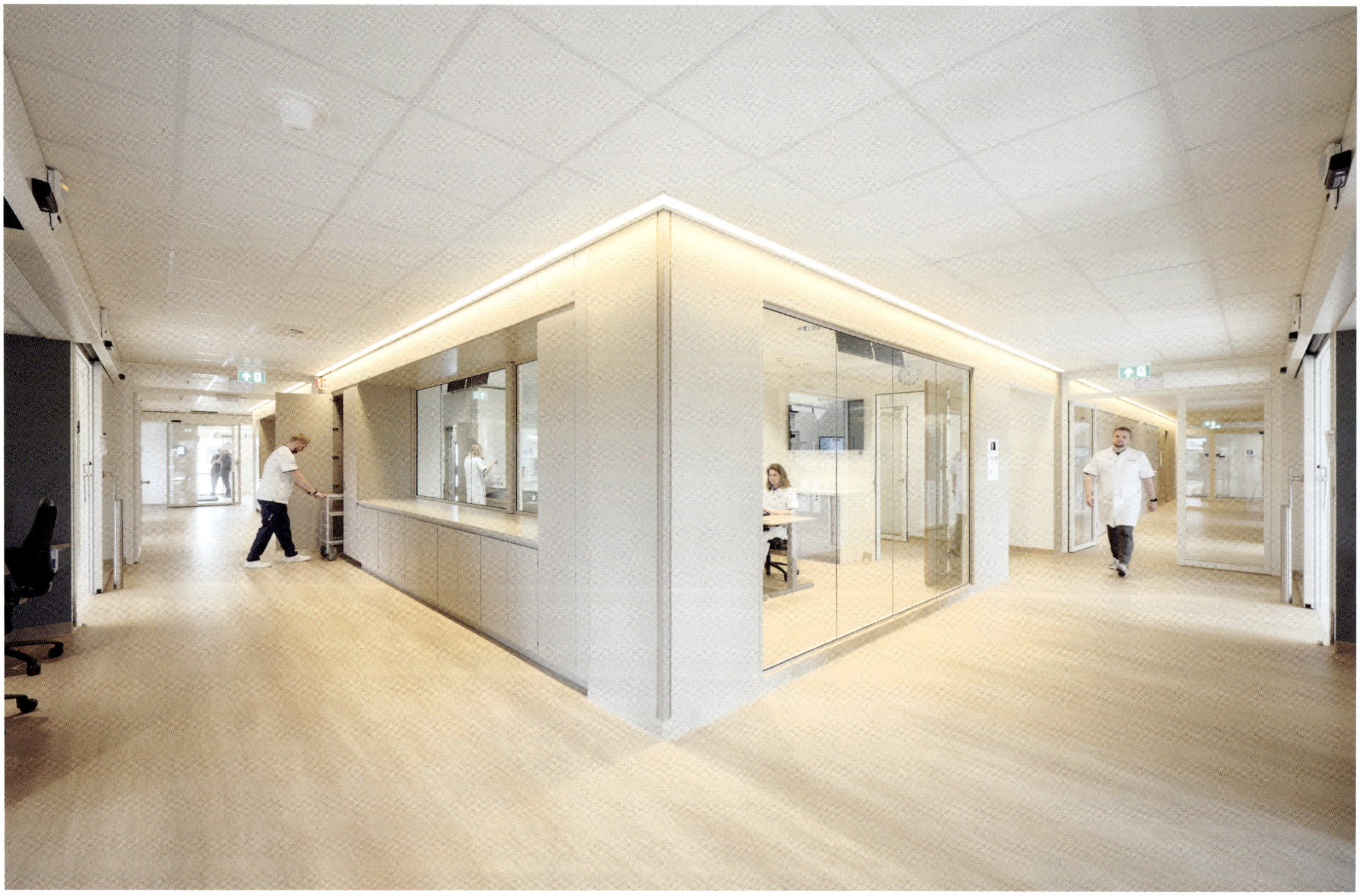

Central nursing station in the ICU.

Typical ICU floor plan.

Section.

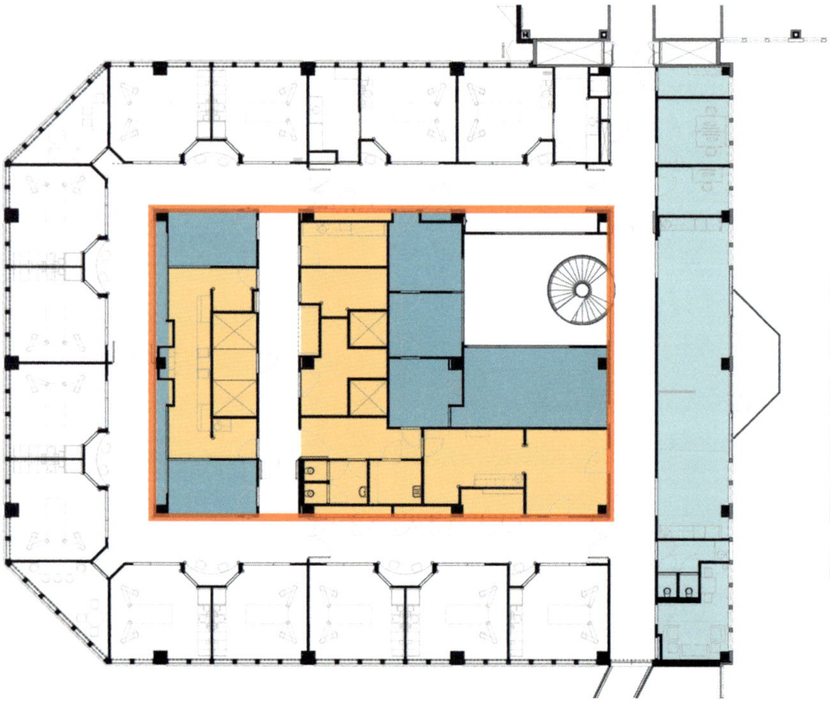

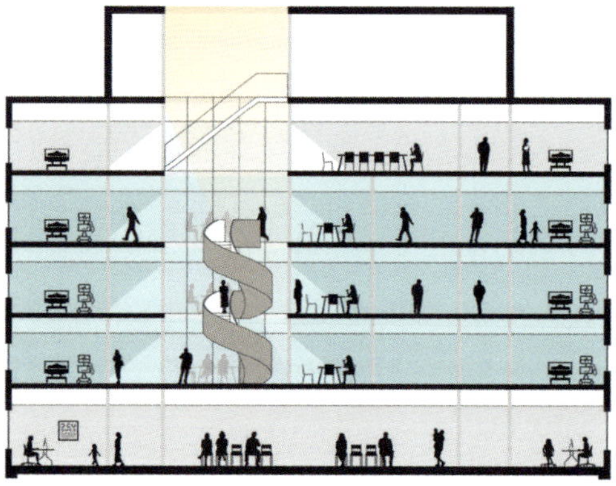

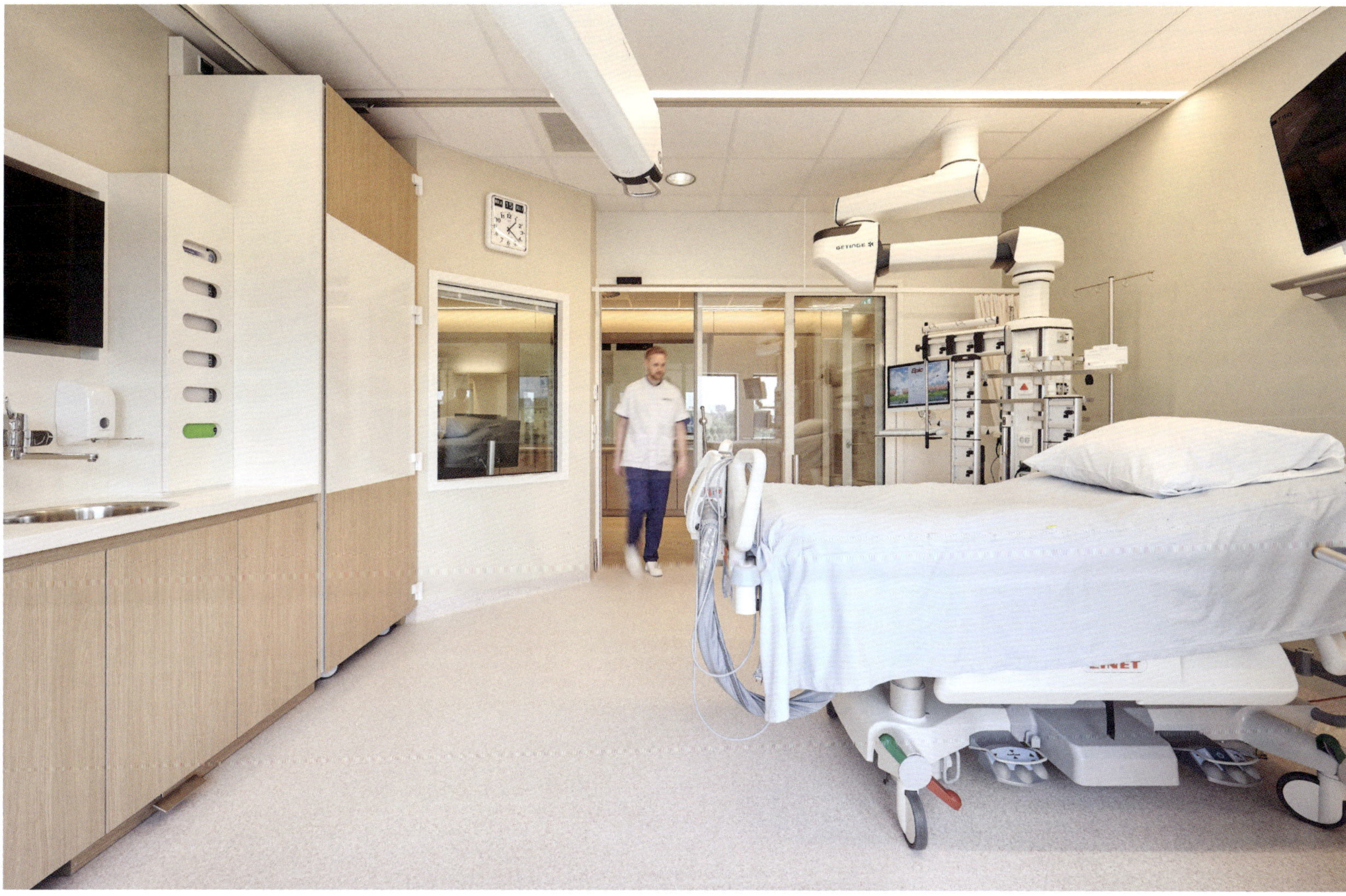

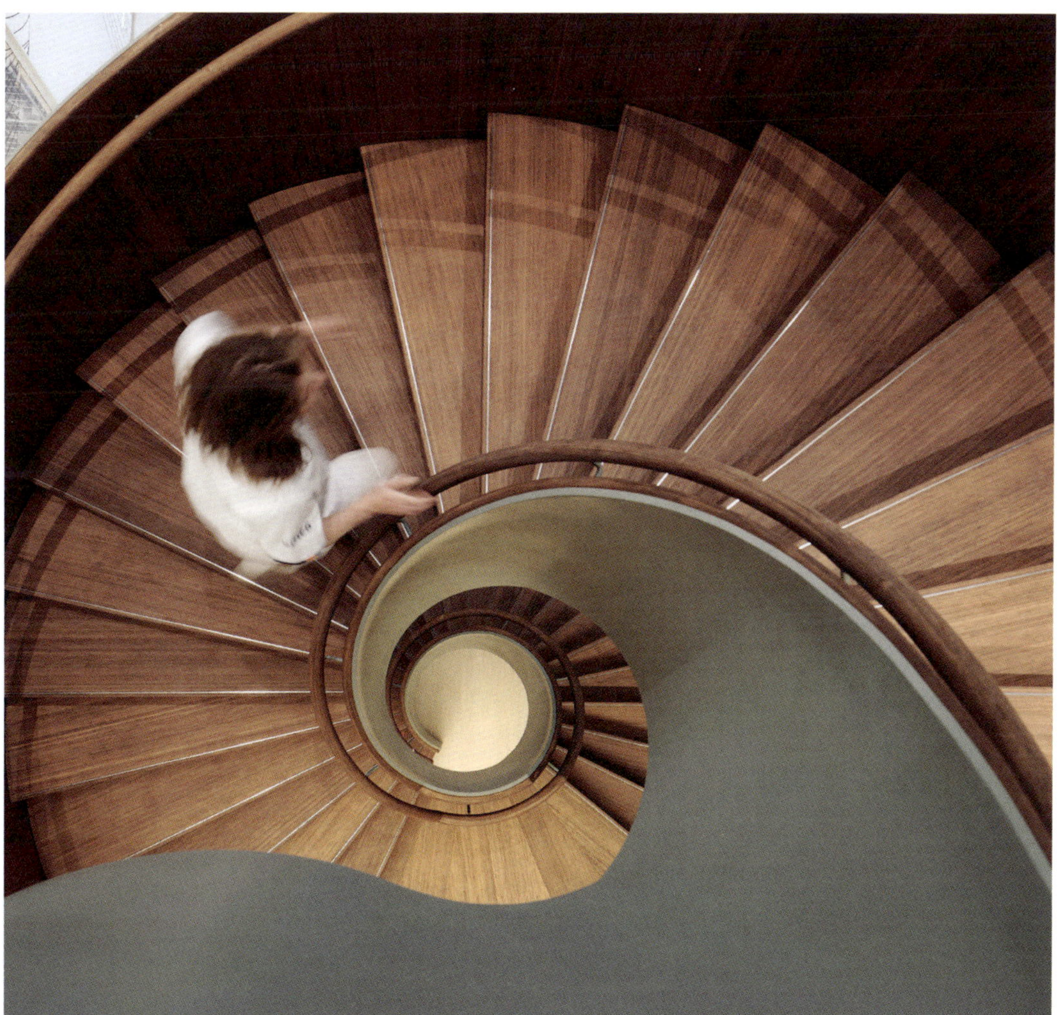

The patient room is literally designed from the patient's perspective.

The wooden spiral staircase in the atrium.

WIT Design & Research

Shenzhen
China

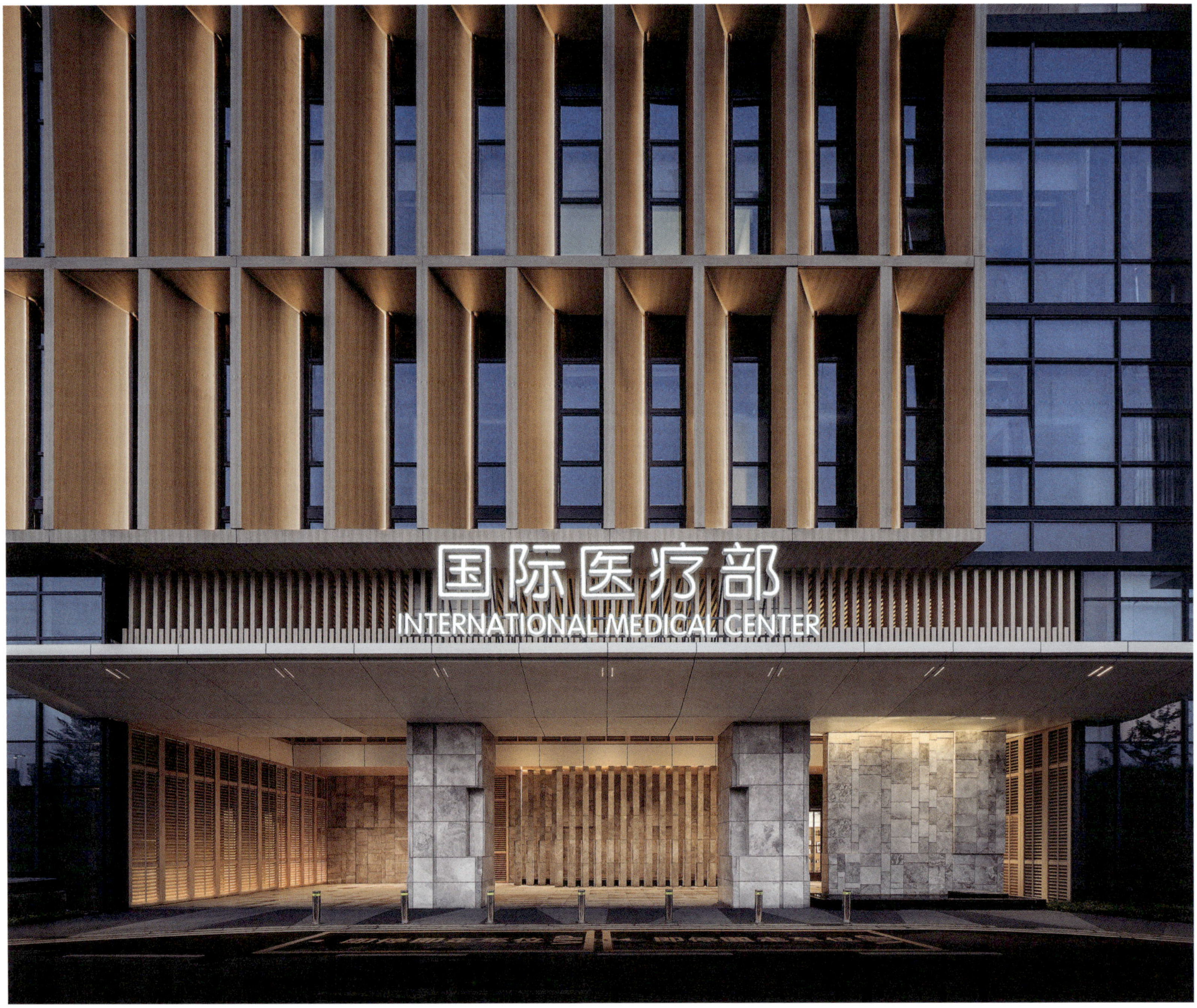

International Medical Center's main entrance.

Hospital ward's lobby area.

Spacious and well lit reception area.

Taikang Hospital International Medical Center

The International Medical Center of Qianhai Taikang Hospital in Shenzhen is designed to balance efficiency with emotional clarity. The spatial strategy emphasizes seamless circulation, a sense of privacy, and calming light atmospheres – creating a setting that supports recovery and reduces patient anxiety. Built around the idea of an 'art hospital', the design integrates multiple forms of artistic expression – light, texture, form, and curated installations – offering sensory stimulation and psychological comfort throughout the patient journey. This clinic is tailored to elderly patients, providing advanced technology, integrated care systems, and a calm environment that promotes preventive health and long-term well-being. The hospital has a private entrance sequence with layered screens and garden walls, offering a discreet and composed arrival experience and carefully planned interiors and partitions to define zones.

Address: Unit 201, Qianhai Taikang Hospital, 3099 Menghai Boulevard, Nanshan District, Shenzhen, Guangdong Province, China | **Client:** Taikang Insurance Group Inc. | **Completion:** 2024 | **Size:** 5,000 m^2 | **Sector:** private | **Number of treatment rooms:** 20 | **Number of patient rooms:** 78

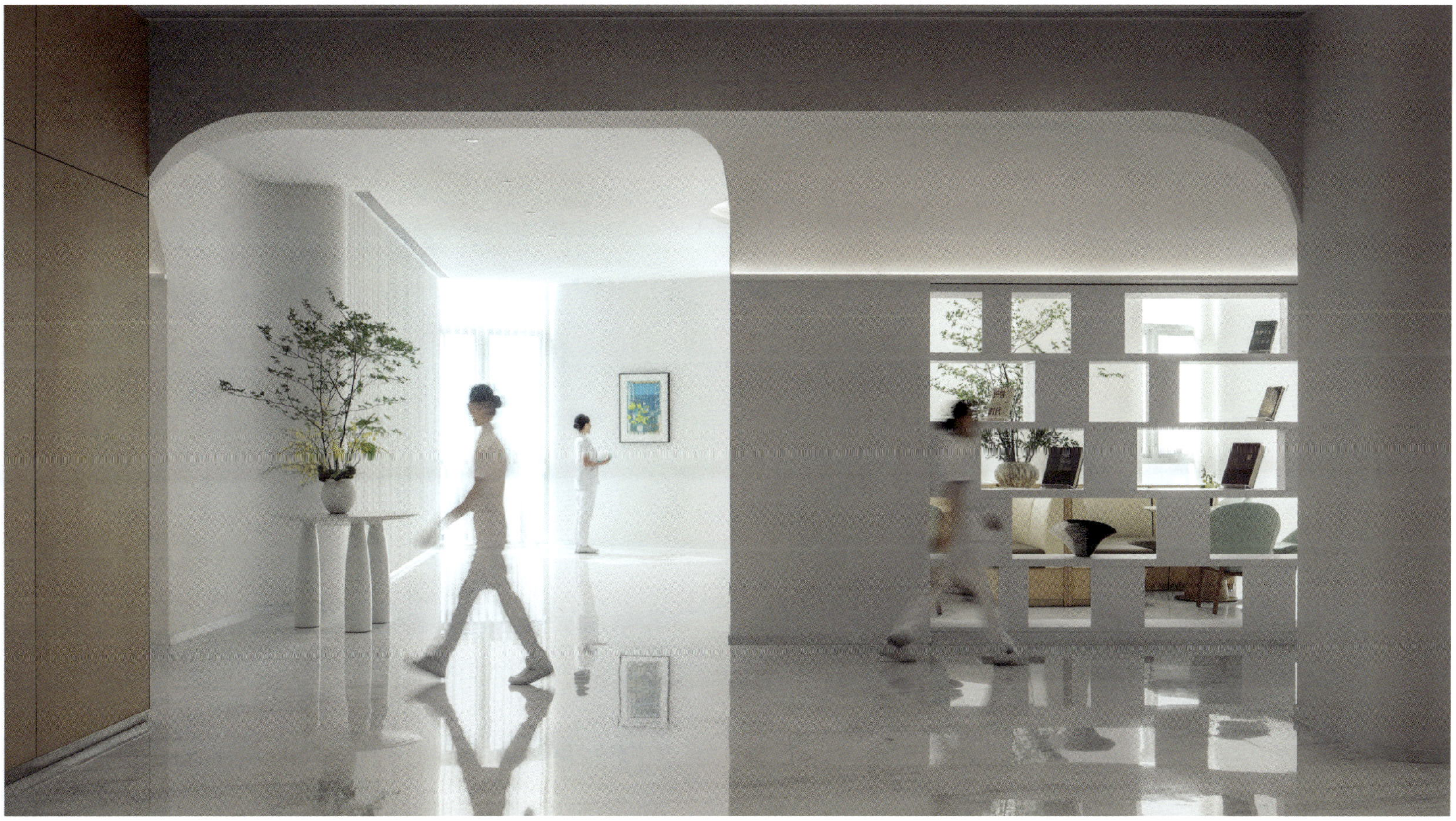

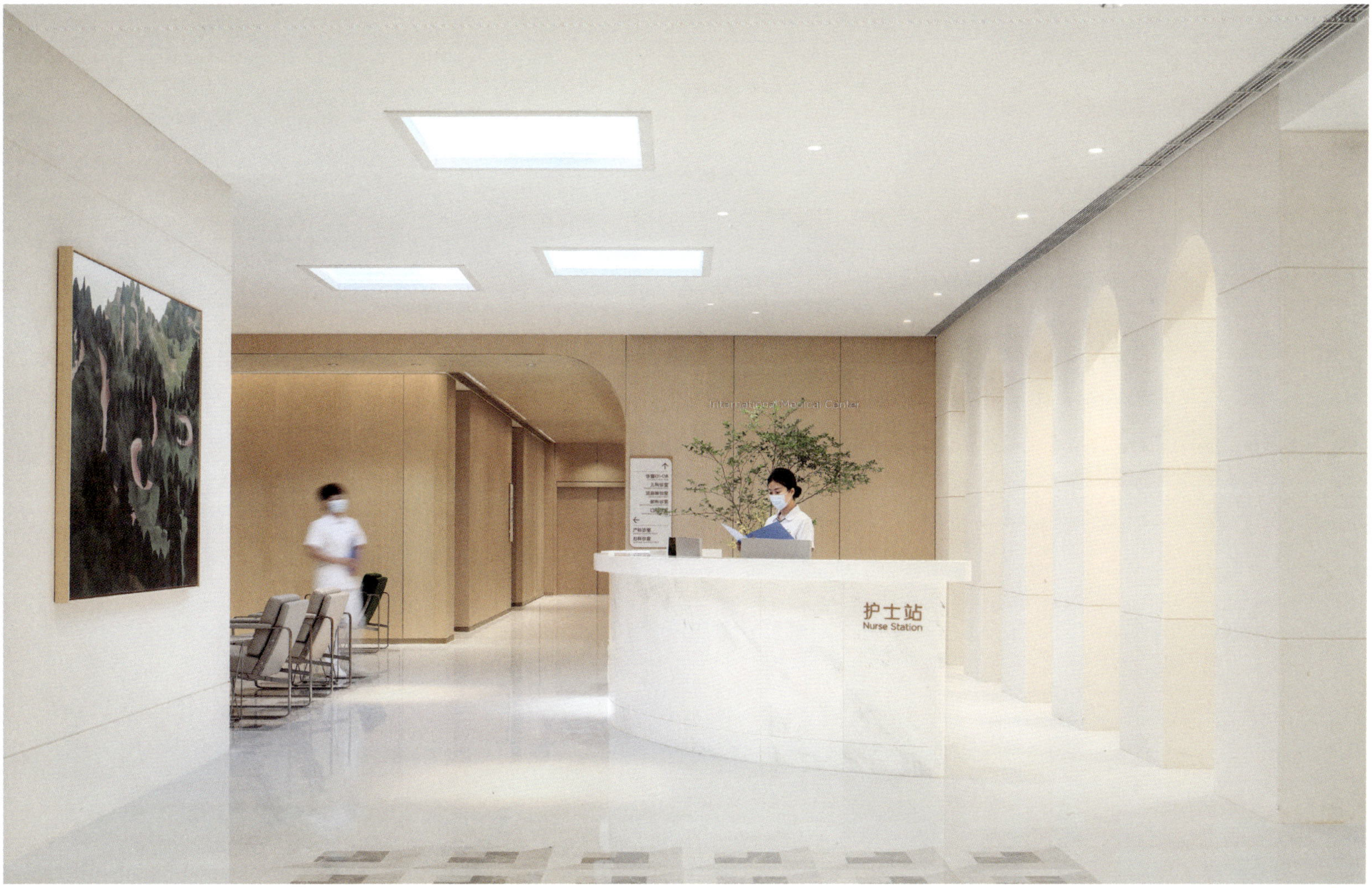

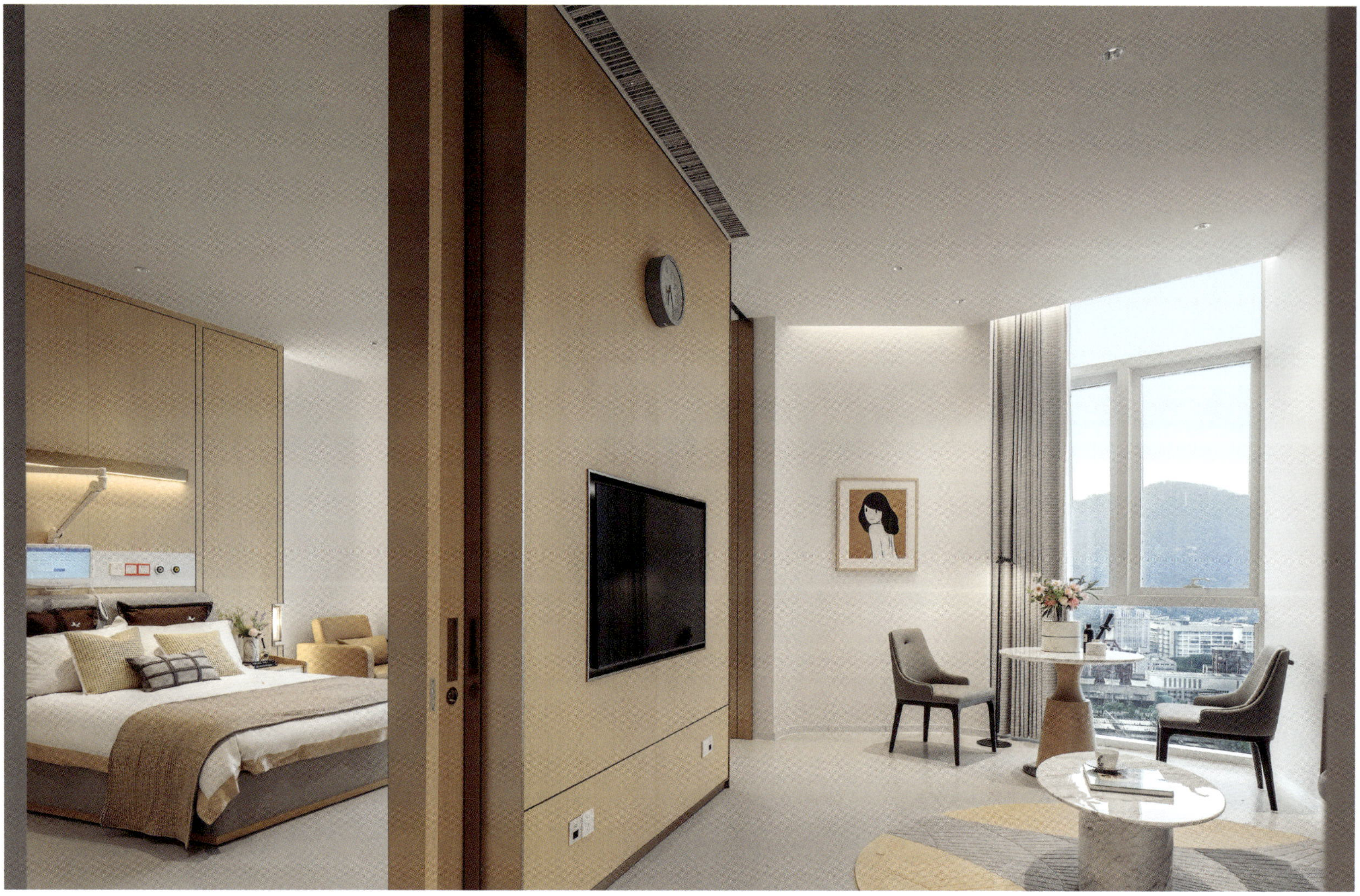

Ward's luxurious suite with elegant interiors and a view.

First floor plan.

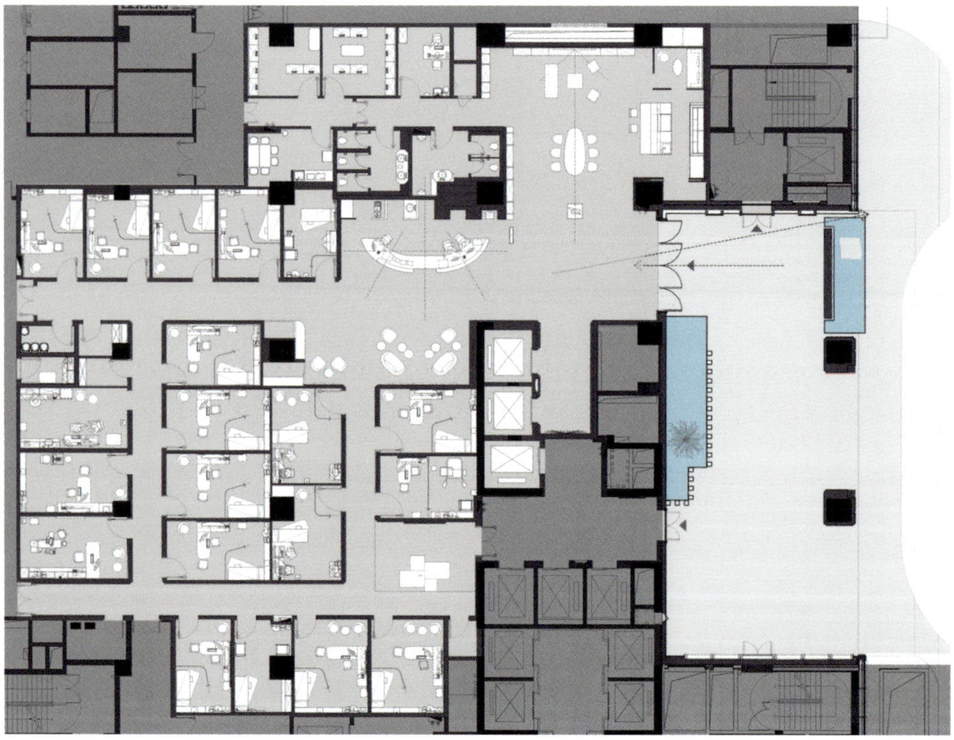

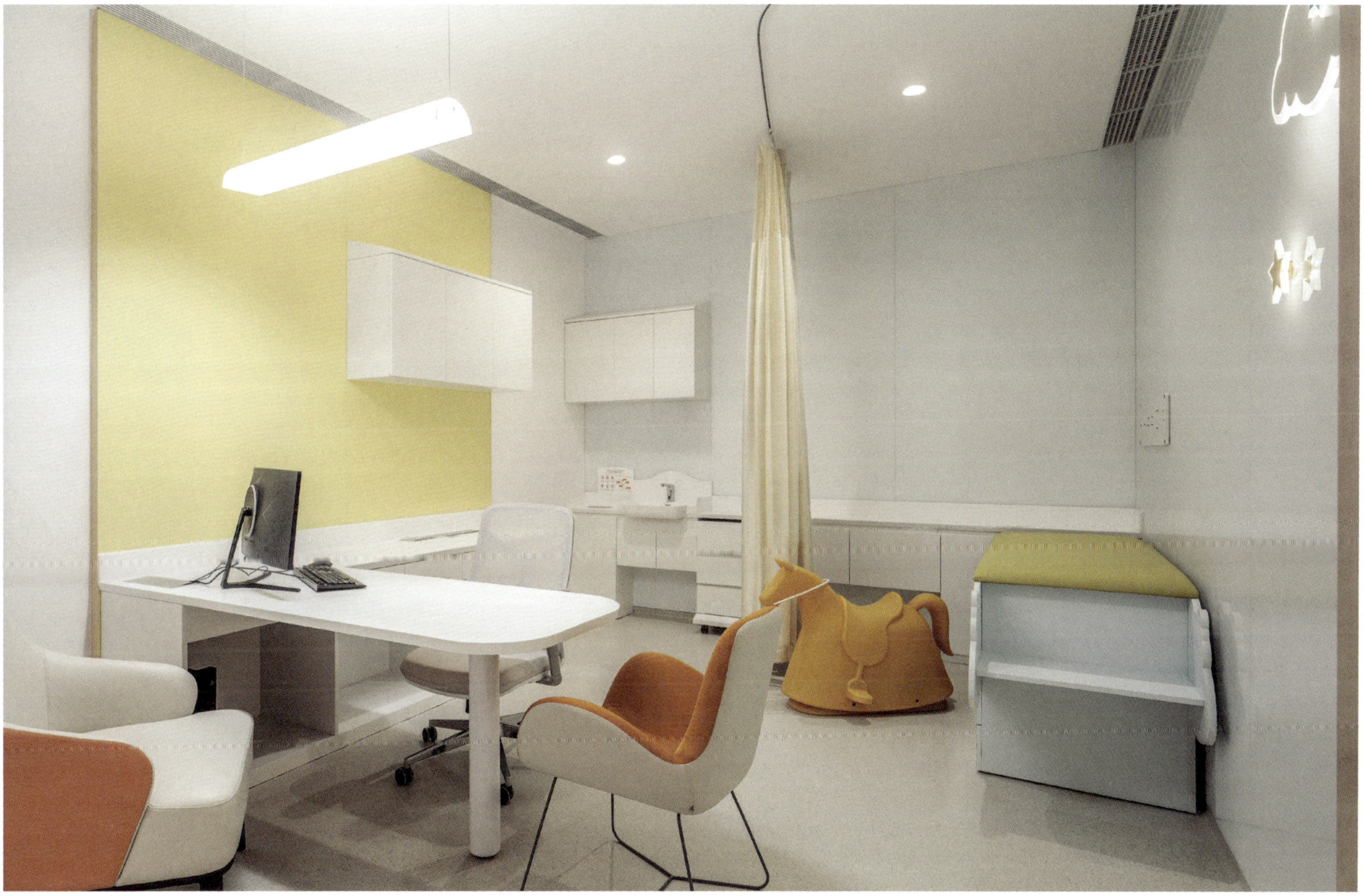

Hospital's pediatric clinic.

22nd floor plan.

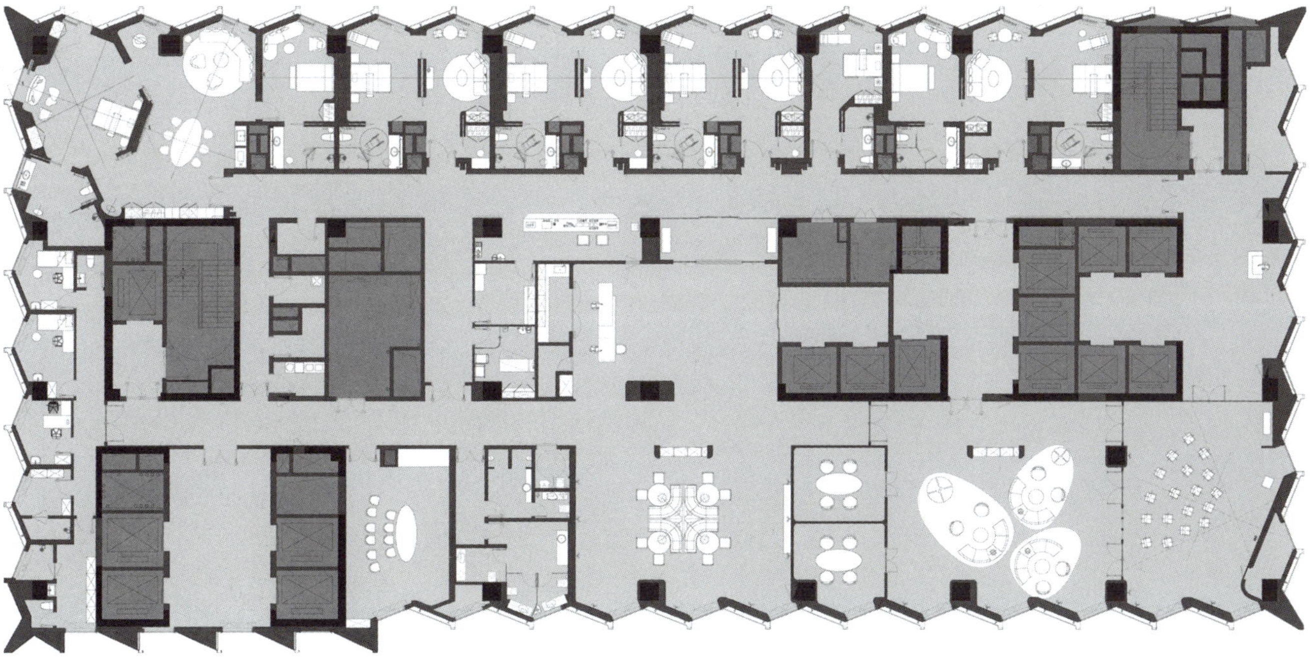

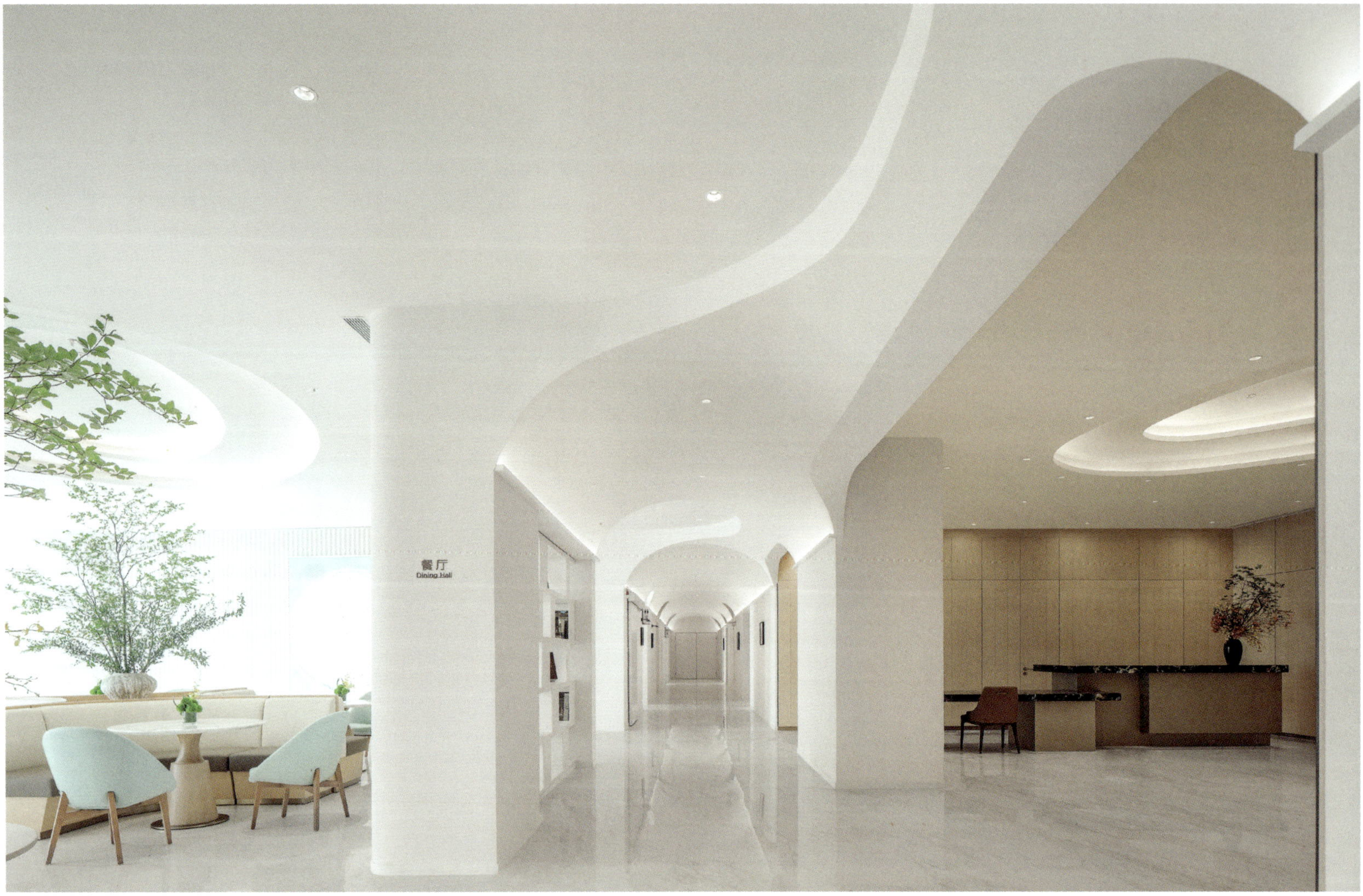

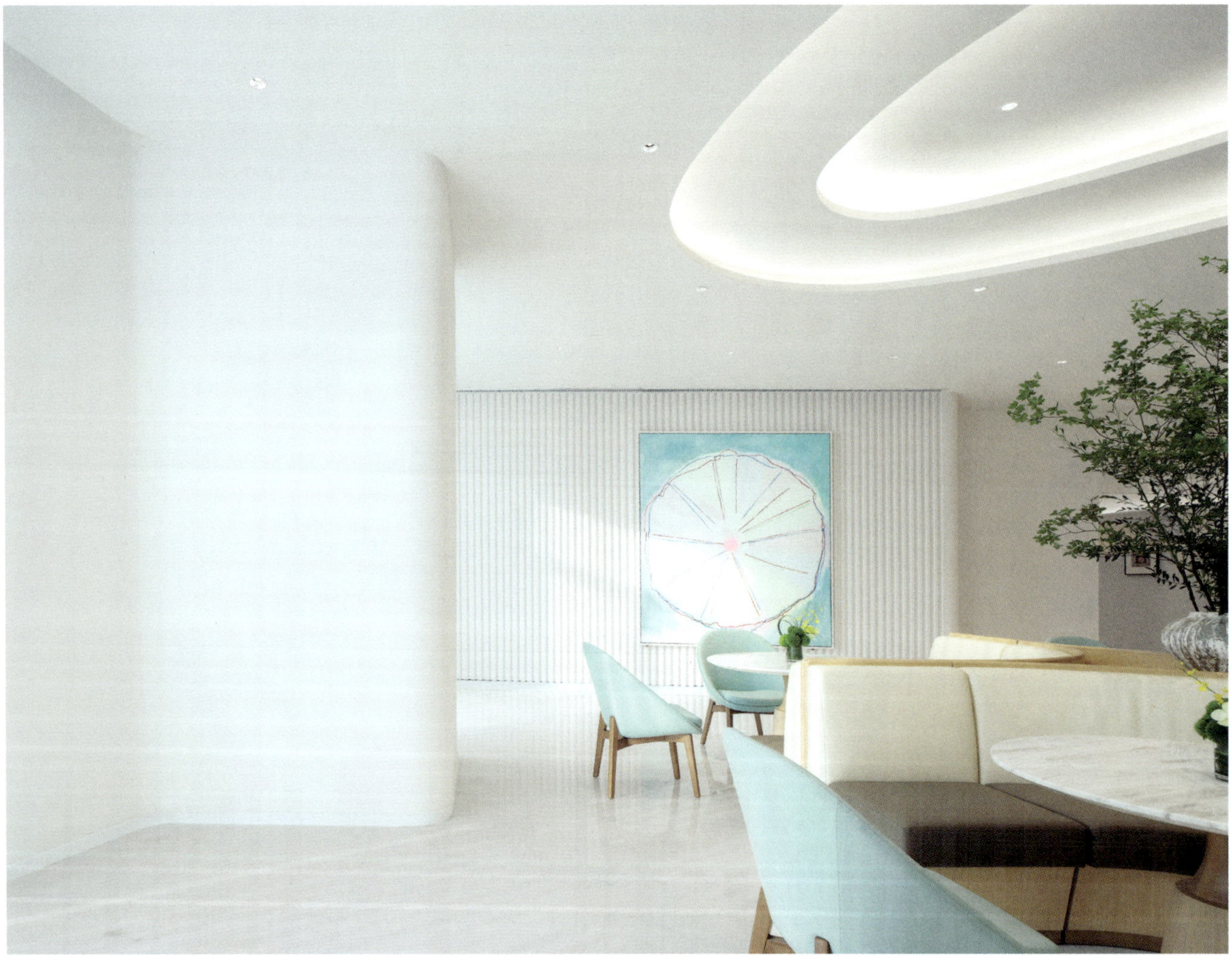

Spacious ward lobby area with soothing colors and interiors.

Lobby area.

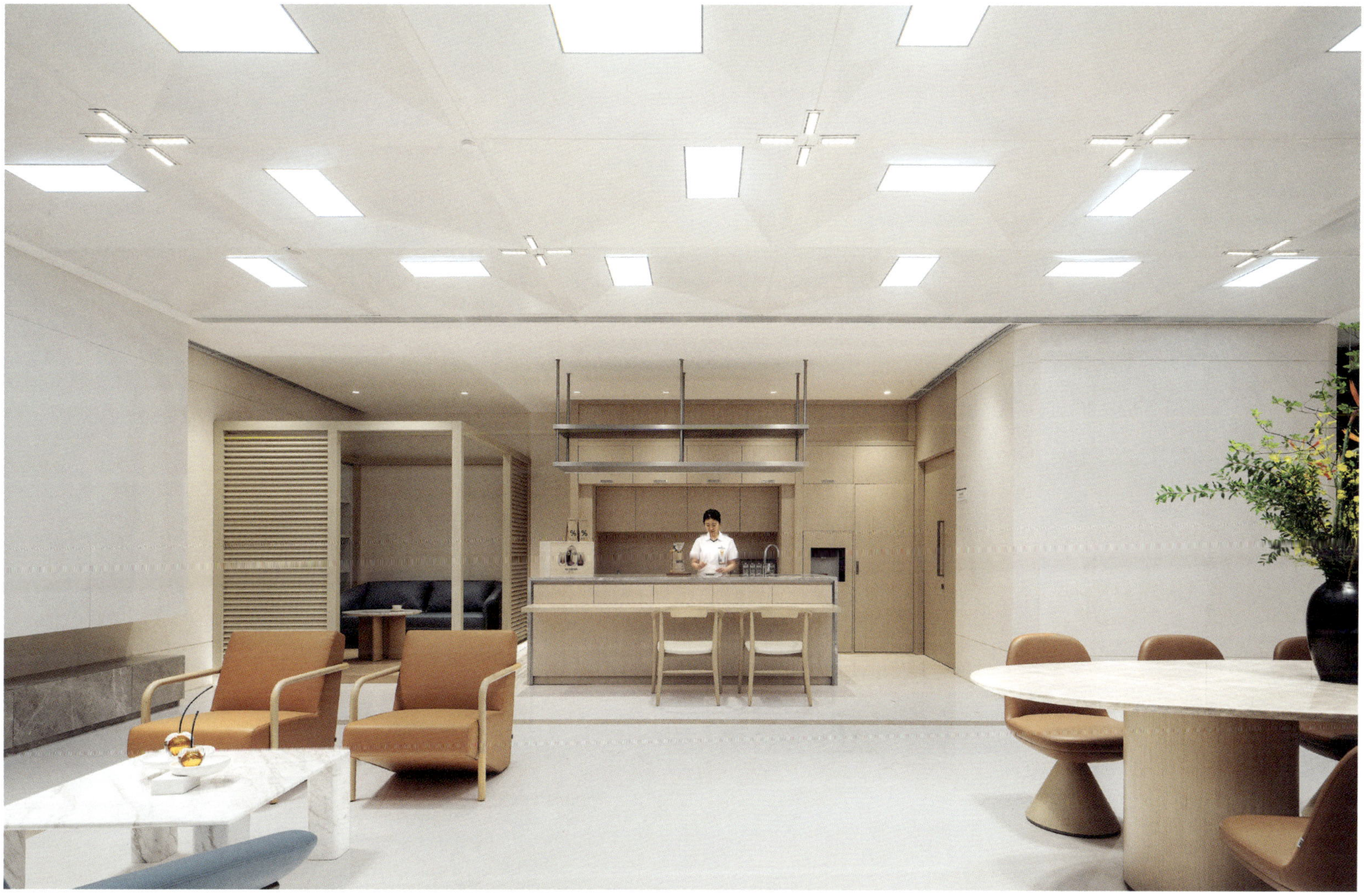

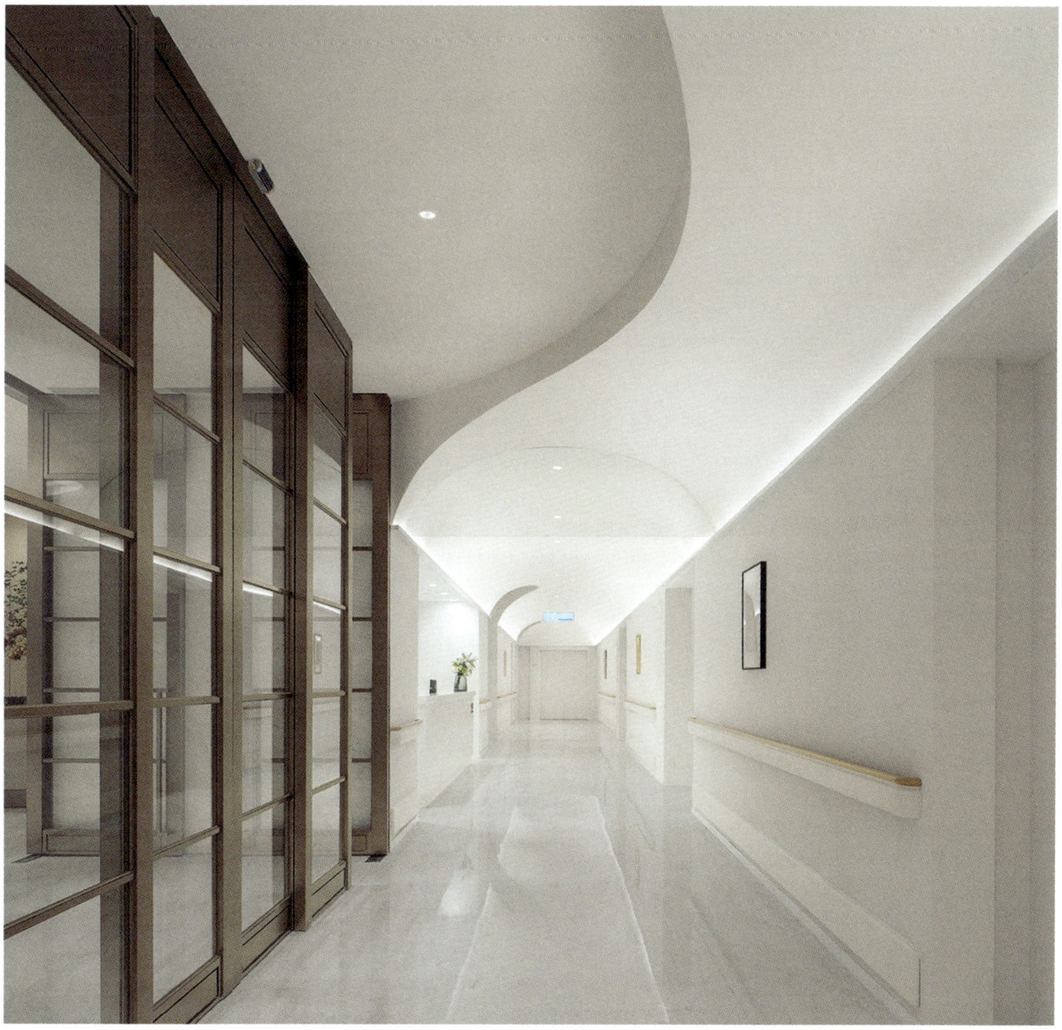

Registration area café

Hospital's ward area corridor.

Davide Macullo Architects

Ashdod
Israel

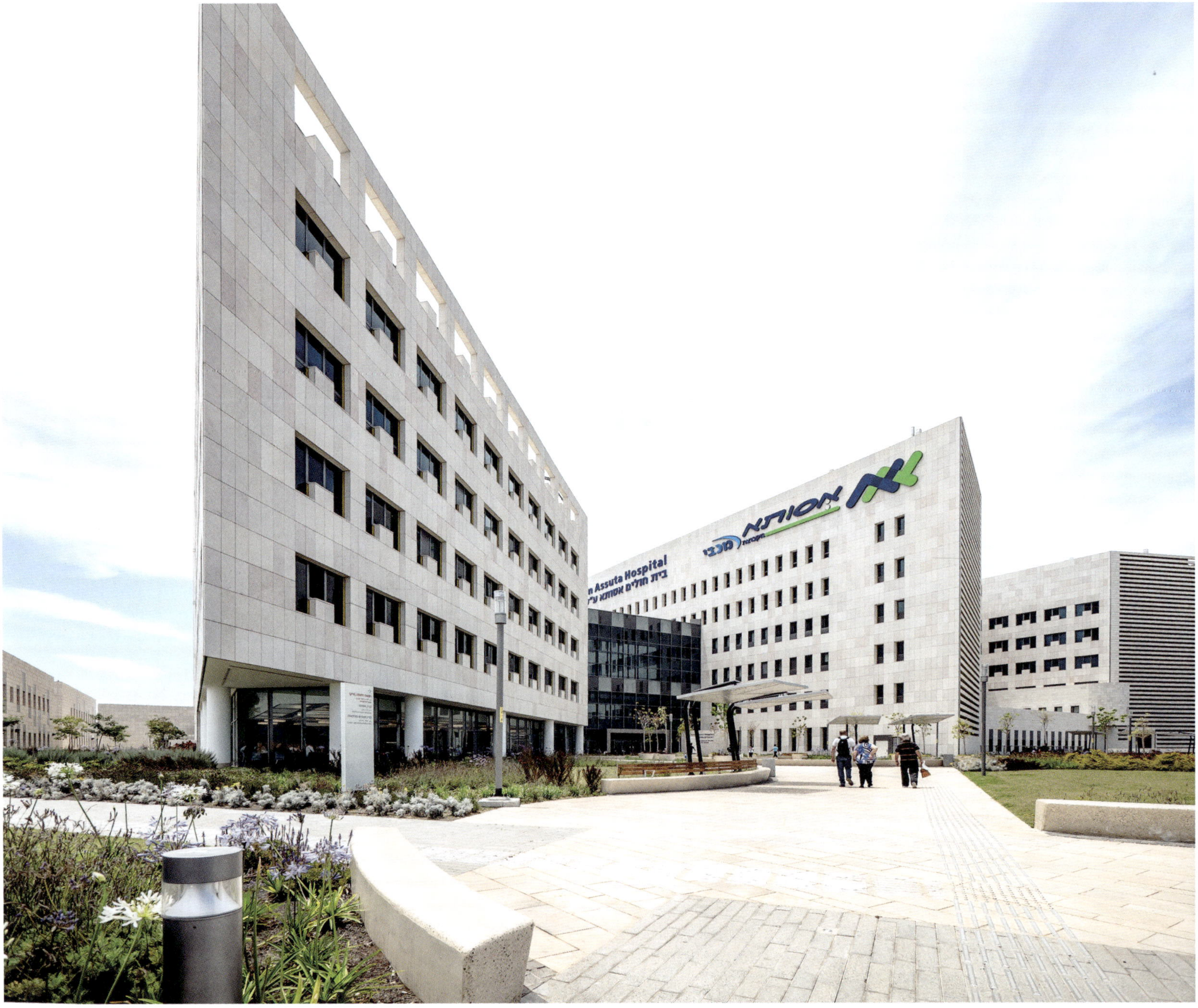

View of the entrance and building volumes.

Elevator area inside the building with floral wall design.

Samson Assuta University Hospital

The Ashdod hospital is born out of the roots and the culture of Israel. The hospital uses a designated flower theme to create a warm and welcoming environment that is appealing to its visitors. The building is approachable through various gardens with indigenous vegetation, each one representing a region of Israel. Inside, the natural oases are transformed into artificial oases. Following an artistic understanding of architecture as the representation of nature, the interior spaces are consequently punctuated and animated by photographic representations of the nature that is outside: the natural landscape of Israel, which is seen as the major element that unites its people. Those who come to the hospital will follow a particular flower, which represents a specific cure. Flowers have been chosen because they express the beauty, harmony, and joy and contribute to the well-being of the patients.

Address: Ha-Refu'a St 7, Ashdod, 7747629, Israel | **Client:** Assuta Ashdod | **Completion:** 2017 | **Size:** 72,000 m² |
Sector: public | **Number of treatment rooms:** 147 | **Number of patient rooms:** 196 | **Interior design:** Davide Macullo |
Nature photographies: Doron Horovitz

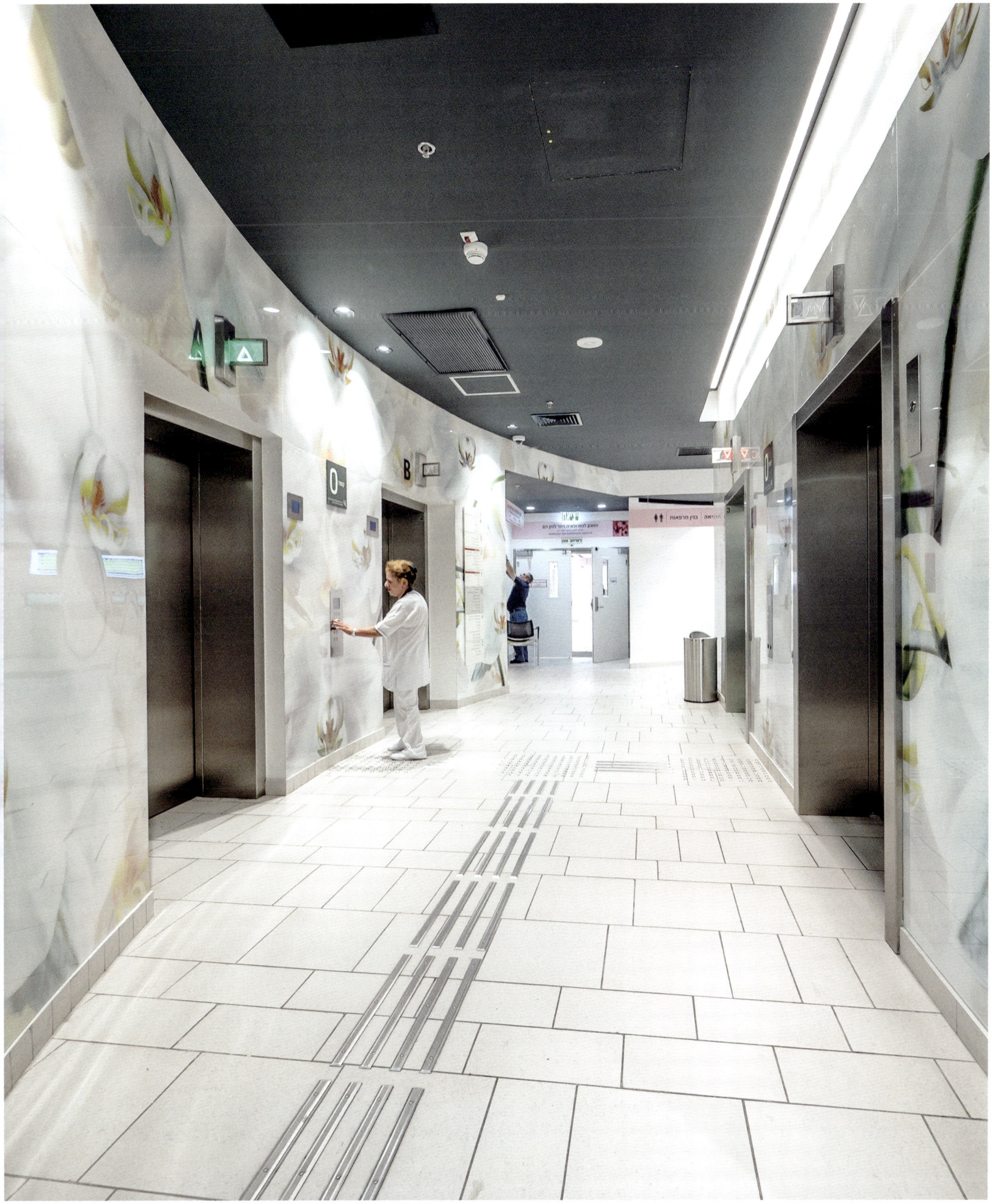

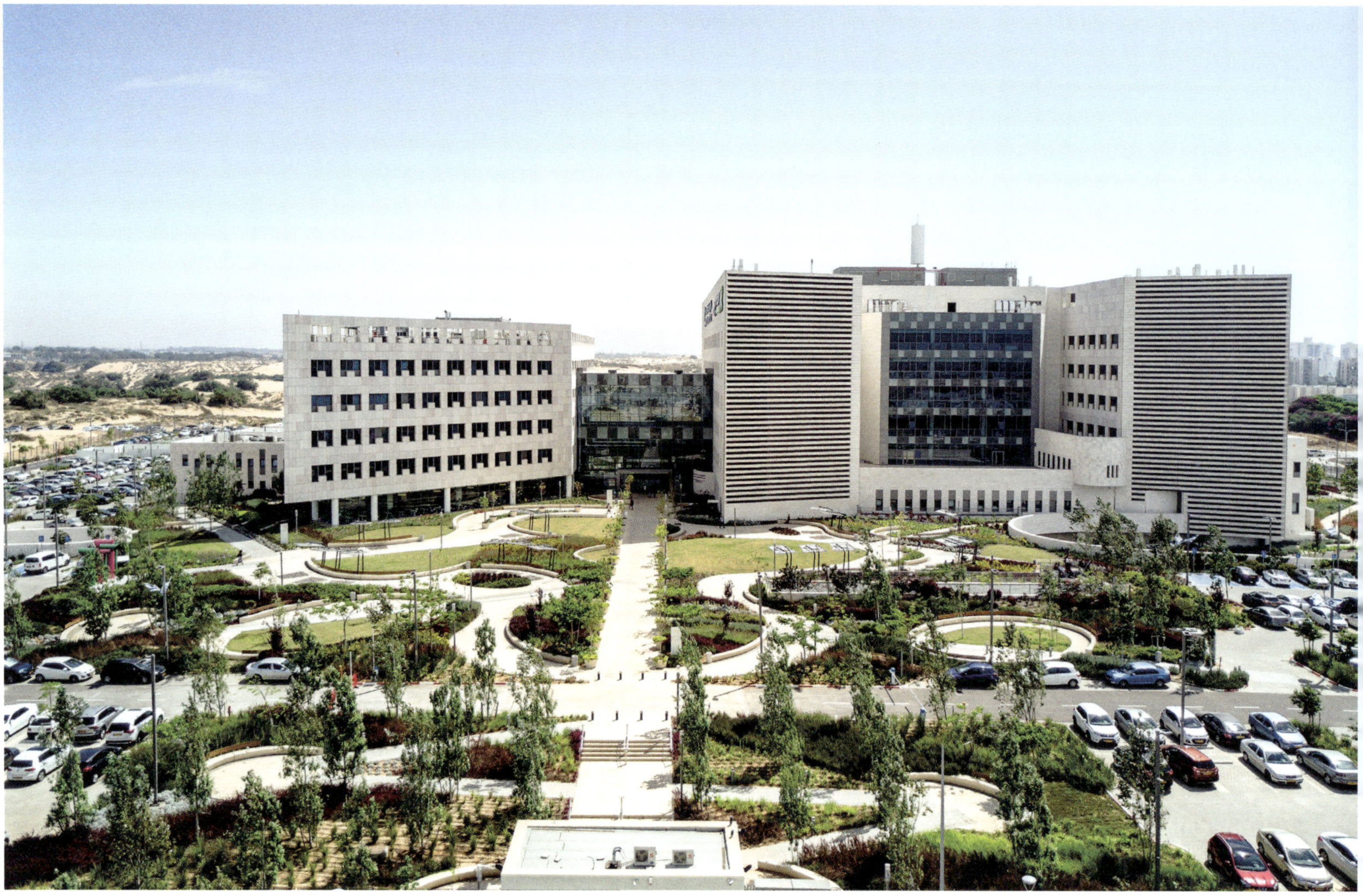

The building's location within the urban context.

Site plan.

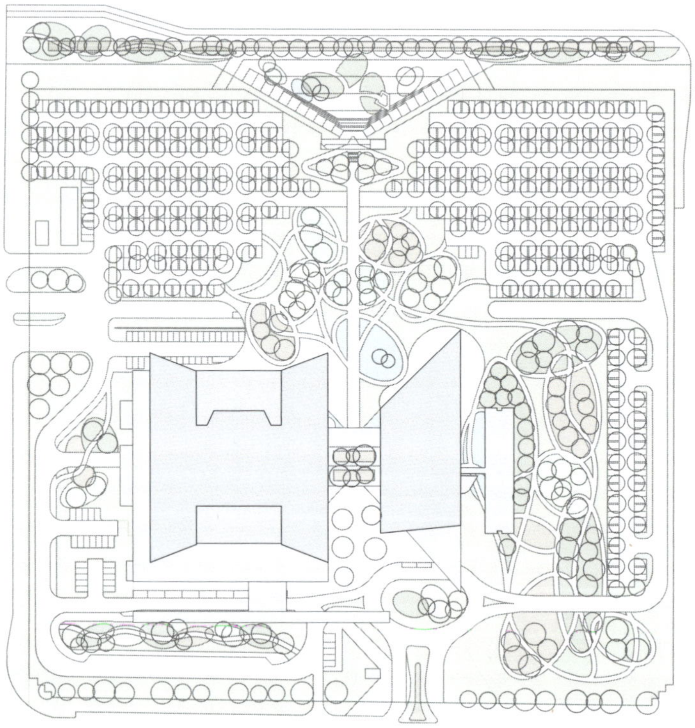

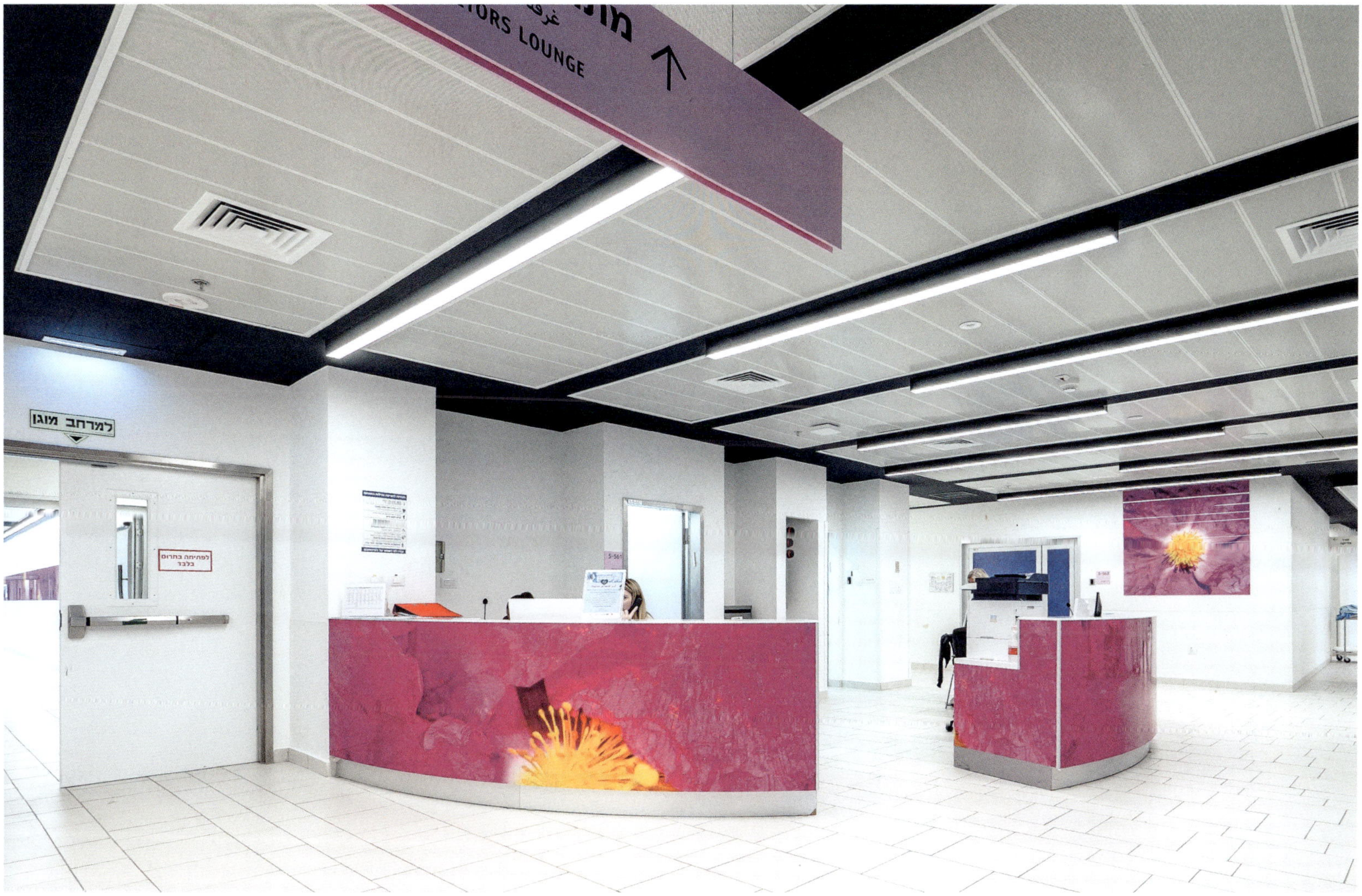

Reception desk with floral design.

Original sketch.

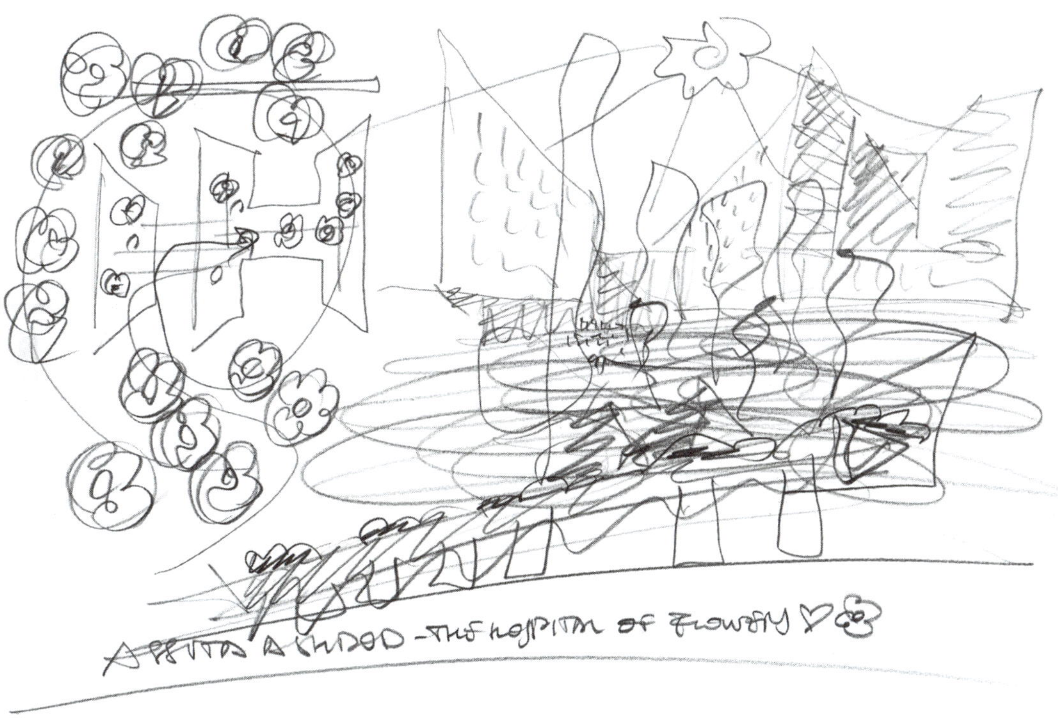

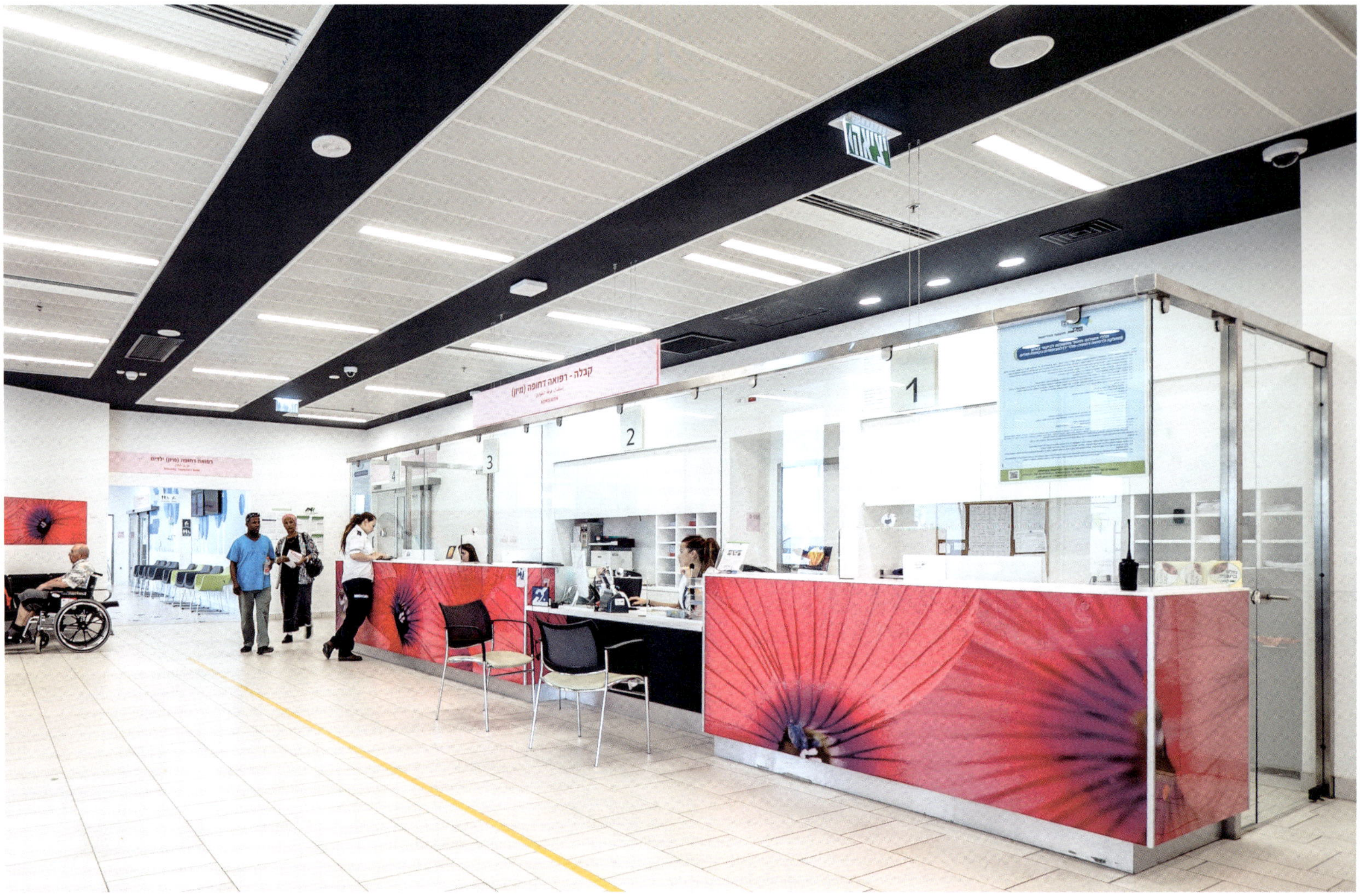

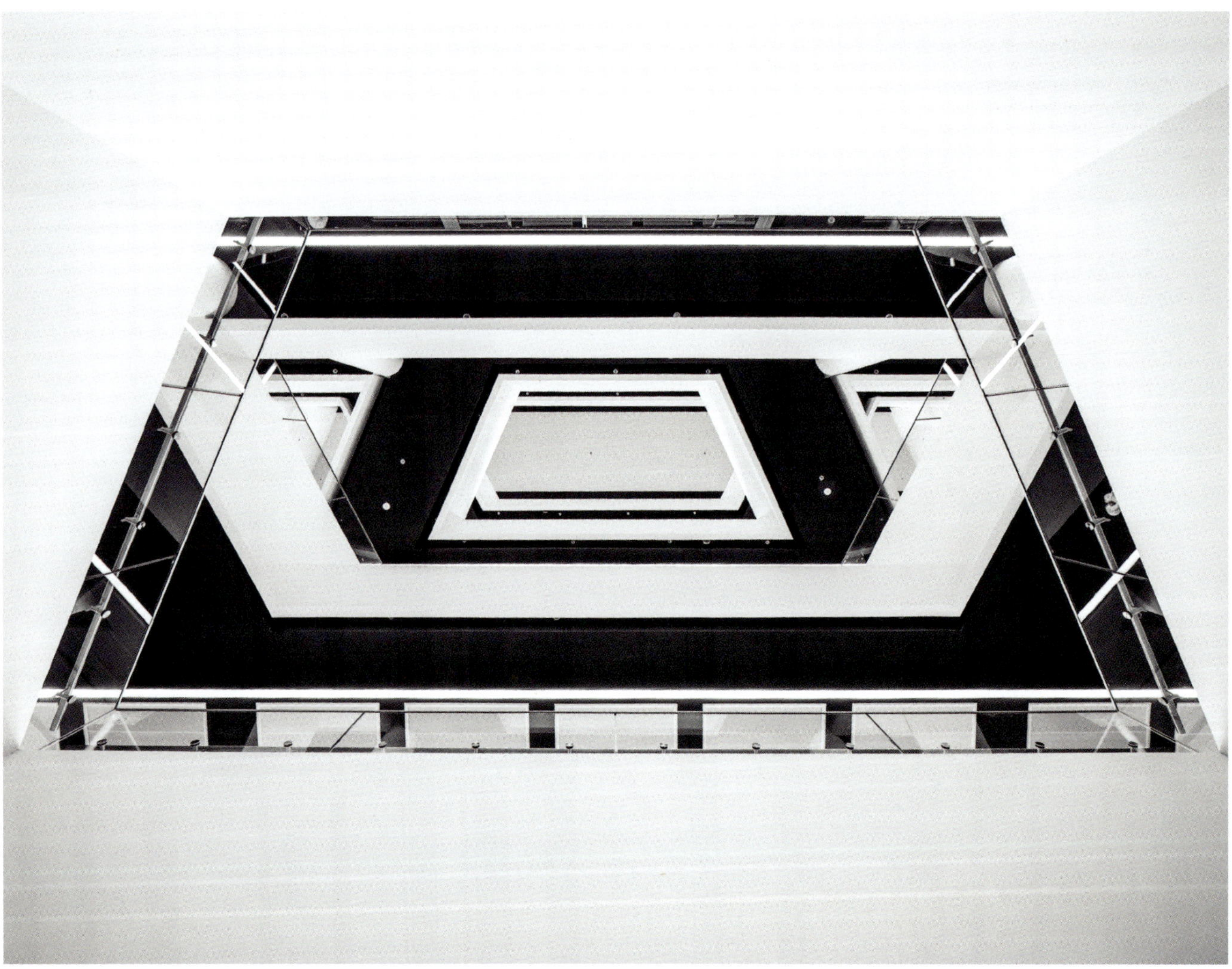

Interior view with floral design.

View into the stairwell.

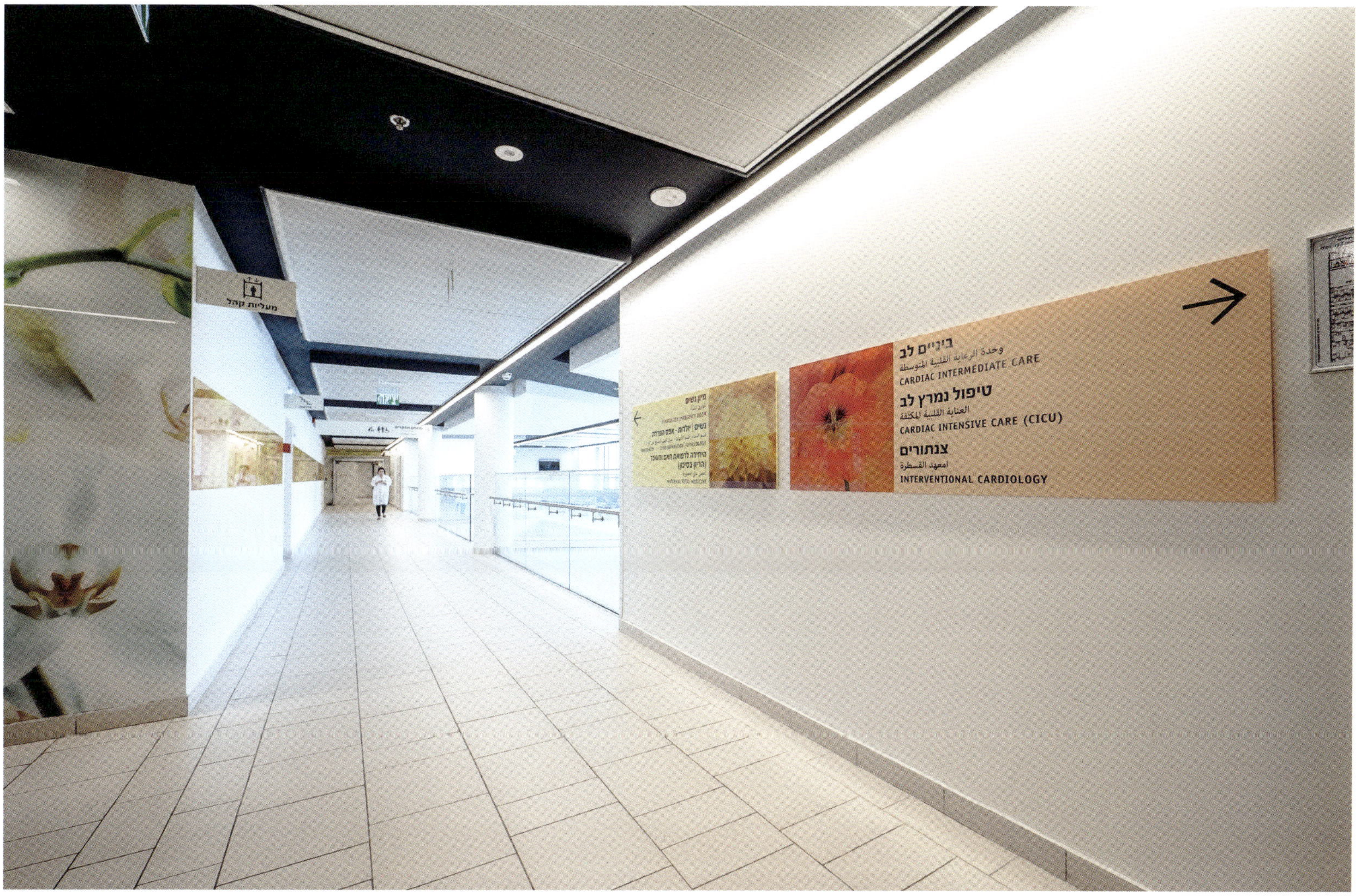

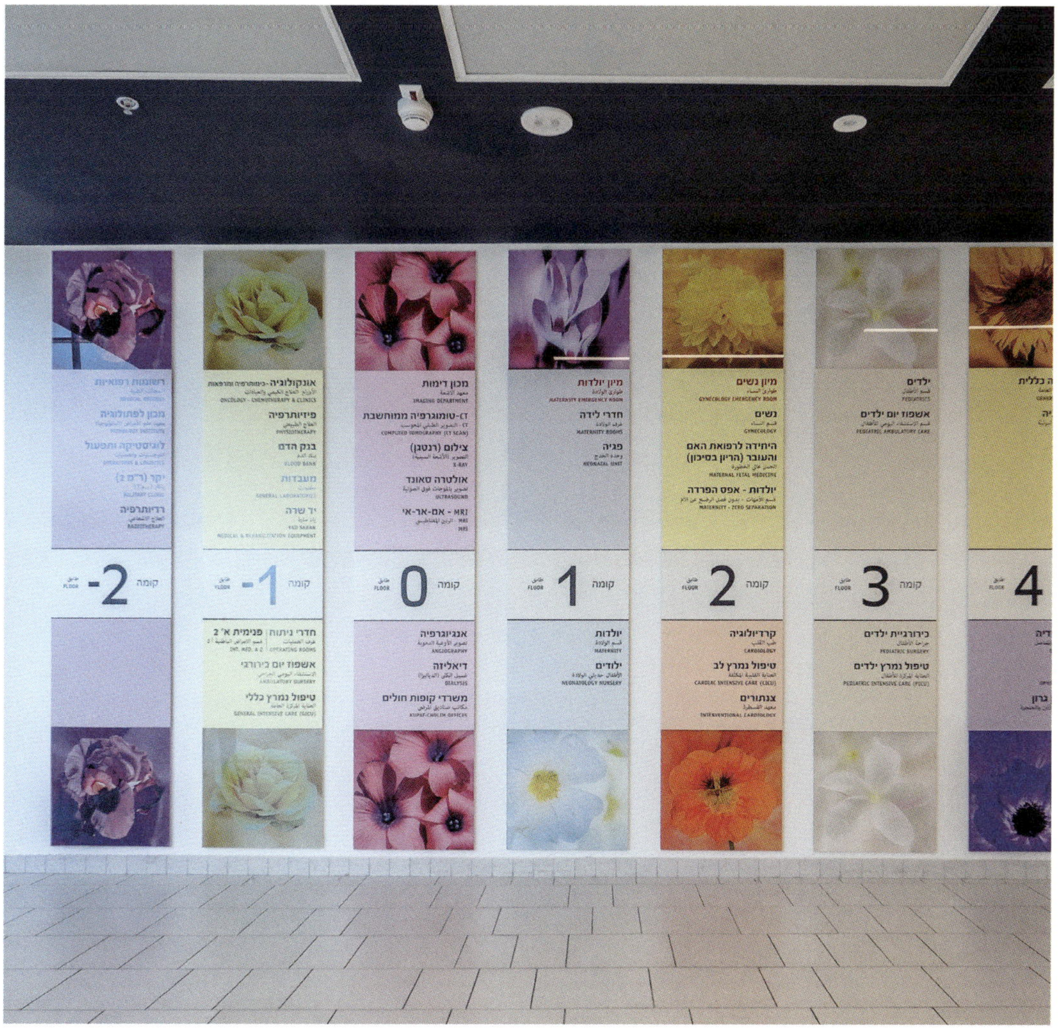

Corridor with colorful signage and floral wall design.

Signage for orientation showing the range of floral design.

Moloney O'Beirne Architects

Dublin Ireland

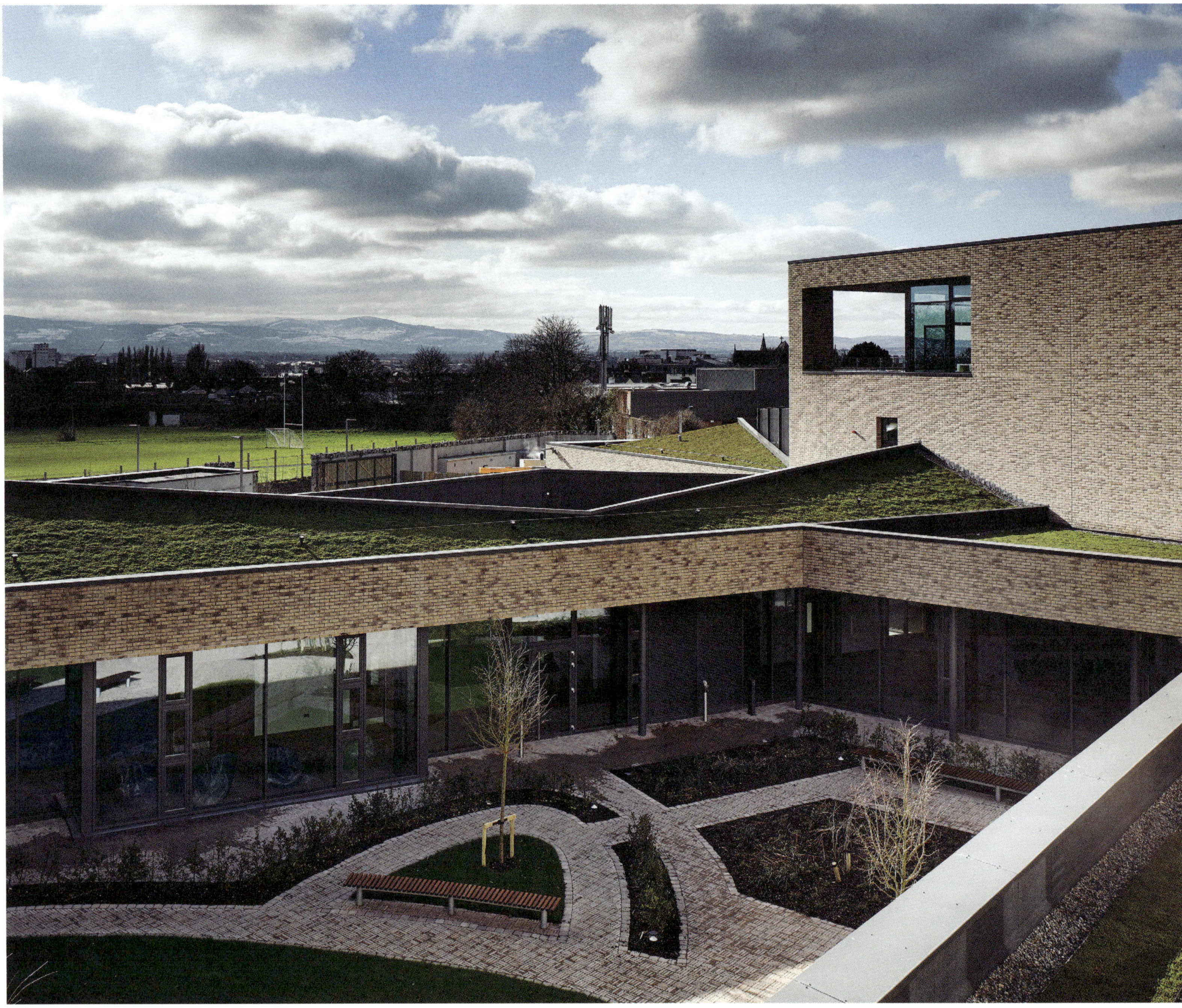

Aerial view of the building, organized around two central courtyards within the surrounding landscape.

Patio framed by the building, with planted and paved surfaces defining the courtyard.

Timber-floored waiting area integrated into a light-filled open space.

Phoenix Care Centre

Set within Grangegorman Campus, Phoenix Care Centre replaces an 1814 psychiatric clinic and provides a 54-bed low secure facility that combines supervision with a non-institutional character. The form and orientation of the building optimize solar penetration, whilst also responding to the master planning requirements. Single-, two- and three-story volumes organize around two courtyards, structuring patient groups and ensuring access to human-scaled outdoor space. At ground level, the higher risk intensive care unit is embedded in a dual-courtyard system, enabling secure external access and clear functional segregation. Orientation maximizes southern daylight and solar gain; green roofs and planting extend landscape into the building fabric. Light clay brickwork and restrained detailing soften institutional expression, while interior colors drawn from gardens reinforce a calm atmosphere.

Address: North Circular Road, Grangegorman, Dublin 7, Ireland | **Client:** Grangegorman Development Agency | **Completion:** 2014 | **Size:** 7,800 m² | **Sector:** state | **Specialization:** mental health | **Number of patient rooms:** 54

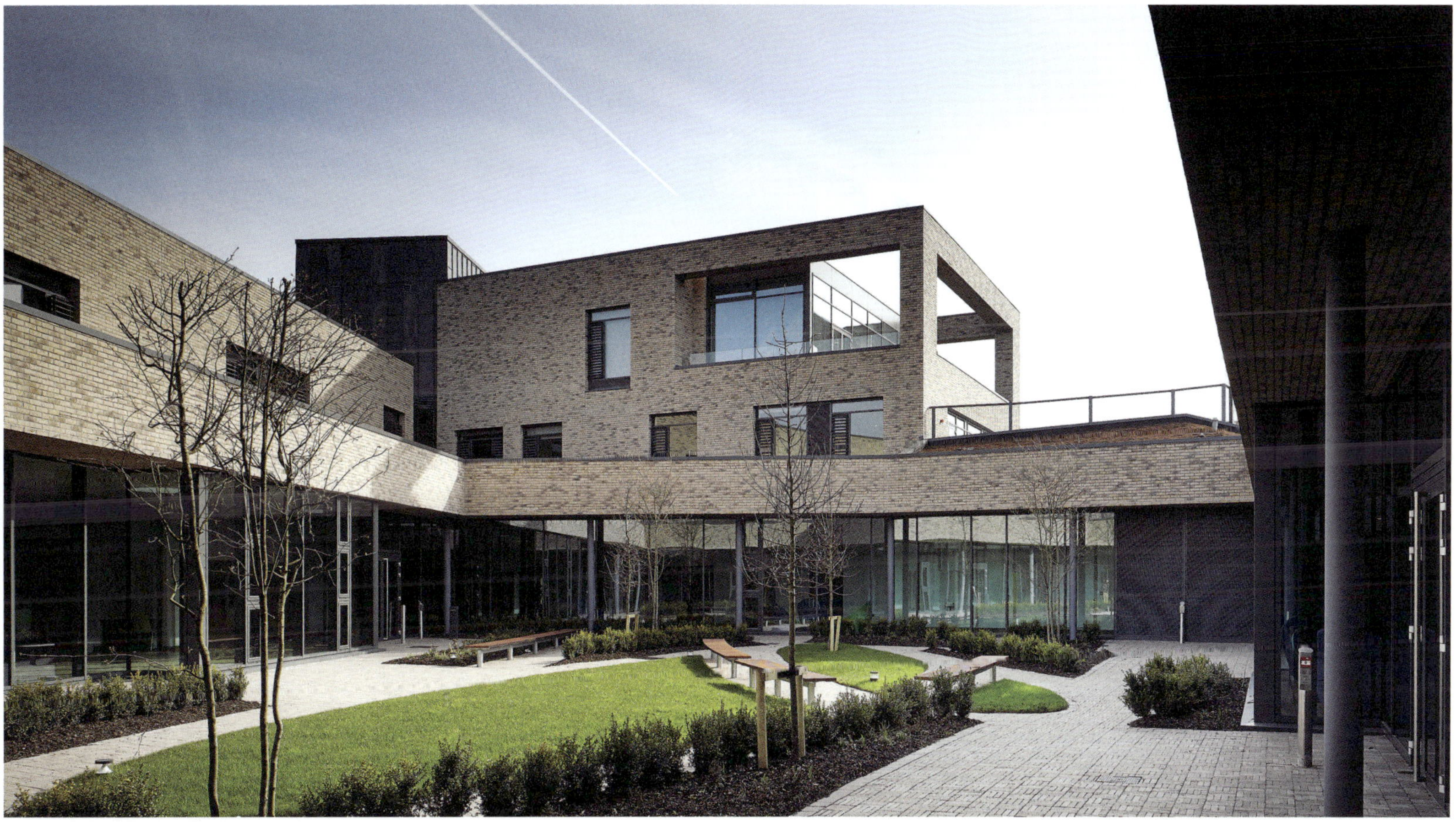

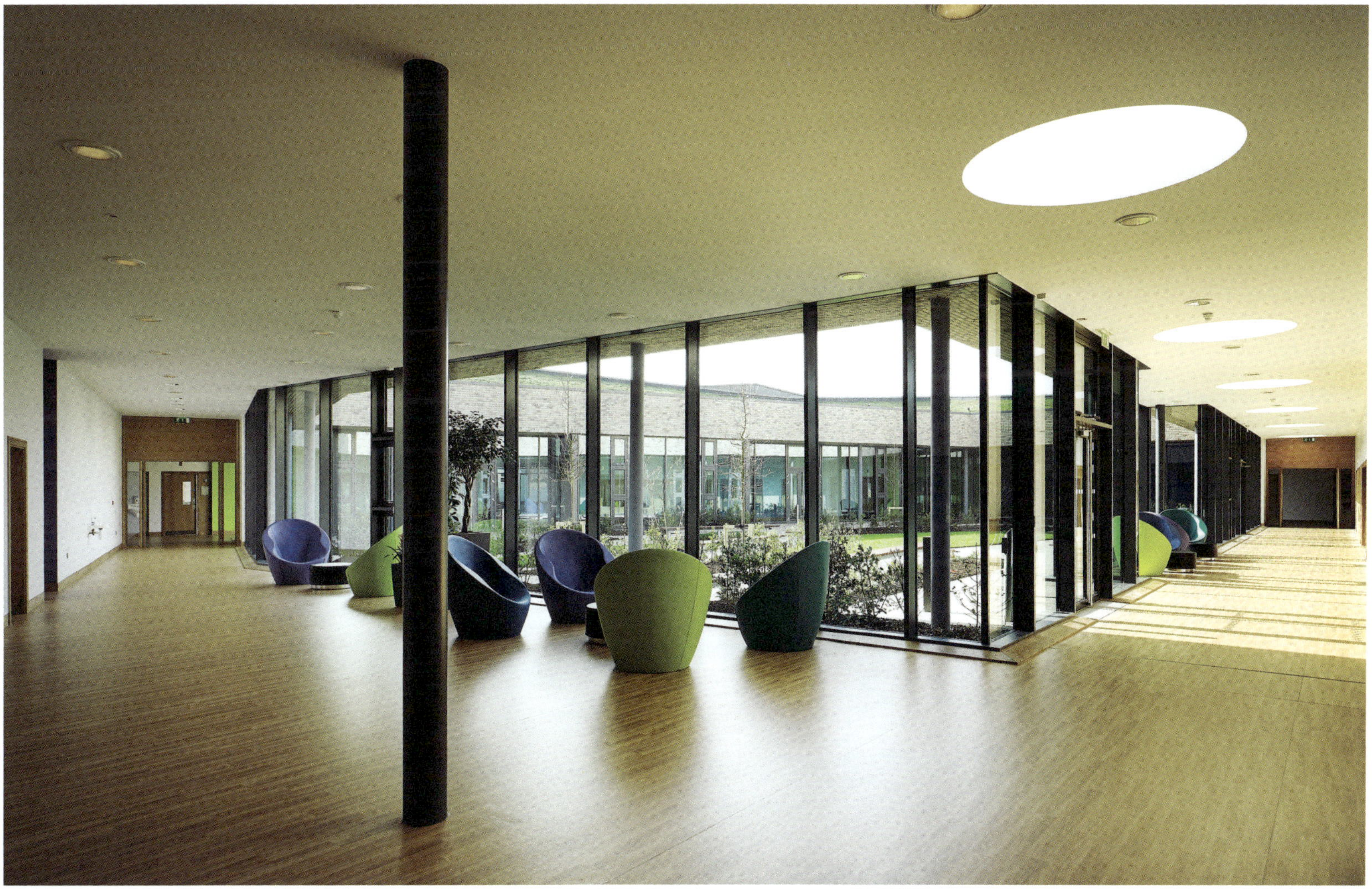

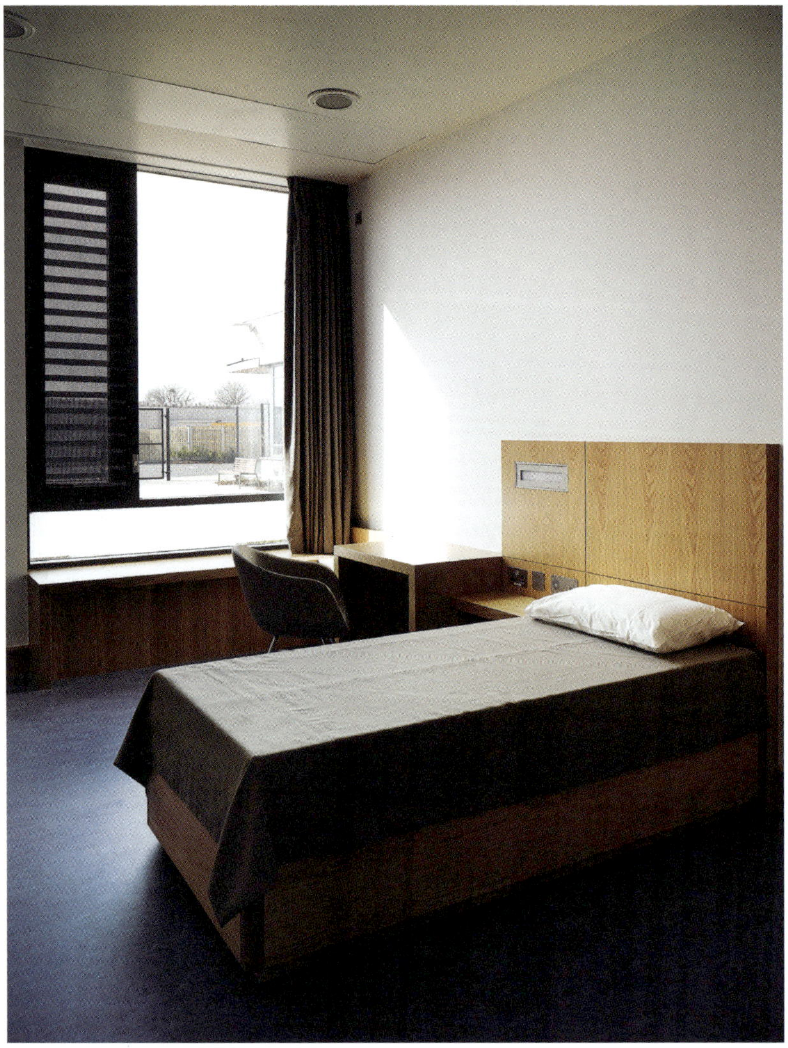

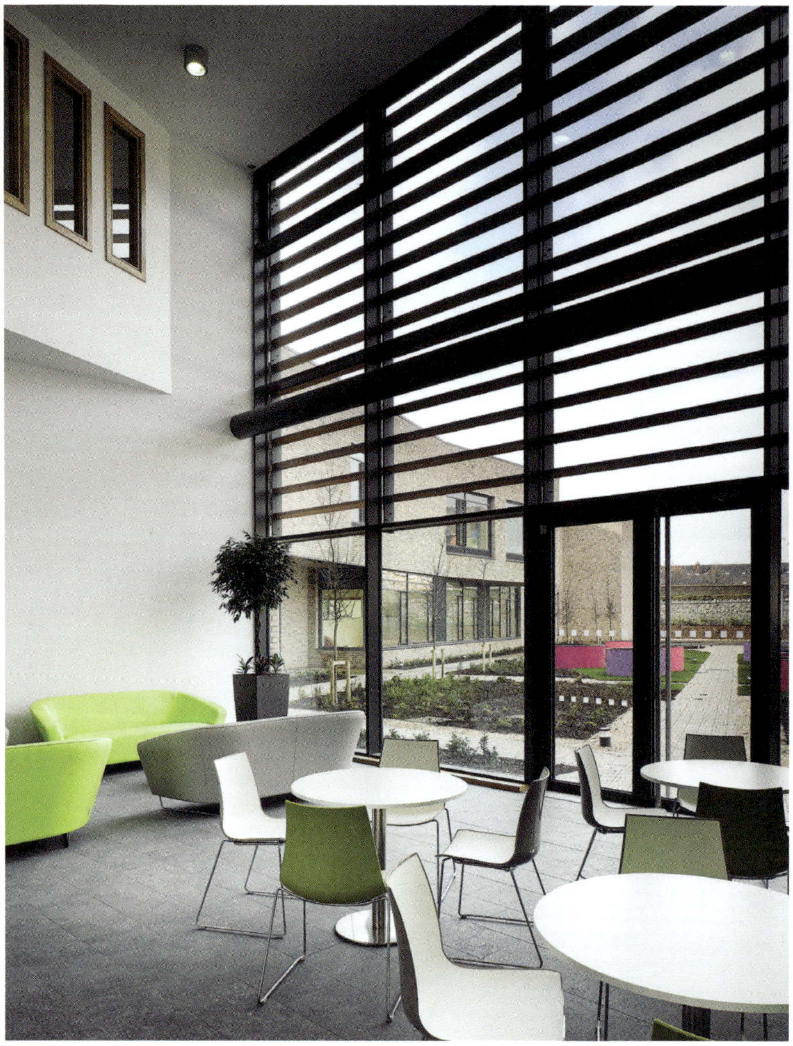

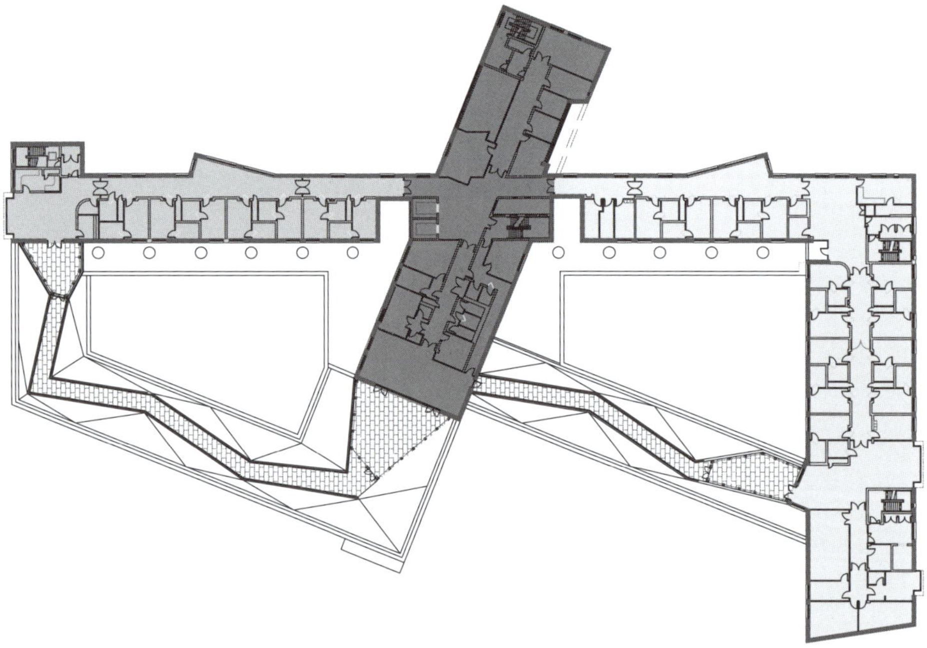

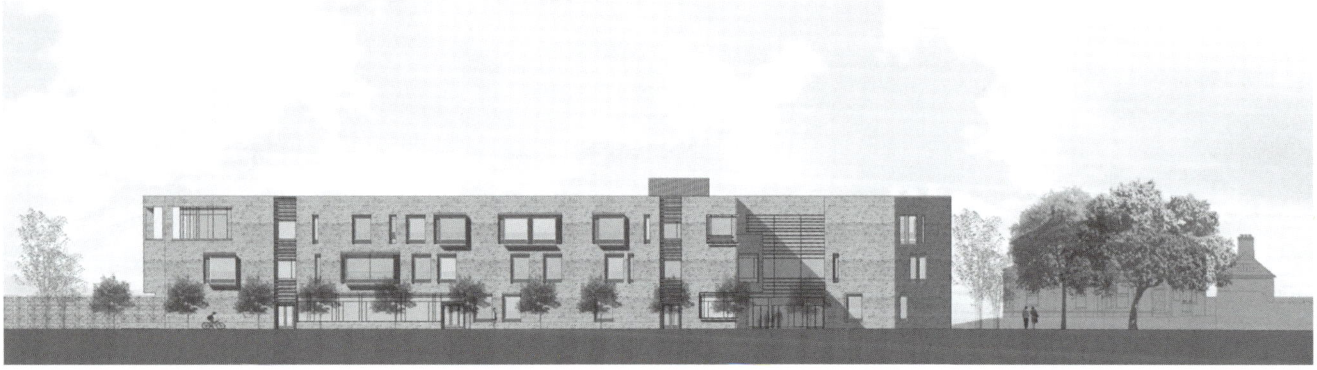

Single-bed patient room with natural color palette and wood finishing.

Dining room with tall windows, defined by a clean aesthetic and expansive glazing.

First floor plan with female, shared, and male areas.

Elevation.

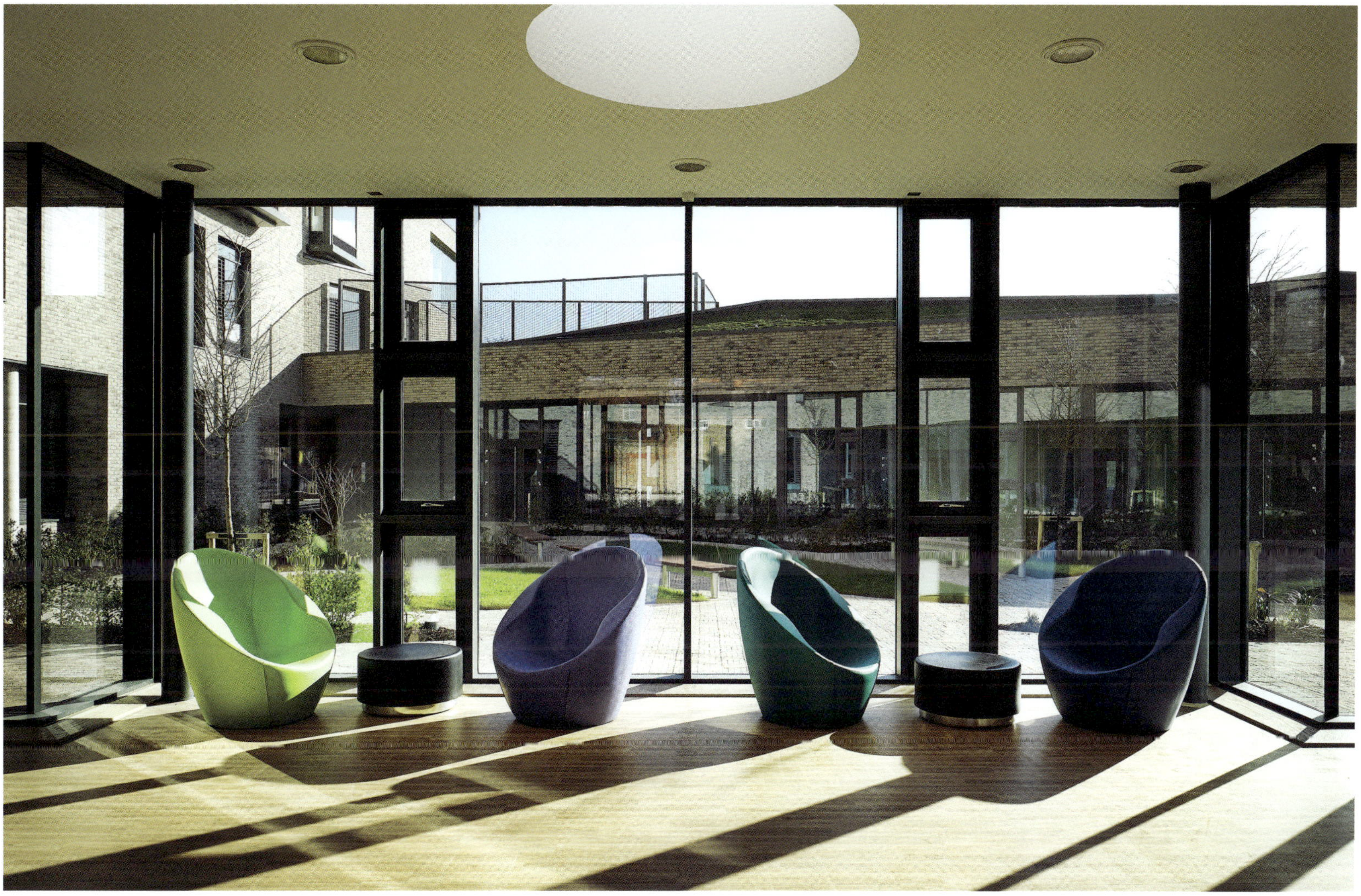

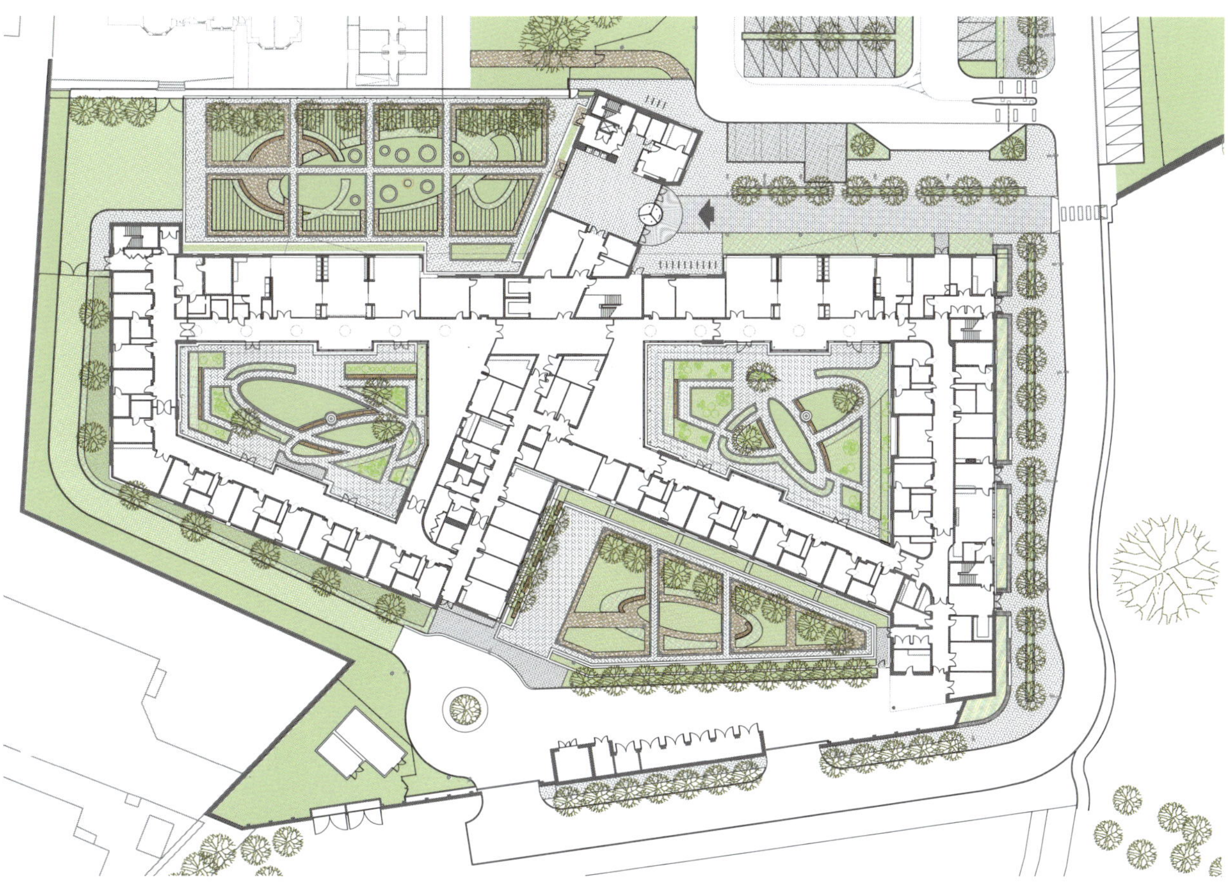

Colored seating with view towards the patio, designed for patients' and visitors' comfort.

Landscape plan.

Sweco Architects

Stuttgart
Germany

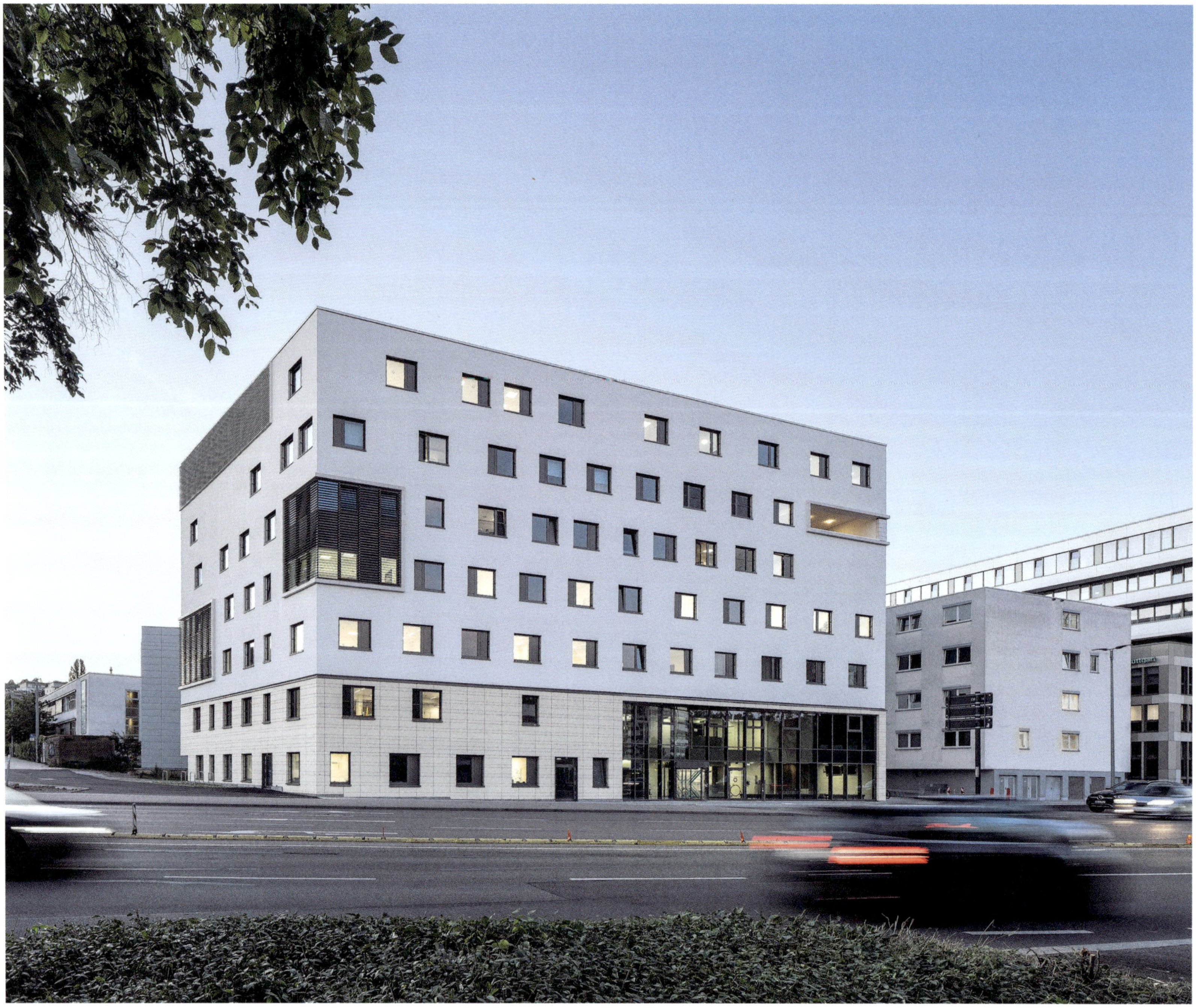

Hospital's façade detail in twilight.

Hospital with the Tower of Linden-Museum, Stuttgart.

Hospital's façade in the heart of the city.

New Stuttgart Cancer Center – Eva Mayr-Stihl Tumor Center (SCC)

The Stuttgart Cancer Center – Eva Mayr-Stihl Tumor Center (SCC) is setting new standards in patient-centered cancer care. The new Stuttgart University Hospital – Building G brings together modern diagnostic and therapeutic services such as chemotherapy, radiation therapy, and nuclear medicine, as well as outpatient and inpatient care. Precise functionality and architectural clarity define the building: An understated base made of ceramic panels blends harmoniously into the surroundings. The interplay of mullion-transom glazing and irregularly arranged perforated windows lends the light-colored plastered upper floors a timeless structure and maximizes natural light. The interior design deliberately avoids a traditional hospital aesthetic, creating a pleasant atmosphere and promoting orientation, tranquility, and efficiency.

Address: Kriegsbergstraße 60, 70174, Stuttgart, Germany | **Client:** Klinikum der Landeshauptstadt Stuttgart | **Completion:** 2024 | **Size:** 14,615 m² | **Sector:** state | **Specialization:** cancer center, oncology clinic | **Number of treatment rooms:** 85 | **Number of patient rooms:** 31 | **Interior design:** Sweco

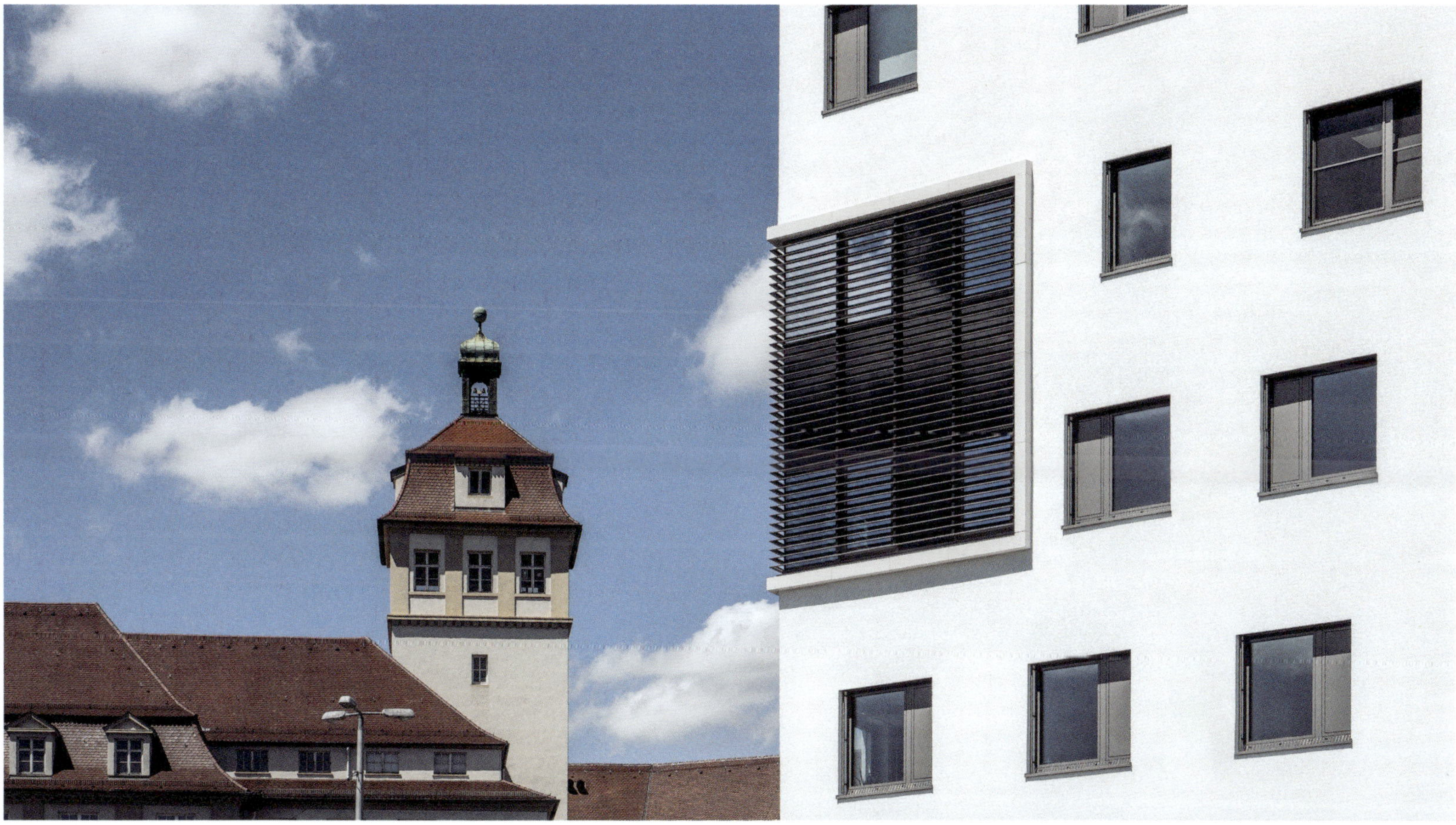

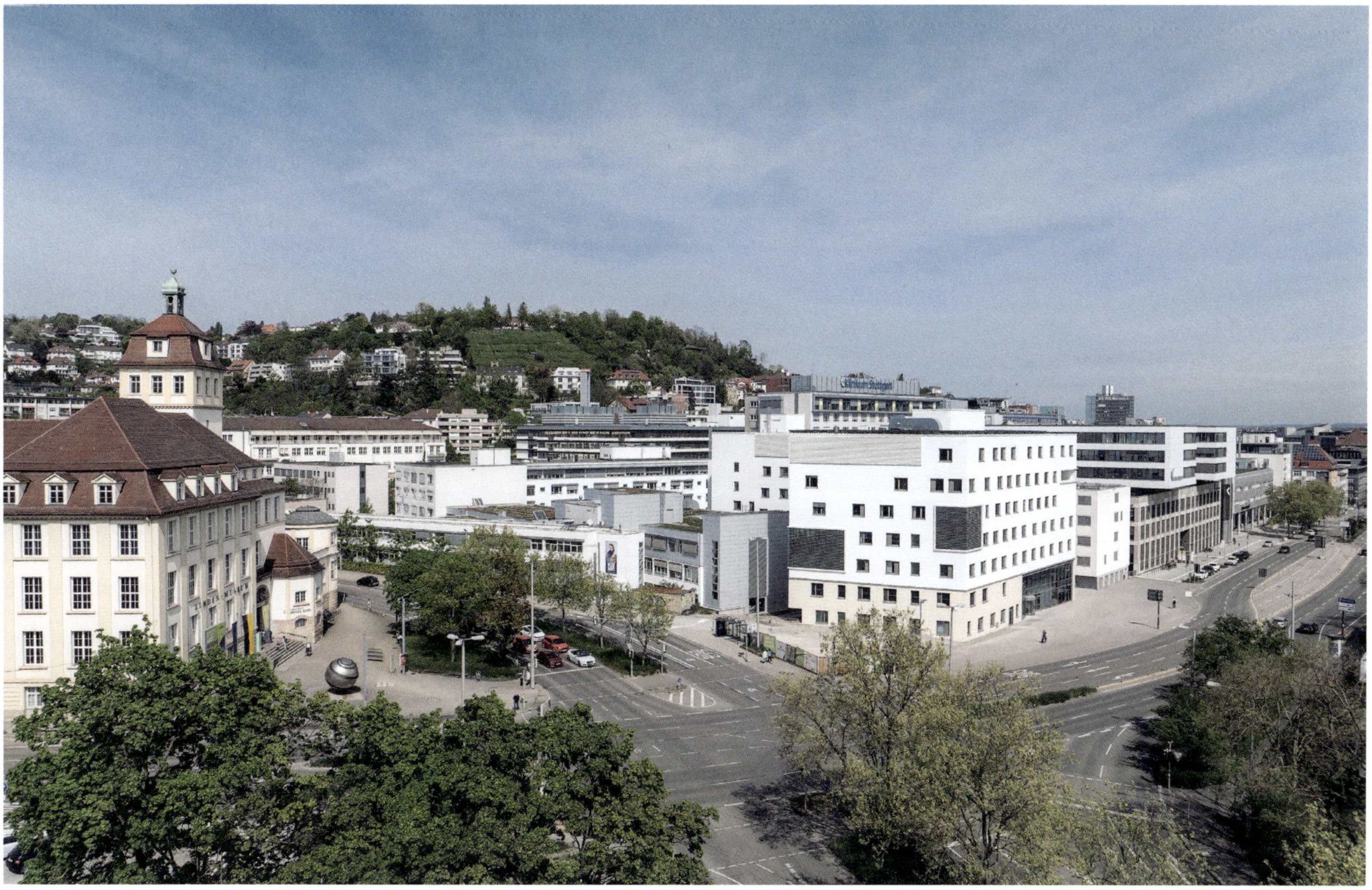

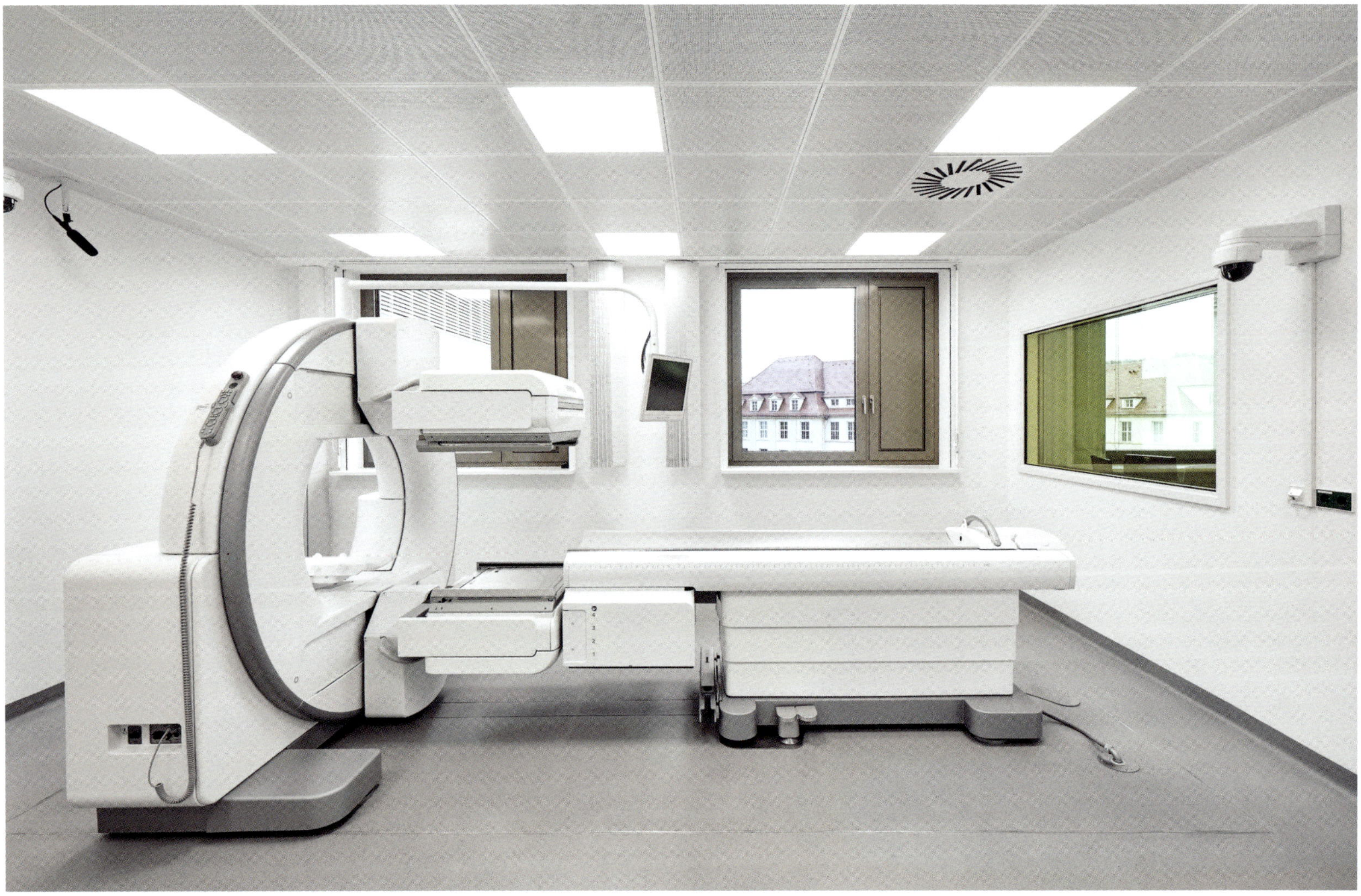

PET-CT scanning room.

Entry level and fourth floor plans.

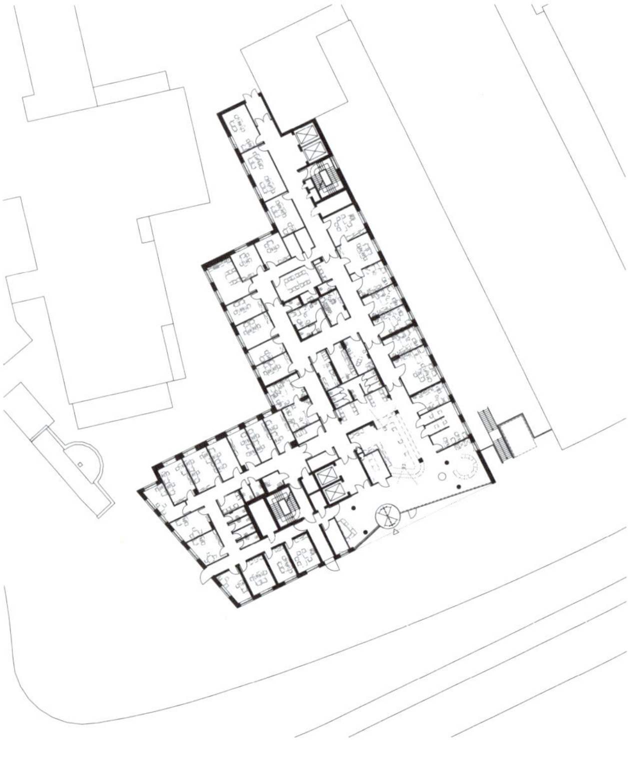

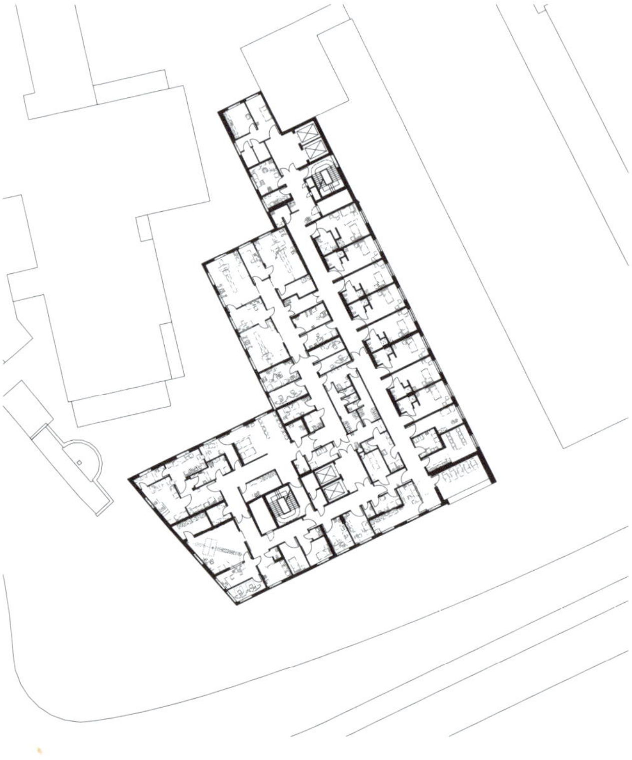

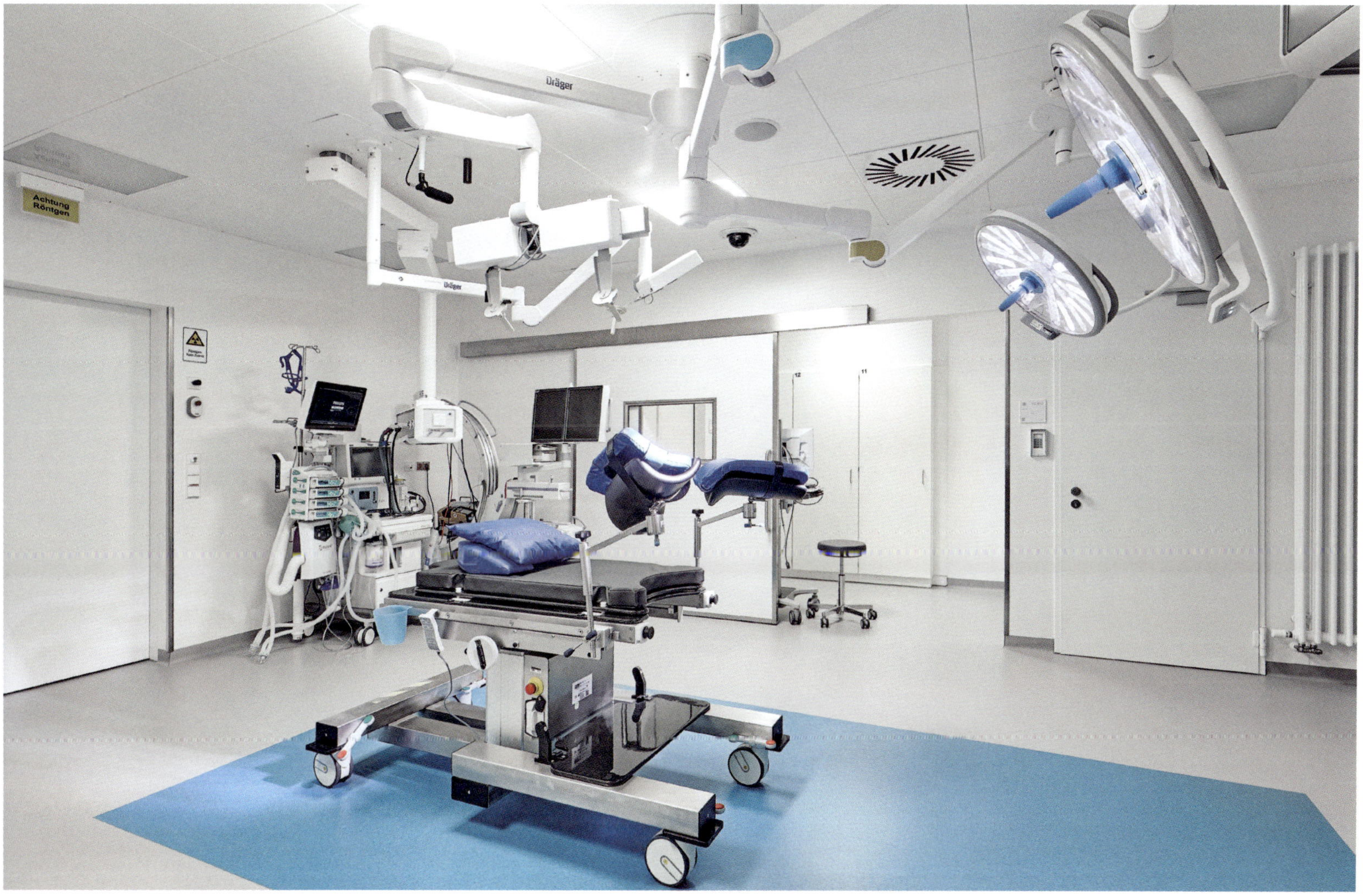

Examination room.

Site plan.

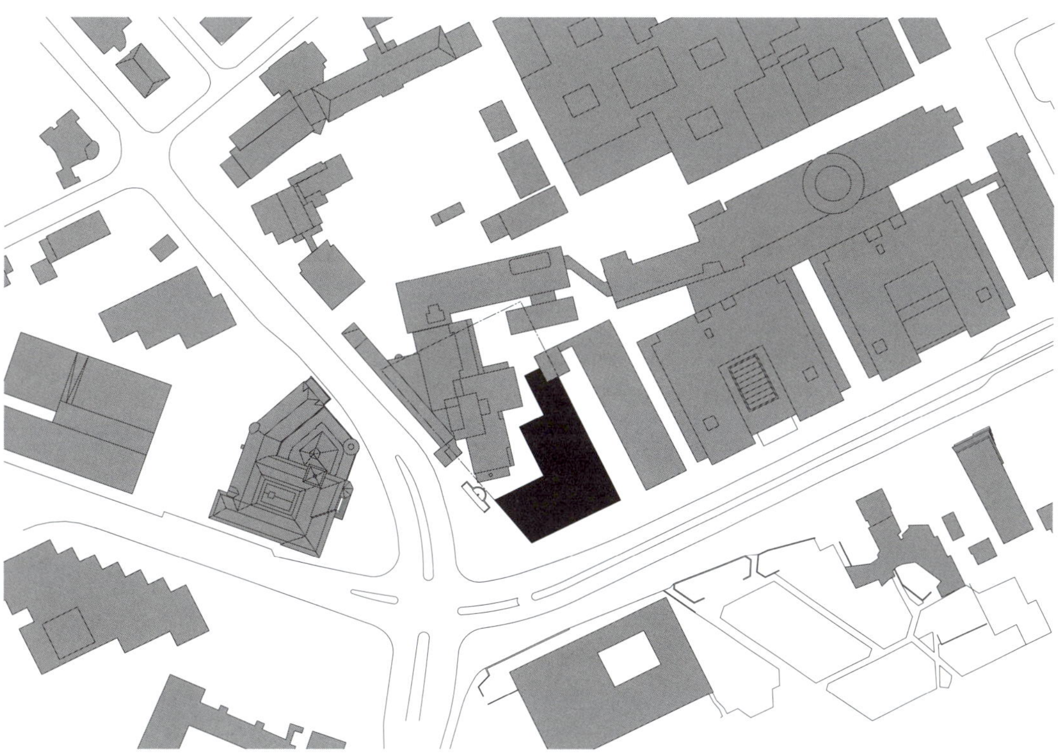

Silvia Gmür Reto Gmür Architects

St. Gallen Switzerland

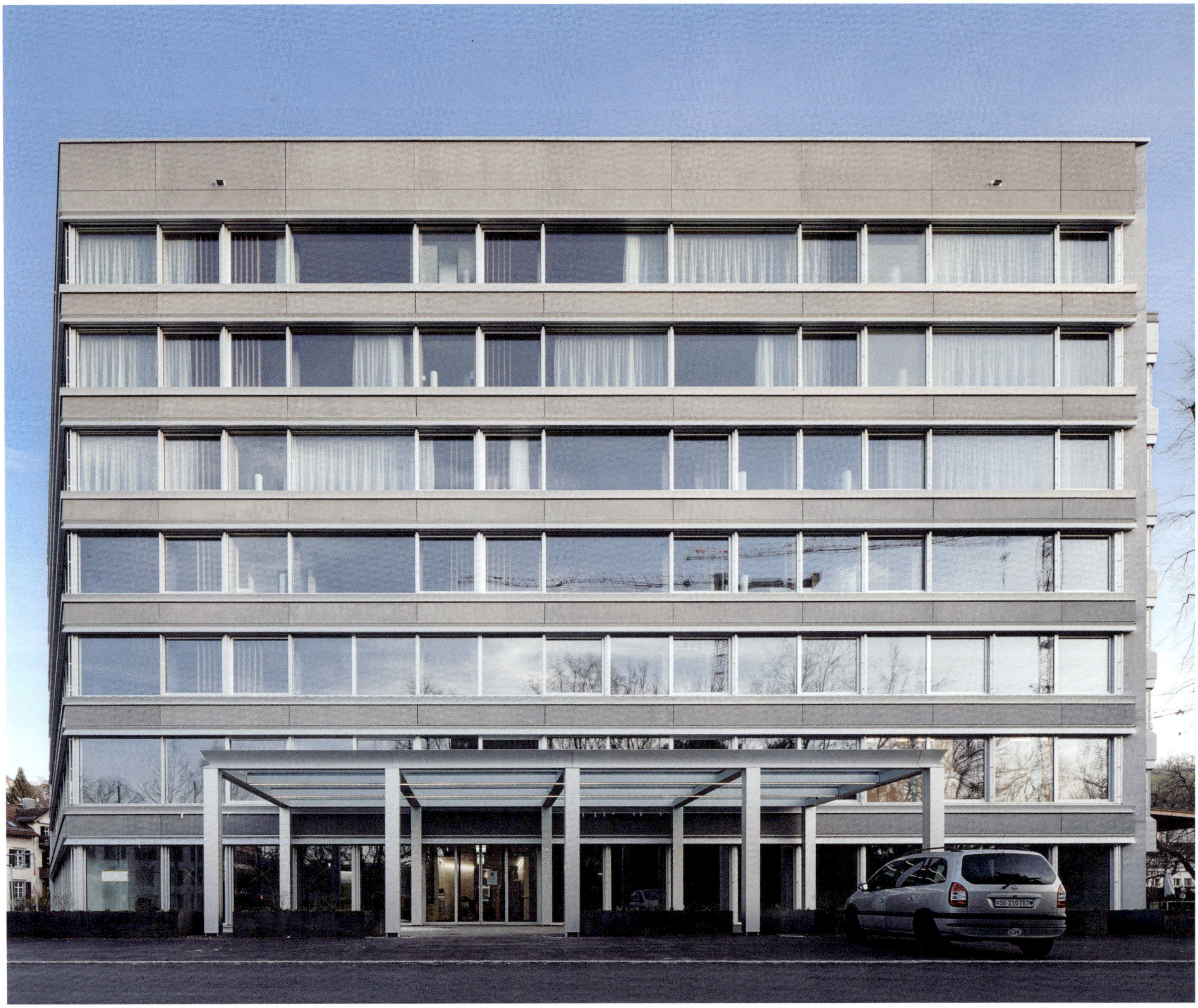

The renovated Geriatric Clinic building with its glass façade.

The expanded patient's room.

Rooms with large windows provide natural light and view towards nature.

Geriatric Clinic

The existing geriatric clinic building was constructed in 1980 by Bärlocher and Unger as an addition to the completion of the 19th and 20th century Bürgerspital ensemble and had not undergone any significant renovation or refurbishment since then. In 2011 and 2012, a selective process was conducted to find a renovation and expansion option for the clinic. The original structure of the existing building was supplemented by a layer of rooms on the north side, thus preserving the basic urban design of the building and maintaining the linear conclusion of the Bürgerspital ensemble. The result is a rational three-bay typology in which the additional space is optimally integrated with the existing building. The design of the room and the layout of beds and wardrobes along with large windows have all been arranged in a way so that patients can find peace and relaxation, perceiving the room as a protective cocoon.

Address: Rorschacher Strasse 94, 9000, St. Gallen, Switzerland | **Client:** Ortsbürgergemeinde, St. Gallen | **Completion:** 2020 | **Size:** 11,673 m² | **Original building:** Geriatric Clinic, Bärlocher and Unger, 1980 | **Sector:** public | **Specialization:** geriatric hospital | **Number of treatment rooms:** 22 | **Number of patient rooms:** 59

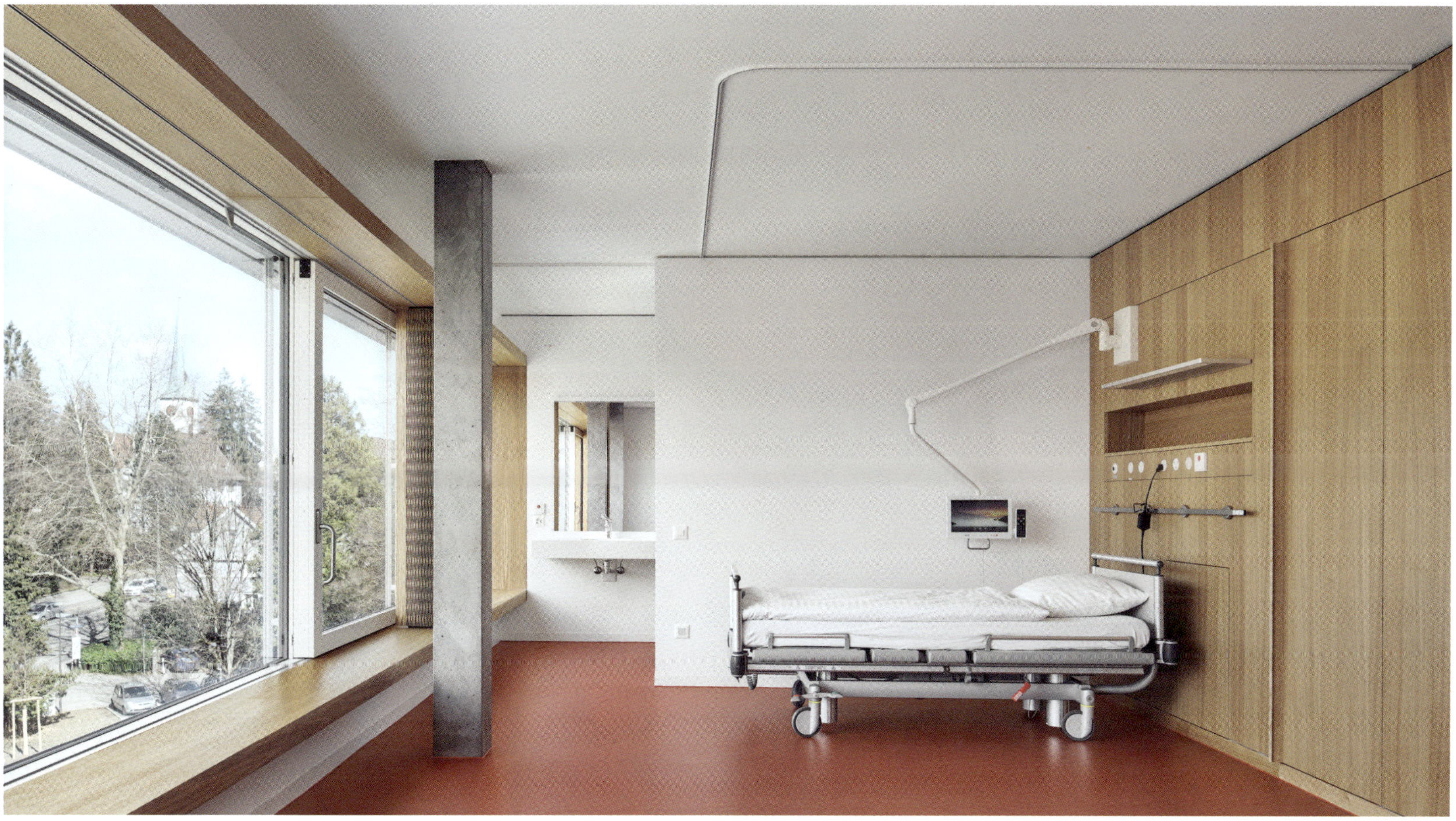

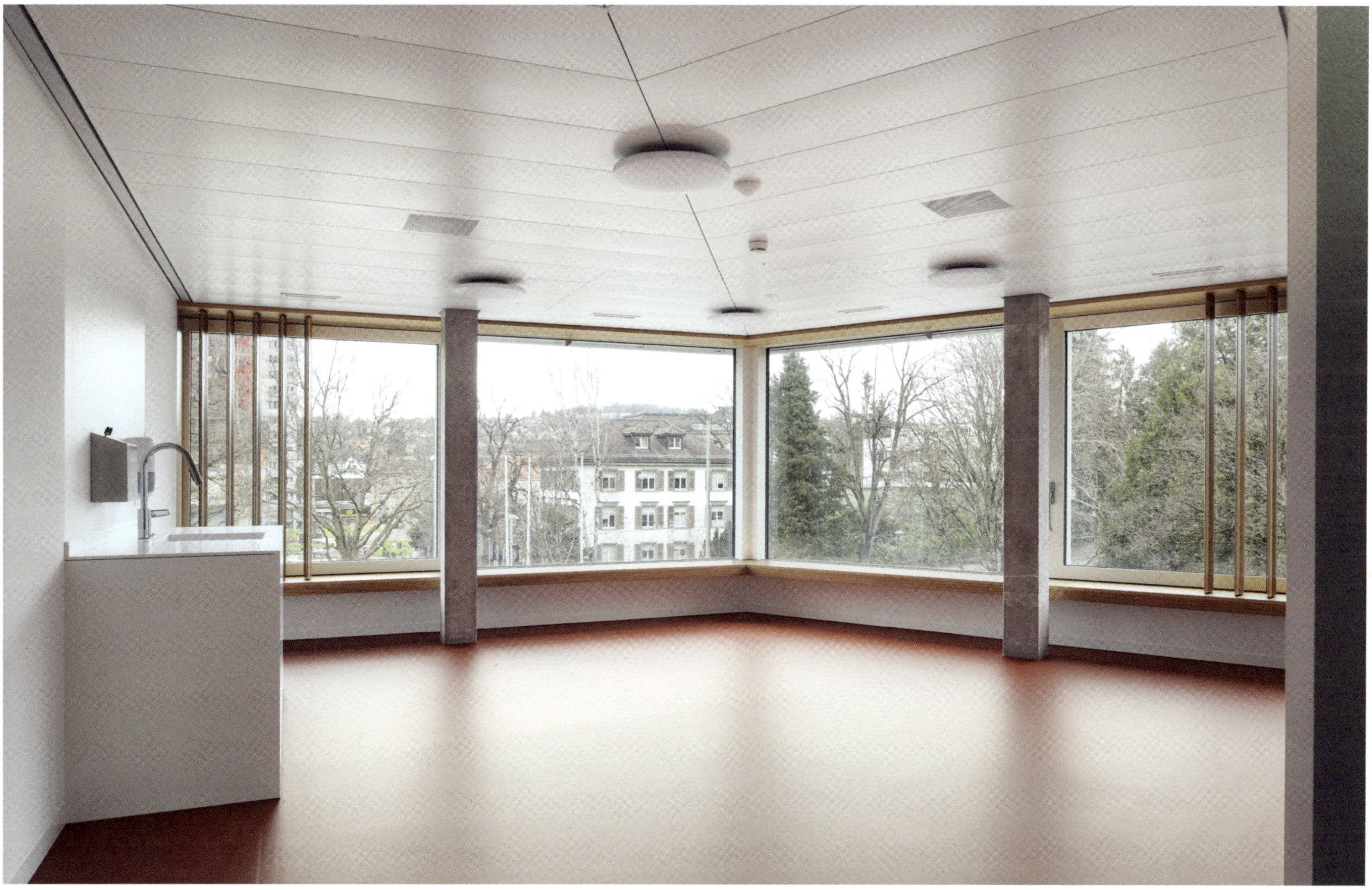

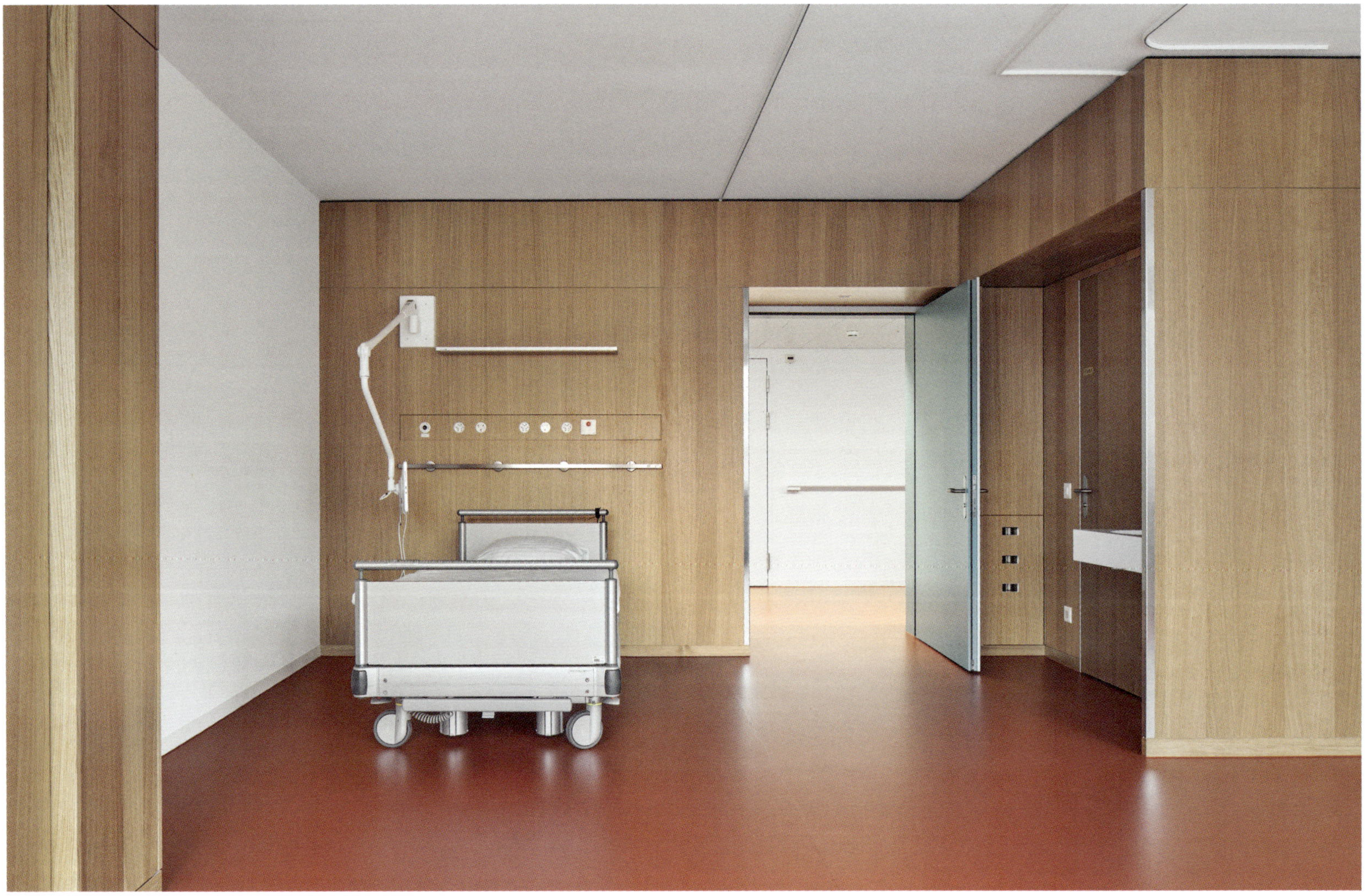

Patient room after renovation.

Floor plan after renovations and extension.

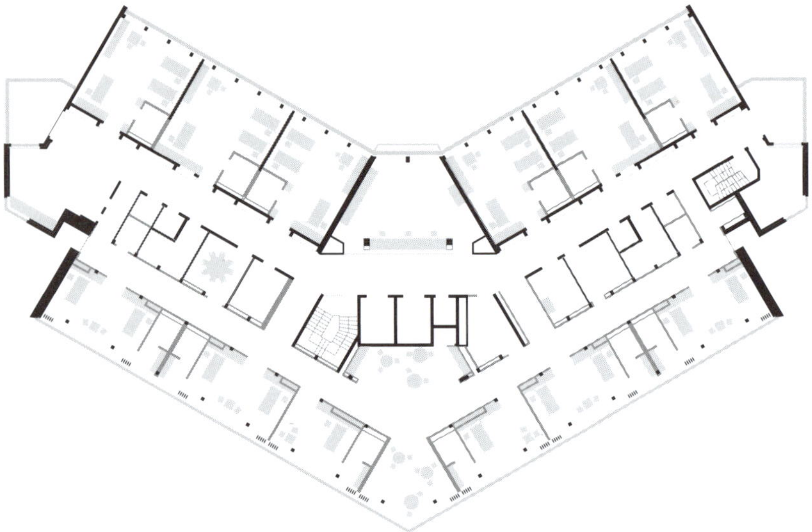

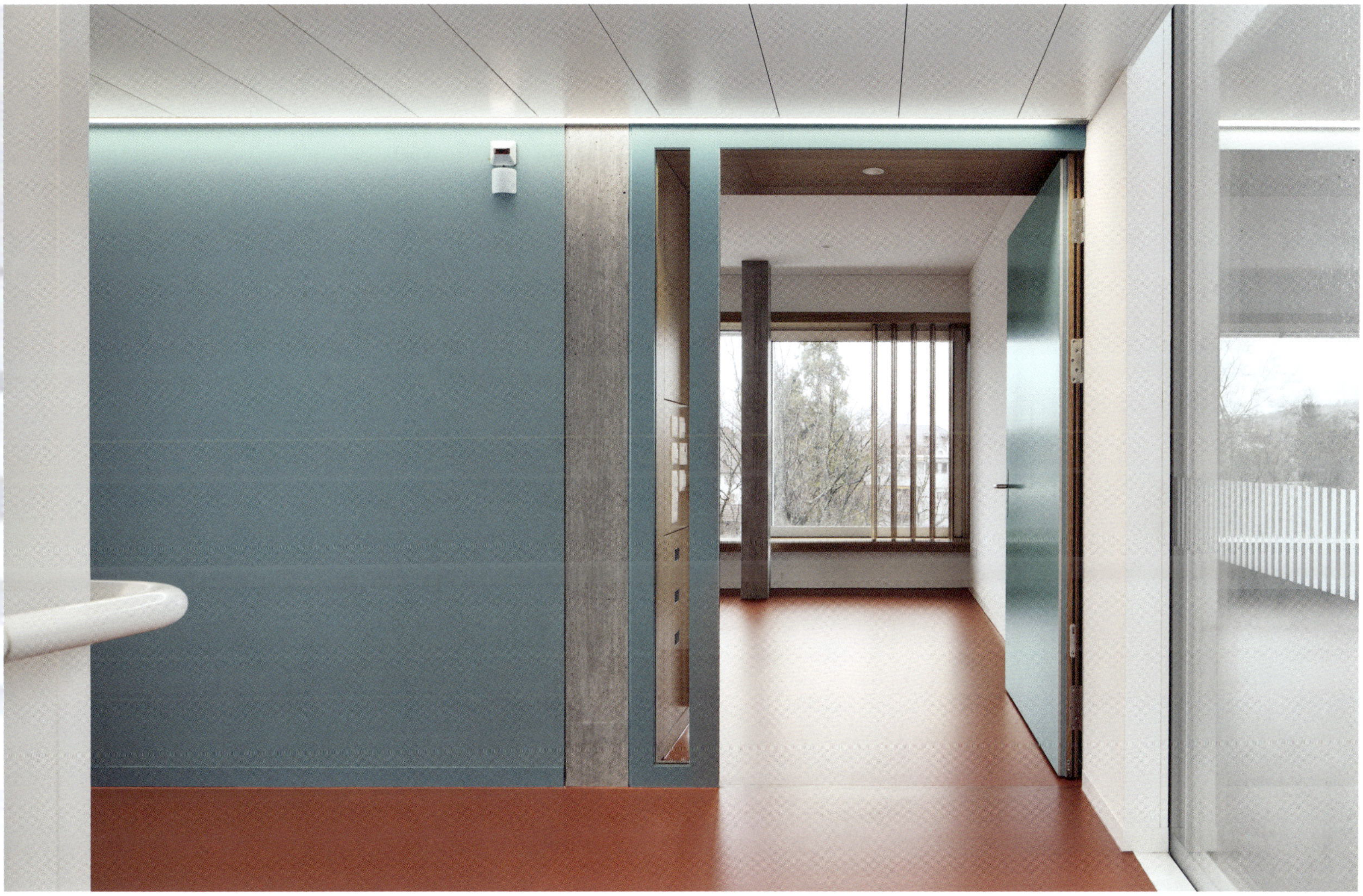

View from corridor renovation to room extension.

Floor plan of the new patient rooms.

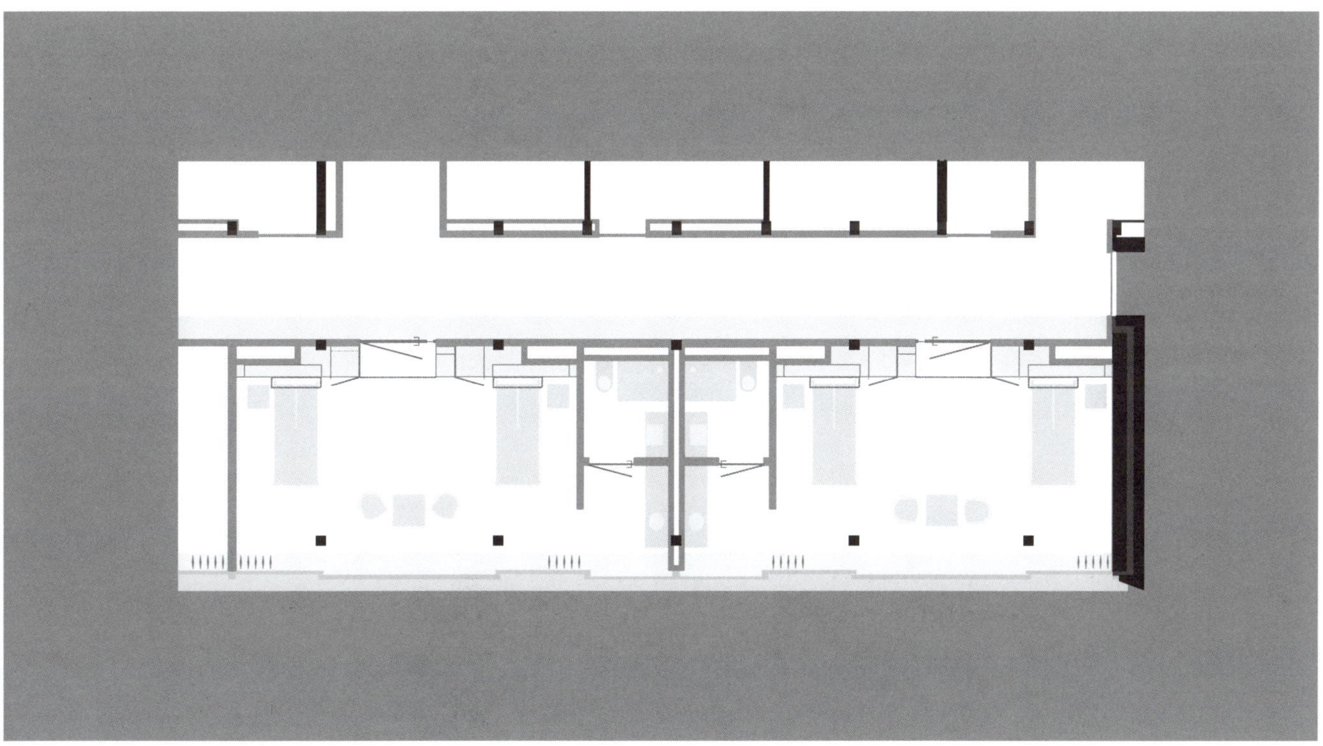

Gortemaker Algra Feenstra Architects

Elst
The Netherlands

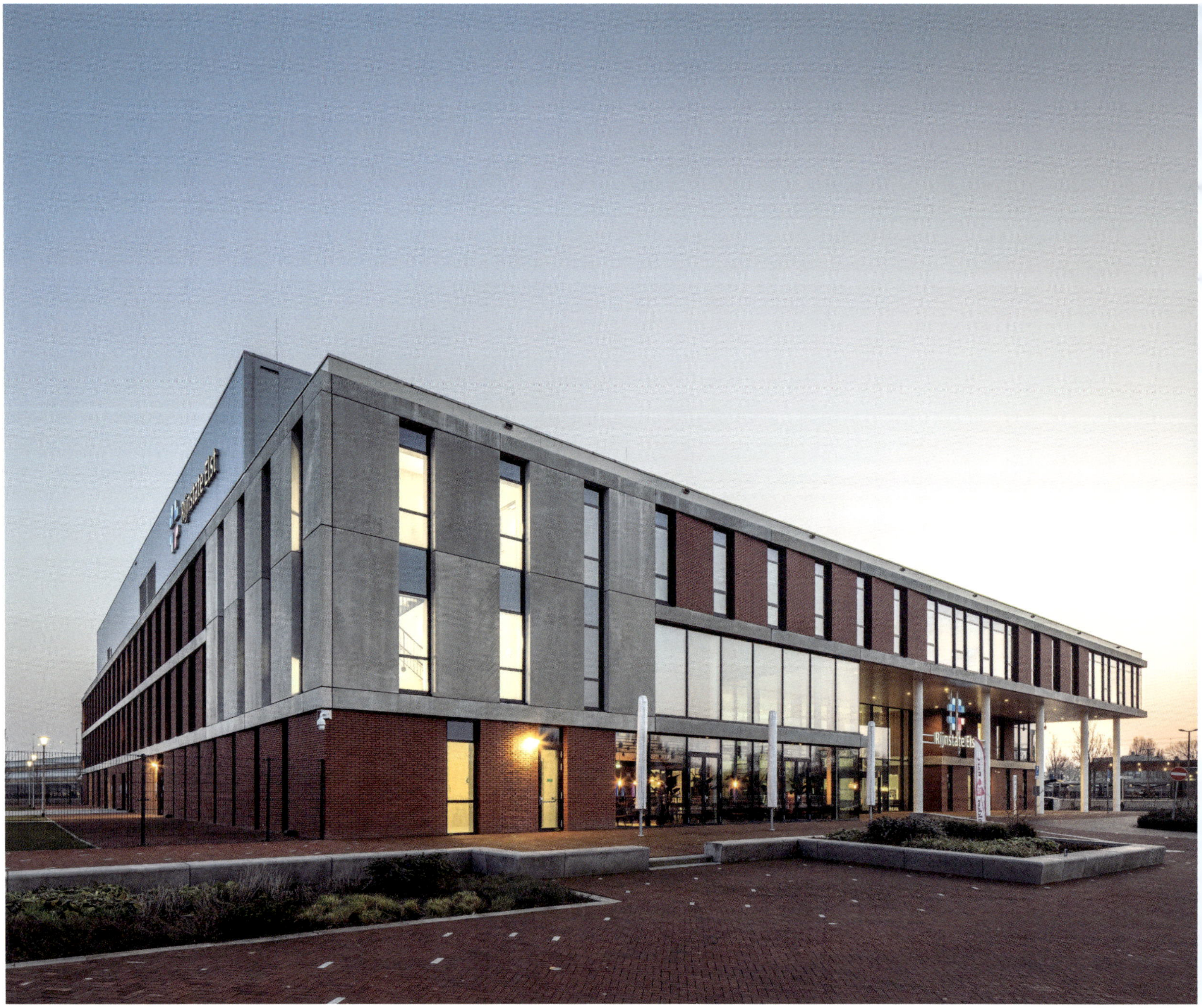

Rijnstate Elst is integrated between the station and the neighborhood.

Instead of a waiting room, patients can relax in the restaurant or take a walk, and are notified of their appointment.

Rijnstate Hospital Elst

Rijnstate Elst is an innovative Health Hub that transforms traditional hospital care into a fully outpatient and patient-centered approach. The small-scale, flexible building relieves hospitals and supports a neighborhood-oriented model of care. Several wings are situated around a central atrium, which serves as a public reception area. Sustainability and innovation are integrated into the design: The gas-free, fully electric building with solar panels and a hydrogen tank reduces CO_2 emissions by approximately 90 percent. Smart building technology also enhances the patient experience by automatically recognizing visitors upon arrival and minimizing waiting times. While waiting, patients, local residents, and train passengers, can use the restaurant and other facilities. Rijnstate Elst sets a new standard for outpatient healthcare environment focusing on human-centered care, flexibility, and ecological responsibility.

Address: Stationsplein 2, 6662 NC Elst, The Netherlands | **Client:** Rijnstate Hospital | **Completion:** 2023 | **Size:** 13,056 m² | **Sector:** private | **Number of treatment rooms:** 120

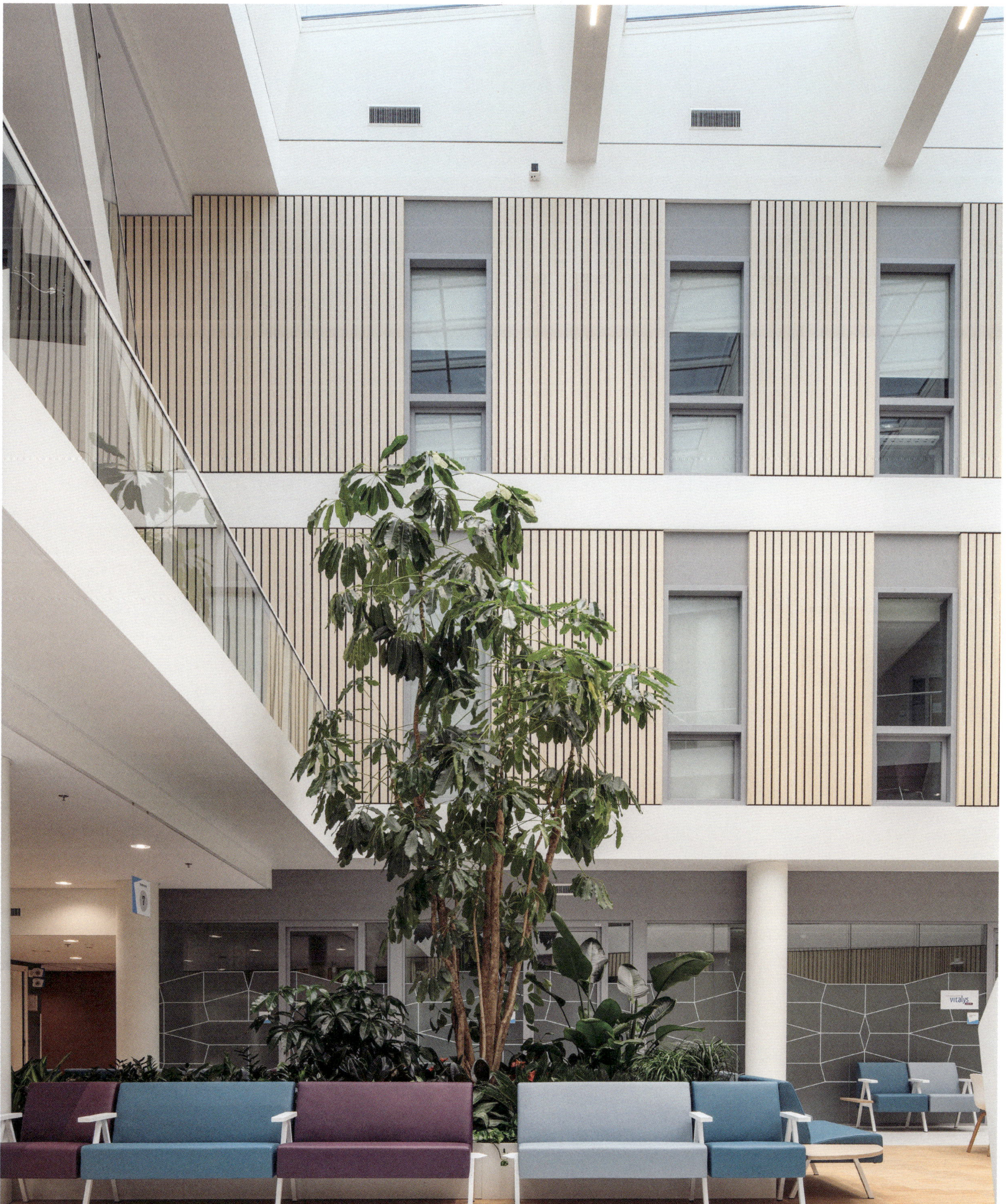

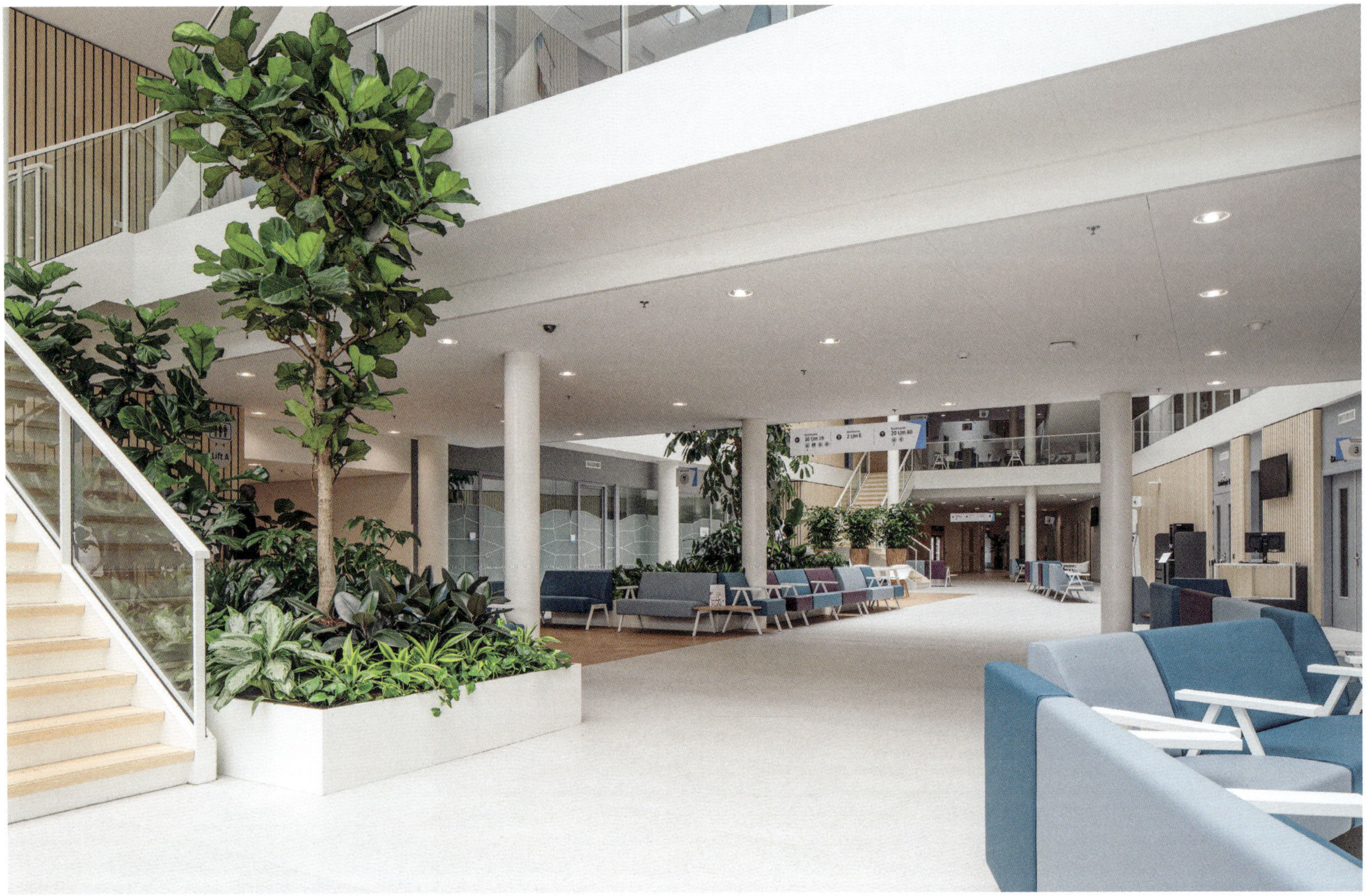

A healing environment with a green atrium, fruit trees, and plenty of daylight support wellbeing.

First floor plan.

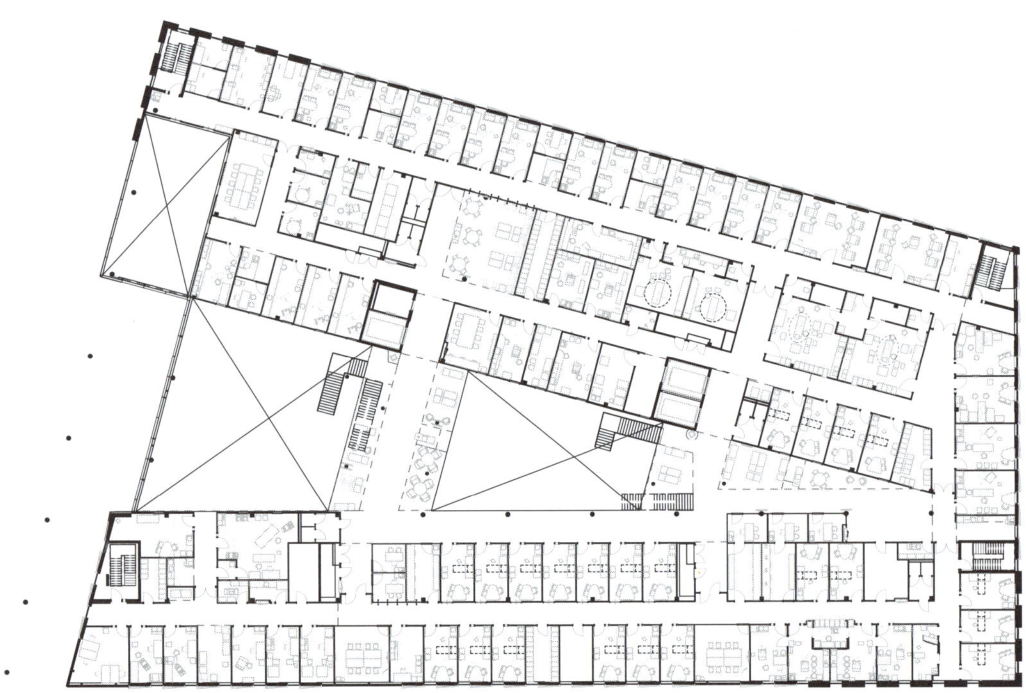

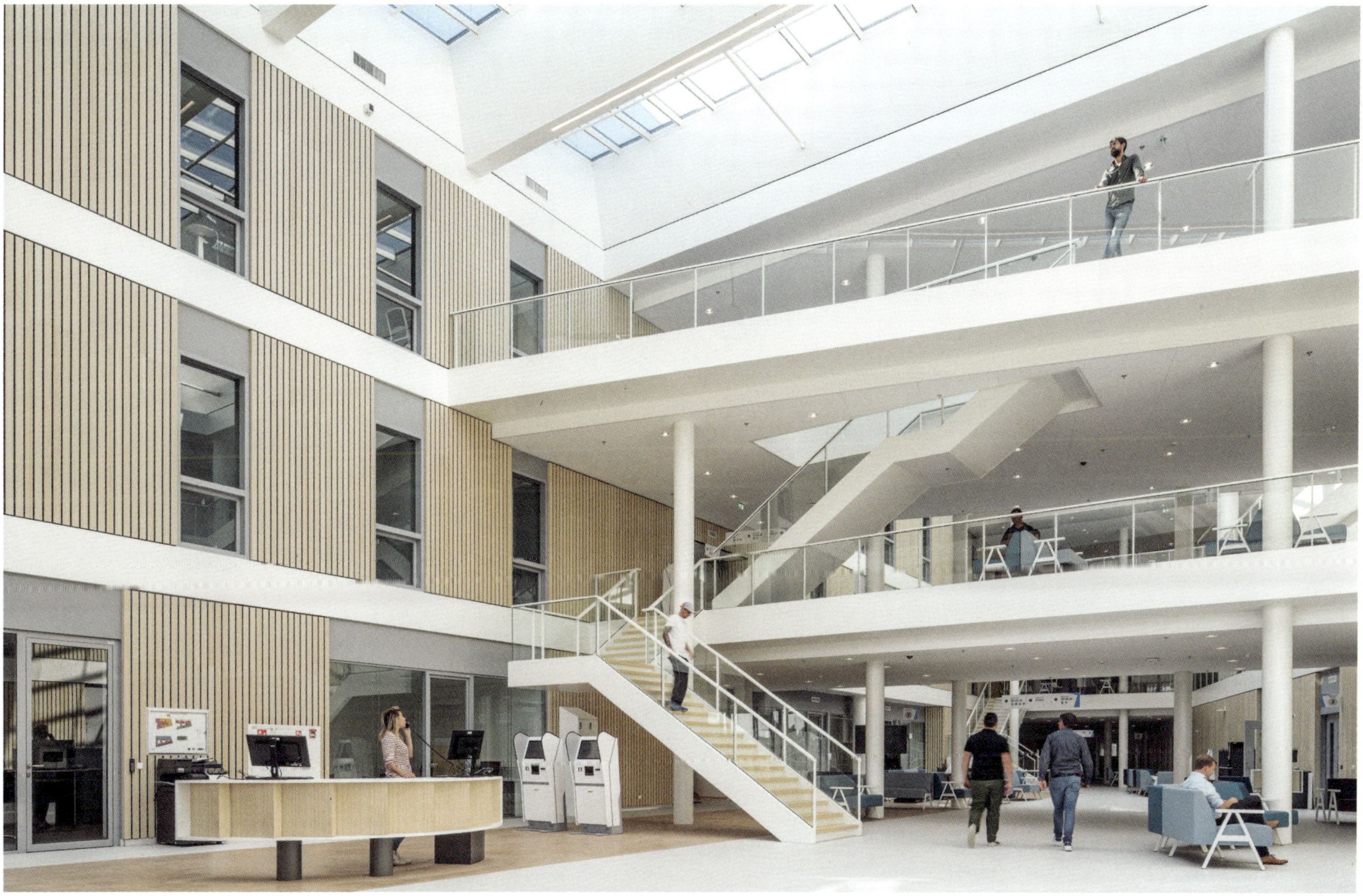

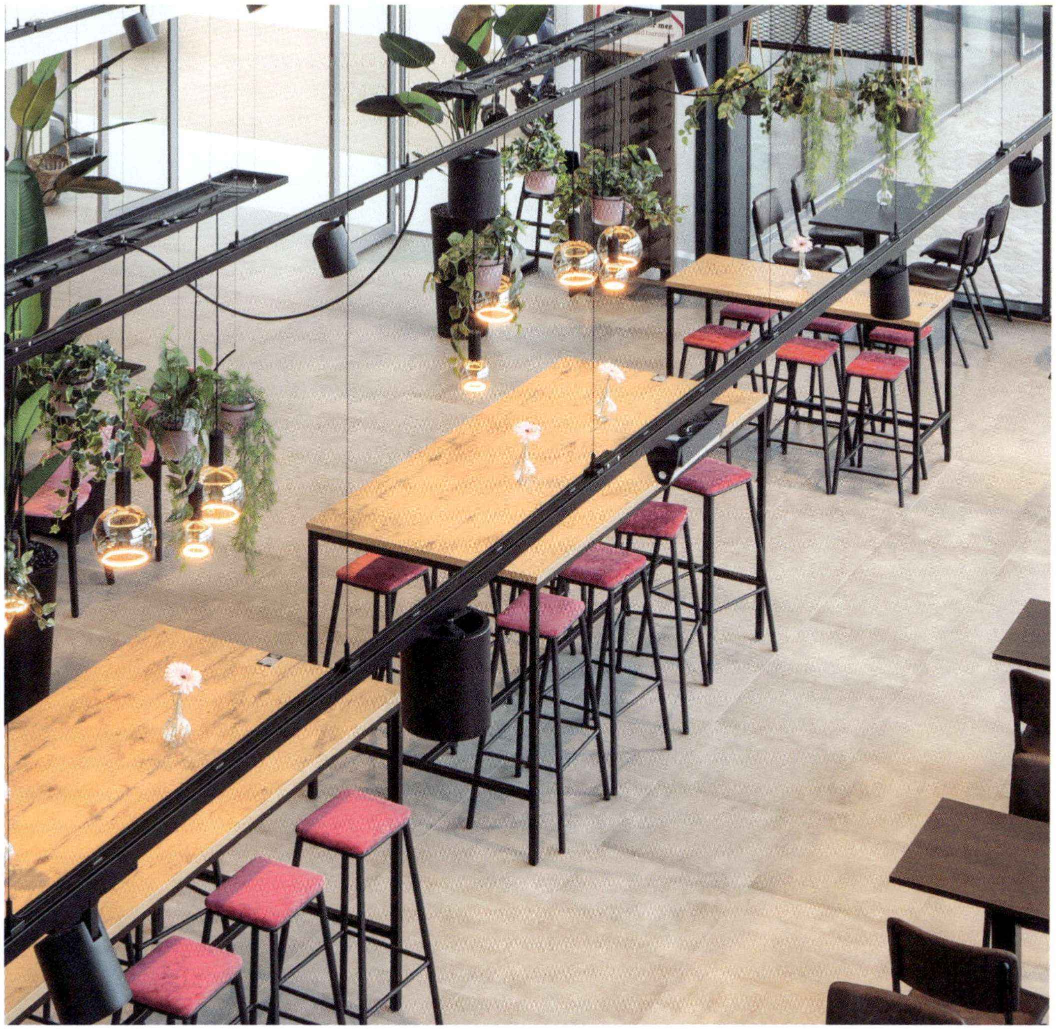

The central atrium functions as a public reception area, surrounded by wings that can be closed off separately.

The restaurant is attractive to local residents and travelers.

ARGE Health Team Vienna: Albert Wimmer ZT & Architects Collective ZT

Freiburg im Breisgau Germany

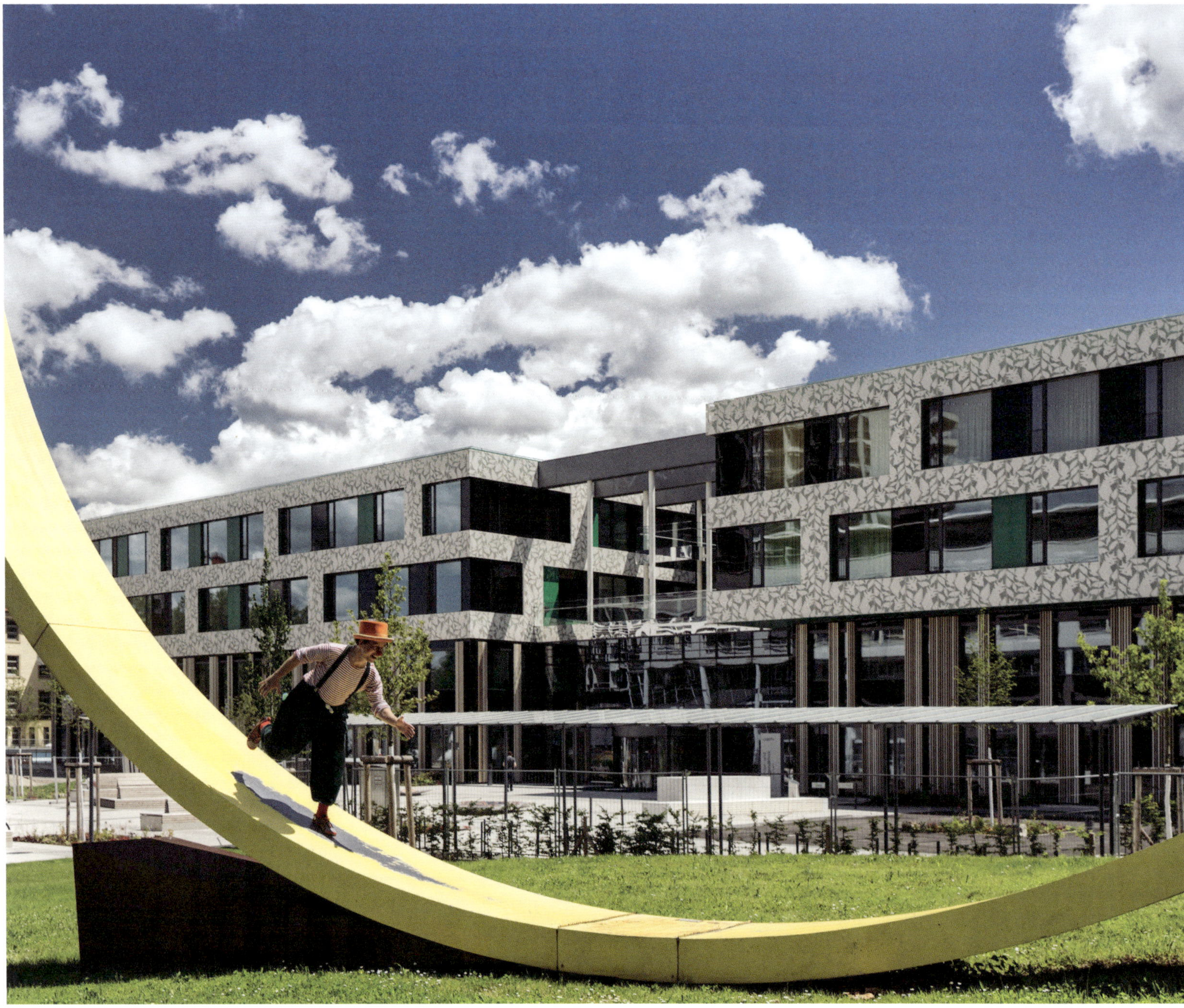

Forecourt of the Children´s Hospital Freiburg with clown doctor.

The main entrance at the forecourt.

Entrance hall with light ceiling by artist Paul Schwer.

Children´s Hospital Freiburg

The Children's Hospital Freiburg is an award-winning project that blends medical excellence with the patient-centered concept of Healing Architecture – as evidence-based design approach – into a holistic healthcare model. It embodies an exemplary vision of healthcare design, thoughtfully creating a healing, stress-reducing environment that promotes recovery and well-being for patients, staff, and relatives. Healing Art as integral part of the therapeutic approach, natural materials, and the color concept support orientation and atmosphere. The intuitive layout ensures easy navigation, while greenery and terraces strengthen the connection to nature. Certified with DGNB Platinum standards, the hospital features a 1.2 million liter cold storage tank and photovoltaics, supporting a climate concept developed with the University of Chemnitz.

Address: Breisacher Straße 62, 79104 Freiburg im Breisgau, Germany | **Client:** Land Baden-Württemberg, Vermögen und Bau Baden-Württemberg | **Completion:** 2024 | **Size:** 32,000 m² | **Sector:** state | **Specialization:** pediatrics | **Number of treatment rooms:** 76 | **Number of patient rooms:** 104 | **Number of beds:** 156 | **Ren-cluster and anti-waiting room interior concept:** Kopvol architecture & psychology | **Landscape design:** SETUP Landschaftsarchitektur partG mbB bdla

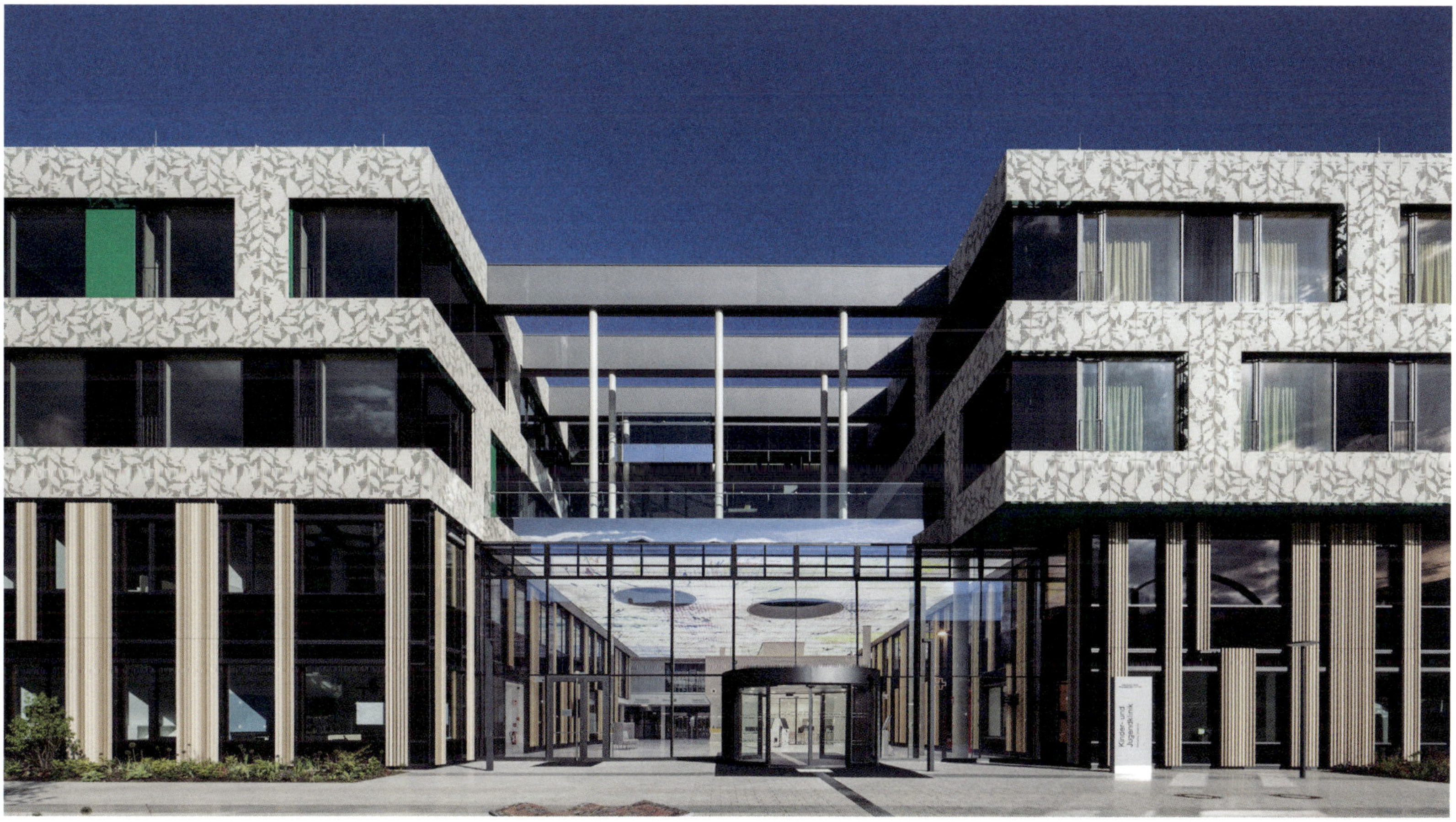

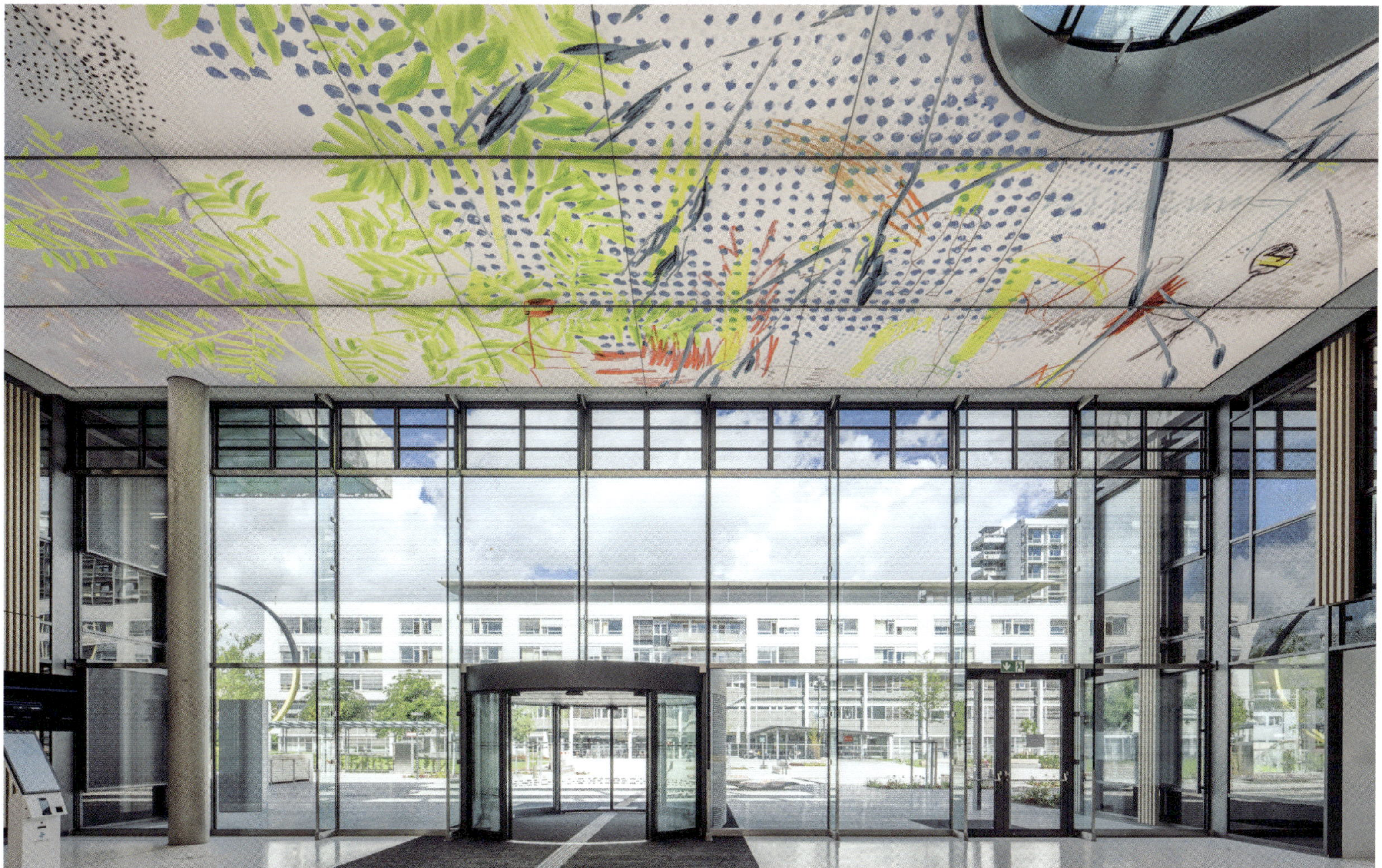

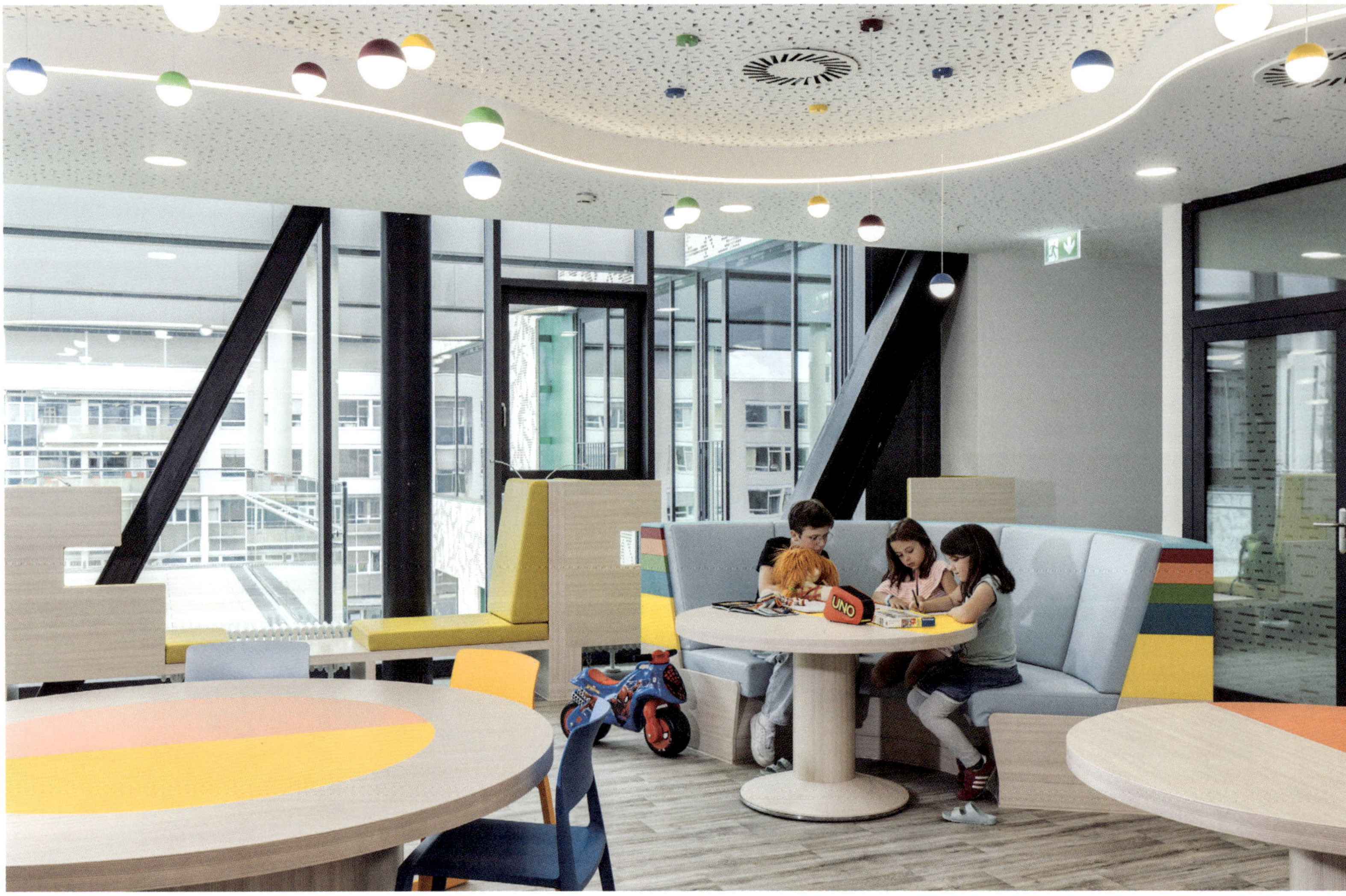

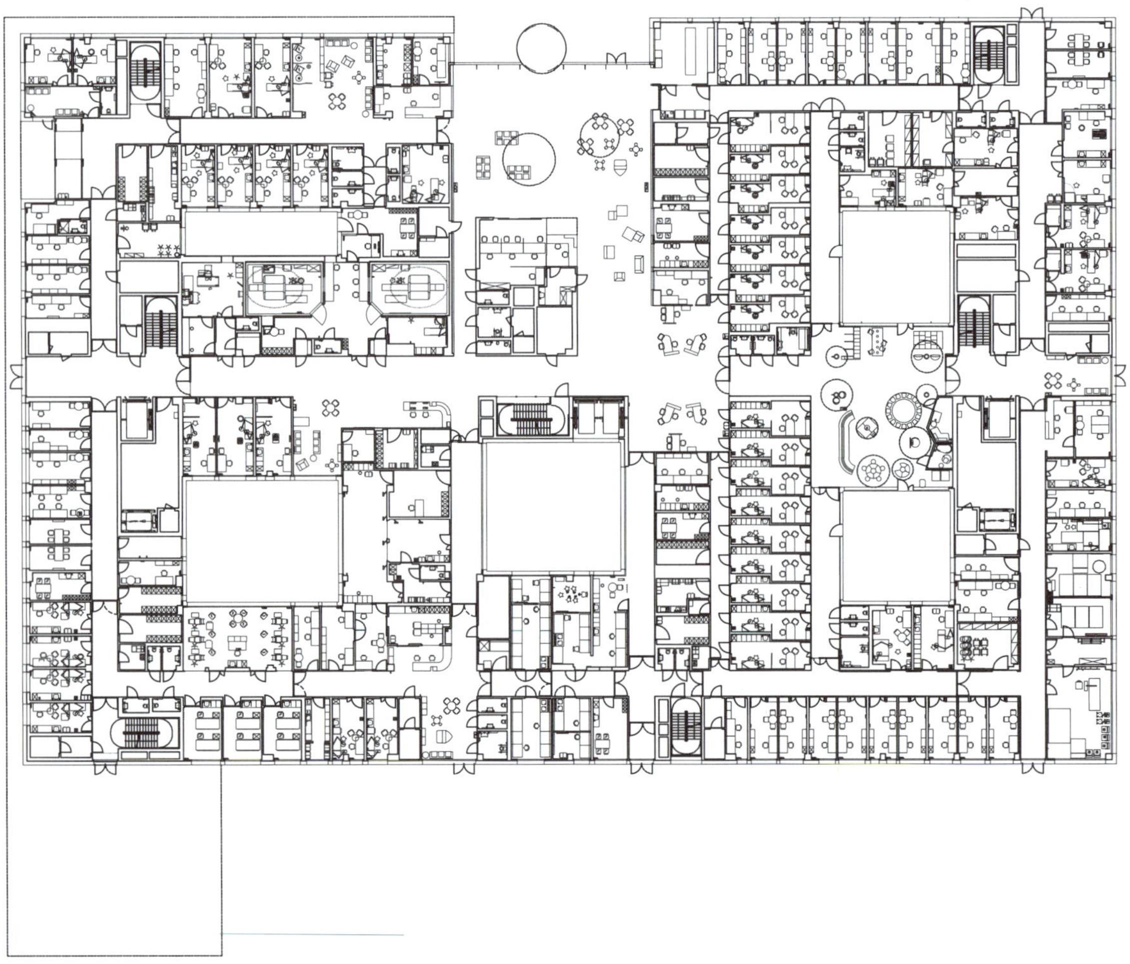

Ren-cluster, a room for development, upgrowth and normality.

Ground floor plan.

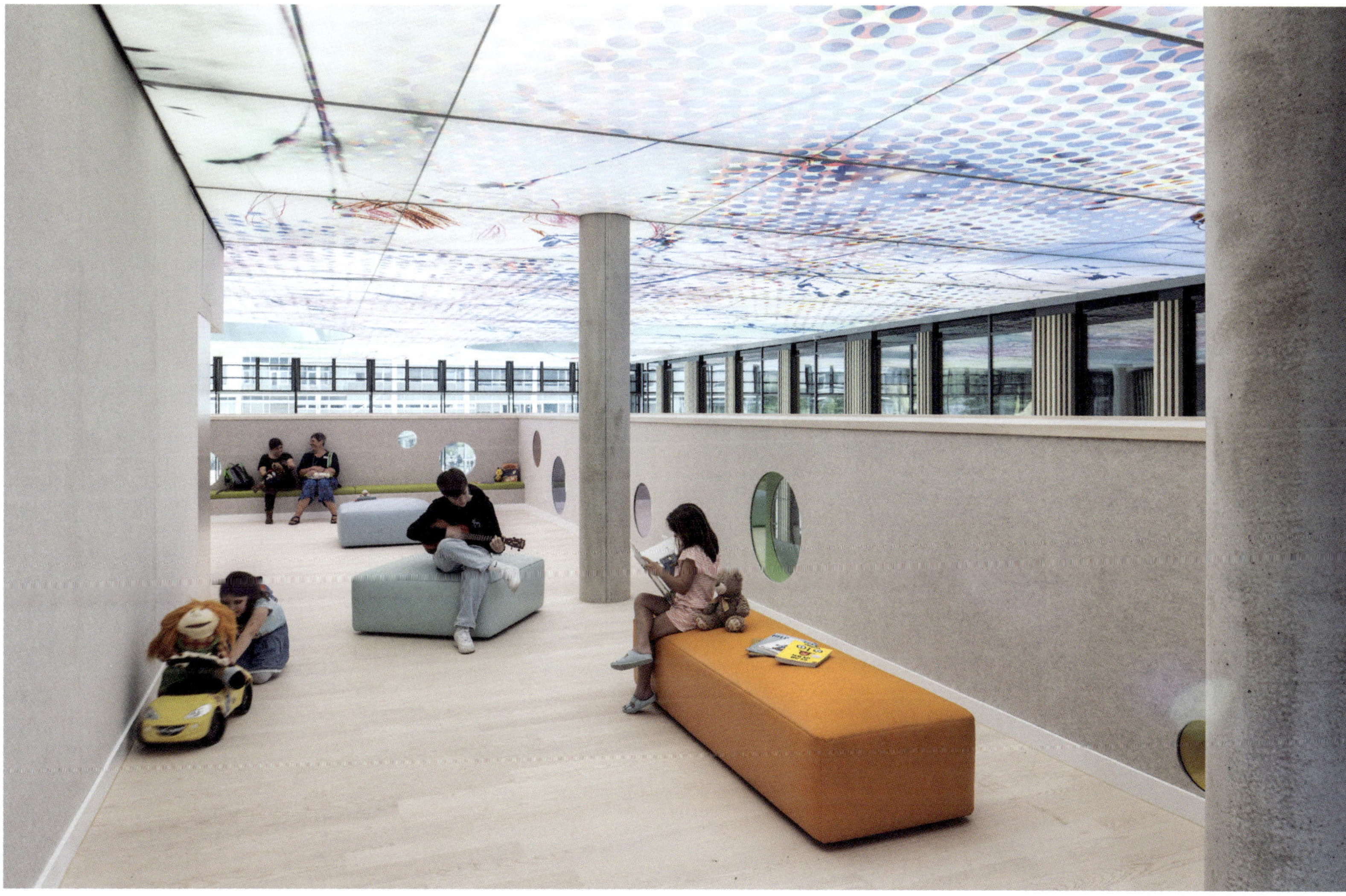

Library with light ceiling by artist Paul Schwer.

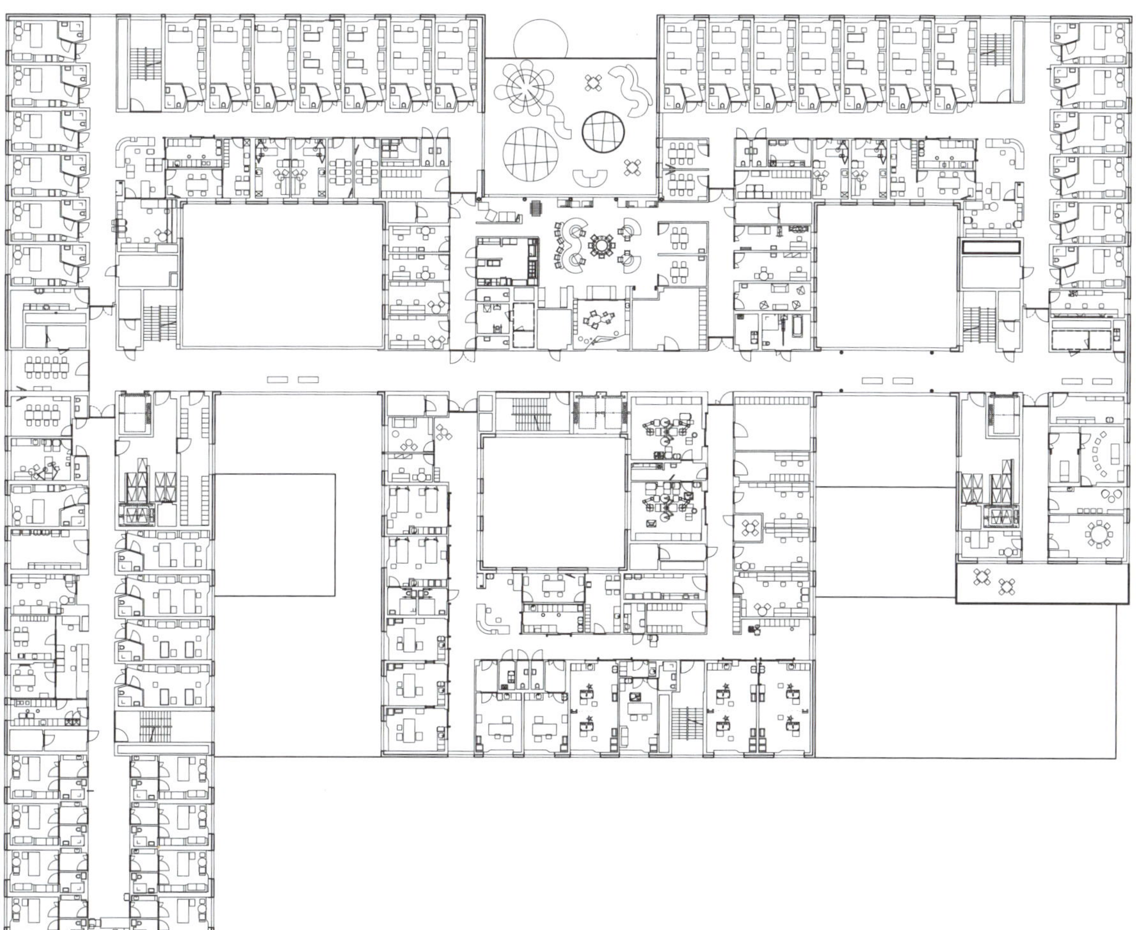

First floor plan.

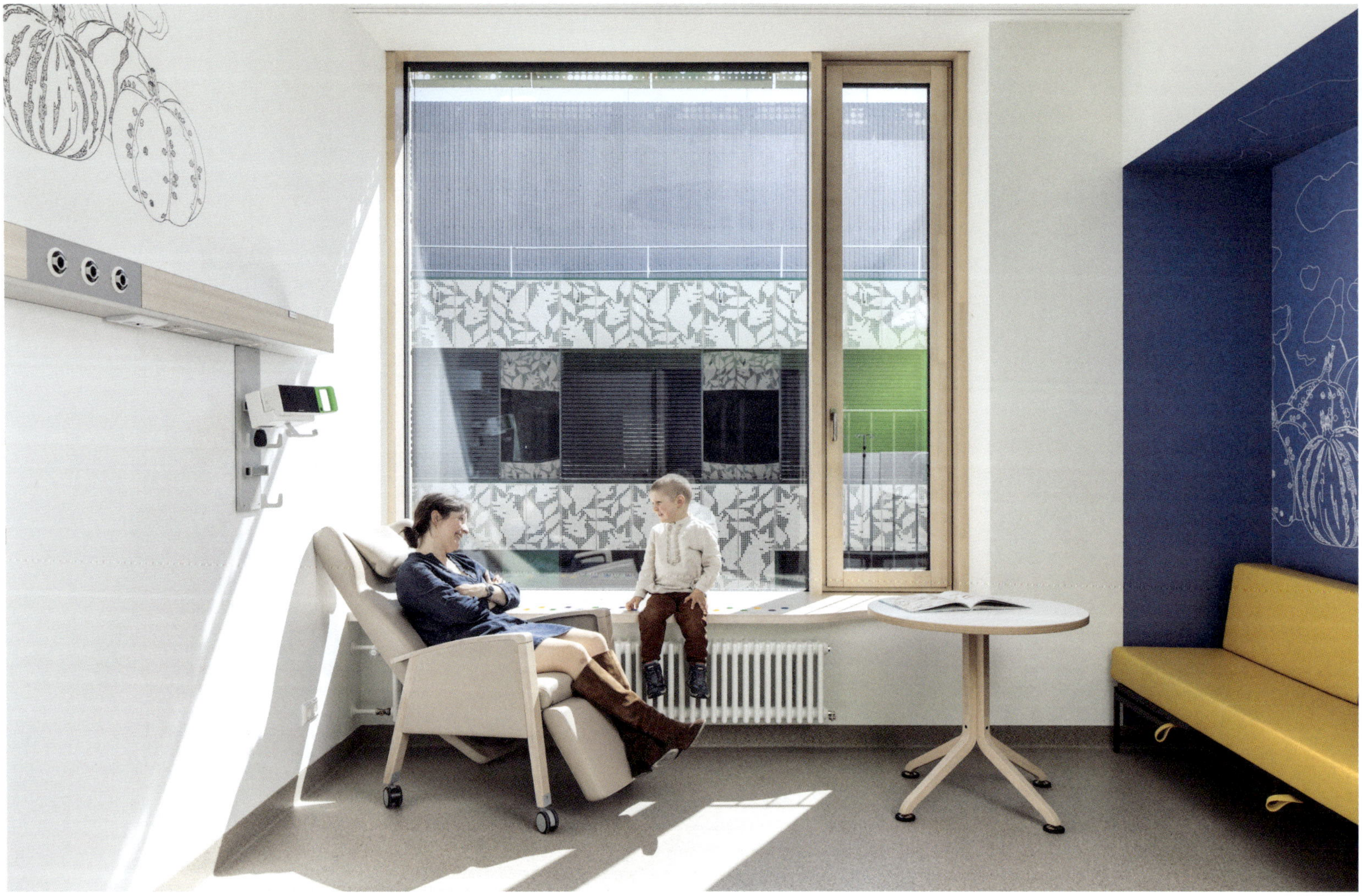

Patients room with rooming-in furniture and murals by Jack Broeders.

Site plan.

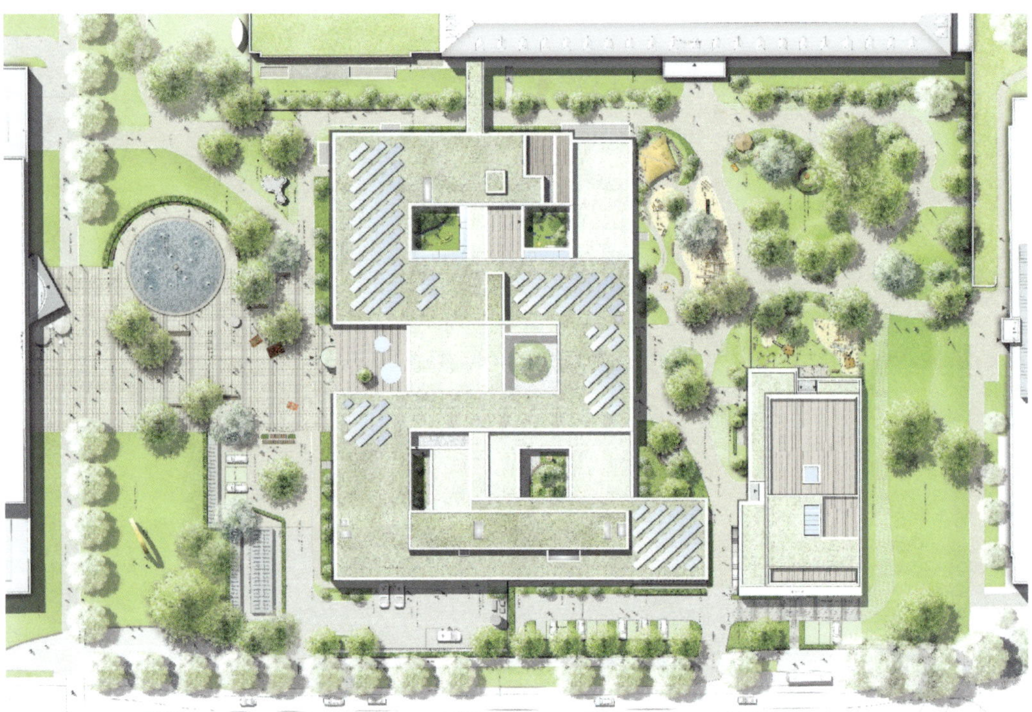

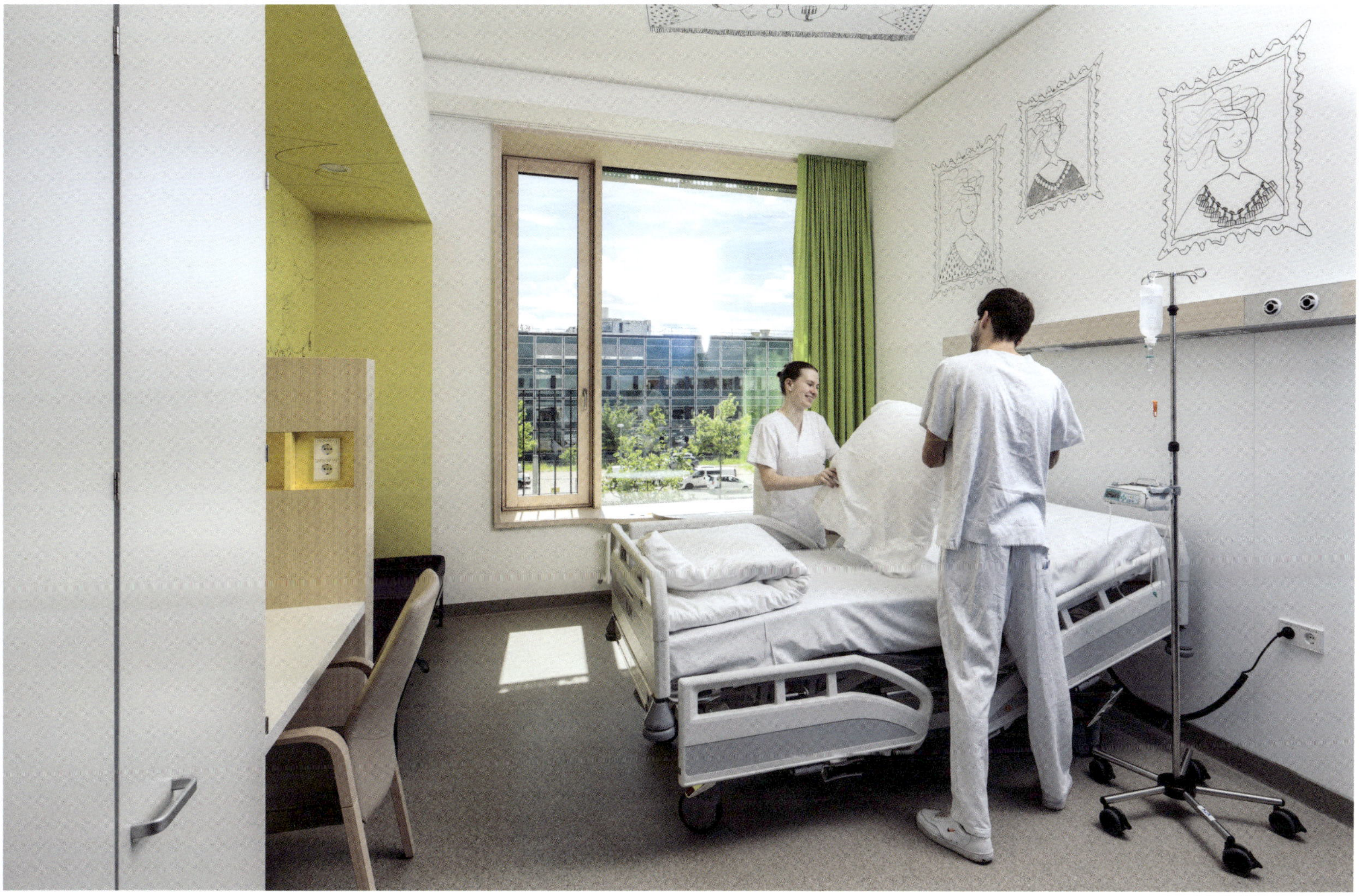

Patients room with desk and murals by Jack Brooders.

Functional areas diagram.

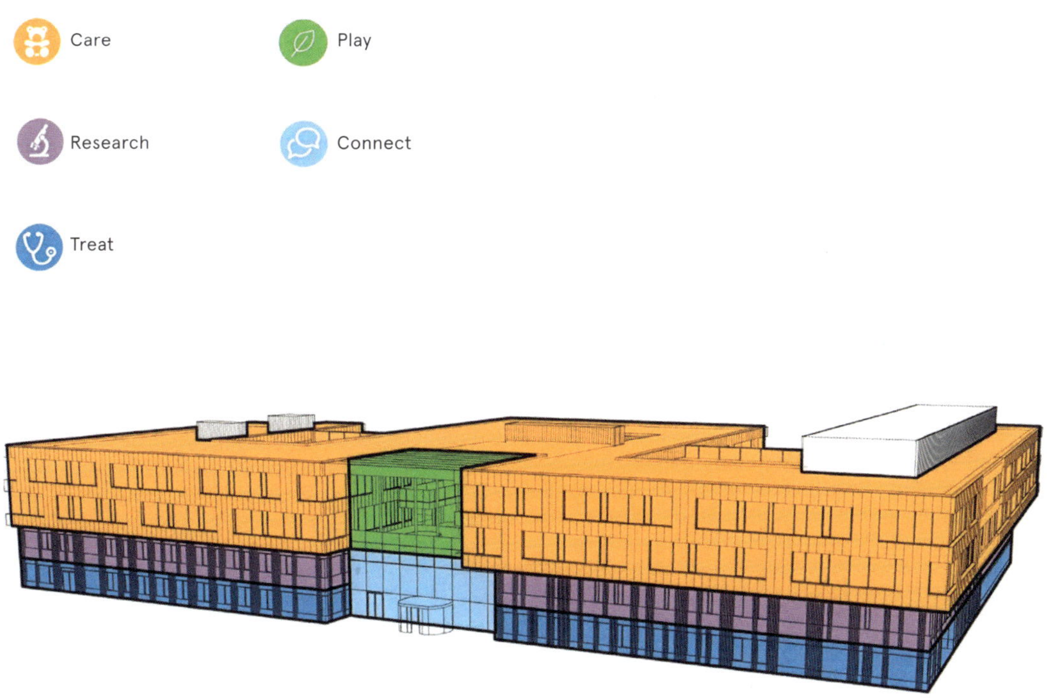

C.F.Møller Architects
ARCO Architecture Company

Tampere
Finland

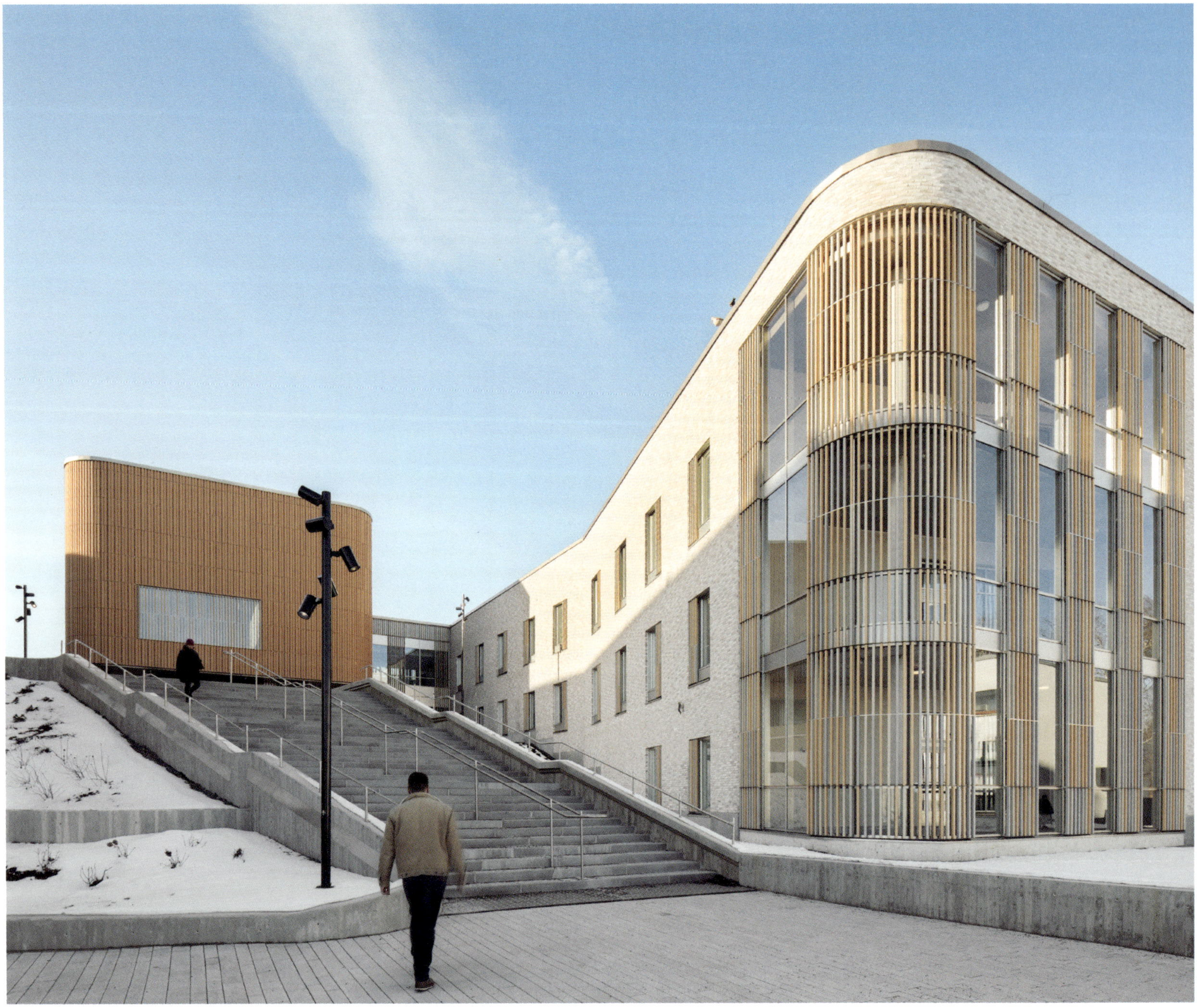

Façade and entrance staircase framed by warm brick architecture.

Greenhouse and outdoor garden space, supporting therapeutic activities and daily interaction with nature.

Lounge area with warm materials, natural daylight, and views towards the surrounding landscape.

Tampere Psychiatric Clinic

Positioned at the edge of Tampere University Hospital and embedded within a pine forest setting, the Tampere Psychiatric Clinic re-imagines mental healthcare through a close relationship between architecture, nature, and wellbeing. Three U-shaped ward buildings form a semi-circle around a central activity hub and courtyard, creating a balance between privacy, safety, and community. The 180-bed facility is organized into specialized units, while individual rooms maximize daylight and views of nature. Brick and wood, inspired by Tampere's industrial heritage, give the architecture a warm, human-scaled character. Gardens, courtyards, balconies, and direct outdoor access support recovery through continuous contact with nature. Shared functions and flexible planning strengthen staff collaboration and operational efficiency, presenting a contemporary approach to mental healthcare architecture.

Address: Tampere University Hospital, Arkkiatrinkuja 1, 33520 Tampere, Finland | **Client:** PSHP, Pirkanmaan Sairaanhoitopiiri | **Completion:** 2024 | **Size:** 30,000 m^2 | **Sector:** state | **Specialization:** psychiatry | **Number of patient rooms:** 180 | **Landscape design:** Rambøll

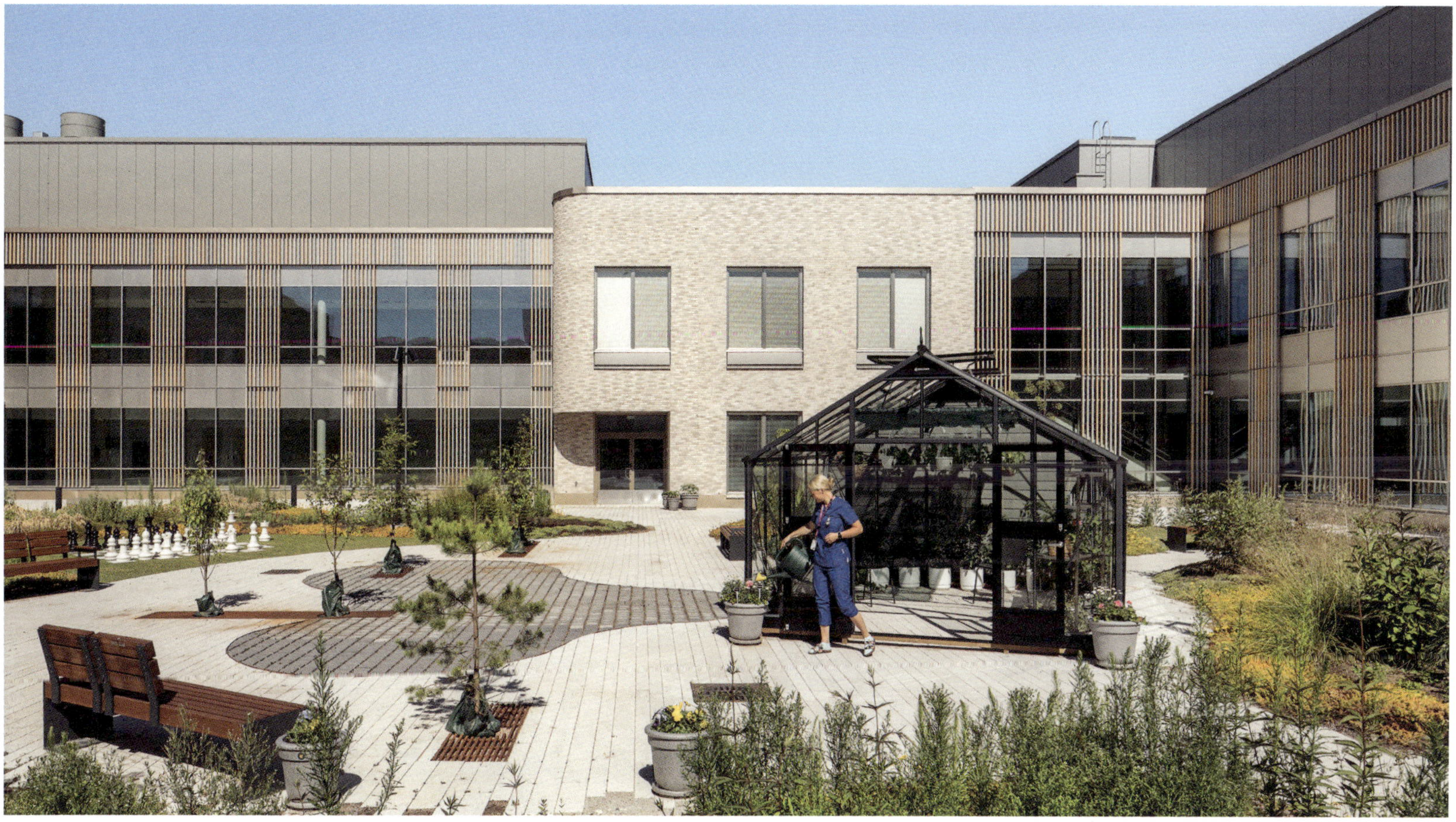

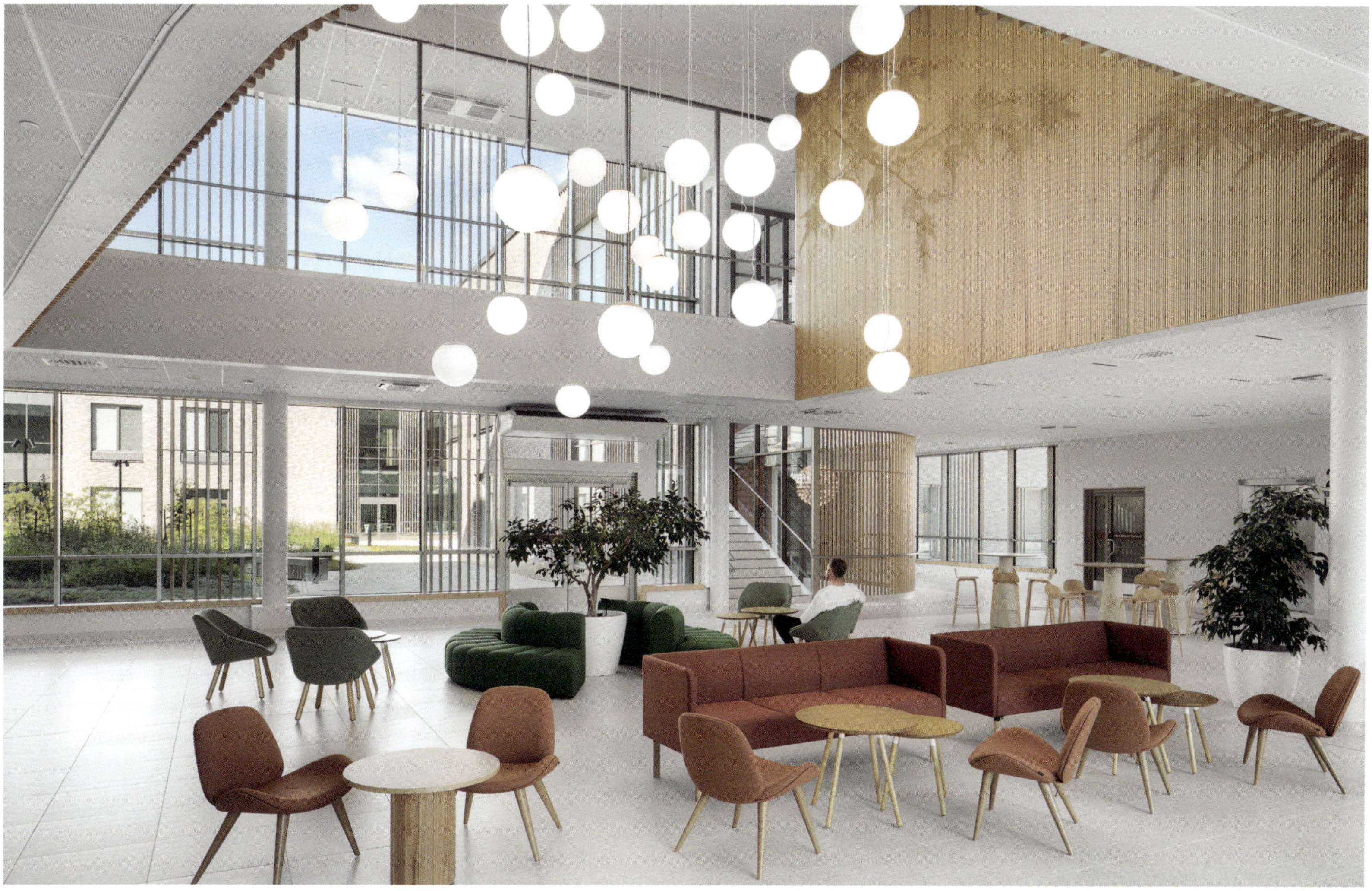

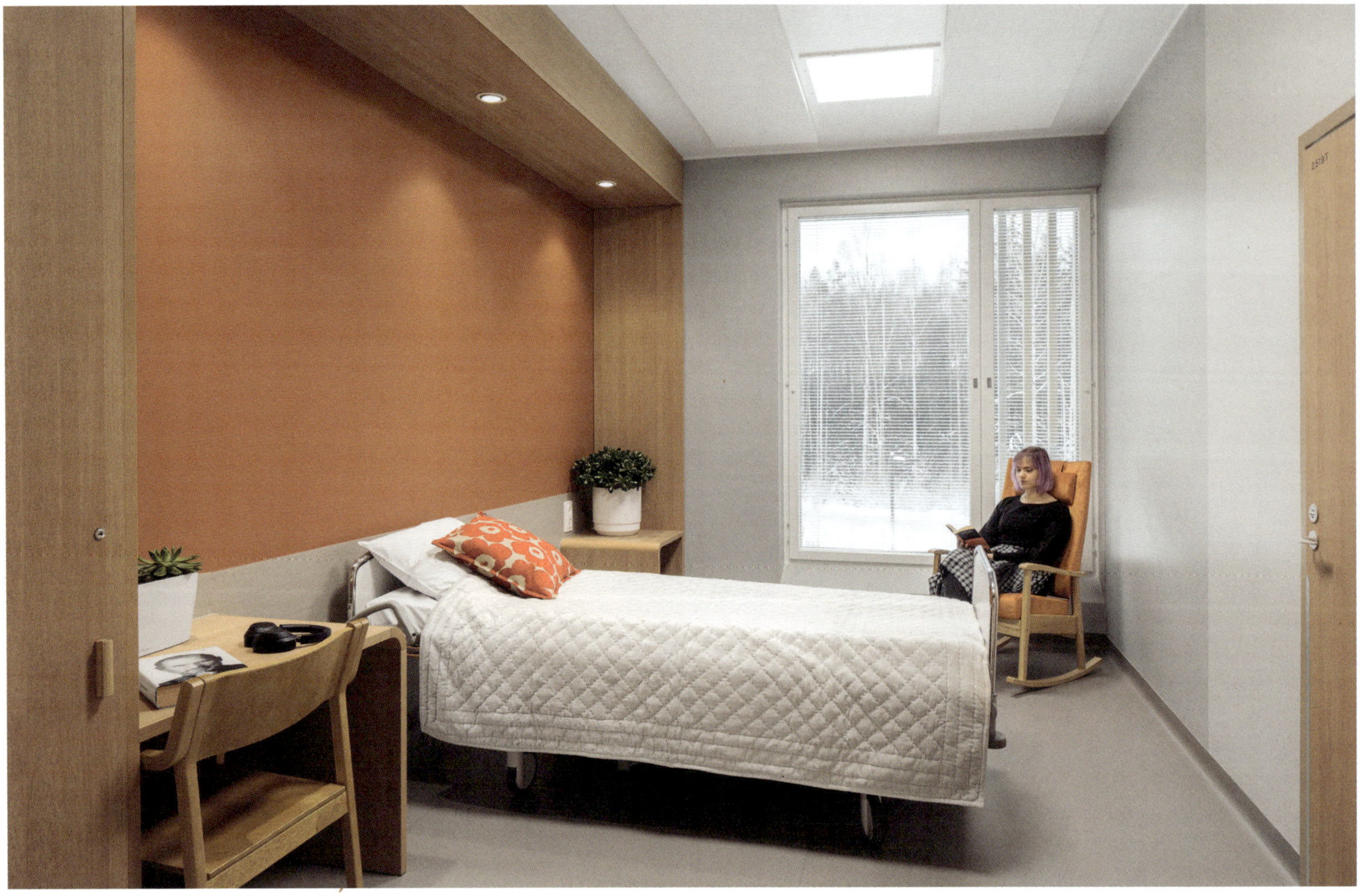

Patient room with natural daylight, warm materials, and views of the surrounding forest.

Ground floor plan.

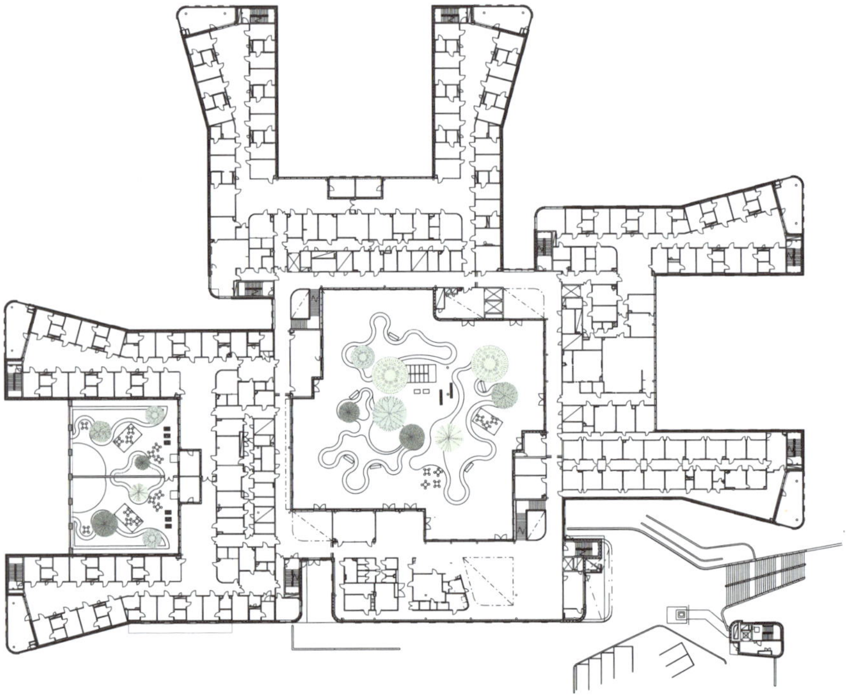

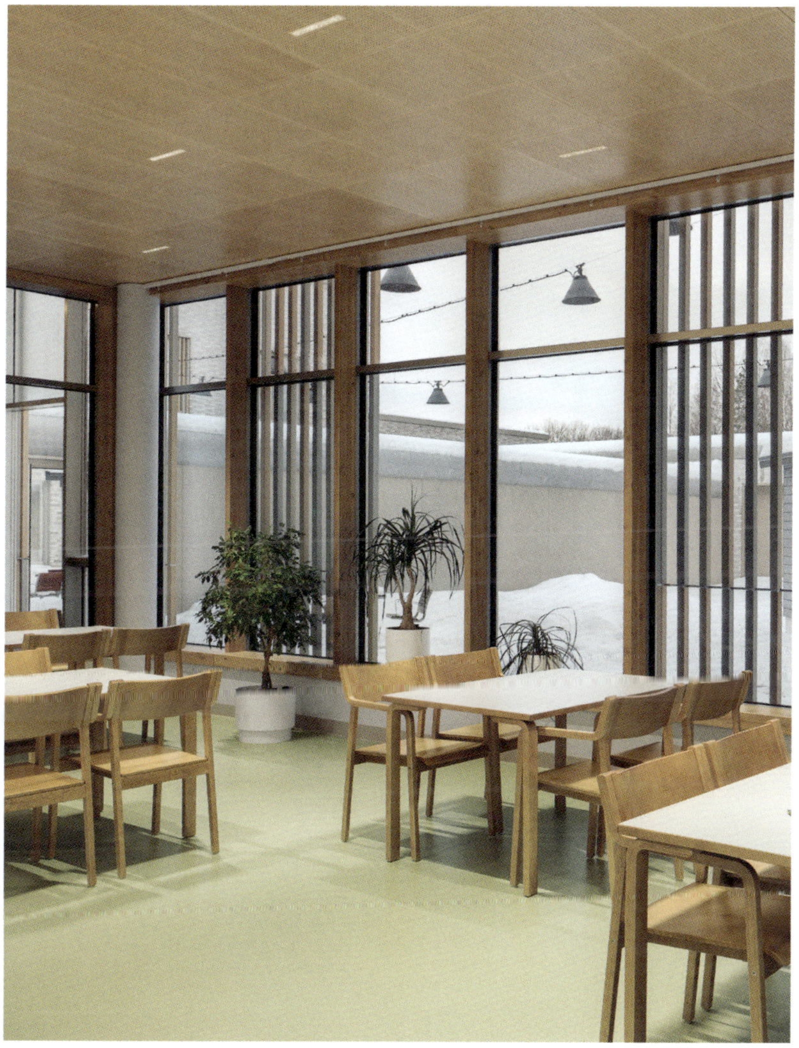

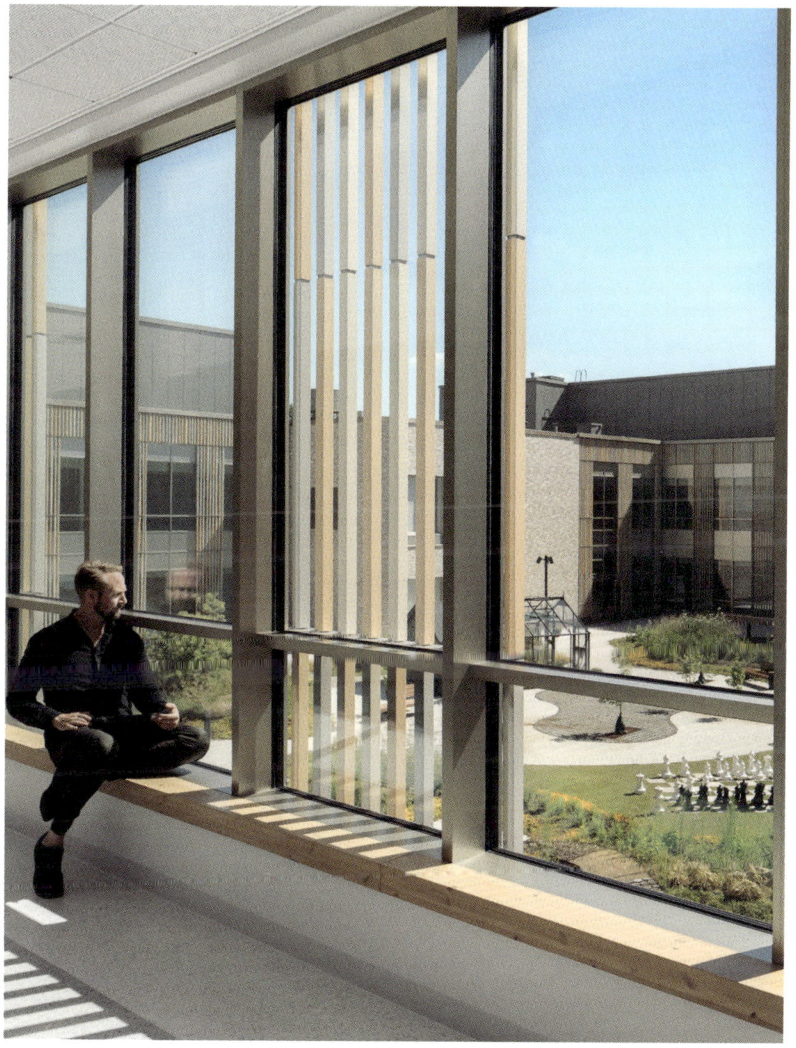

Canteen with extensive timber surfaces, creating a warm and welcoming atmosphere.

Corridor with large windows and abundant natural light, enhancing spatial clarity and supporting the recovery process for patients.

Courtyard and ward section.

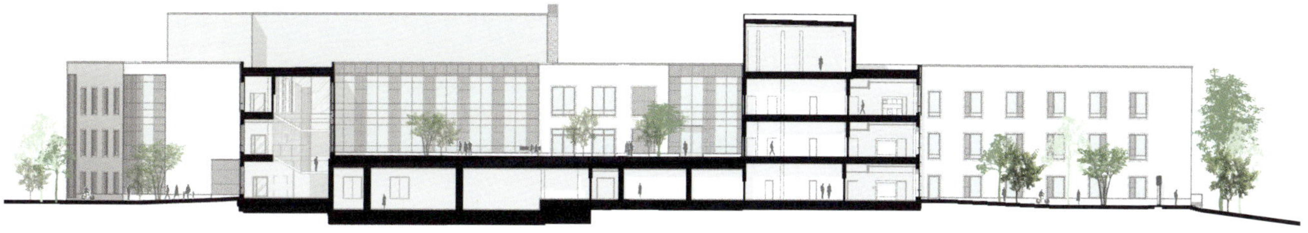

Dost Architektur

Zurich
Switzerland

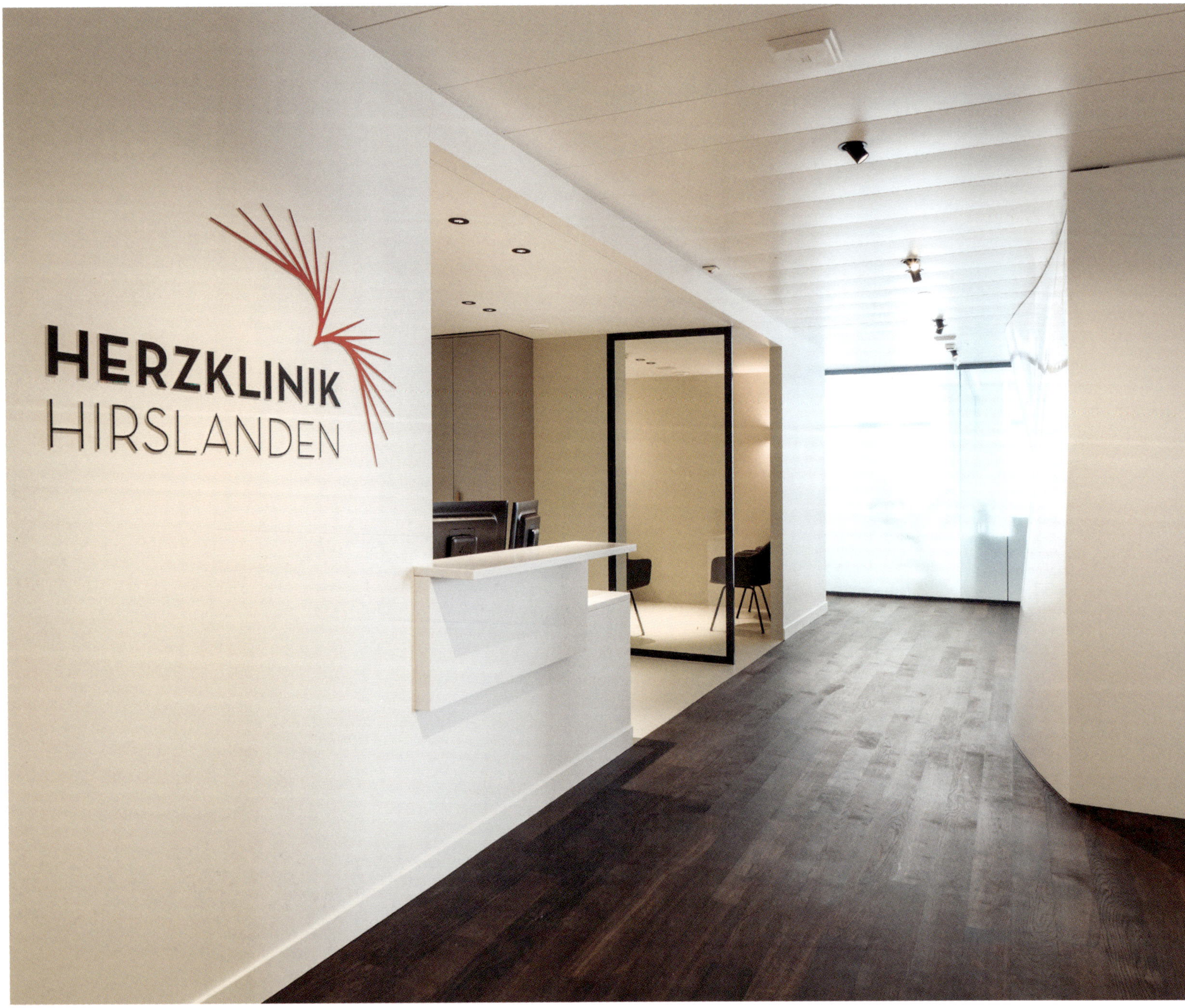

Reception area of the 2023 expansion.

Second waiting area of the basic design, 2013.

Design and Extension of the Hirslanden Heart Clinic

When cardiology and cardiac surgery were brought together at the Hirslanden Clinic in 2013 their close collaboration shaped the design: two distinct wings are linked by a shared reception, waiting, and examination area, with a central green space as a defining landmark. Mirrored lintels and base areas create a visual transition between floor and ceiling, while at turning points the orthogonal grid dissolves and corners rise from the floor to mark changes in direction. The wayfinding system was developed specifically by Büro Fax. The facility was gradually expanded in the following years. For its tenth anniversary in 2023, the clinic received additional space from the Hirslanden Group. The new design adopts the basement's narrative logic in a contemporary way: wave-shaped walls reinterpret the raised corners as flowing movement, while familiar elements maintain spatial continuity and recognizability.

Address: Witellikerstrasse 40, 8032 Zurich, Switzerland | **Client:** Herzklinik Hirslanden | **Completion:** 2013 / 2023 | **Size:** 825 m² / 320 m² | **Original building:** Schmid & Schnebeli Architekten, 2013 | **Sector:** private | **Specialization:** heart clinic | **Number of treatment rooms:** 22 | **Signage and Corporate identity:** Büro Fax

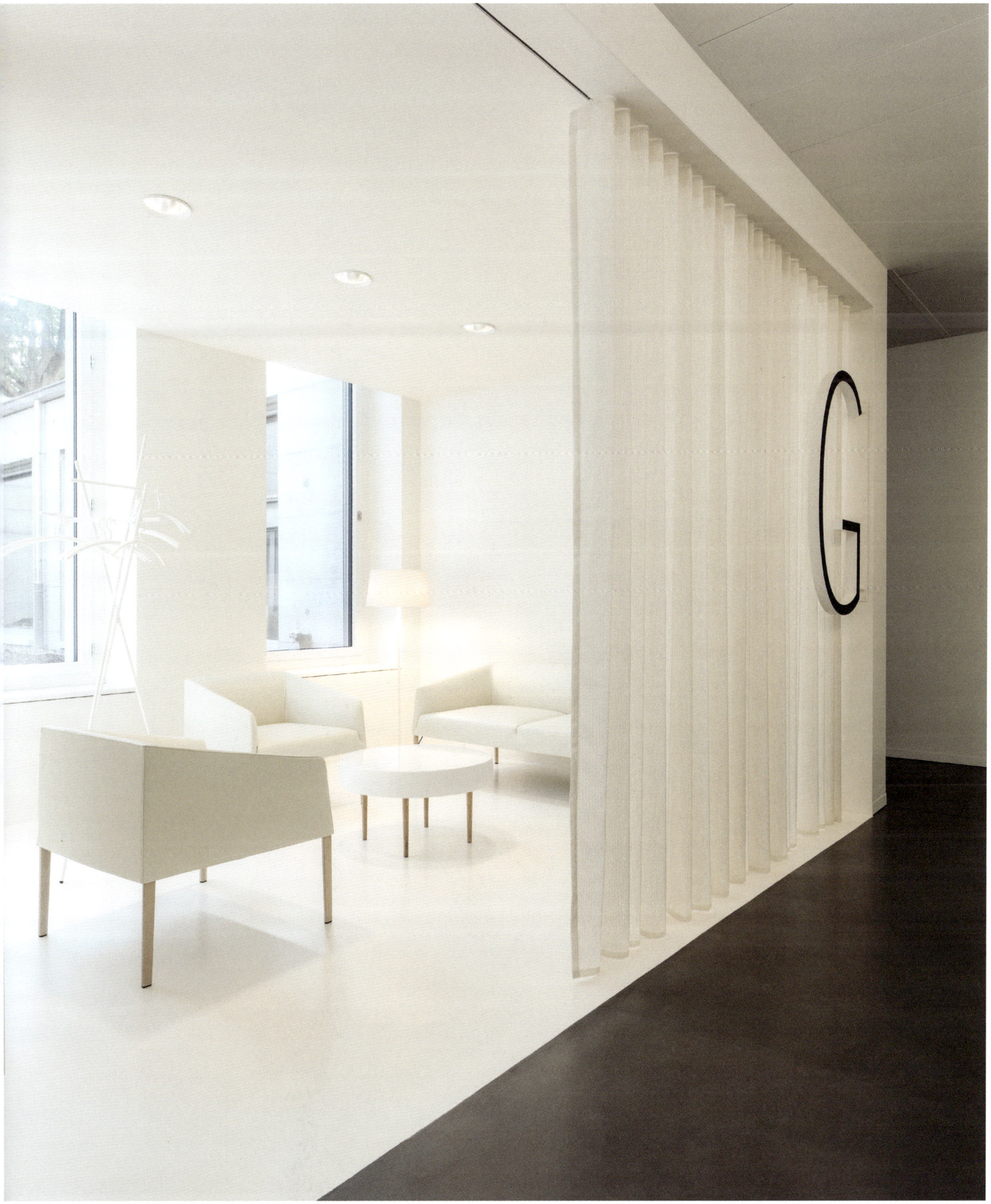

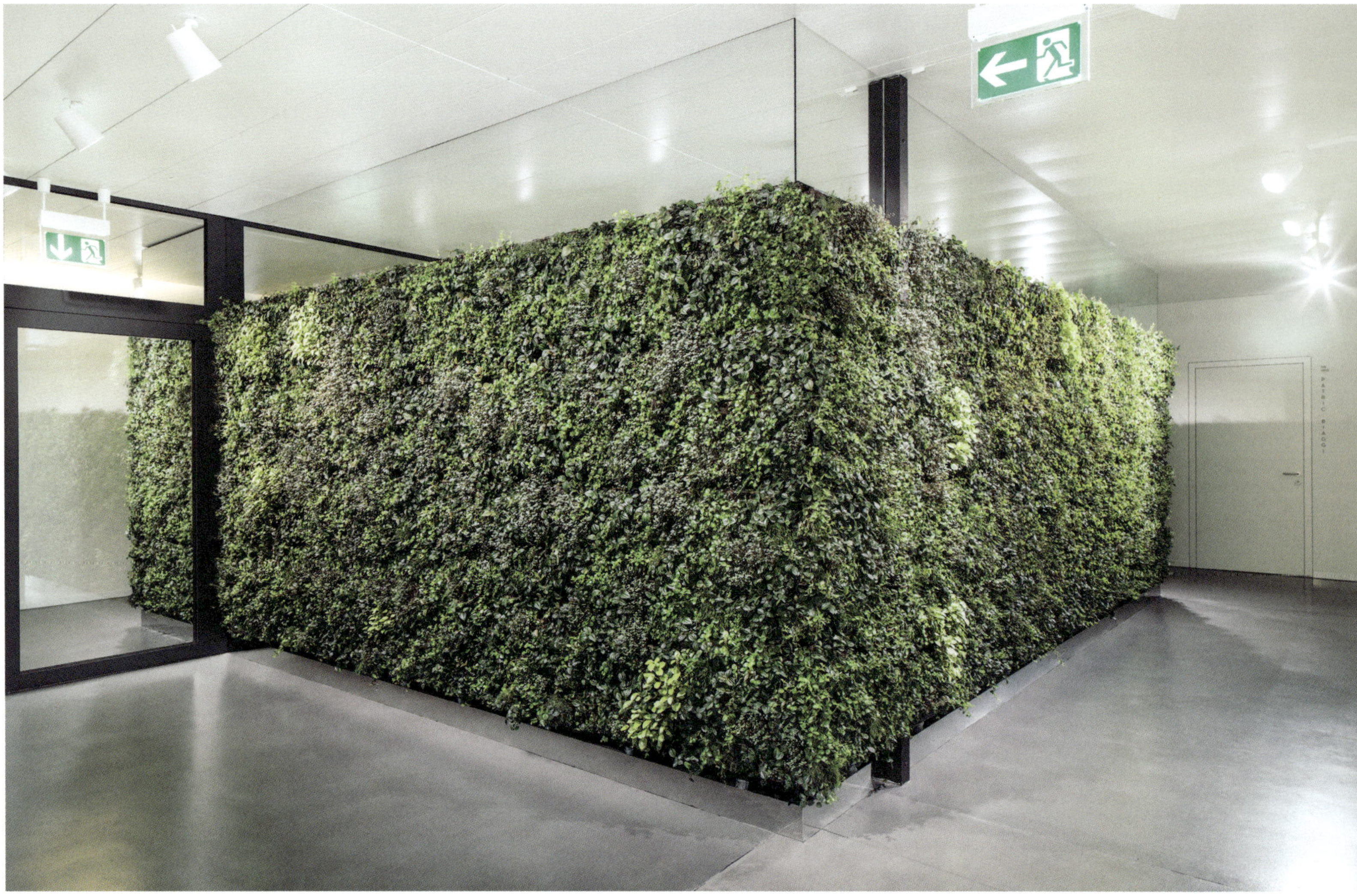

Greened spatial volume as a point of orientation.

Floor plan of the 2013 project.

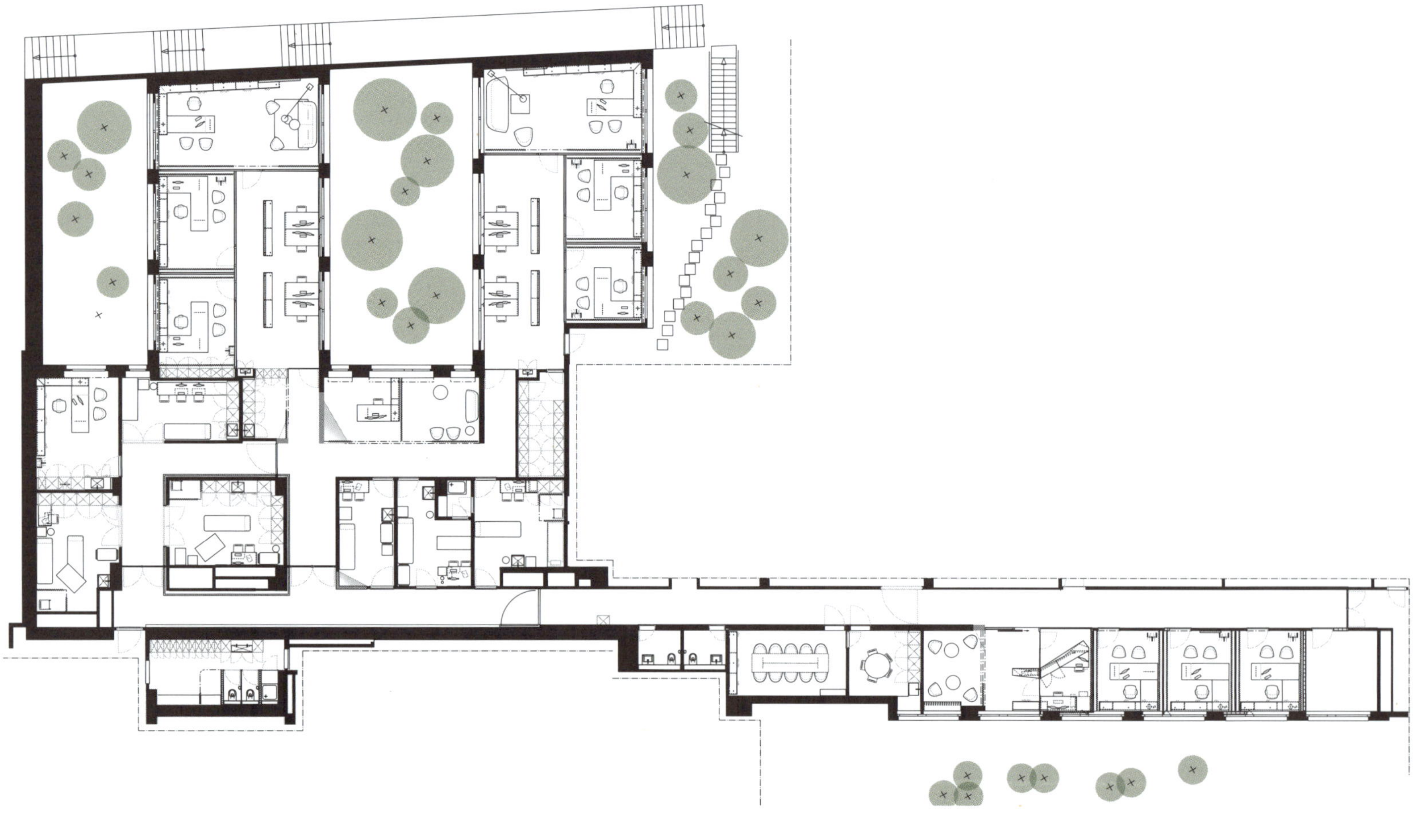

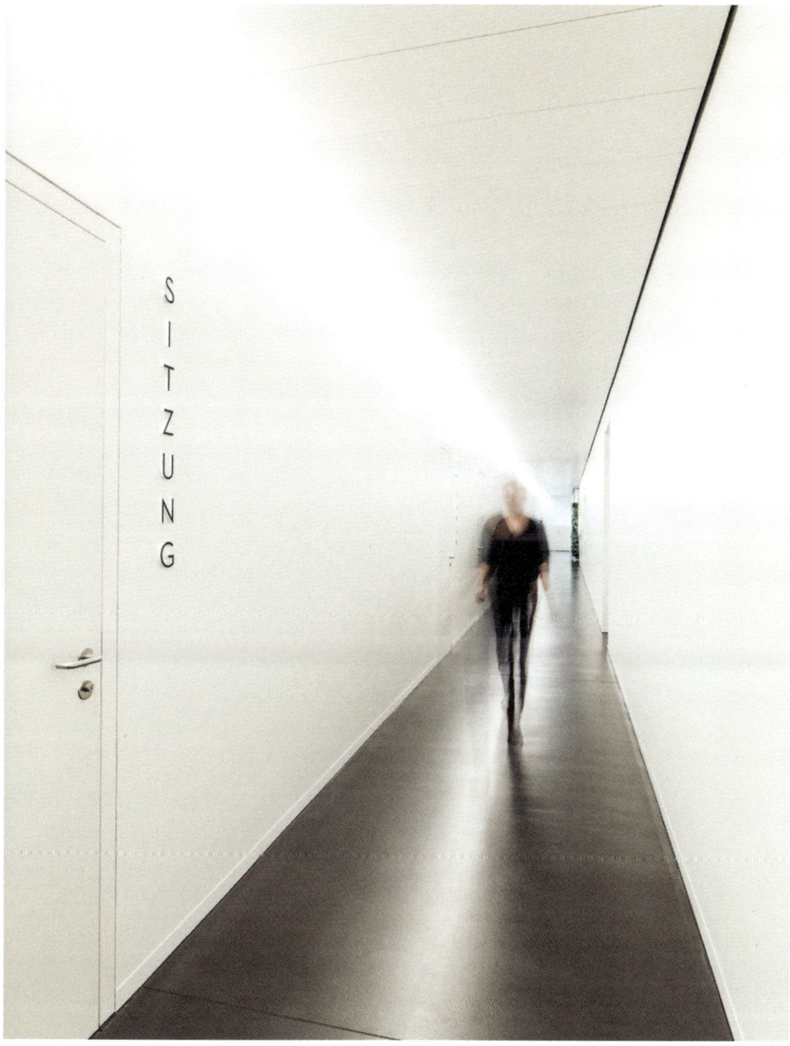

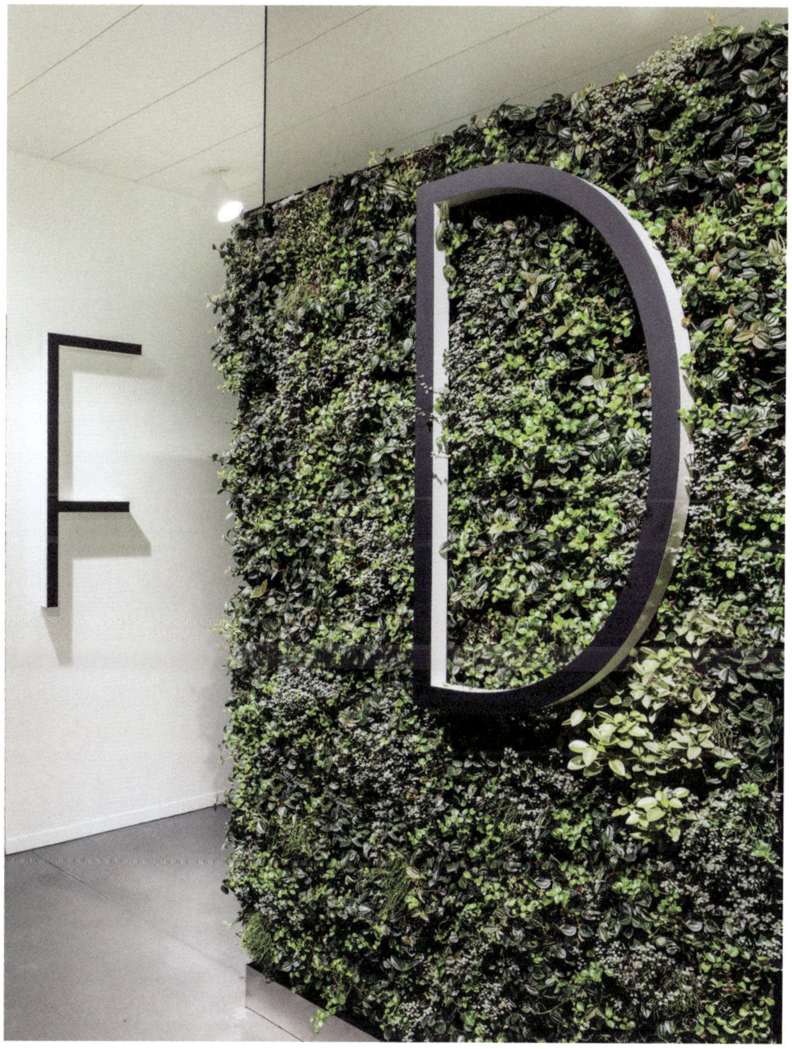

Corridor in the 2013-basic design with signage detail.

Freshly developed signage provides orientation.

Floor plan of the 2023 extension.

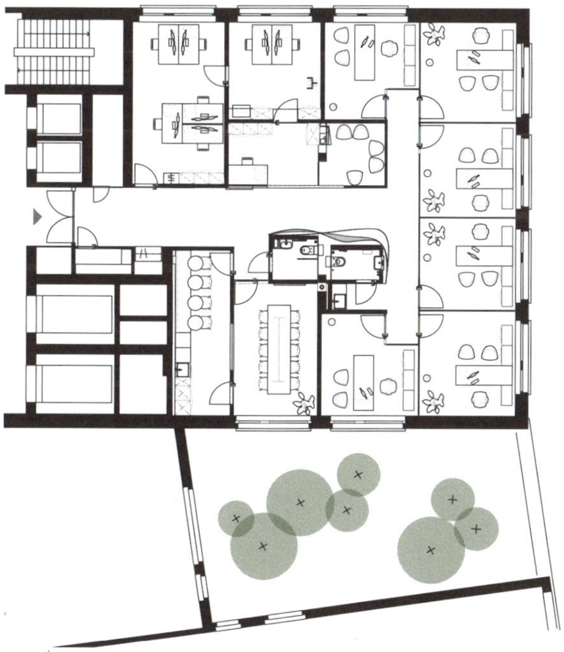

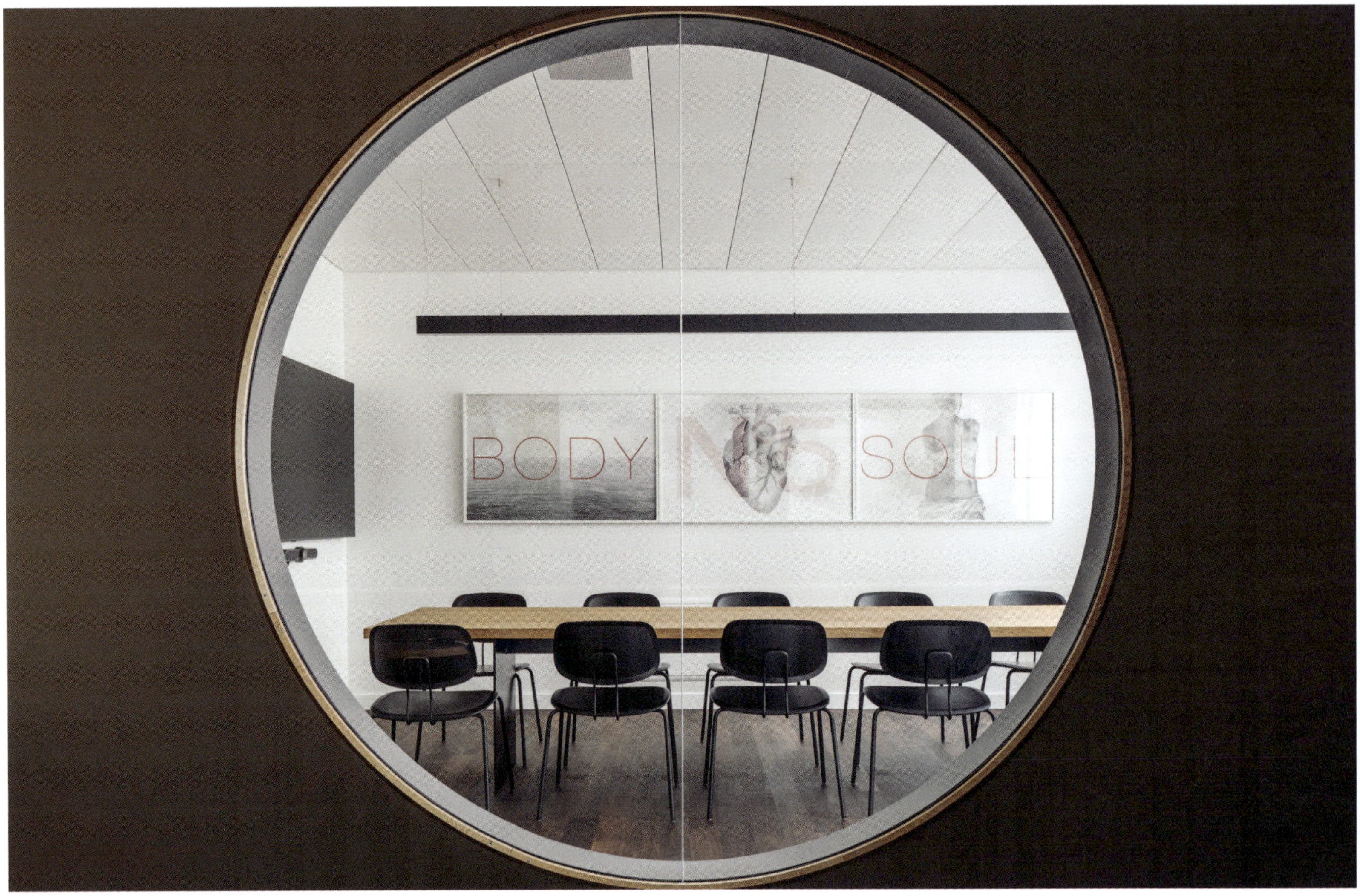

Meeting room as part of the basic design from 2023.

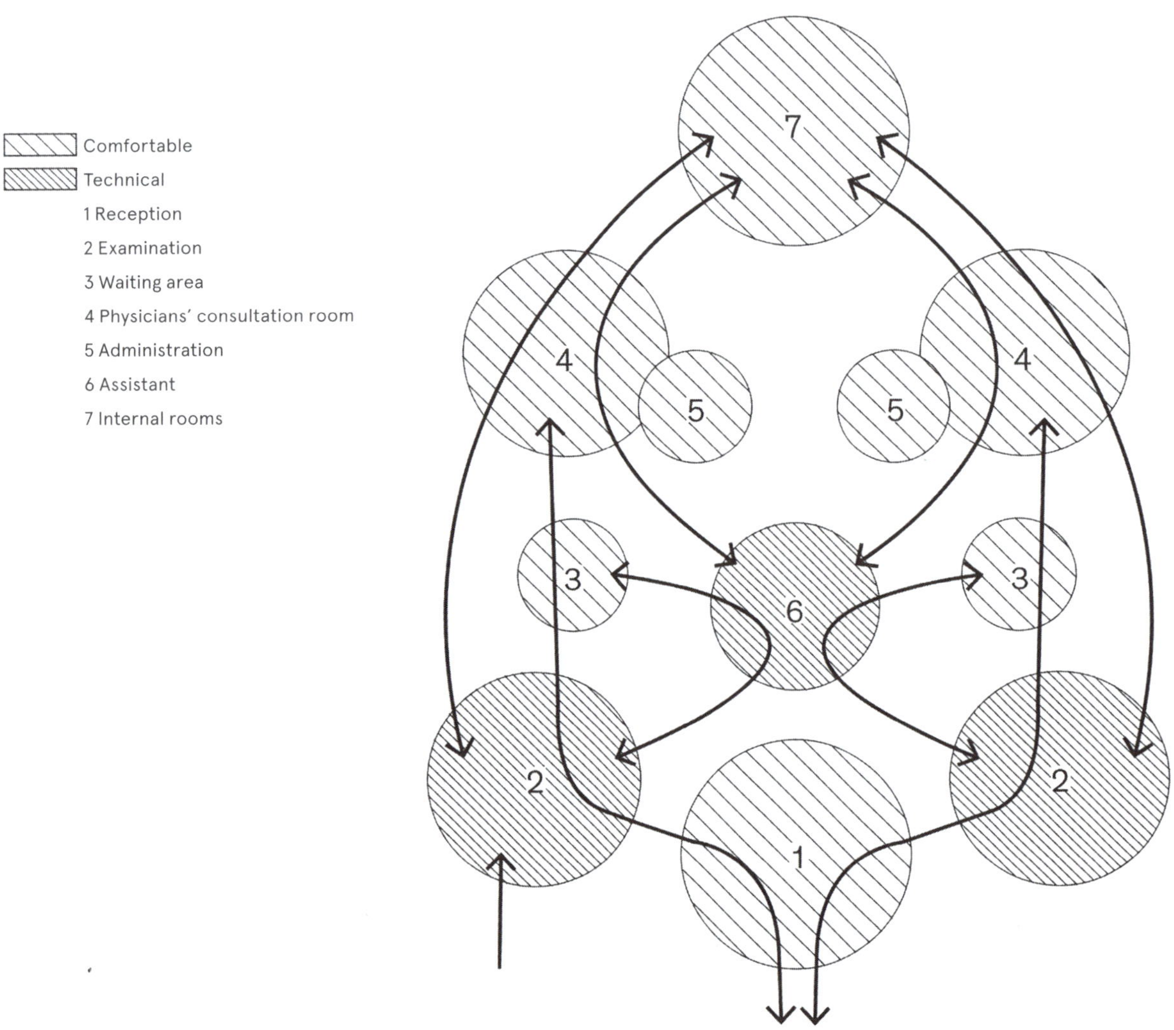

Workflow diagram of 2013s project.

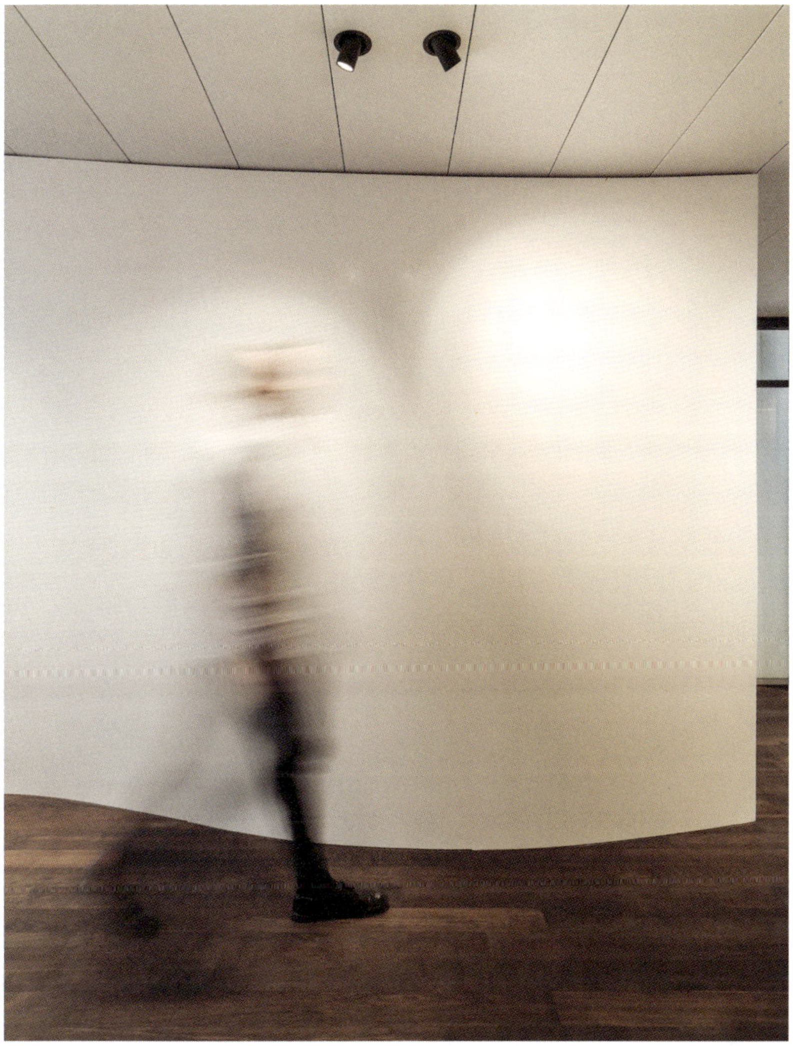

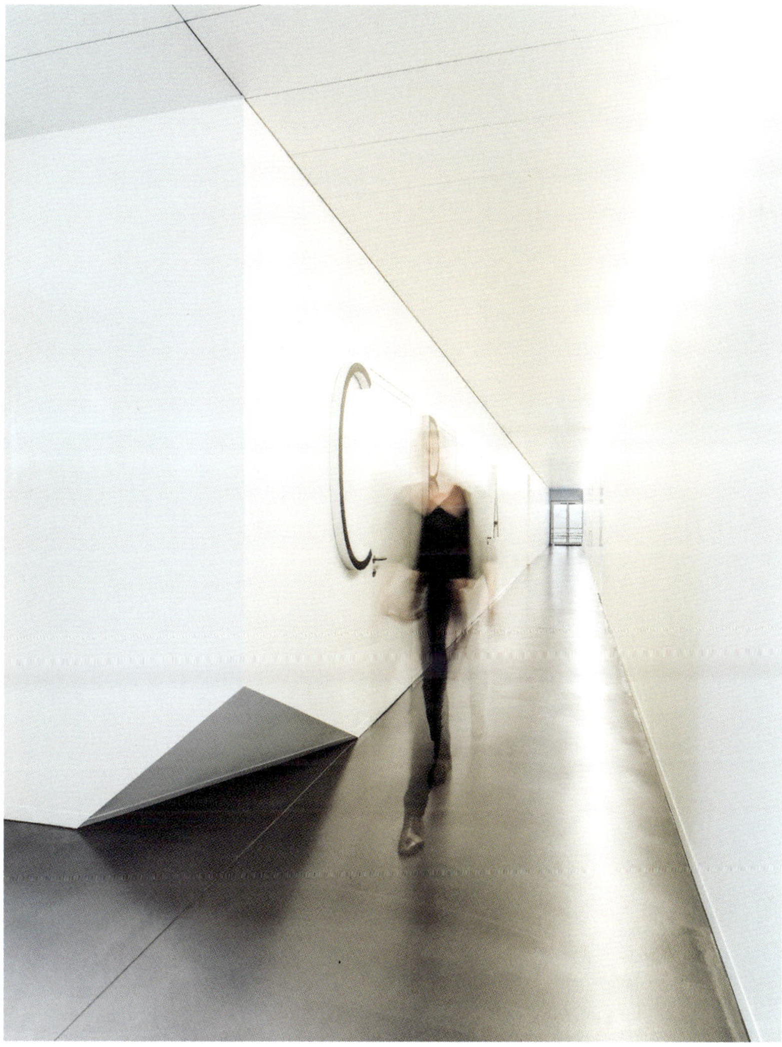

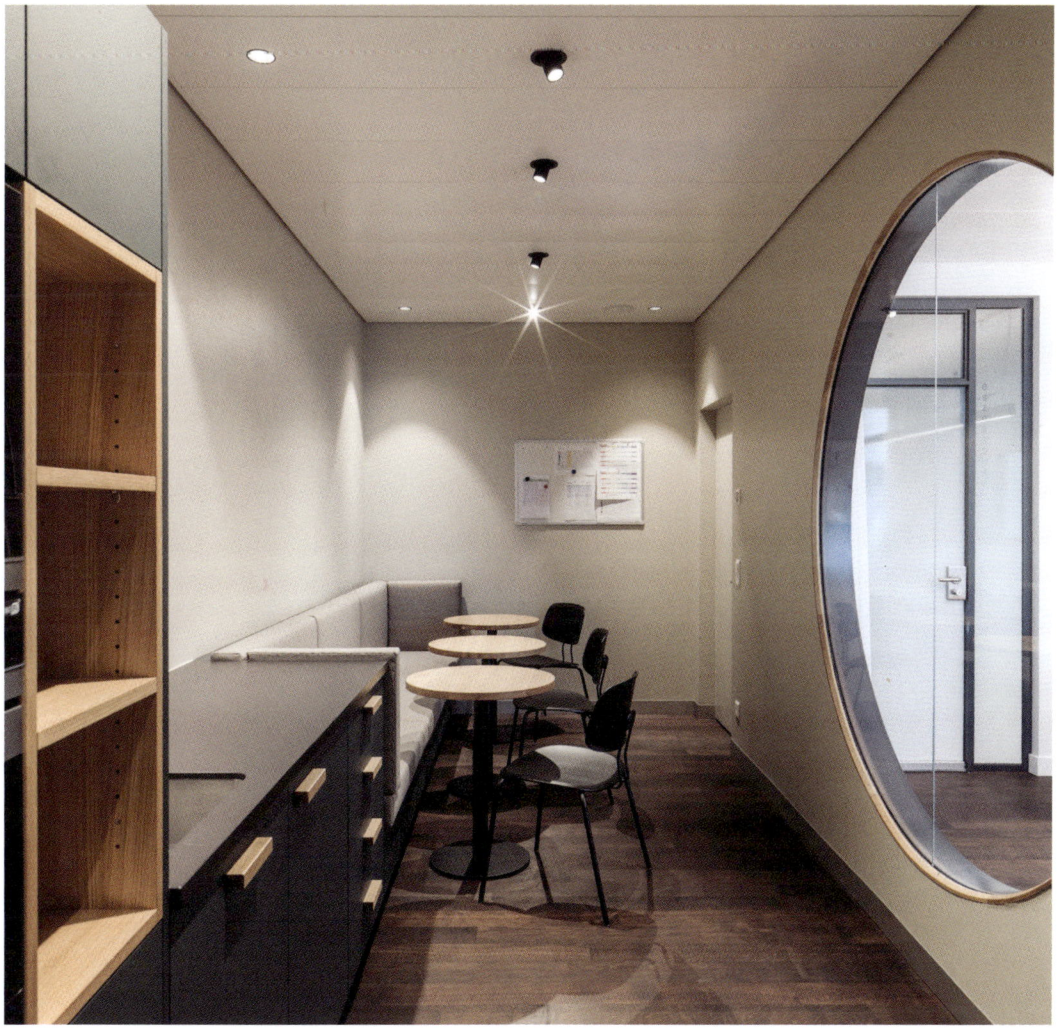

Curved wall as an interpretation of the raised corners, expansion 2023.

Corners rise from the floor and mark changes in direction of the original project.

Lounge area of the expansion, 2023.

AVR Development

Lviv
Ukraine

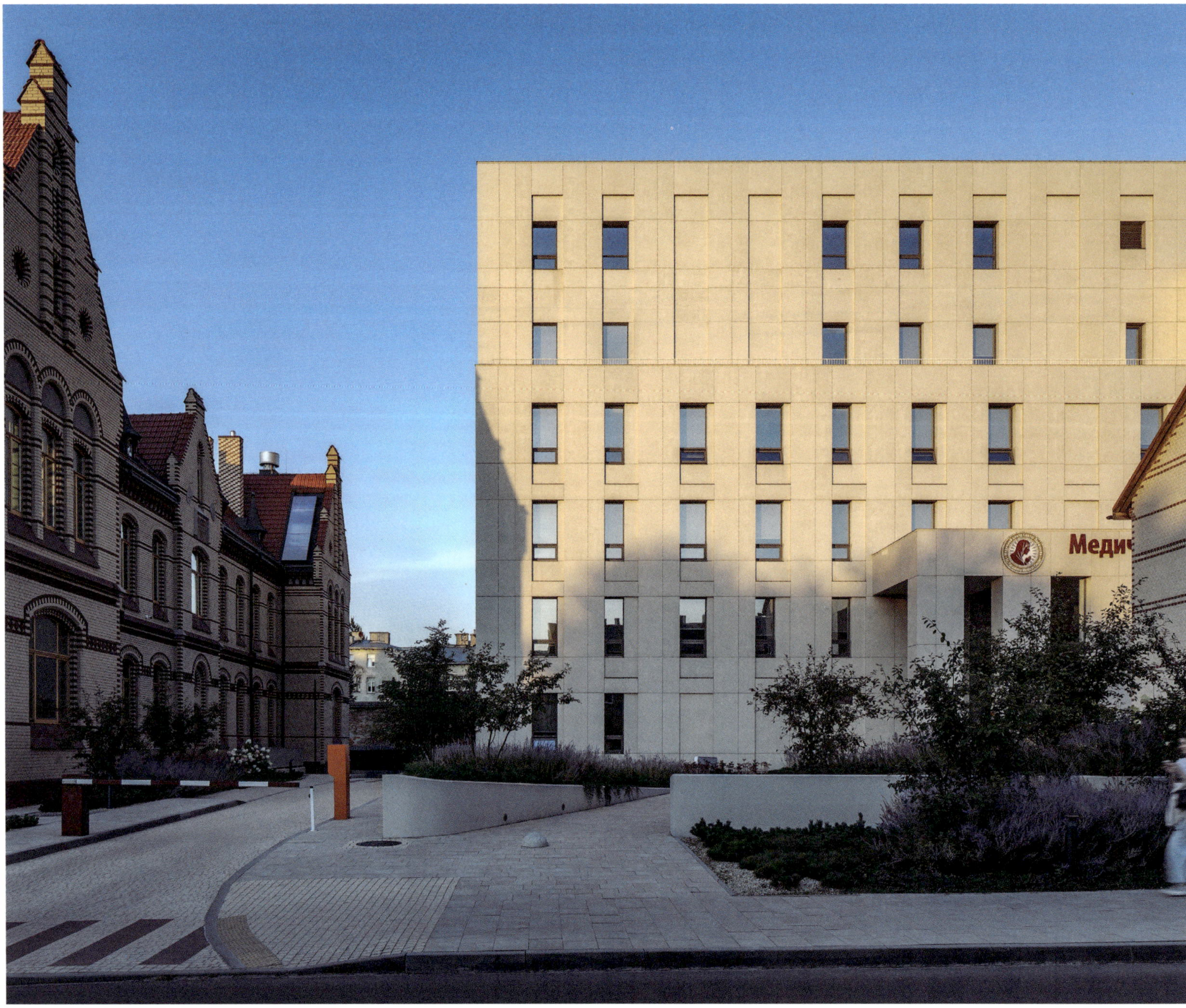

St. Paraskeva Medical Center and its urban surroundings seen from the south.

Protruding structure marking the main entrance.

St. Paraskeva Medical Center

The project is integrated into the historical ensemble of the former Anton and Valeria Bilinski Hospital, where 19th century buildings form a rectangular courtyard. The concept combined careful restoration with a new medical block, preserving cultural heritage while creating contemporary healthcare spaces. The new building accommodates reception and outpatient departments, temporary stay wards, three operating rooms, intensive care, diagnostics, endoscopy, sterilization, and administrative facilities. Each department functions as a distinct zone shaped around the patient's journey. Through projections and recesses gains the façade depth and a three-dimensional quality. Although construction was paused in 2022 due to the military aggression of Russia, the center opened in 2023, continuing the long-term development of St. Paraskeva Medical Center in Lviv.

Address: 27, Akademika Ihoria Yukhnovskoho Street, Lviv 79057, Ukraine | **Client:** St. Paraskeva Medical Center | **Completion:** 2023 | **Size:** 14,900 m^2 | **Original building:** Anton and Valeria Bilinski Hospital | **Sector:** private | **Specialization:** multispecialty medical center | **Number of treatment rooms:** 13 | **Number of patient rooms:** 39 | **Interior design:** Hochu Rayu | **Landscape design:** Synergys Power | **Lighting design:** Luminal

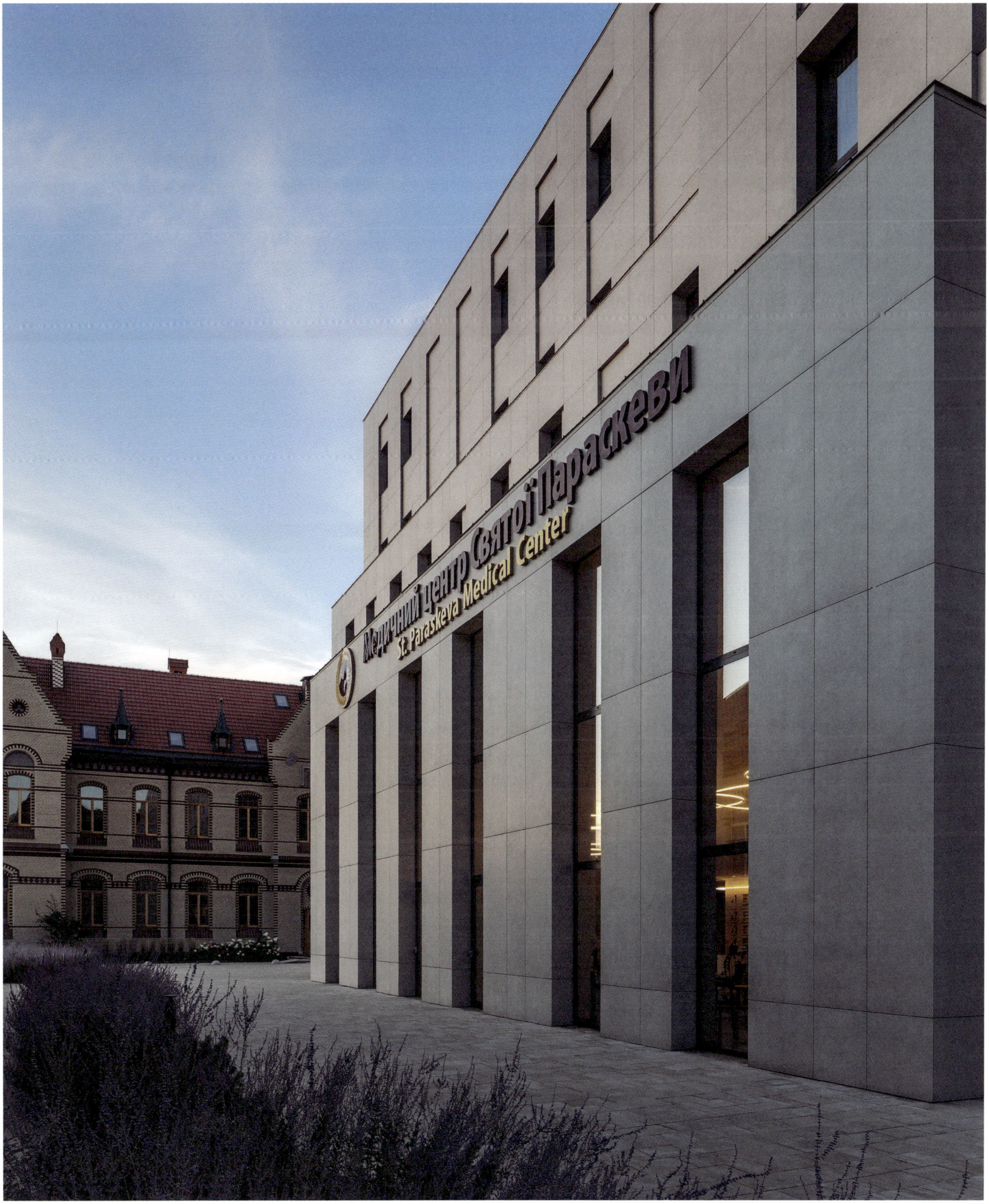

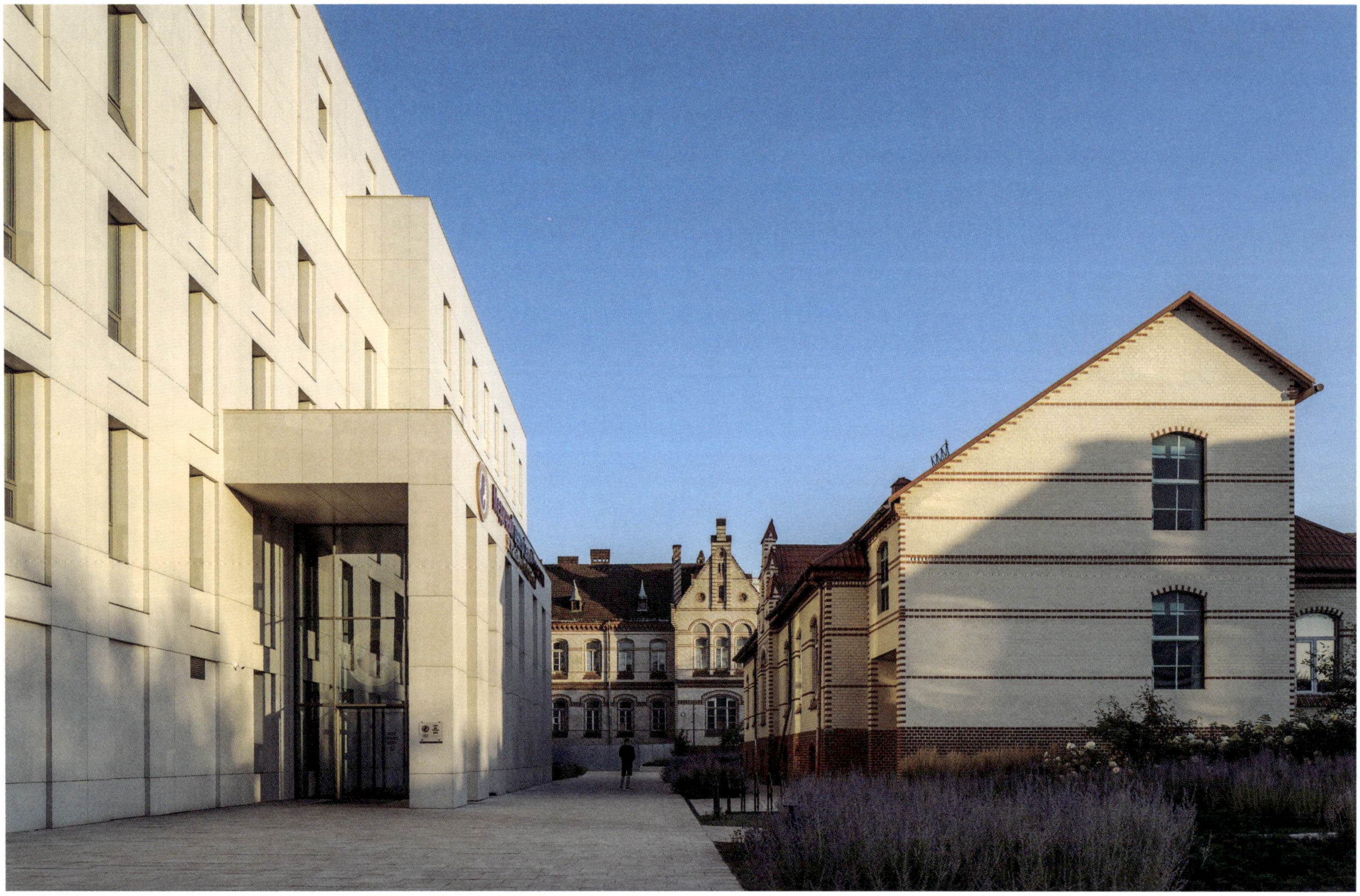

Side view of the main entrance and space between the old and the new building.

Site plan.

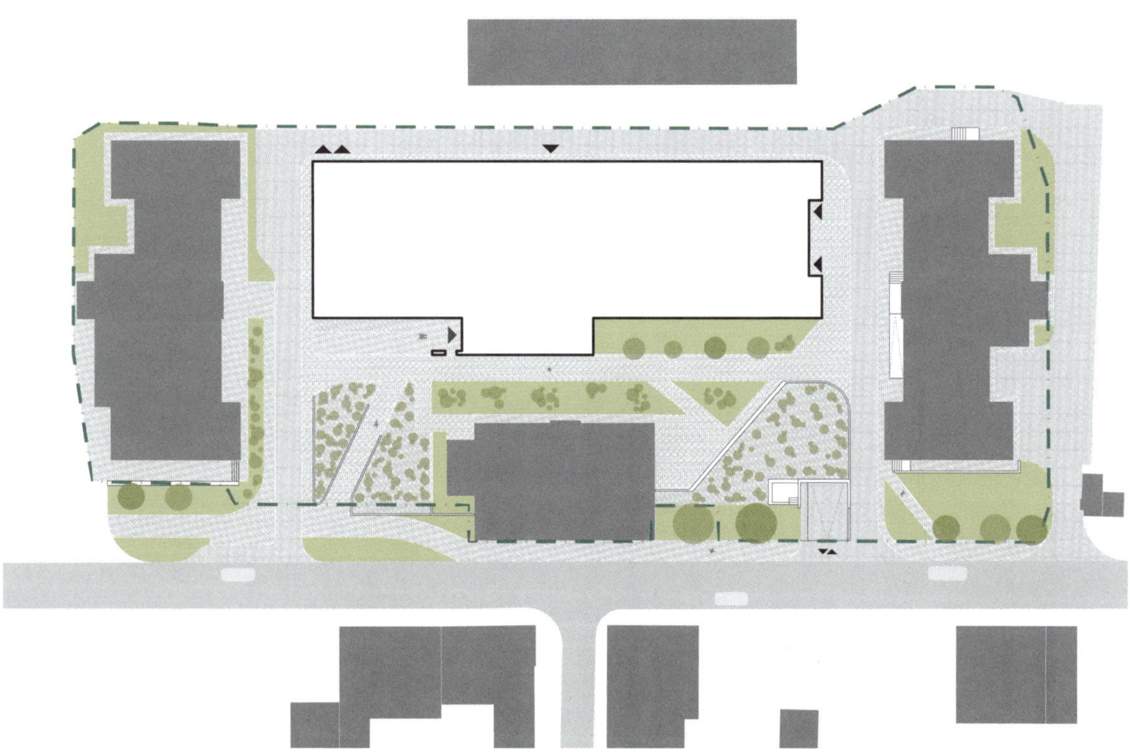

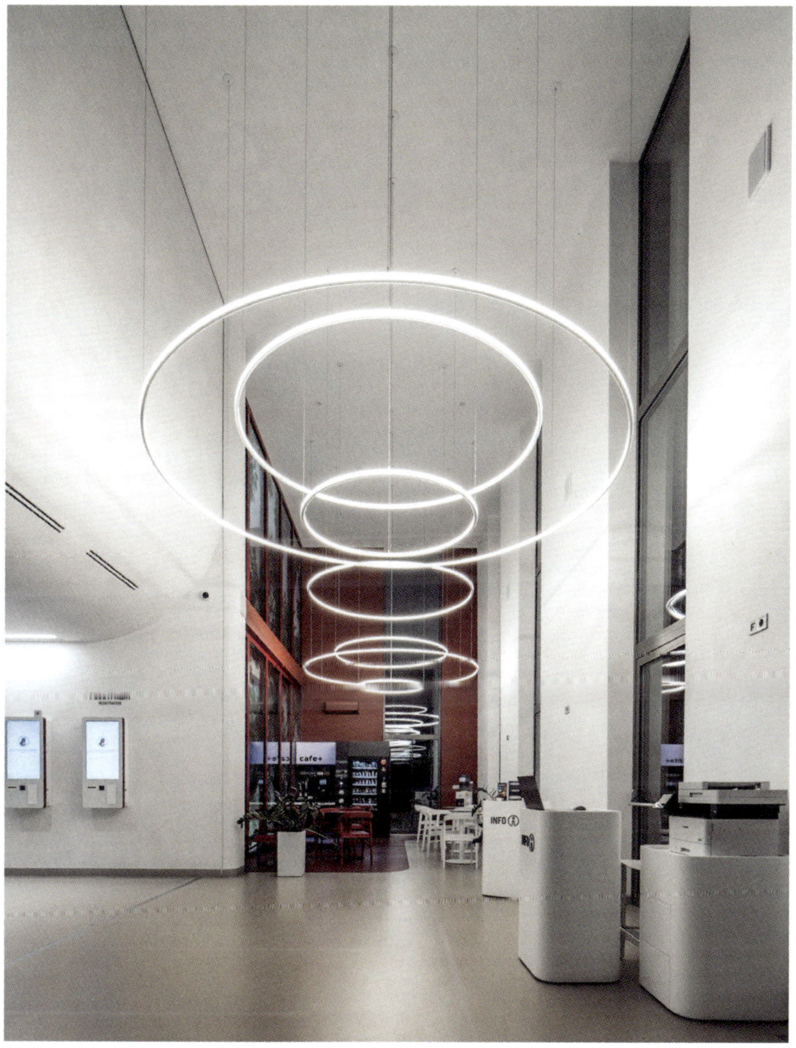

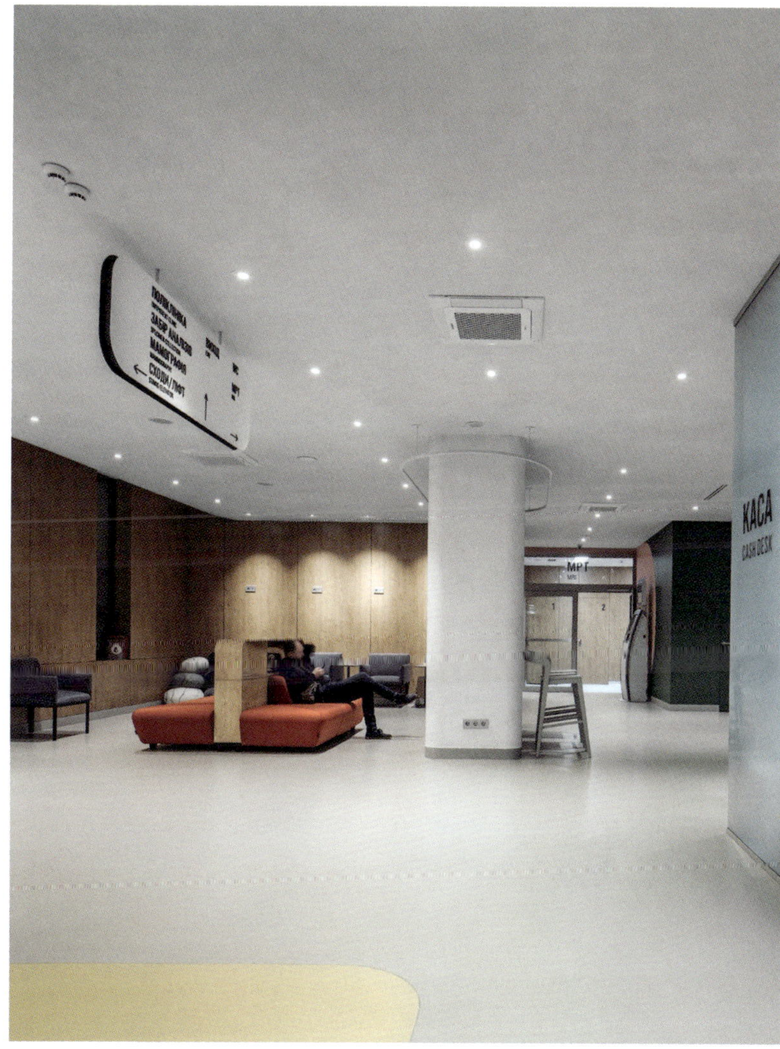

Entrance area with a café corner and circular lights.

Waiting area with signage.

Ground, first and second floor plans.

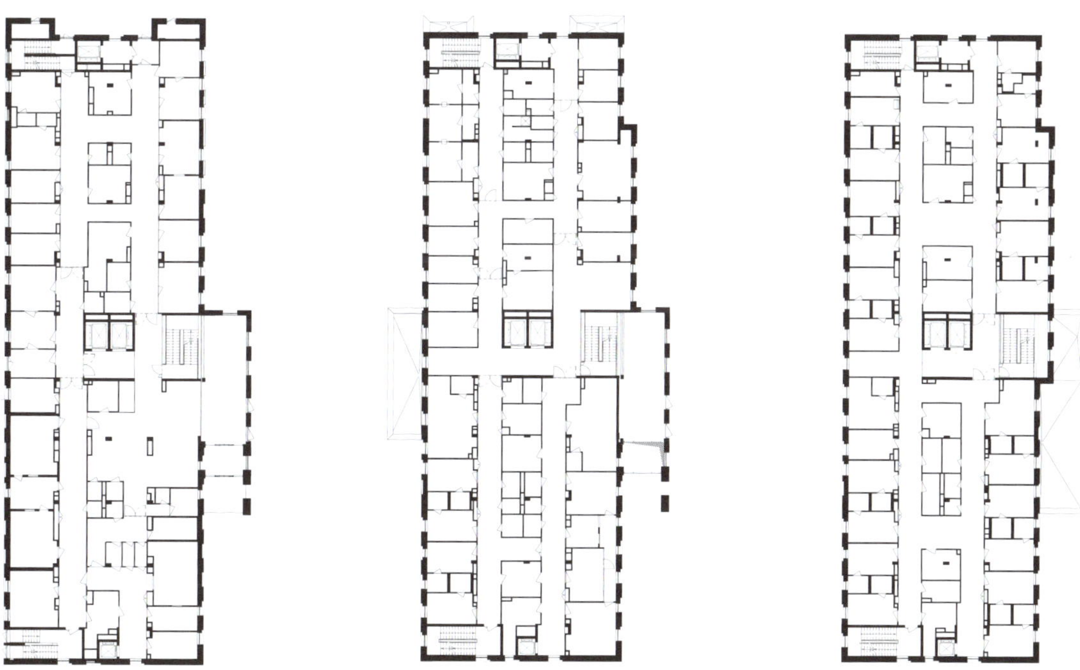

kerstin gierse
architekten

Langenfeld
Germany

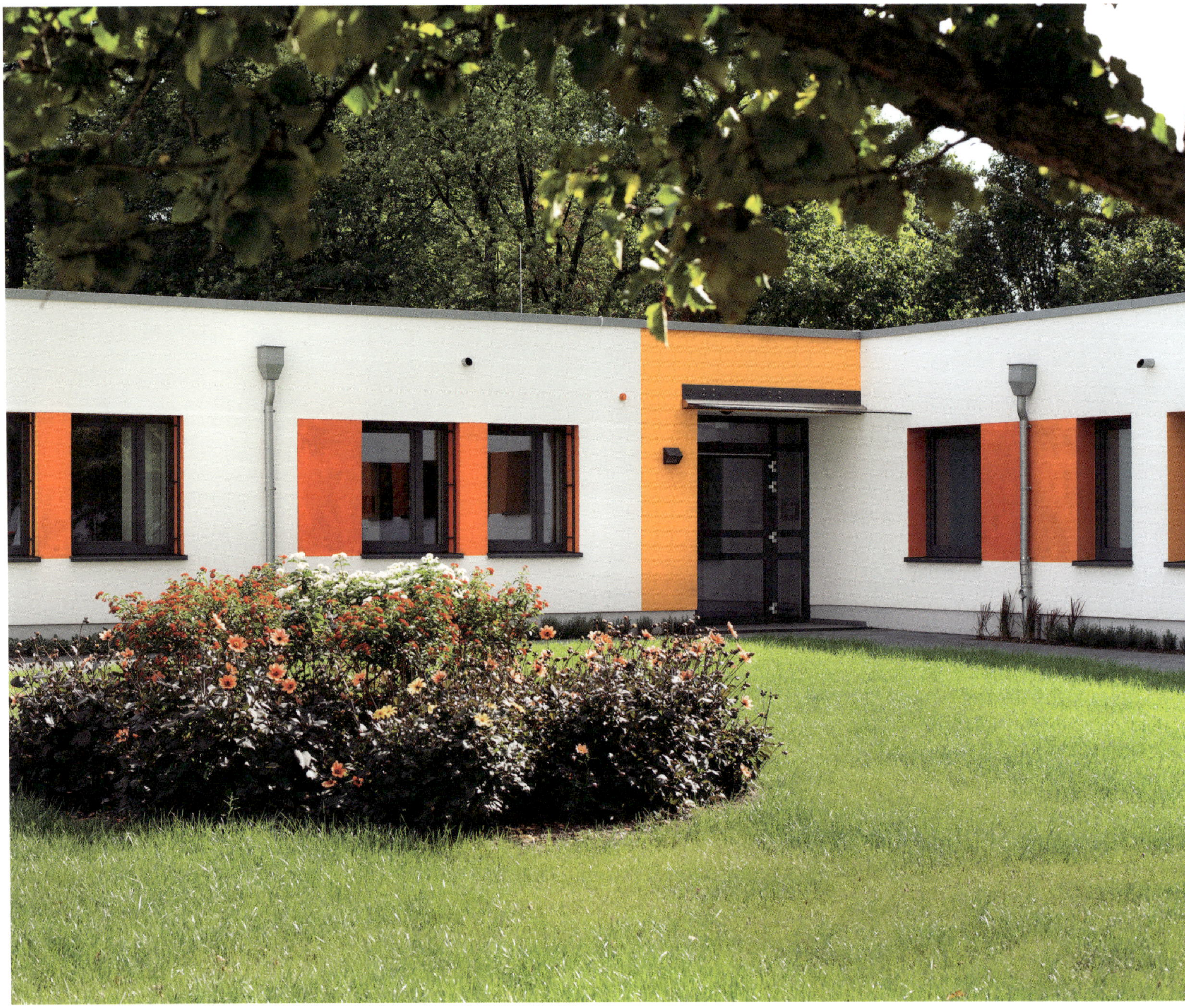

Elective Medical Services LVR Clinic in Langenfeld

The conversion and renovation of a 1950s building created a modern convalescent care facility with a home-like atmosphere. The core of the project was the energy-efficiency and technical modernization of the U-shaped flat-roofed building, as well as the restructuring of the interior spaces. The goal was to offer patients a pleasant atmosphere and a high quality of stay. The result is single and double rooms with private bathrooms, which have a hotel-like feel thanks to warm gray and earth tones, harmonious lighting, and individual decor. Common areas such as the lounge, large rooftop terrace, and landscaped courtyards promote relaxation and social interaction. In the dining room, large-format photo wallpaper featuring nature motifs and modern LED light ceilings create a bright, friendly ambiance. The architects combined functionality, comfort, and modern design into a contemporary overall concept.

As part of the renovation of the single-story 1950s building, a new comfortable ward was created.

Large windows offer an unobstructed view of the garden – and let plenty of natural light into the interior.

Large-format photographic panels illuminated by LED light strips show nature.

Address: Kölner Straße 82, 40764 Langenfeld, Germany | **Client:** LVR-Klinik Langenfeld | **Completion:** 2019 | **Size:** 1,055 m² | **Original building:** 1950s | **Sector:** public | **Number of treatment rooms:** 5 | **Number of patient rooms:** 14

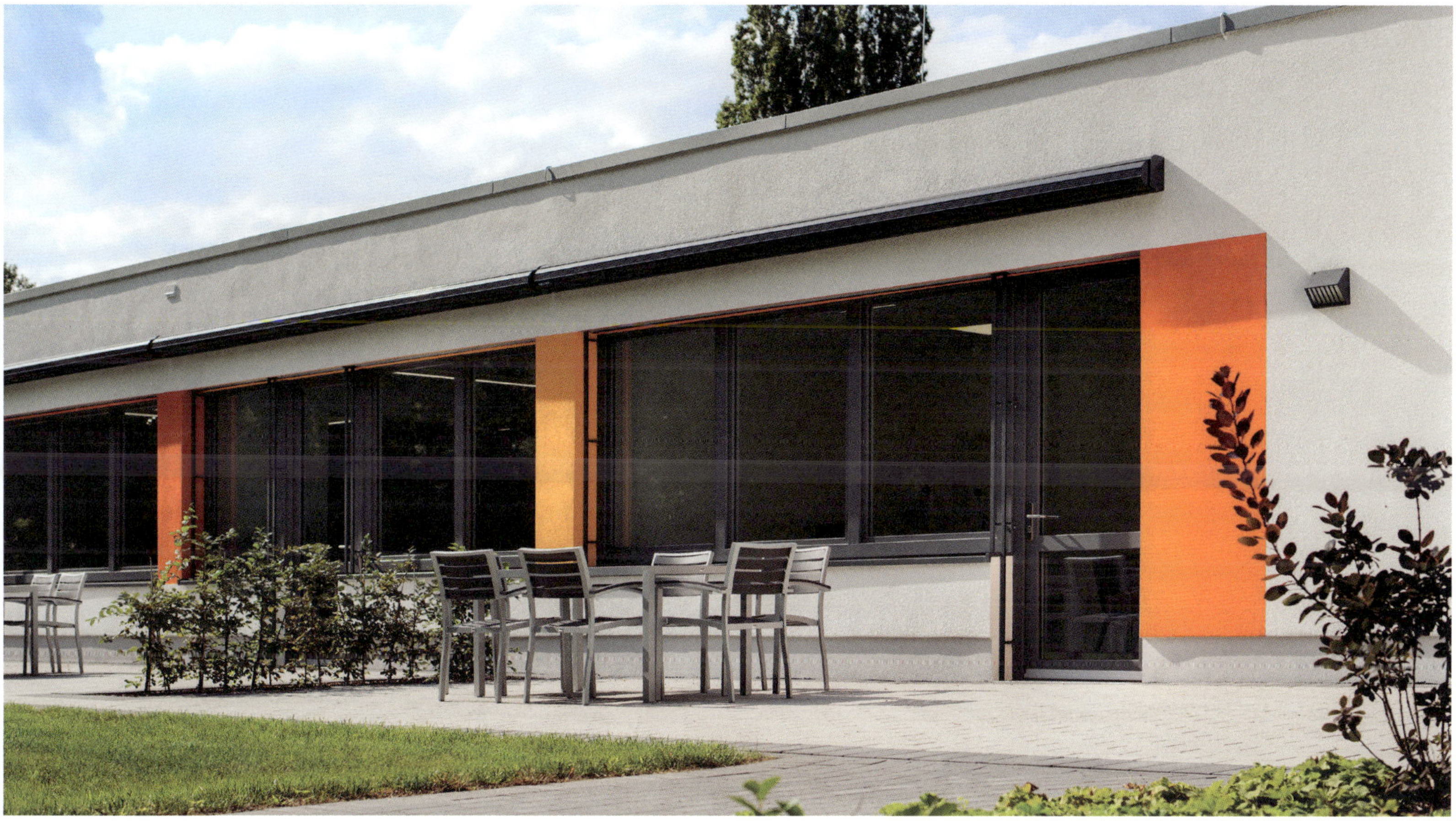

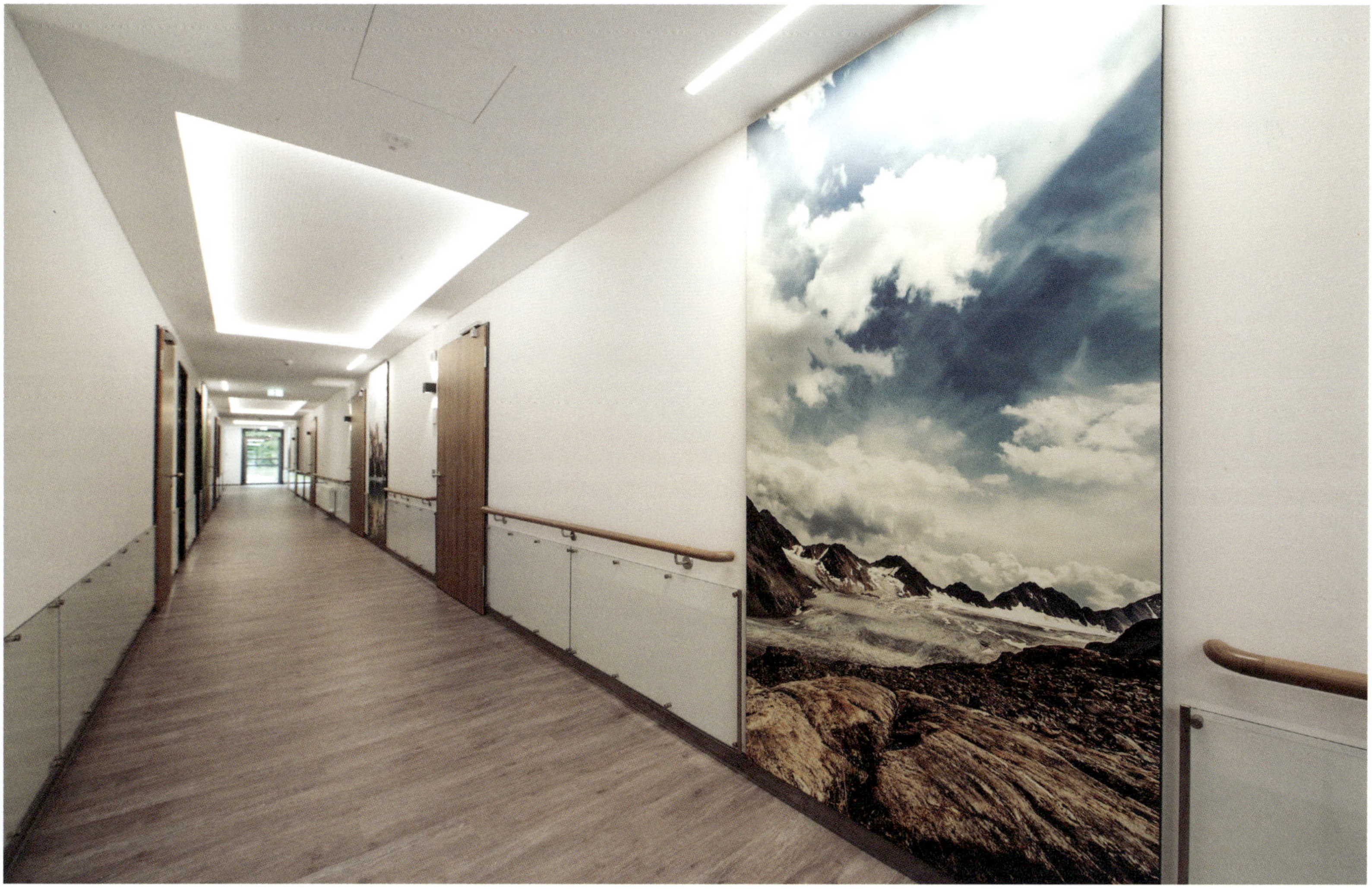

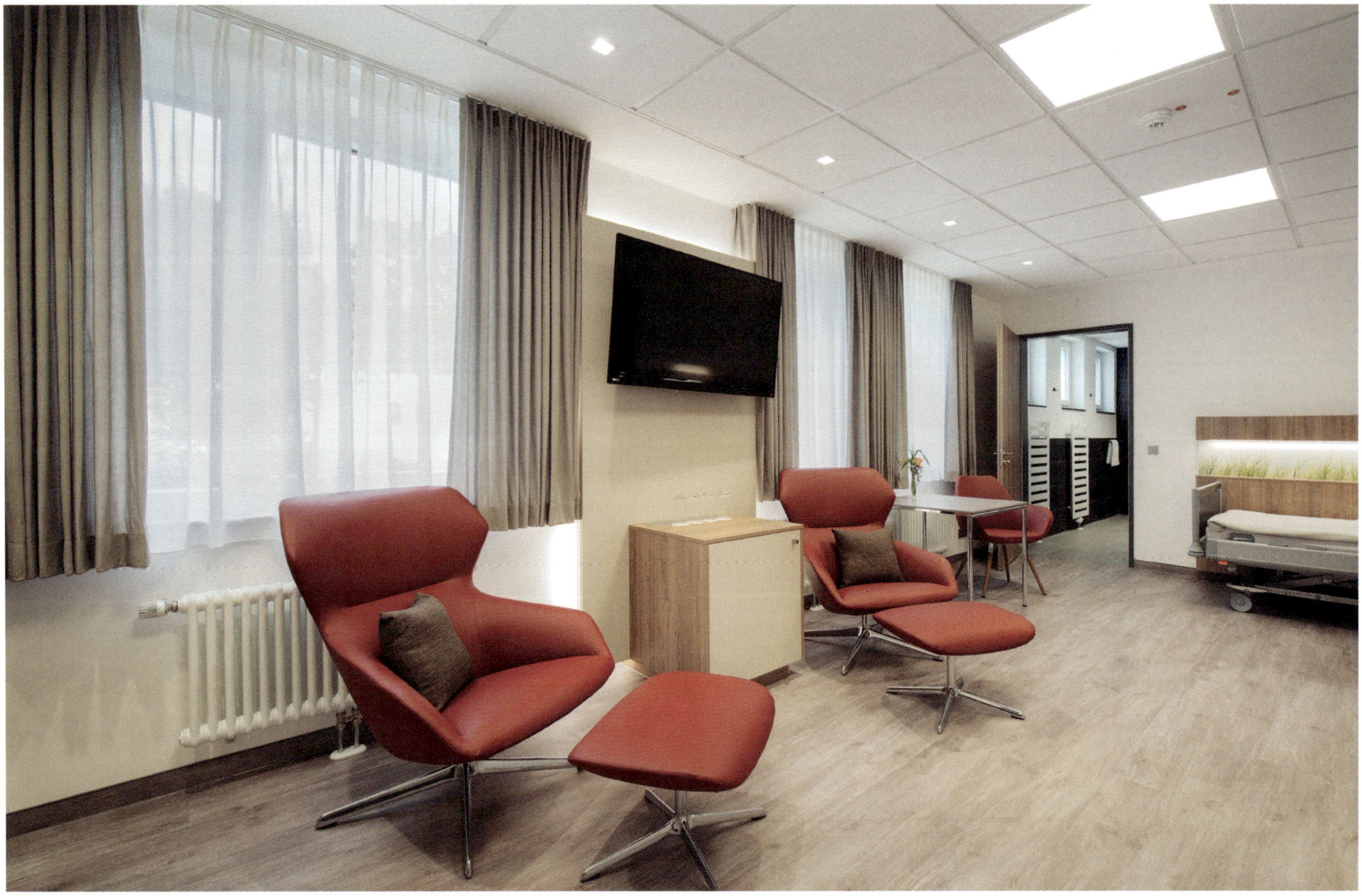

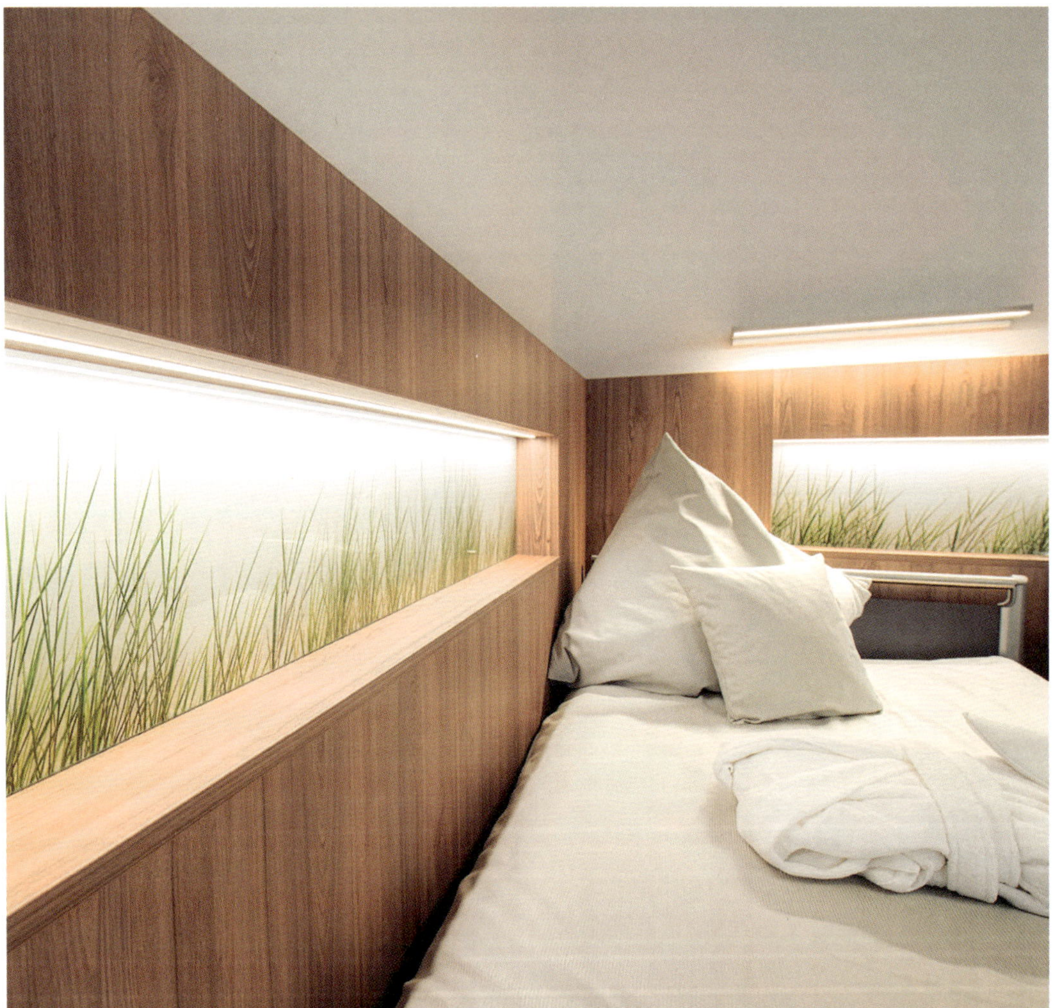

Each of the two side wings houses seven patient rooms with high-end amenities.

Feel good, relax, and recover is the motto of the elective care unit.

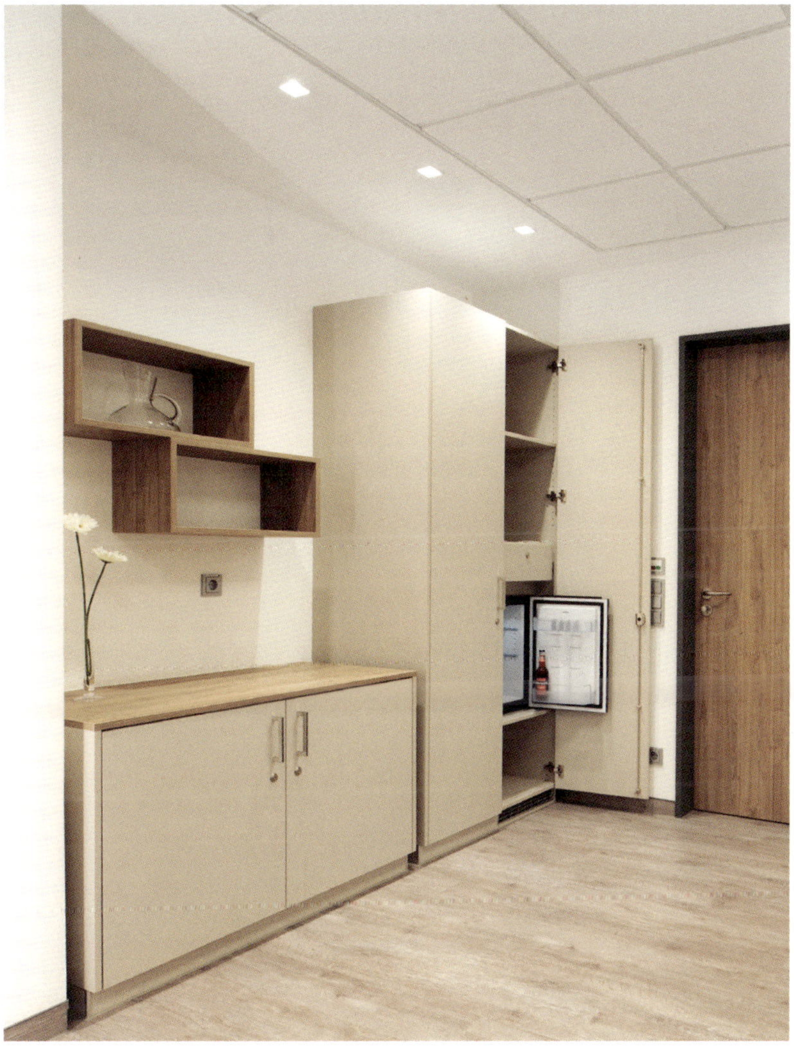

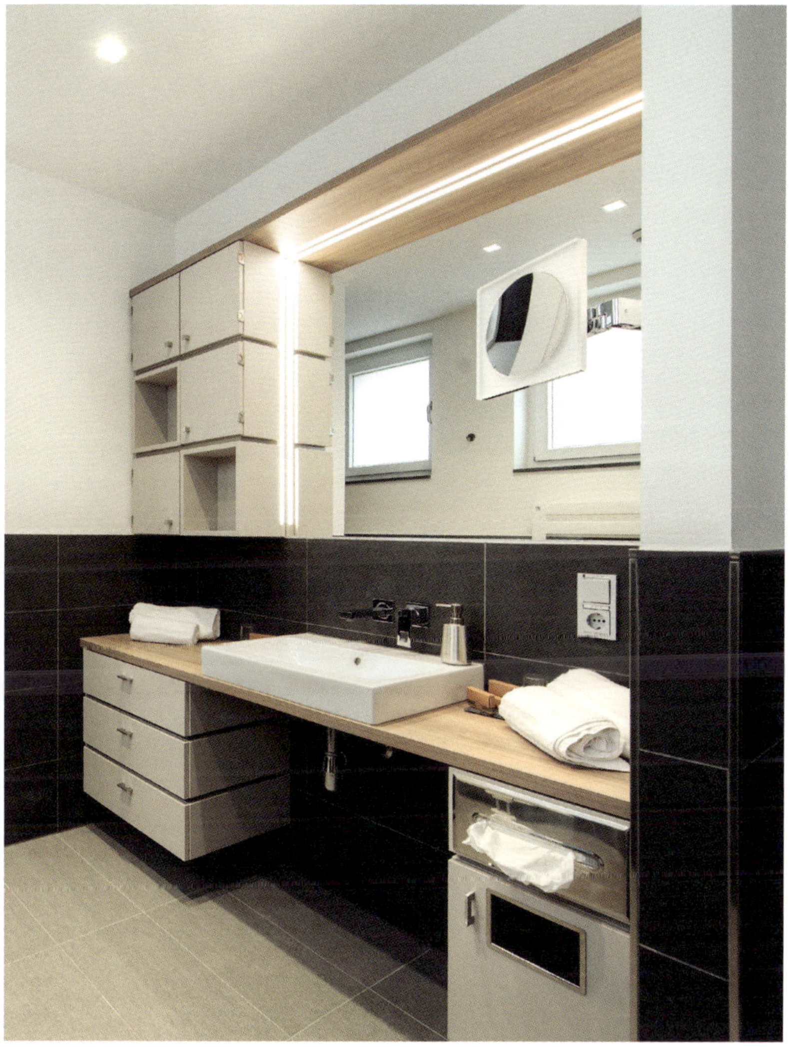

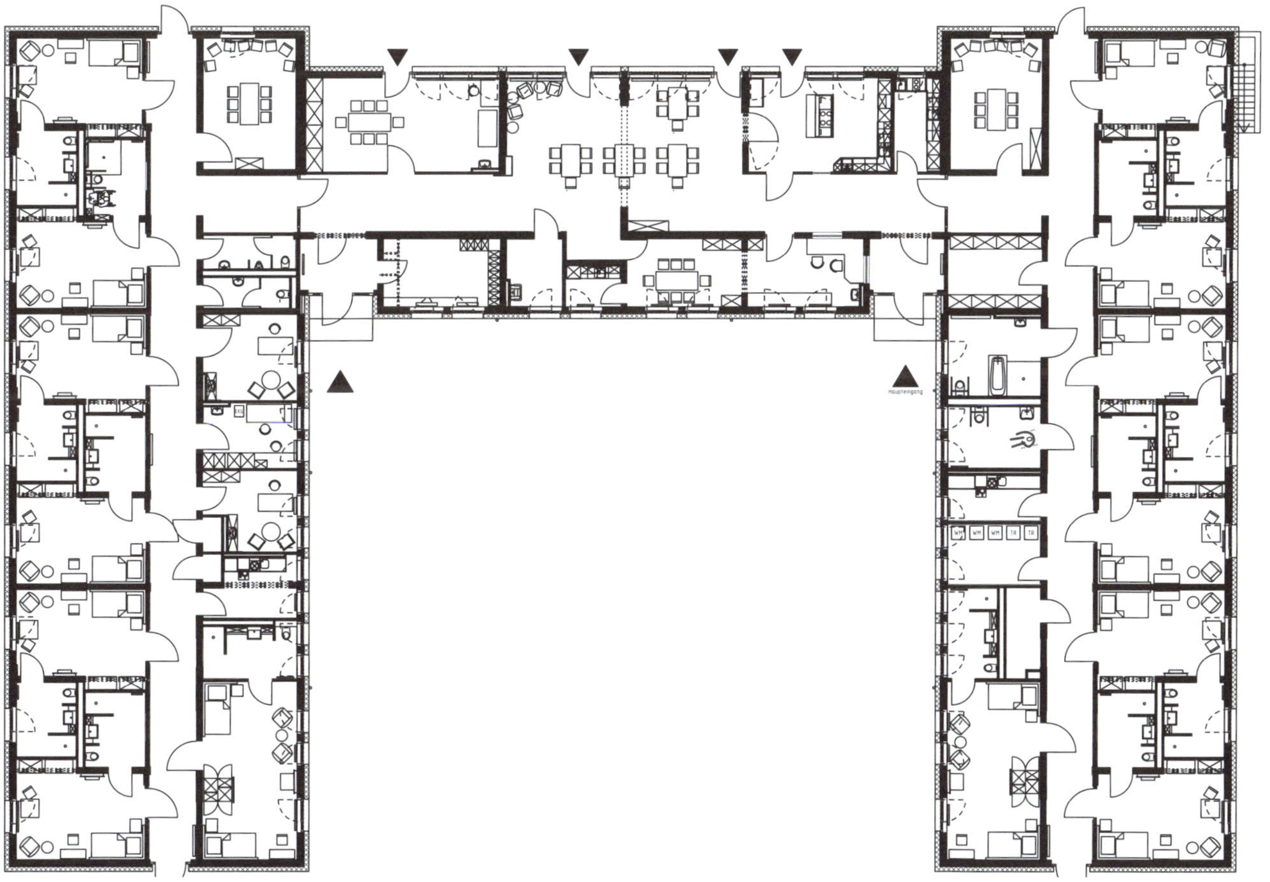

Built-in furniture ensures comfort.

Modern, accessible bathroom with illuminated niches and high-quality fixtures.

Floor plan.

Felix+Jonas Architekten

Kempten im Allgäu
Germany

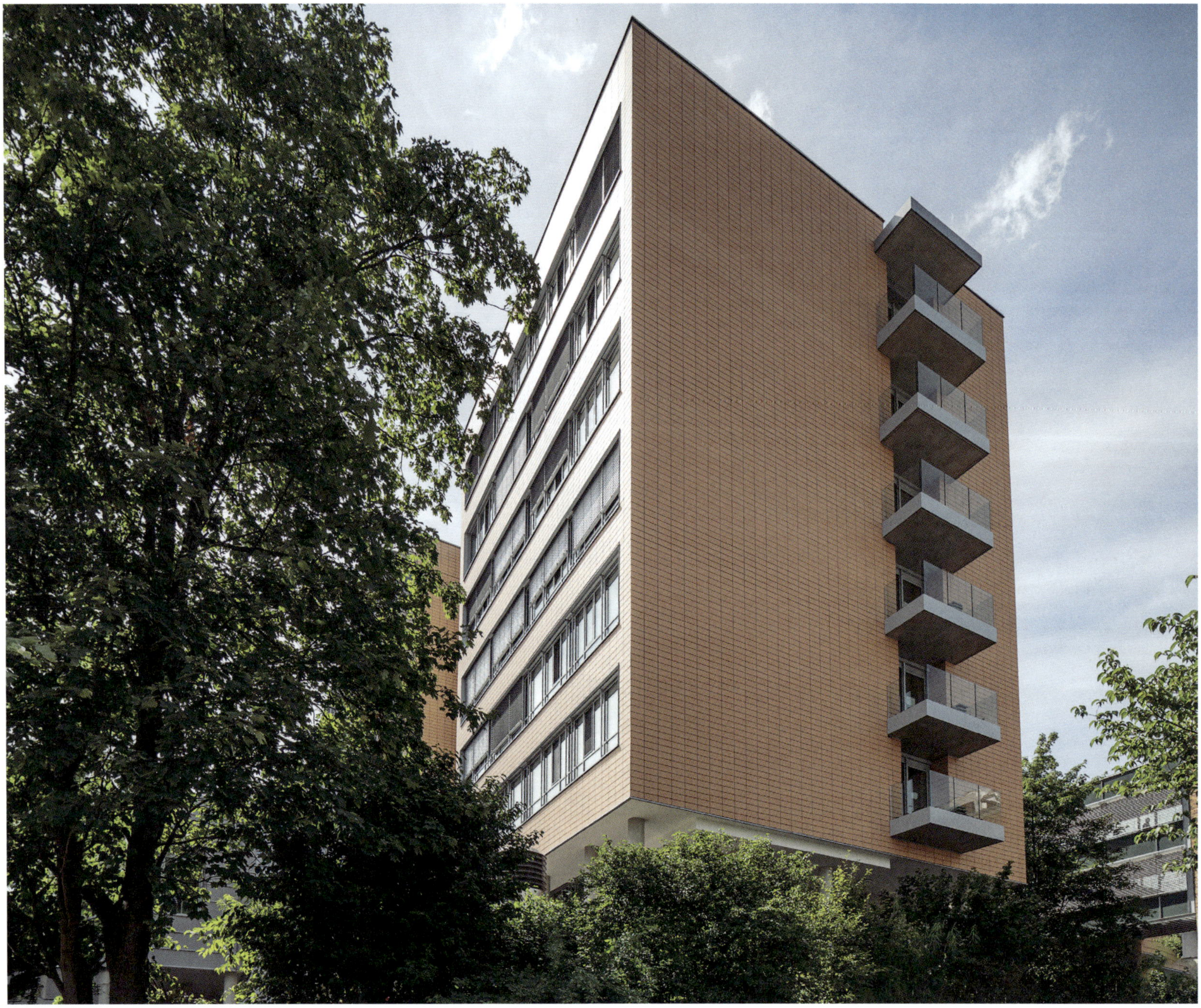

Exterior view of the ward building, seen from the side.

Front exterior view of the eight-story new building.

Kempten Oberallgäu Hospital Ward Building

With the expansion of its inpatient wing, Kempten Hospital is reinforcing its role as the largest hospital in the Allgäu region and a high-performing specialized hospital with 510 beds. The eight-story new building – completed in just under two years – provides modern facilities for 30 patients, including high-quality premium and comfort rooms. At the same time, the existing general care wards were expanded by four rooms per floor and supplemented with functional ancillary rooms. A central element is the new IMC (Intermediate Care) ward, which serves as a link between intensive and general care and meets the growing demands of patient monitoring. In this way, the expansion combines medical progress with thoughtful architecture and creates space for modern patient care.

Address: Robert-Weixler-Straße 50, 87439 Kempten im Allgäu, Germany | **Client:** Klinikverbund Allgäu gGmbH | **Completion:** 2019 | **Size:** 2,510 m^2 | **Sector:** state | **Number of patient rooms:** 24 | **Landscape design:** Schneider Landschaftsarchitekten

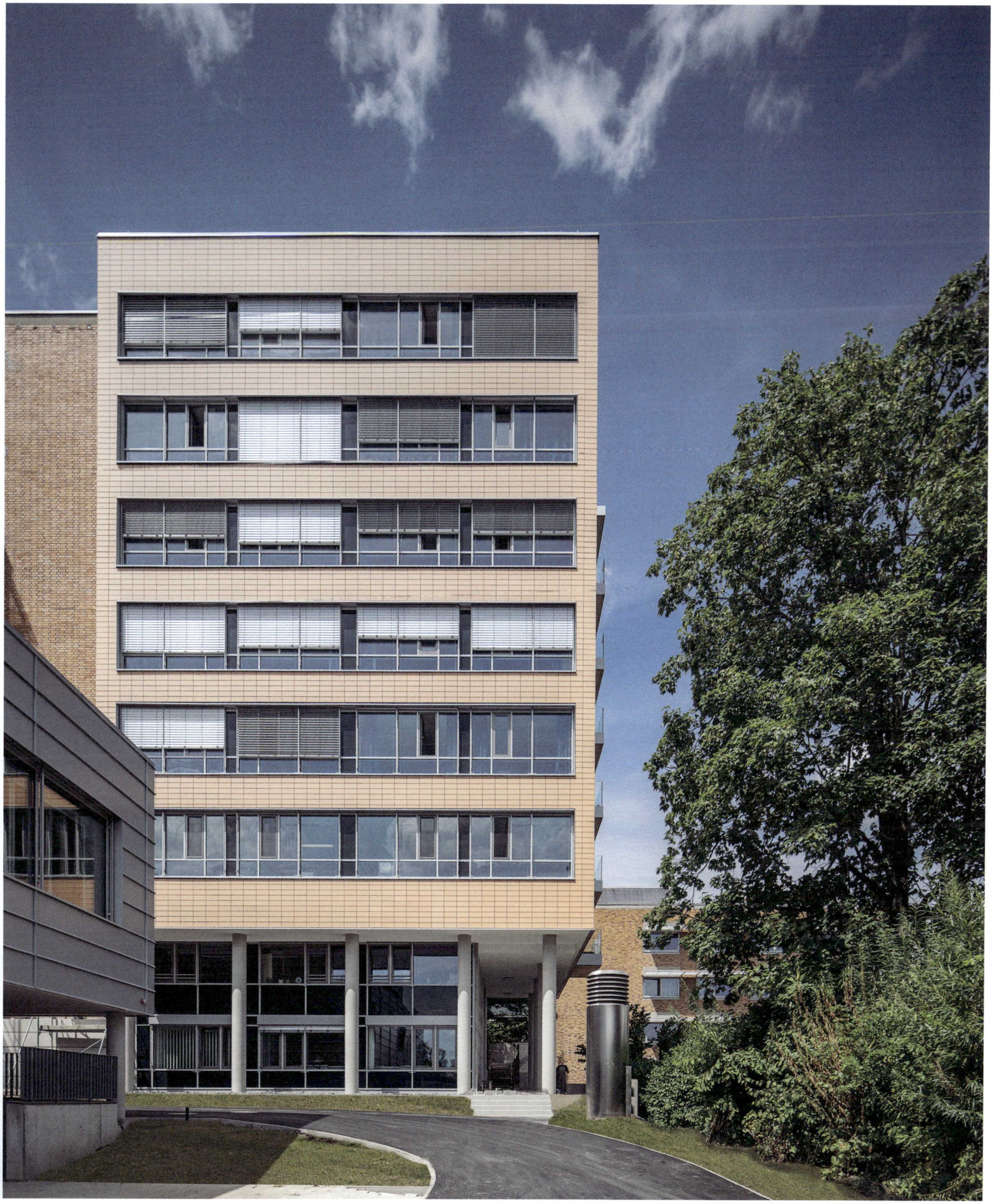

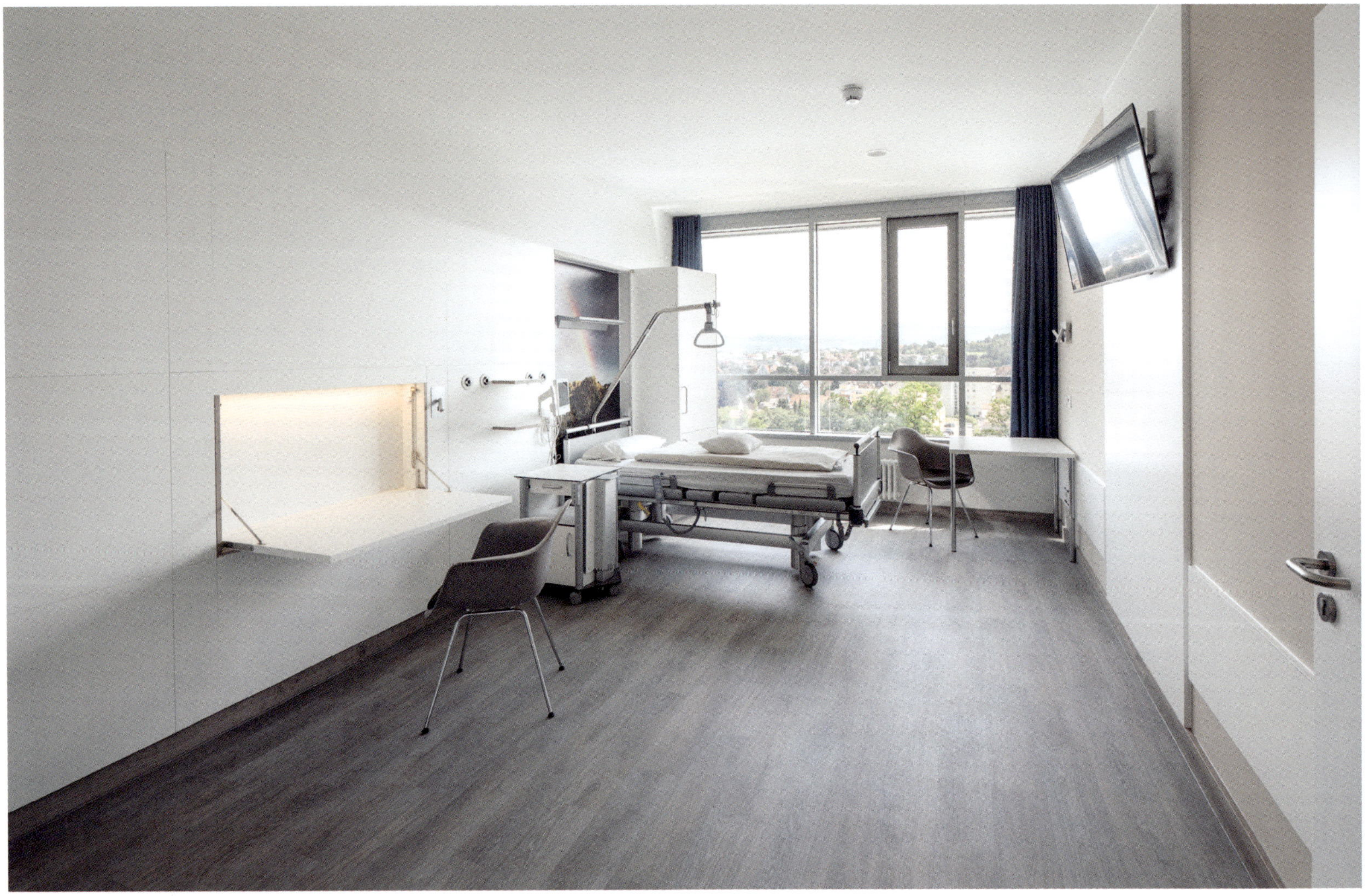

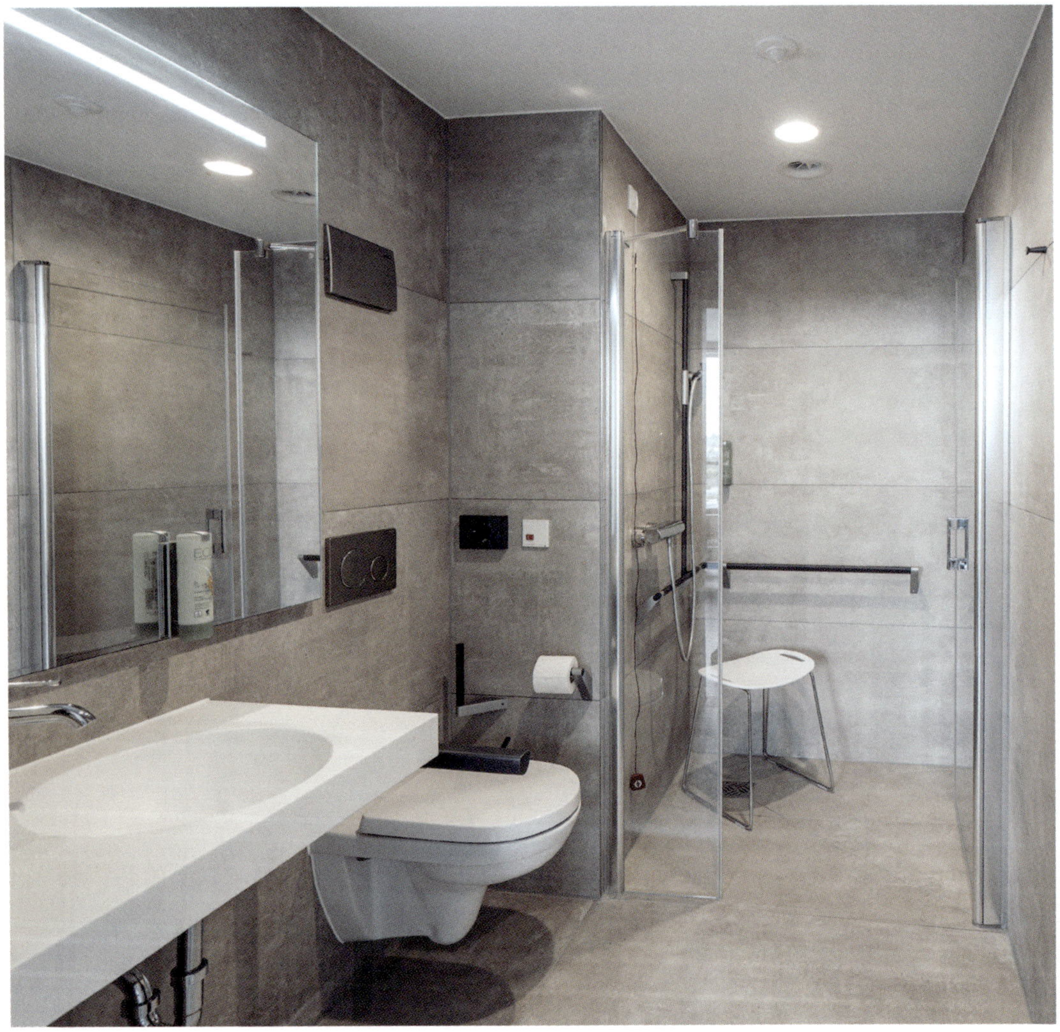

Patient room with a sweeping view of the Allgäu region.

Bathroom with hotel-style amenities designed for accessibility.

Figure-ground plan.

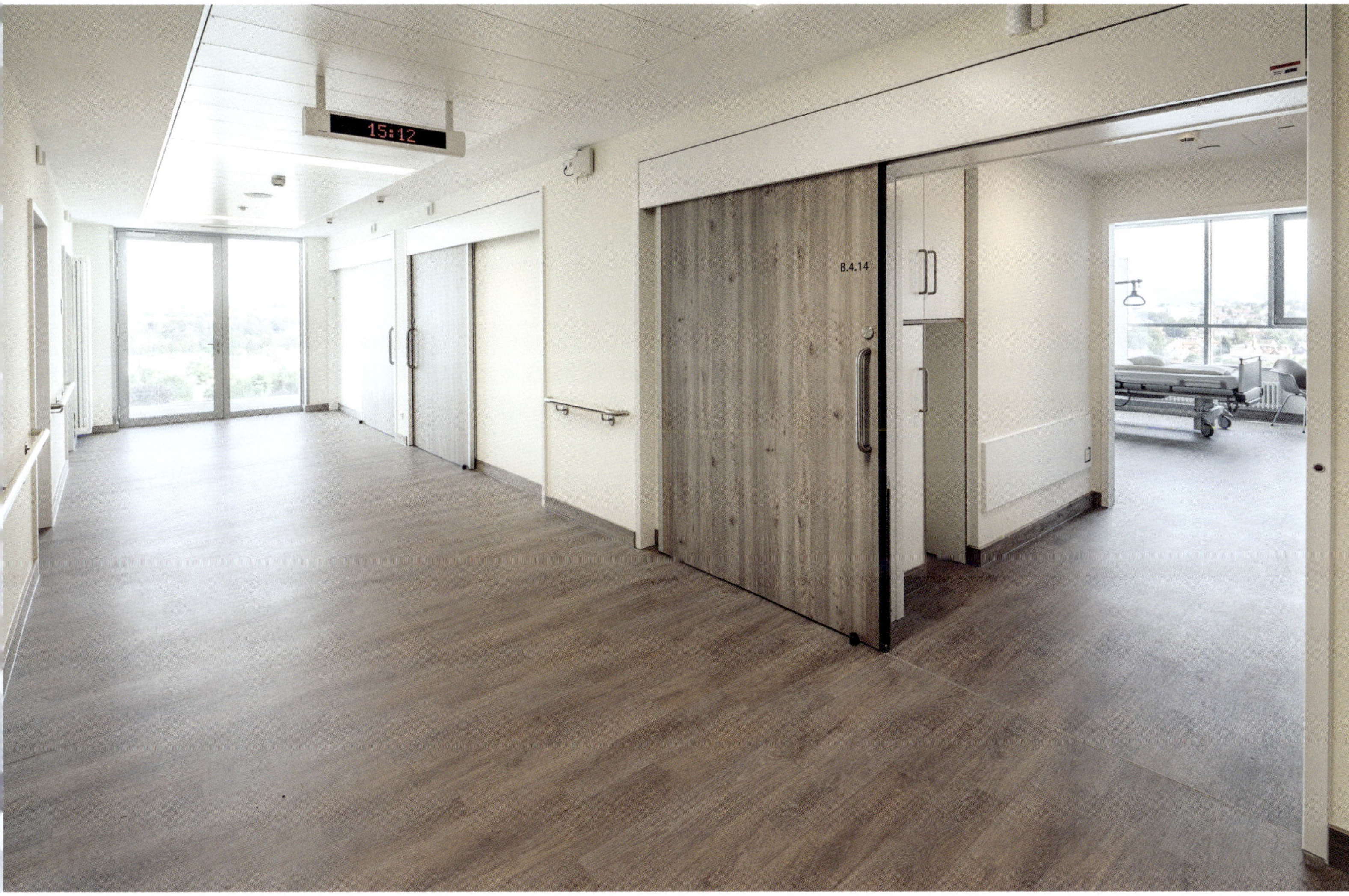

Spacious hallway with sliding doors that open wide.

Typical floor plan.

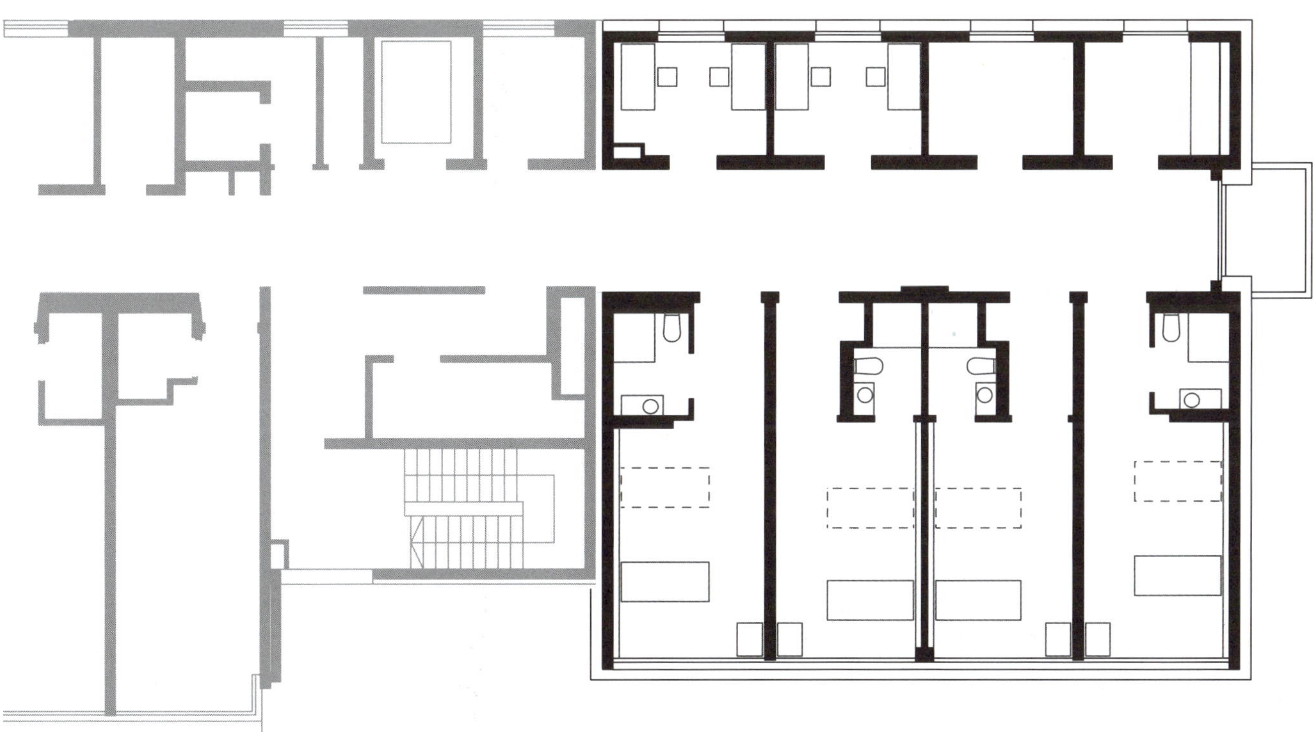

Herzog & de Meuron

Zurich
Switzerland

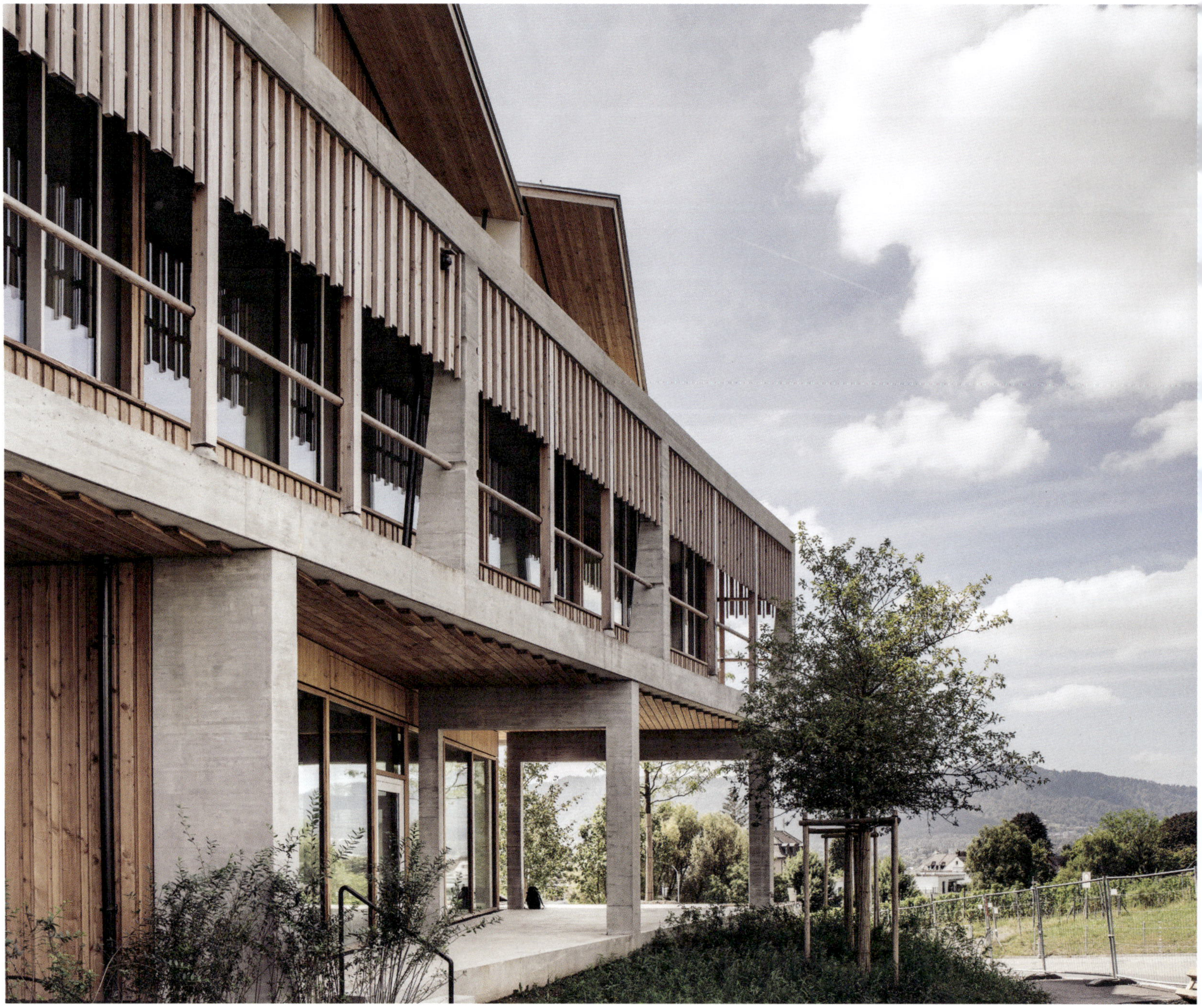

The acute-care hospital consists of a three-story concrete frame with intricate wooden infills that blend into the landscape.

Various green courtyards provide orientation and bring daylight into the building.

University Children's Hospital Zurich

The new University Children's Hospital in Zurich-Lengg is Switzerland's largest hospital for children and adolescents. Designed as a healing environment, the three-story acute-care hospital combines a load-bearing concrete structure with warm wooden elements that blend into the surrounding landscape. Its interior is organized like a small town, with a central main street, courtyards, squares, and neighborhoods that provide intuitive orientation, daylight, and connections to nature. The upper floor accommodates 114 inpatient rooms, each designed as an individual wooden cottage with its own roof, offering privacy, views of greenery, and space for parents to stay overnight. Flexible layouts, natural materials, abundant daylight, and landscaped outdoor areas support patient well-being, while over 250 newly planted trees reinforce the hospital's close relationship with nature.

Address: Lenggstrasse 30, 8008 Zurich, Switzerland | **Client:** Kinderspital Zürich – Eleonorenstiftung | **Completion:** 2024 | **Size:** 96,246 m² | **Sector:** public | **Specialization:** pediatric care | **Number of patient rooms:** 114

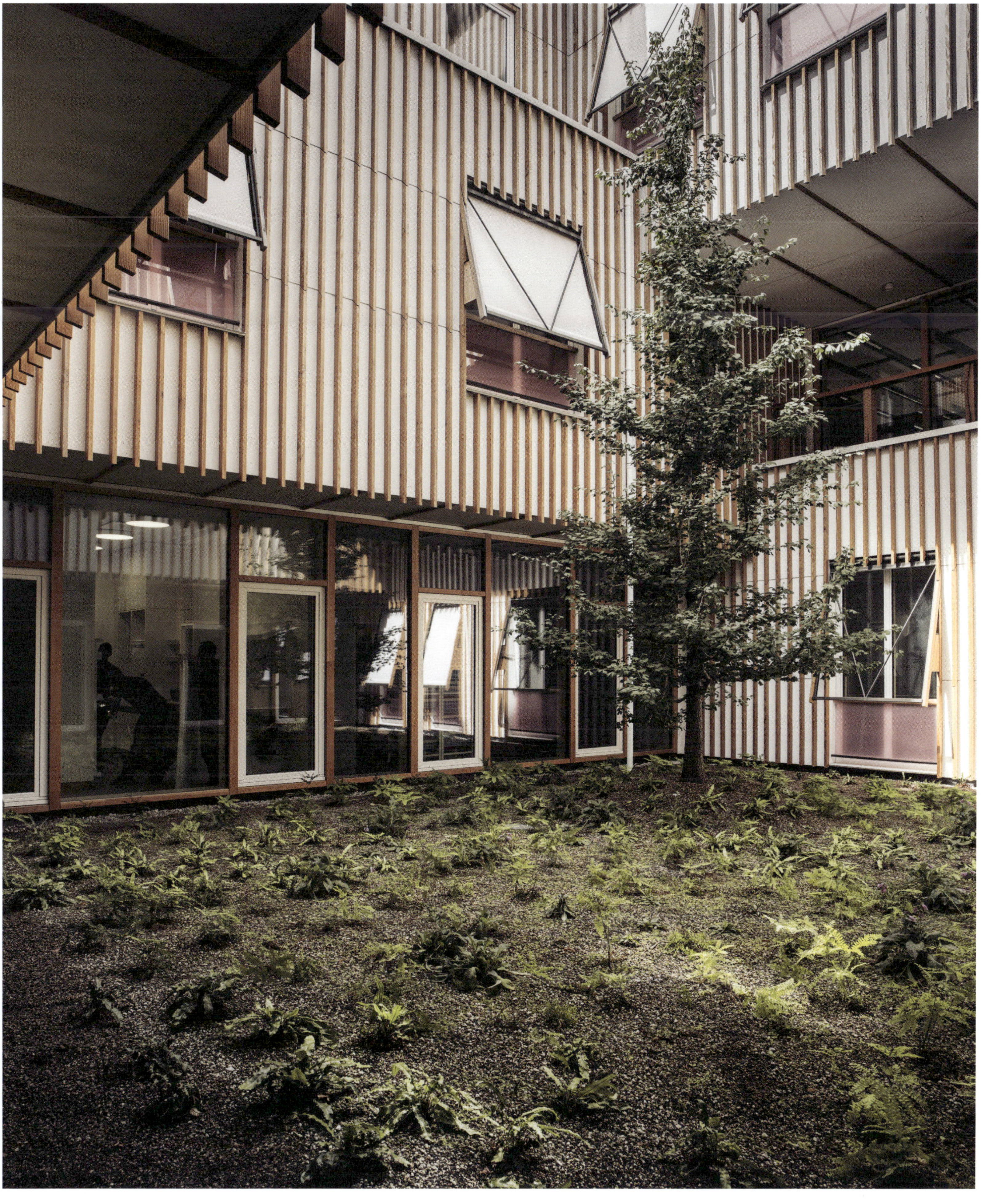

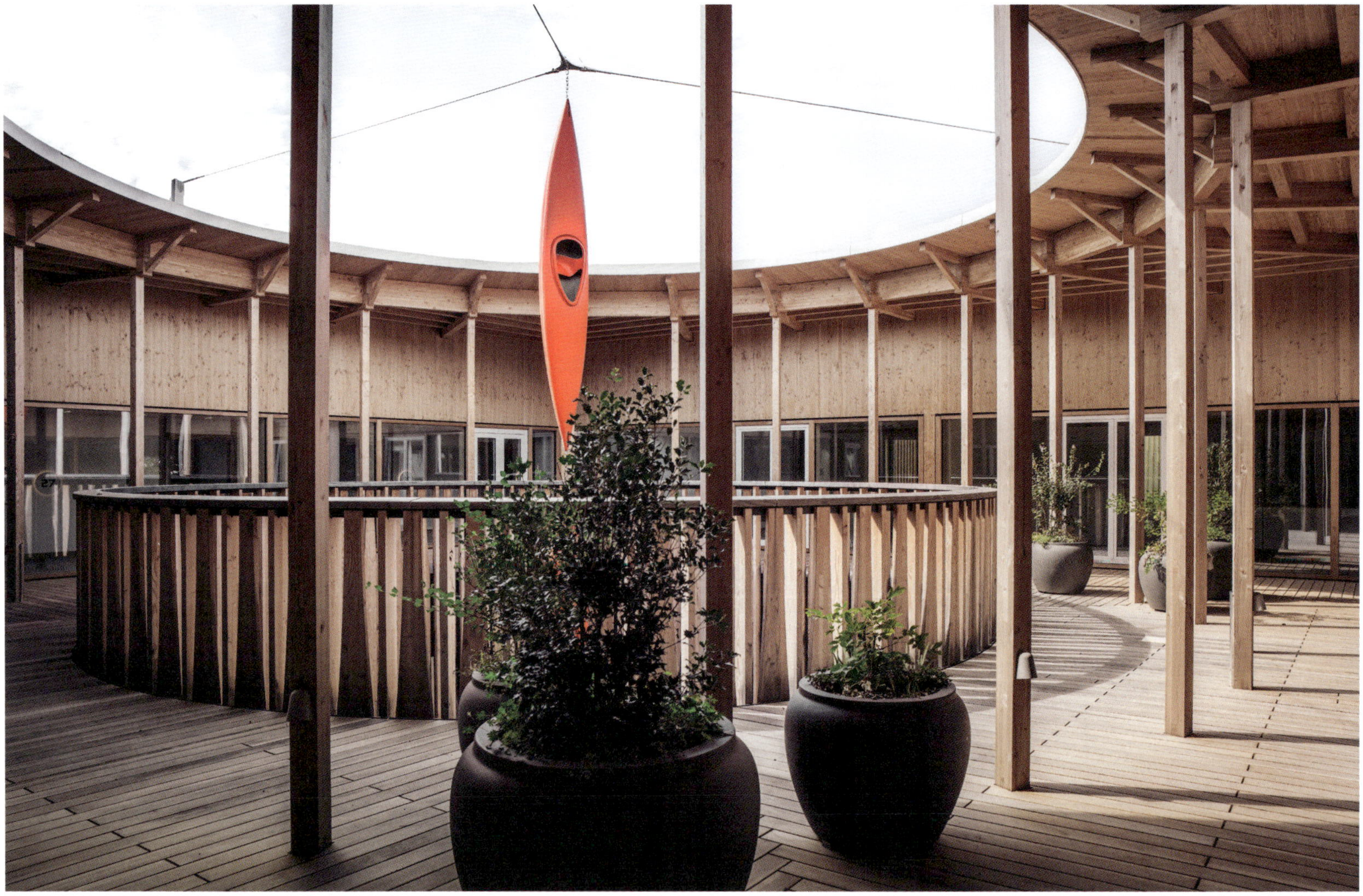

Circular courtyard on the upper floor.

Ground floor plan with land-scaped surroundings.

Boulevards on ground, first and second floor.

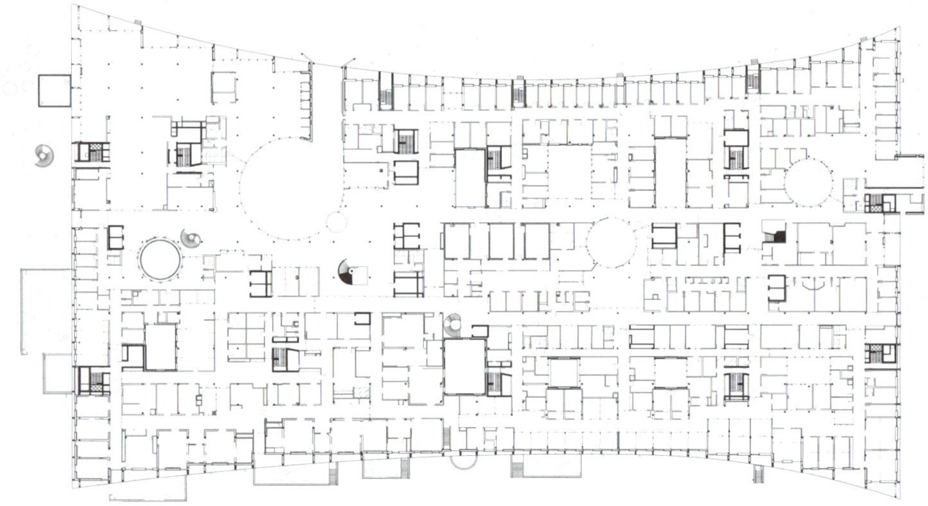

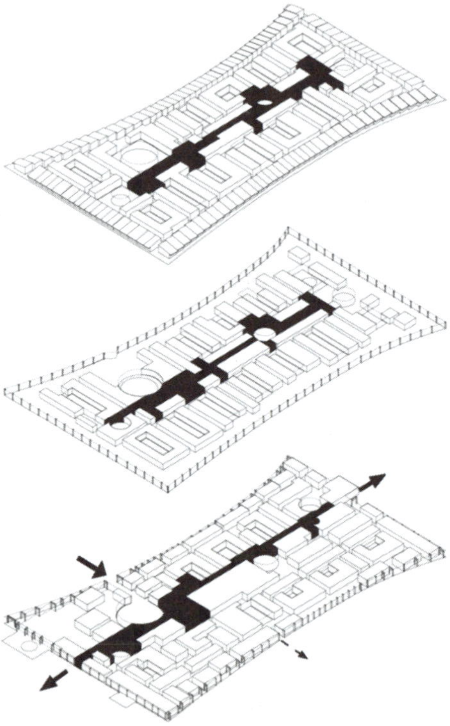

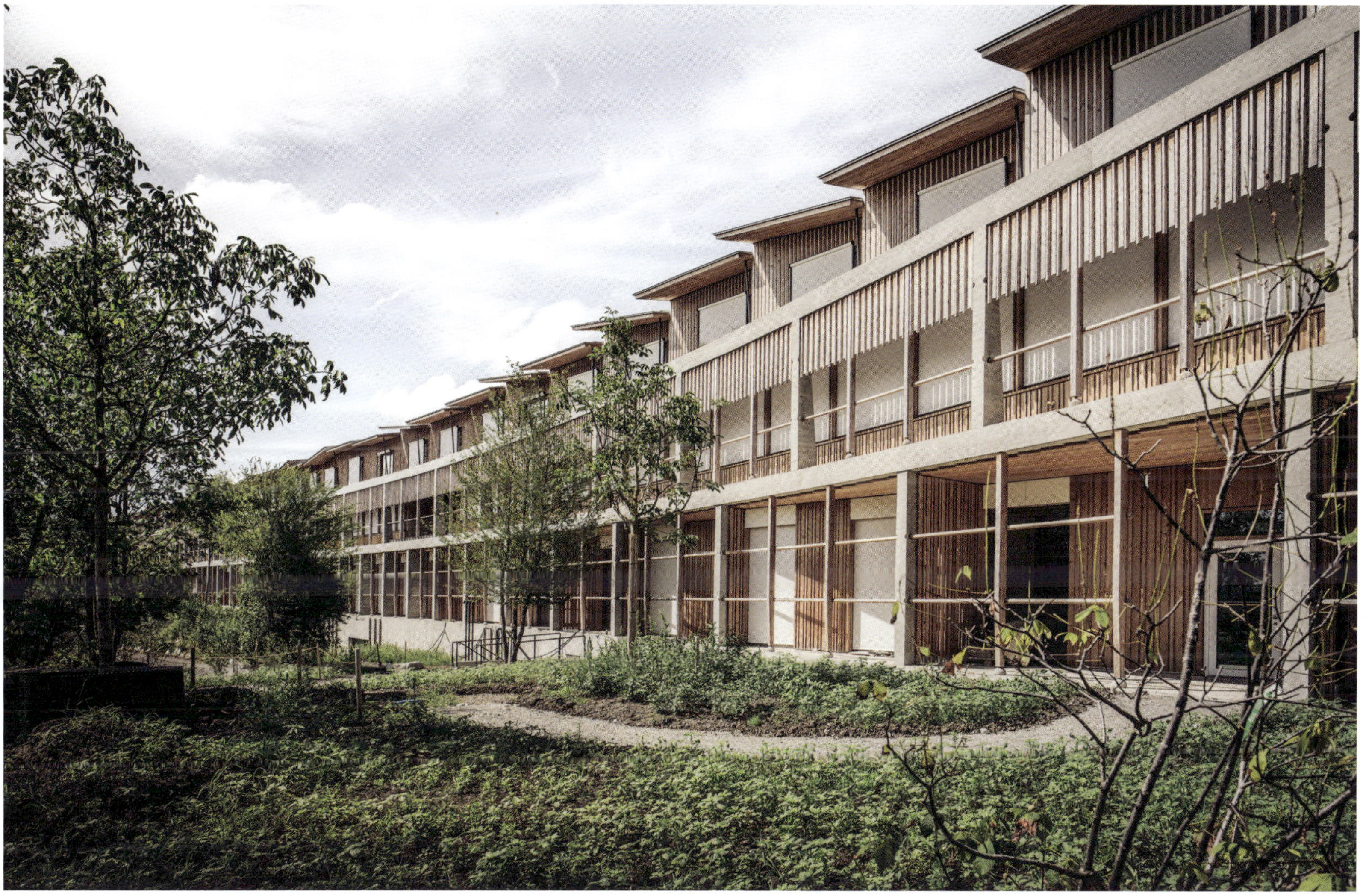

Various green courtyards that provide orientation and bring daylight into the building.

Second floor plan.

Section.

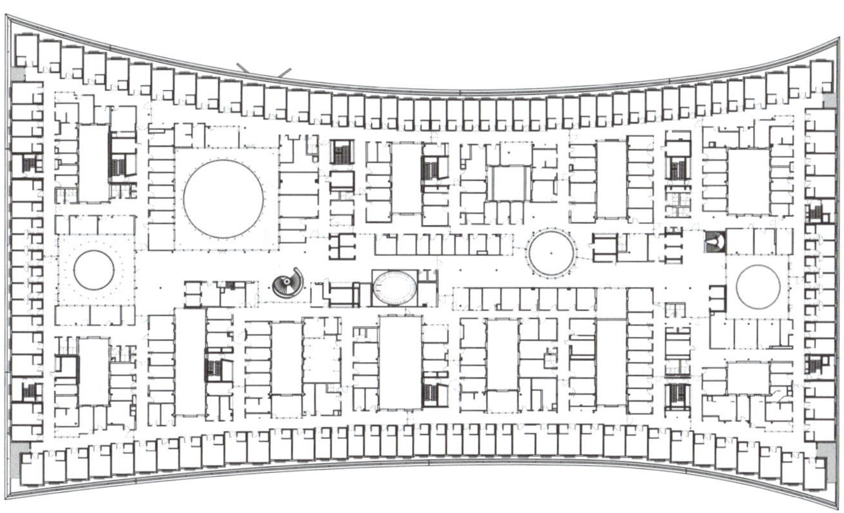

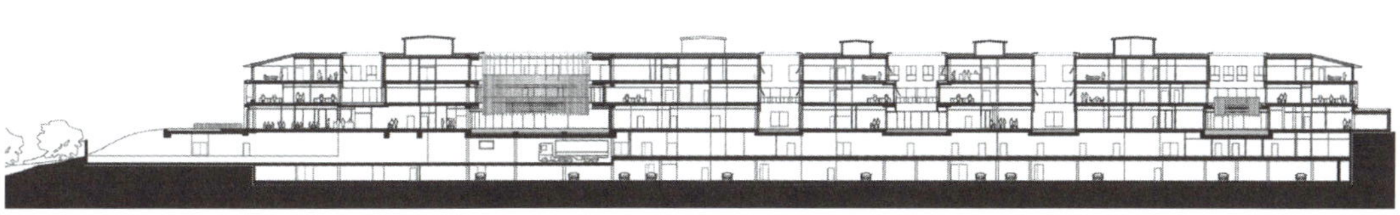

100% interior
Sylvia Leydecker

Cologne
Germany

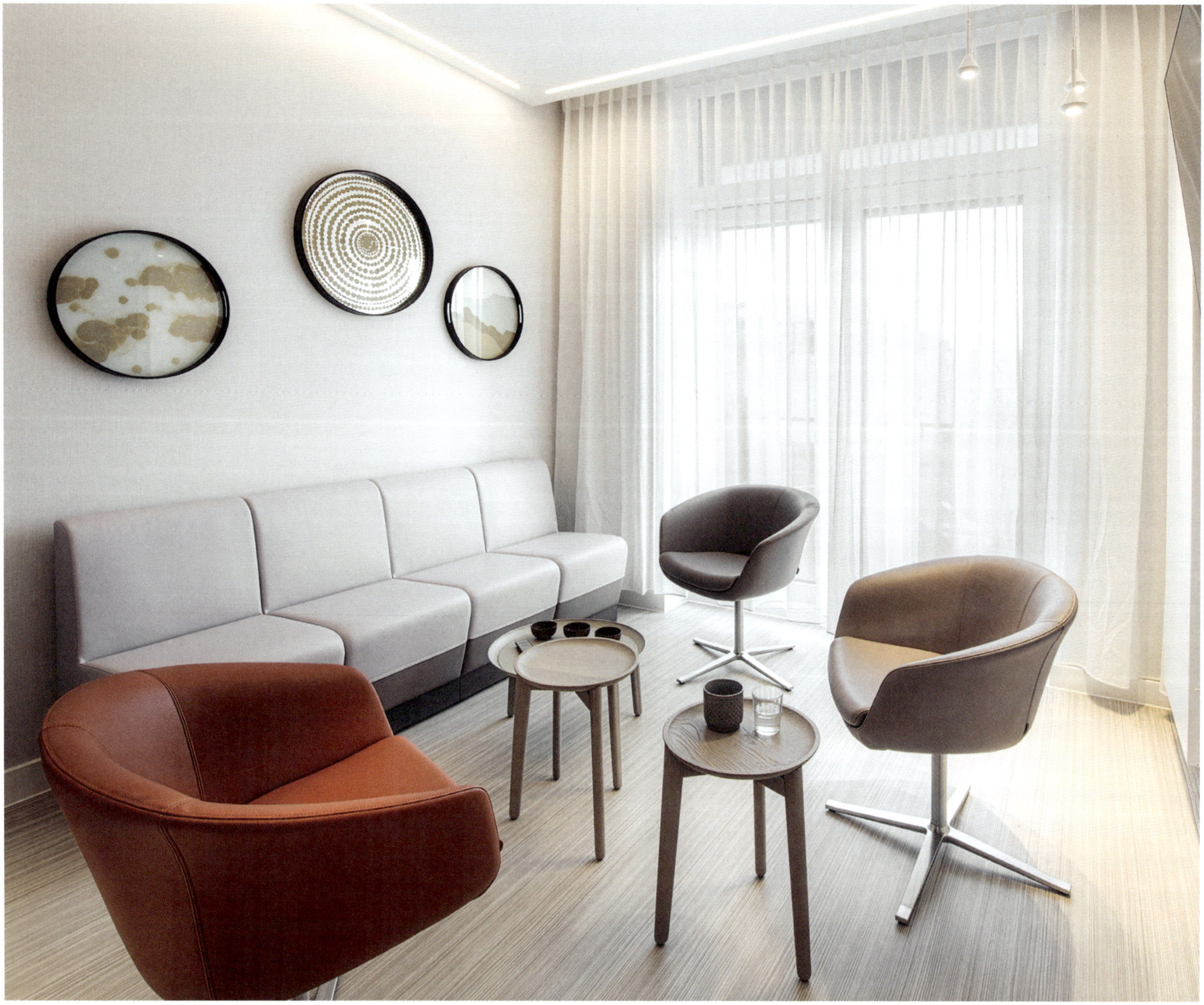

The inviting patient lounge supports a restorative healing environment.

Modern, elegant, and timeless, the comfortable patient room unfolds in natural daylight.

University Hospital Cologne ENT Private Ward

The high standards of cutting-edge medicine at this renowned university hospital, are paired with contemporary architectural concept in the ENT ward. Patients recover here in a future-oriented level of comfort, embedded in an elegantly modern and understated design language. Innovative service duct covers were specially developed for this project. The look and feel of a premium lounge carefully complement the patient rooms, featuring a composition of shades of gray, subtle metallic accents, wood, and natural stone. Closely aligned with the specific clinical profile of otorhinolaryngology, innovations such as acoustically effective transparent textiles enhance the overall patient experience. Medicine and design merge here into a coherent symbiosis, elevating patient safety to a new level and ensuring its appropriate recognition within the architectural and clinical concept.

Address: Gleueler Straße 22Z, 50931 Cologne, Germany | **Client:** medfacilities GmbH | **Completion:** 2024 | **Size:** 800 m^2 | **Original building:** ENT inpatient building, 1961 | **Sector:** public | **Specialization:** clinic and outpatient clinic for otorhinolaryngology | **Number of patient rooms:** 20

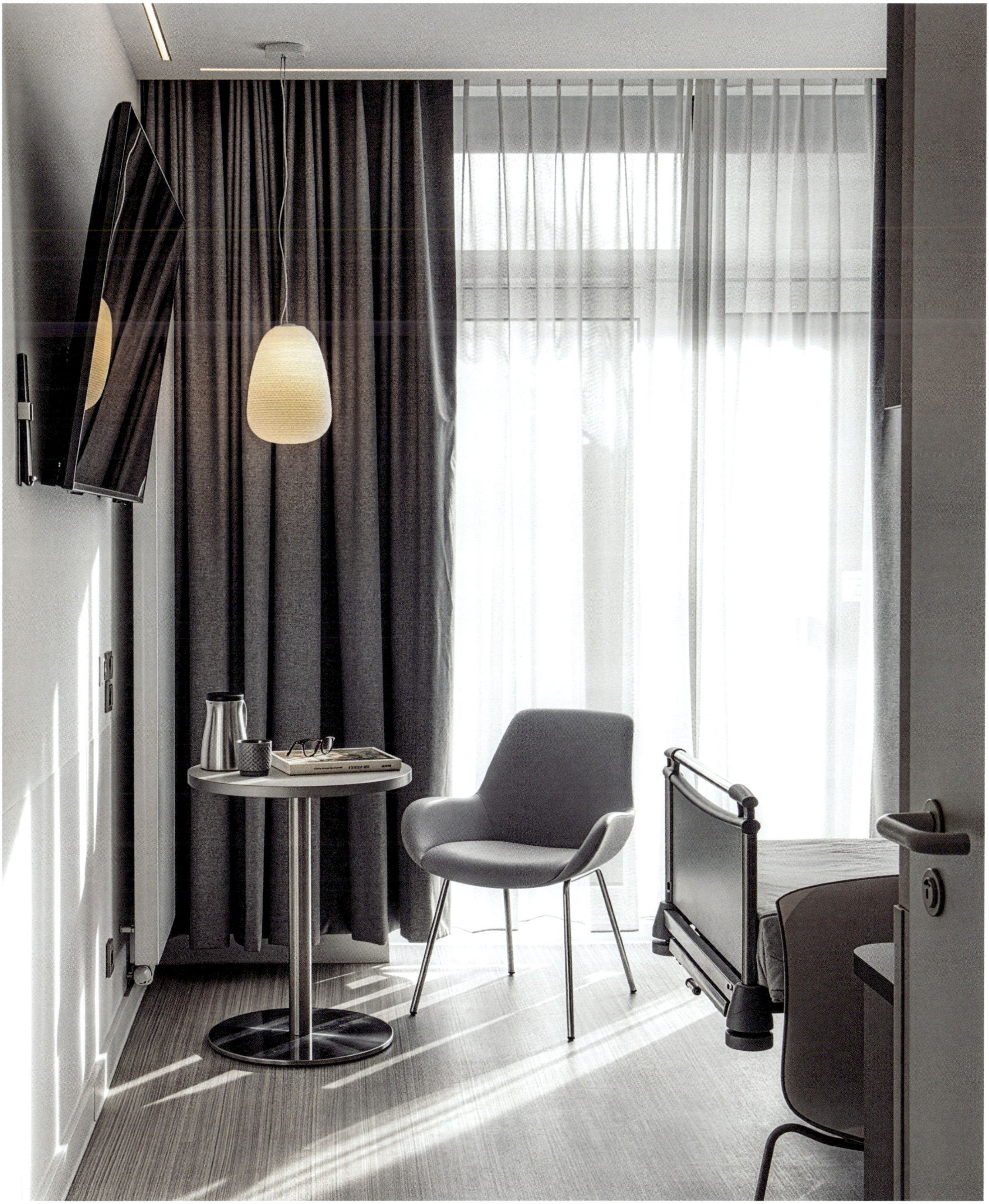

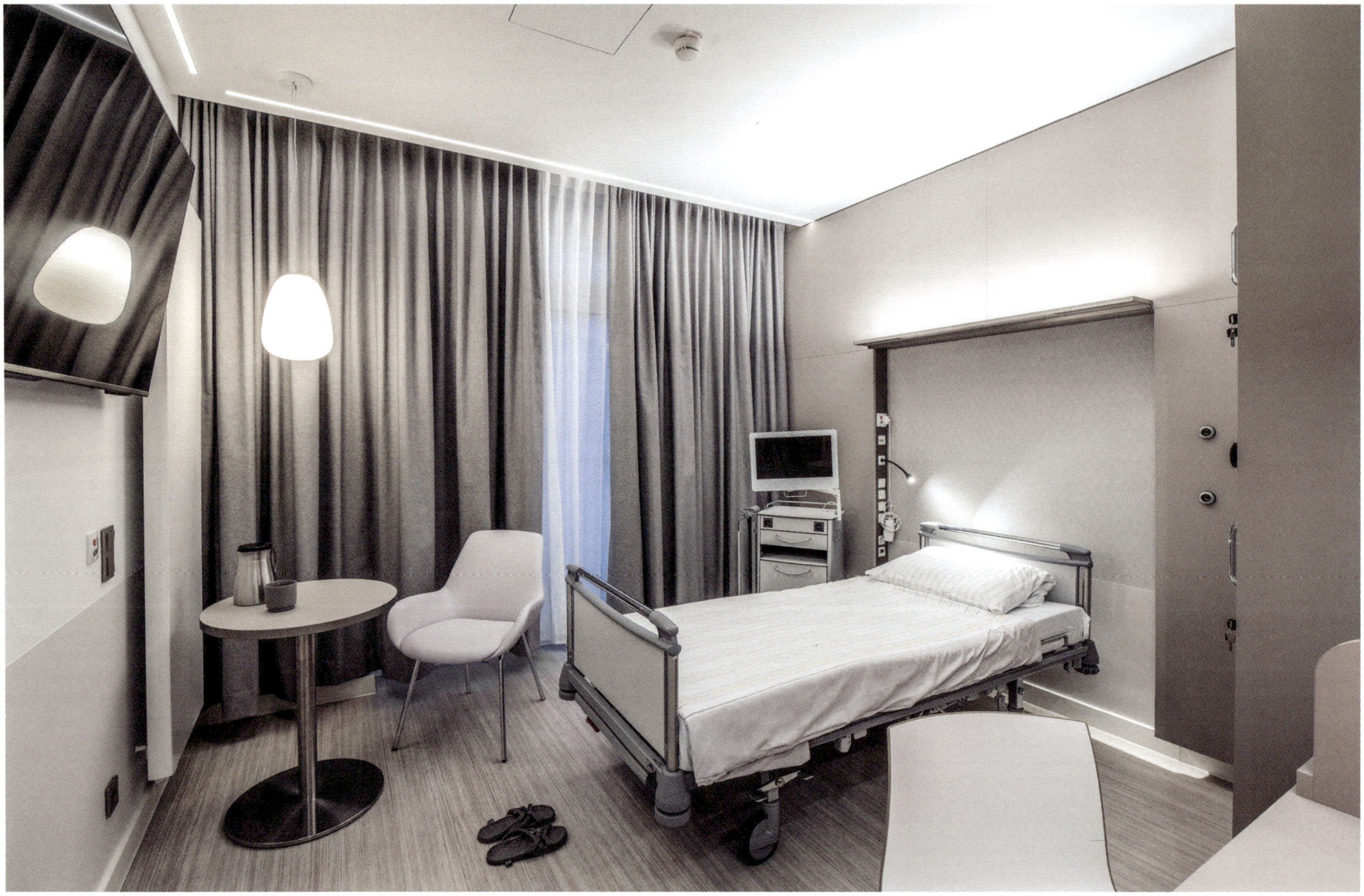

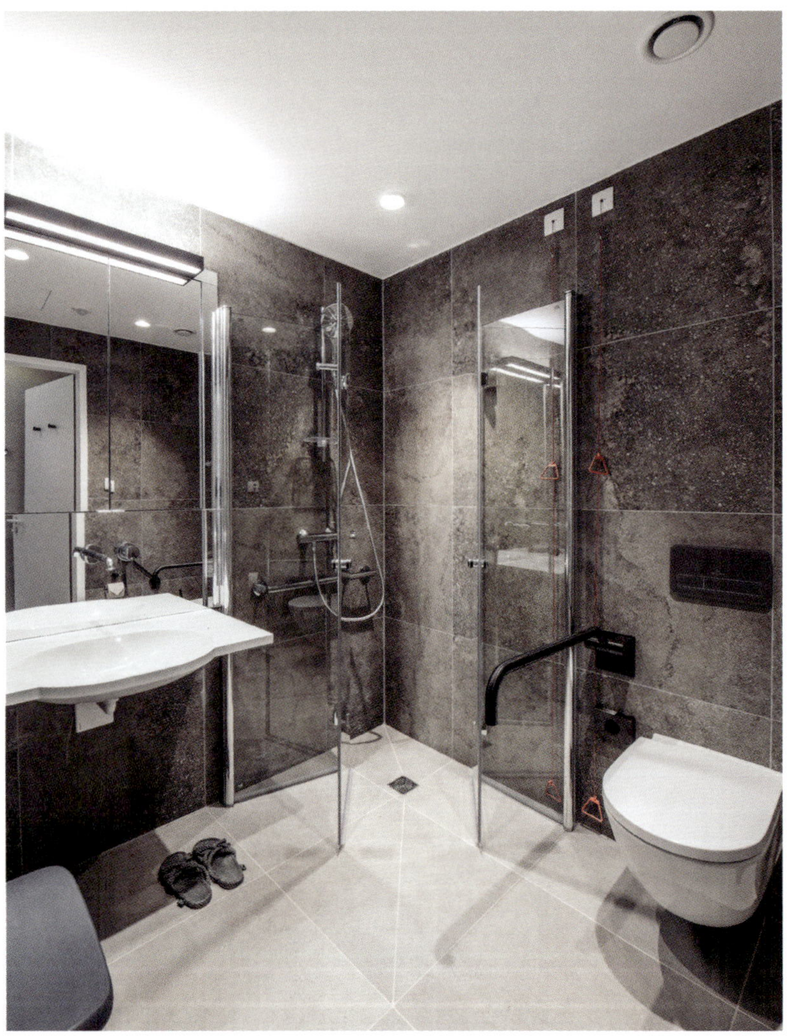

The hygienically immaculate patient room at dusk, with closed curtains and a carefully layered lighting concept.

The bathroom creates an elegant impression and complements the natural color nuances and subtle textures of the patient room.

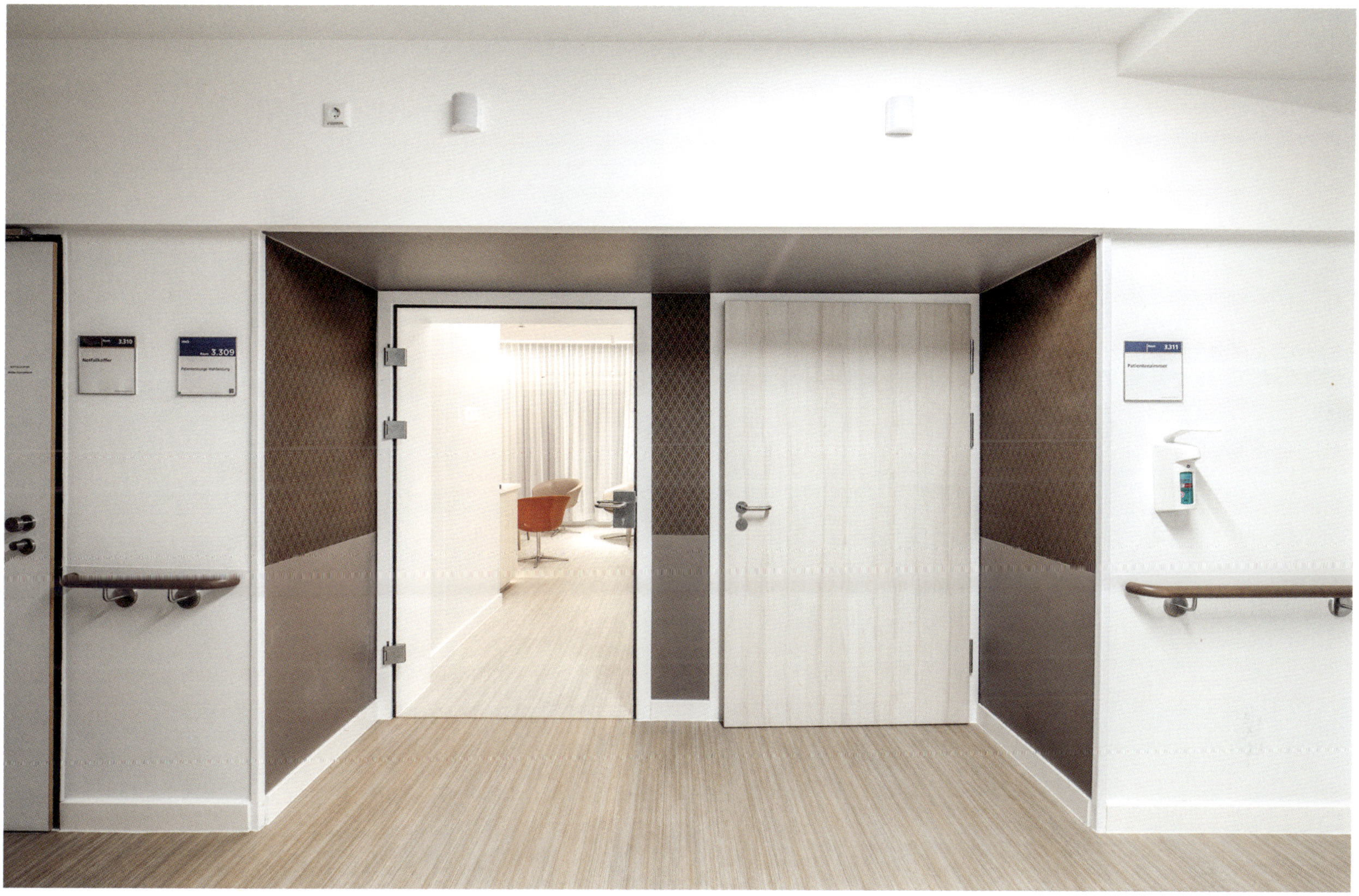

The corridor with its clearly defined design language.

Patient room plan.

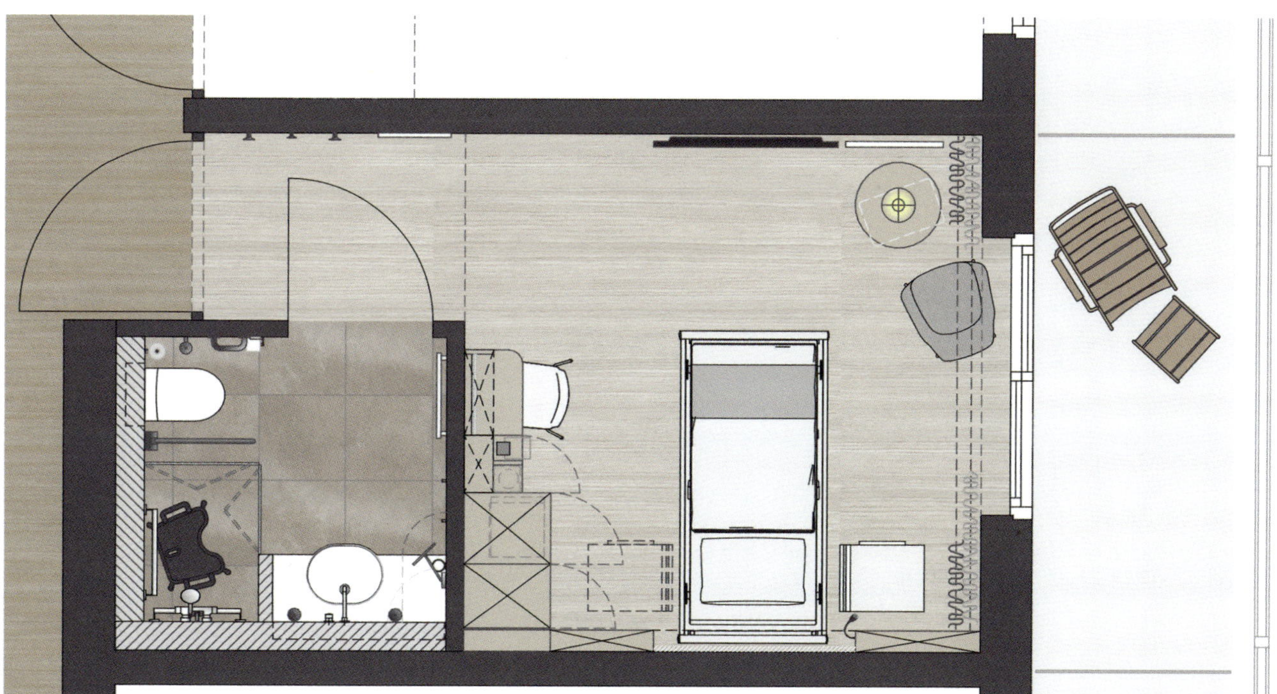

P+HS Architect

Middlesbrough
United Kingdom

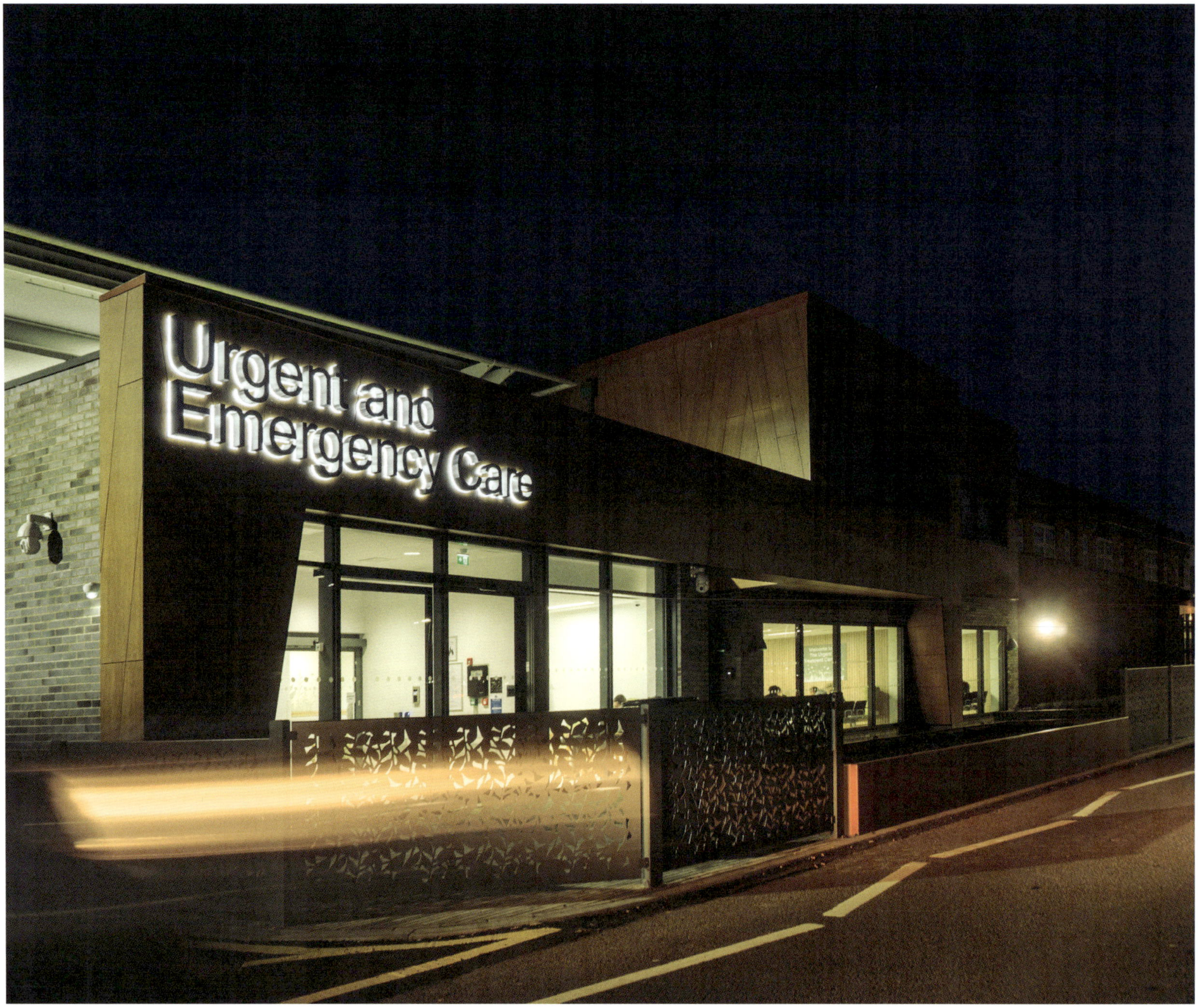

Night view showing clearly visible lettering on the new building.

Daytime view showing the portal-like entrance area in reddish wood.

Lettering on wood at daytime.

James Cook – Urgent Treatment Centre

The James Cook Urgent Treatment Centre (UTC) is a new modular healthcare facility delivered as part of urgent and emergency care services in the Teesside area. Located adjacent to the Emergency Department at The James Cook University Hospital, the UTC improves patient flow, increases capacity and ensures patients receive care through the most appropriate pathway. Designed using modern methods of construction, 27 modules were manufactured off-site, reducing the construction program from 44 to 32 weeks while achieving zero waste to landfill. Natural materials, calming interiors, and intuitive way-finding enhance patient experience, while the flexible modular design allows future adaptation. Within its first six months of operation, the UTC treated more than 30,000 patients and contributed to a 36 percent reduction in accident and emergency attendance.

Address: Marton Road, Middlesbrough TS4 3BW, United Kingdom | **Client:** South Tees Hospitals NHS Foundation Trust | **Completion:** 2024 | **Size:** 982 m² | **Sector:** state | **Specialization:** urgent and emergency care | **Number of treatment rooms:** 11

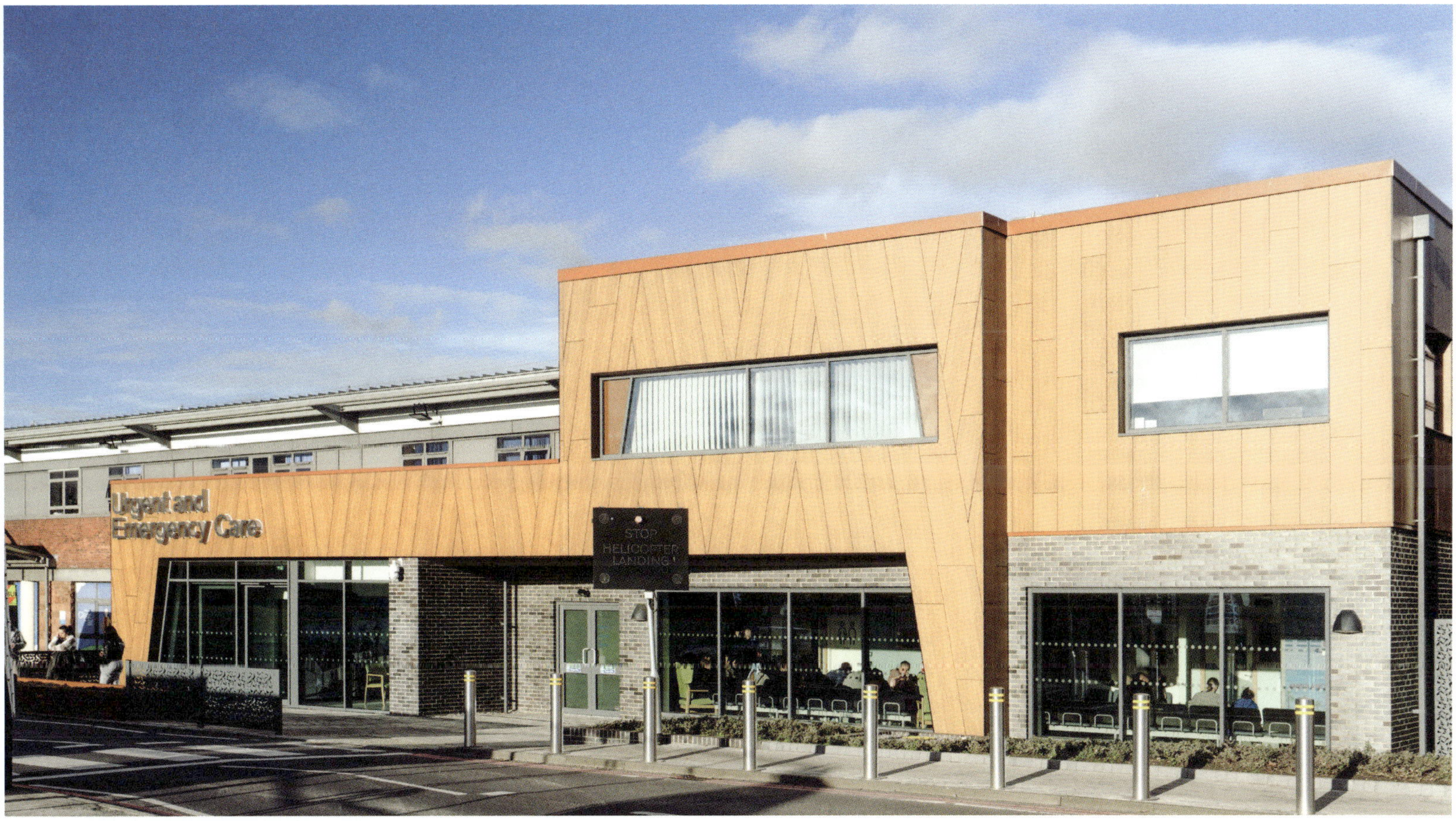

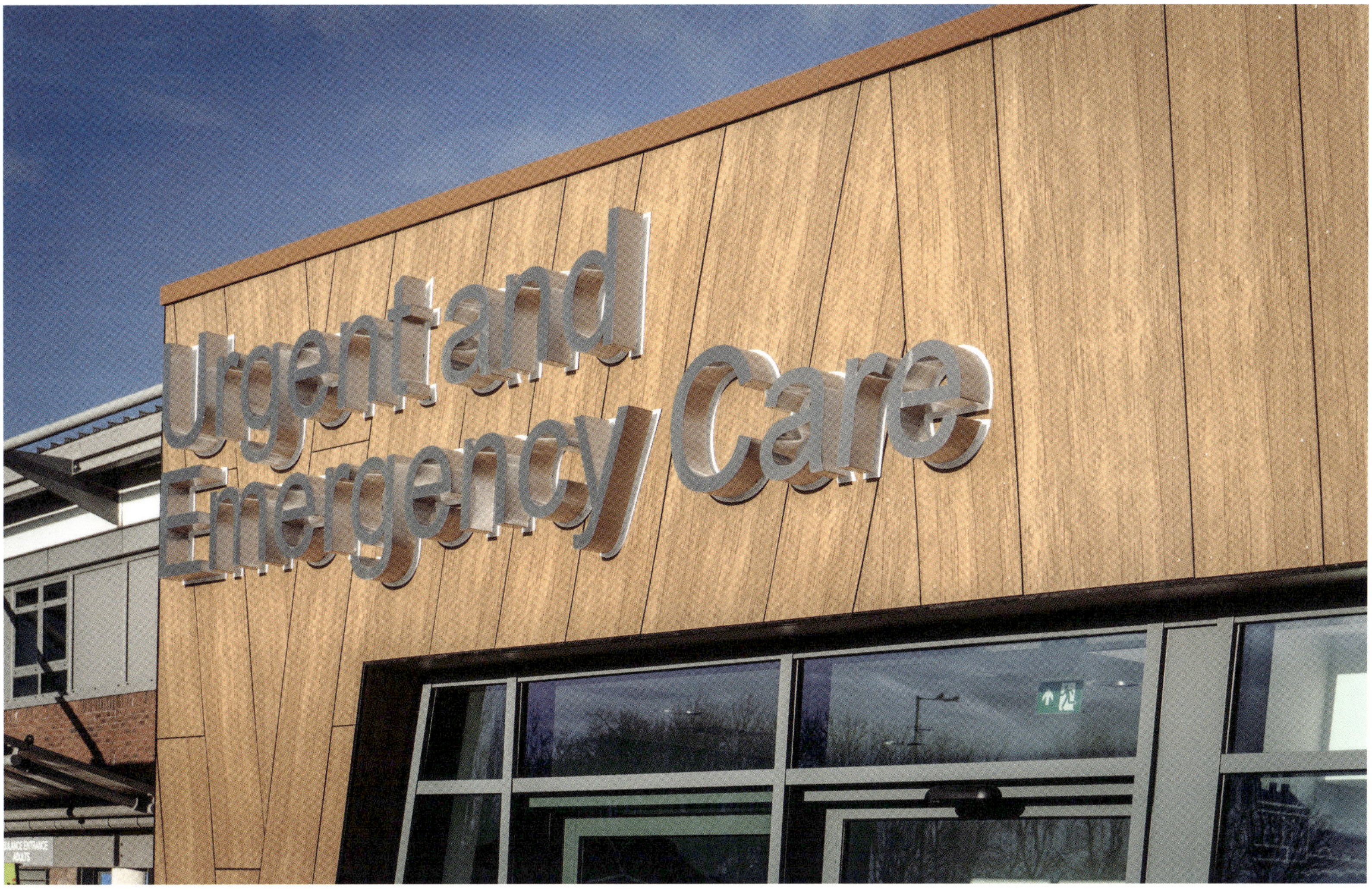

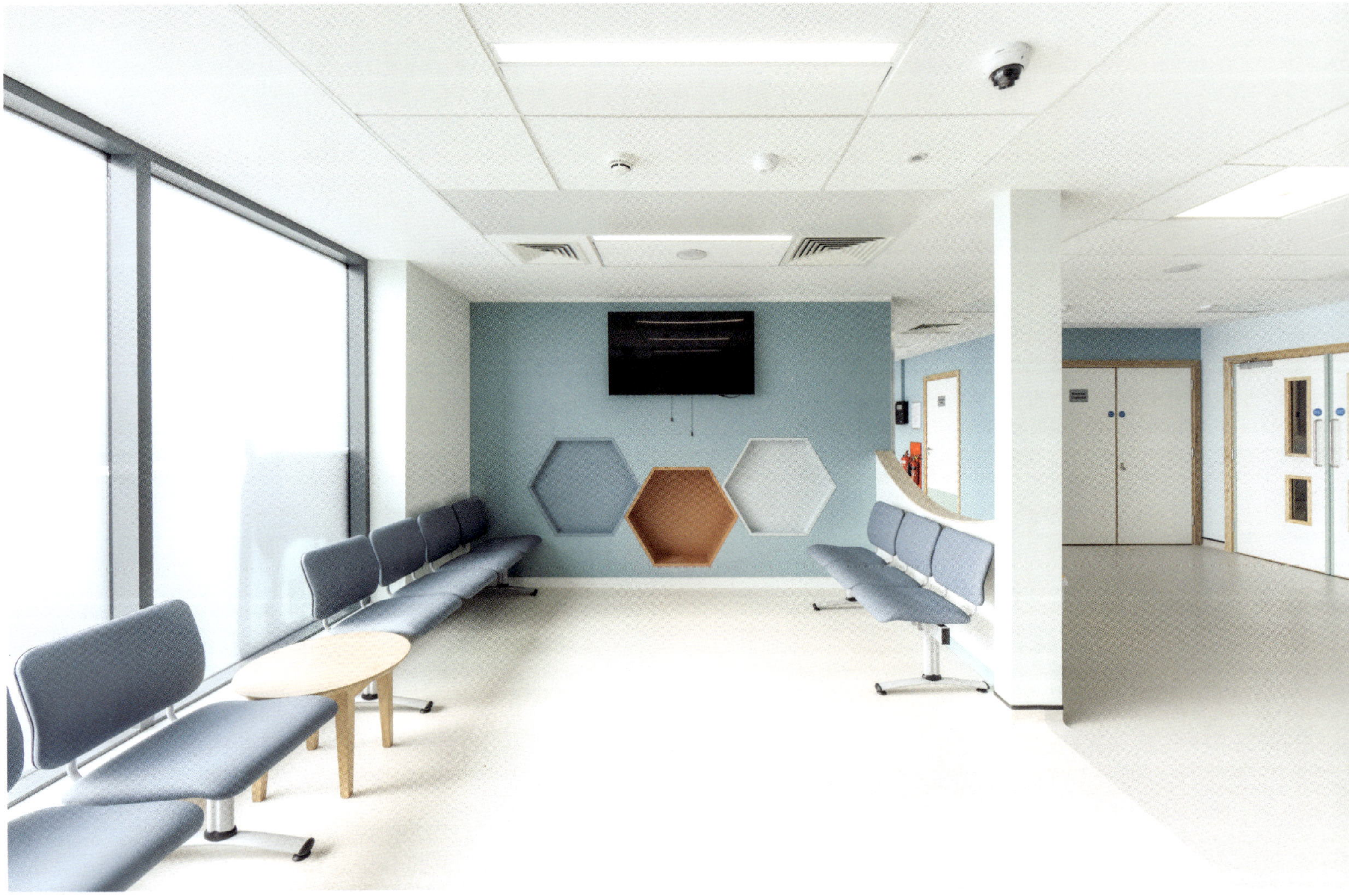

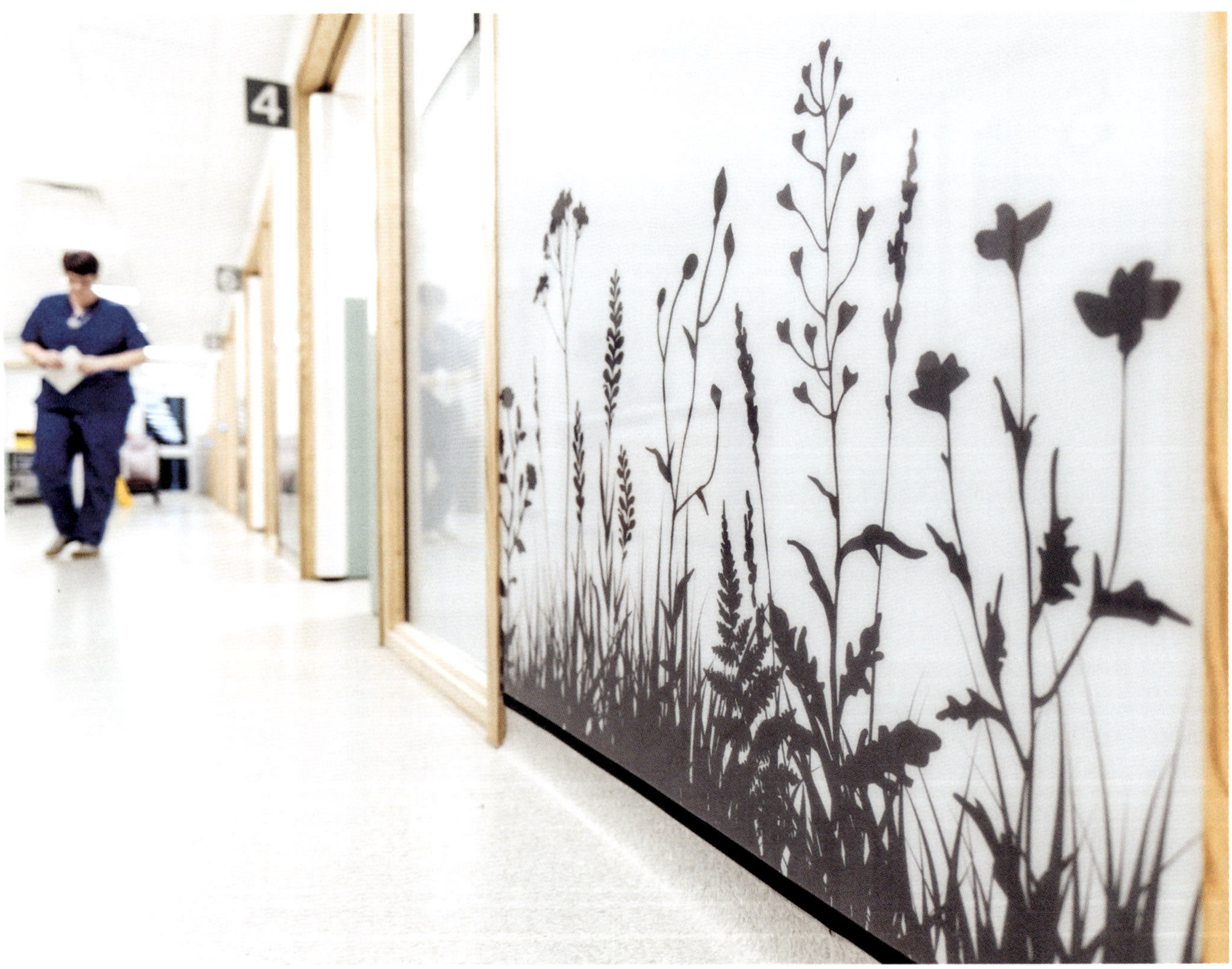

The facility includes separate adult and paediatric waiting areas.

Bright lit corridor to the treatment rooms.

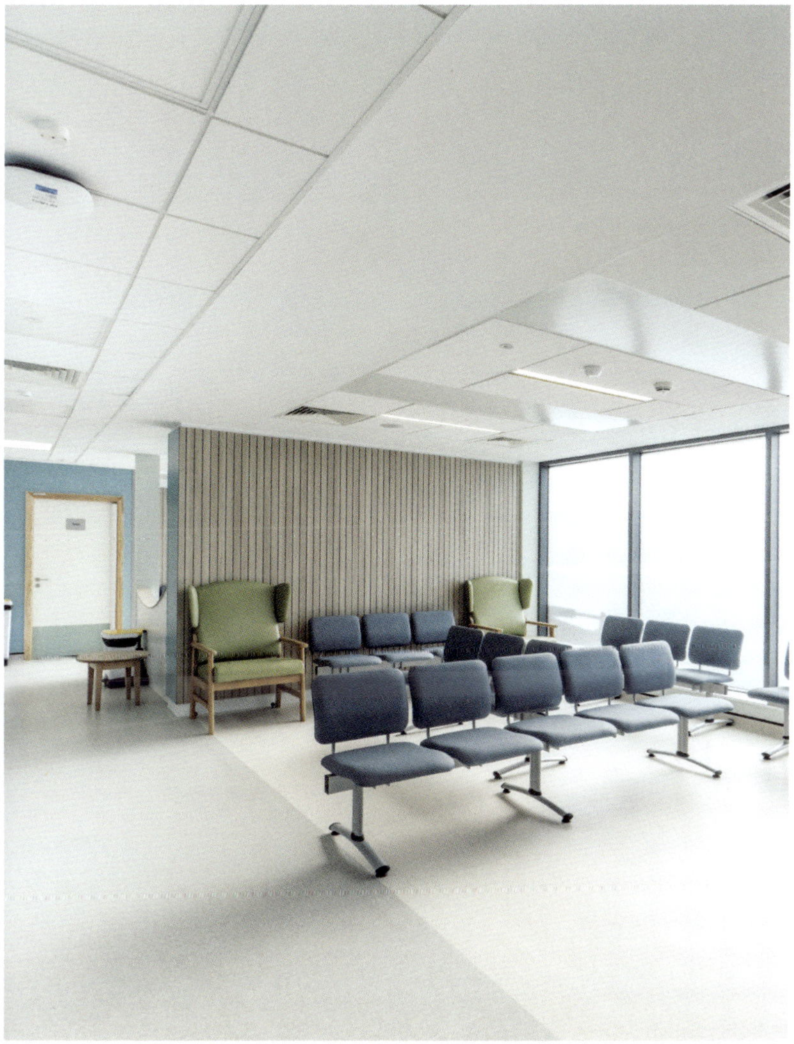

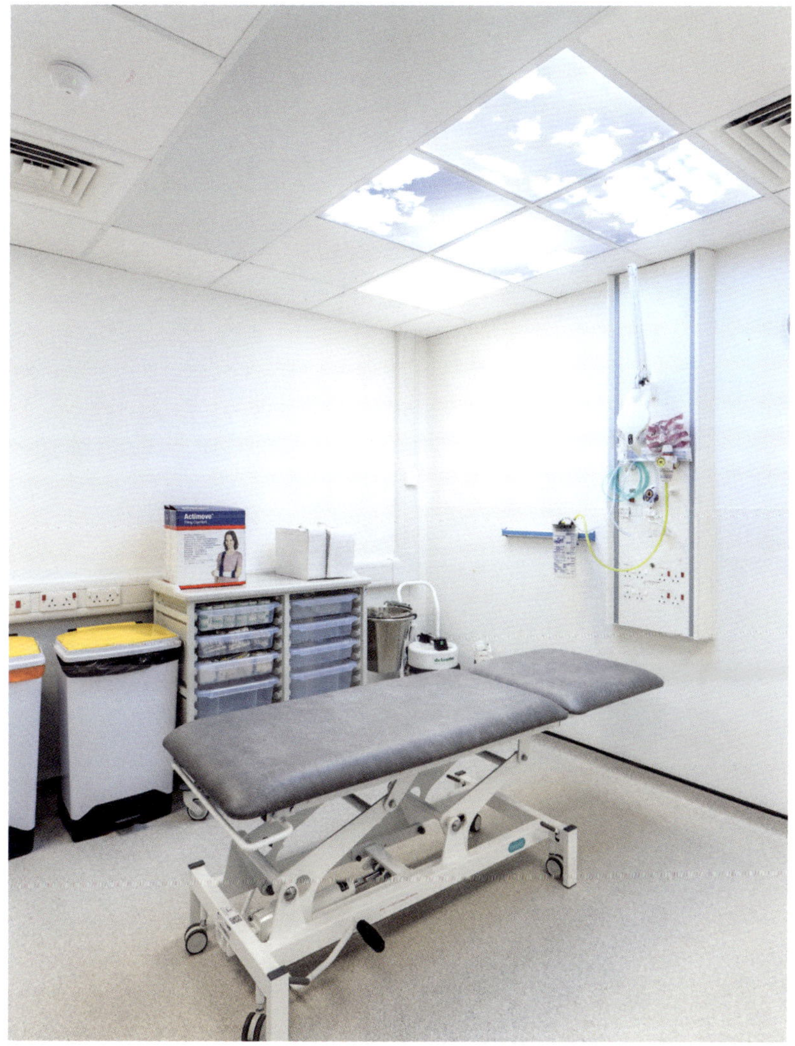

Soft colors and wood dominate the spacious waiting areas.

A cloudy sky helps patients feel calm.

Floor plans.

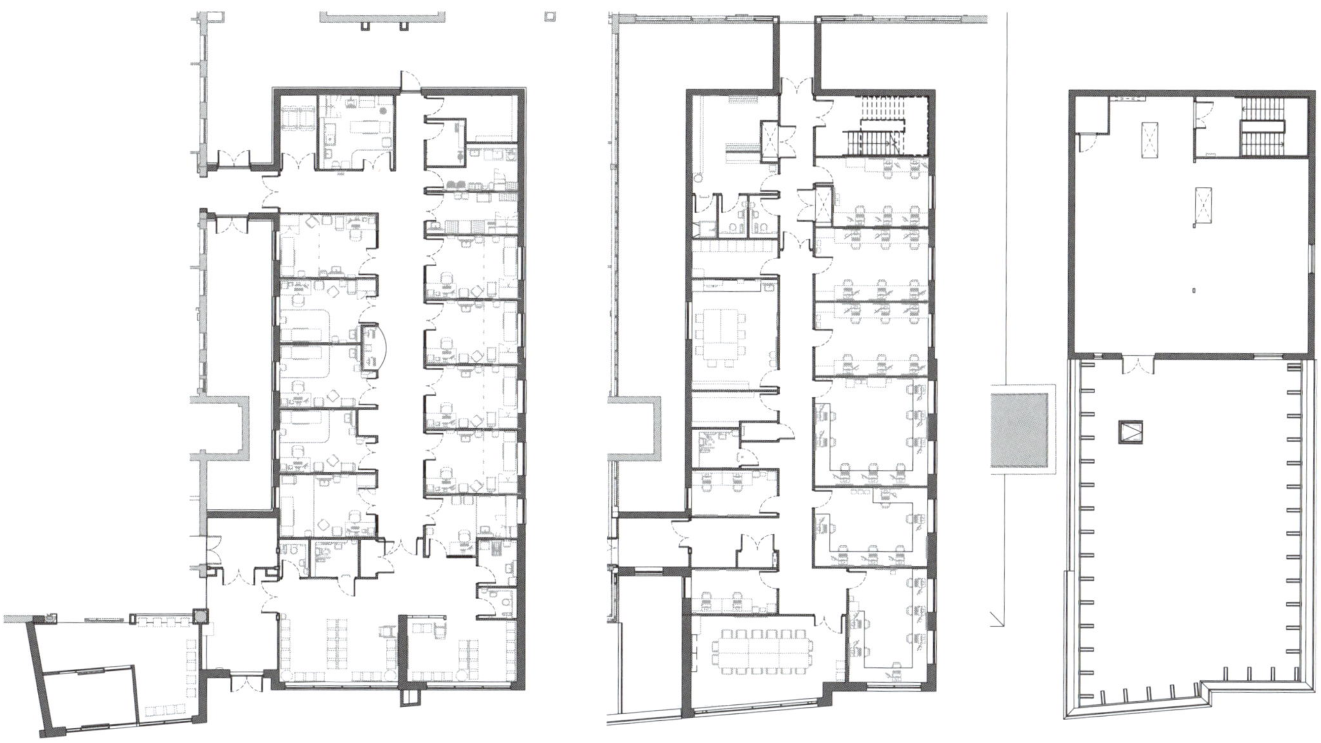

Silvia Gmür Reto Gmür Architects

Solothurn Switzerland

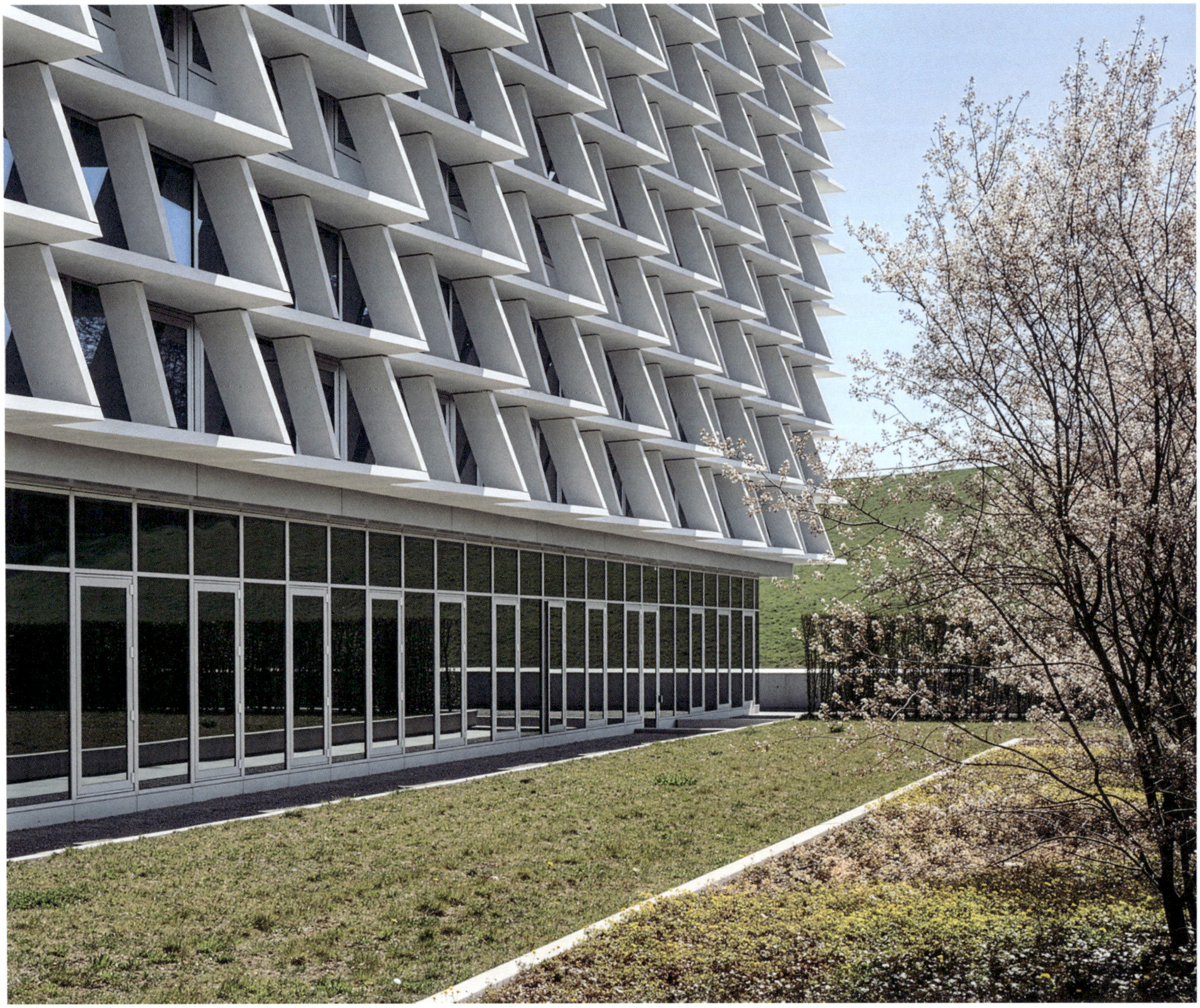

Direct access from the maternity ward to the rooftop garden.

Hospital building with glass façade and fixed sunshades.

New Building for Solothurn Citizens' Hospital

The building is the result of an international competition for a new 290-bed acute care hospital on the site of the current facility. The existing hospital remained fully operational throughout the construction period. The flexibility of the L-shaped new building around the existing structure ensures that the new hospital is future-proof. Once completed, the old buildings will be replaced by a spacious park – a central feature around which the new hospital is oriented. Inner courtyards not only provide natural daylight but also facilitate movement in natural daylight, as well as orientation and a connection to the outside world. This is further ensured by the fixed sunshade system, which nonetheless offers views whether standing, sitting, or lying down. In the patient rooms, the perpendicular bed placement provides both a high degree of privacy and sufficient flexible space.

Address: Schöngrünstrasse 42, 4500 Solothurn, Switzerland | **Client:** Solothurn Building Authority | **Completion:** 2021 | **Size:** 57,000 m² | **Sector:** public | **Number of patient rooms:** 155 | **Color design:** Gido Wiederkehr

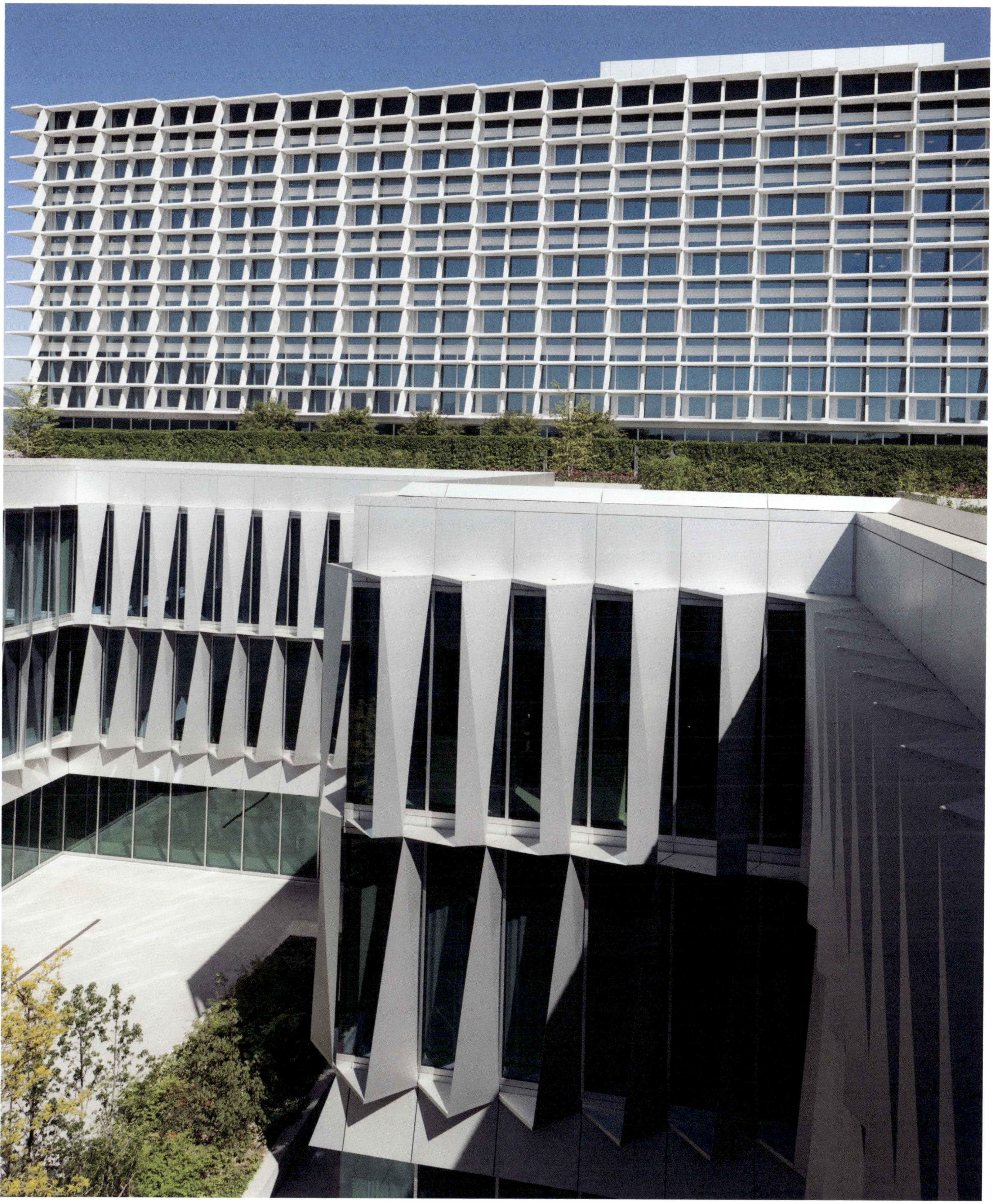

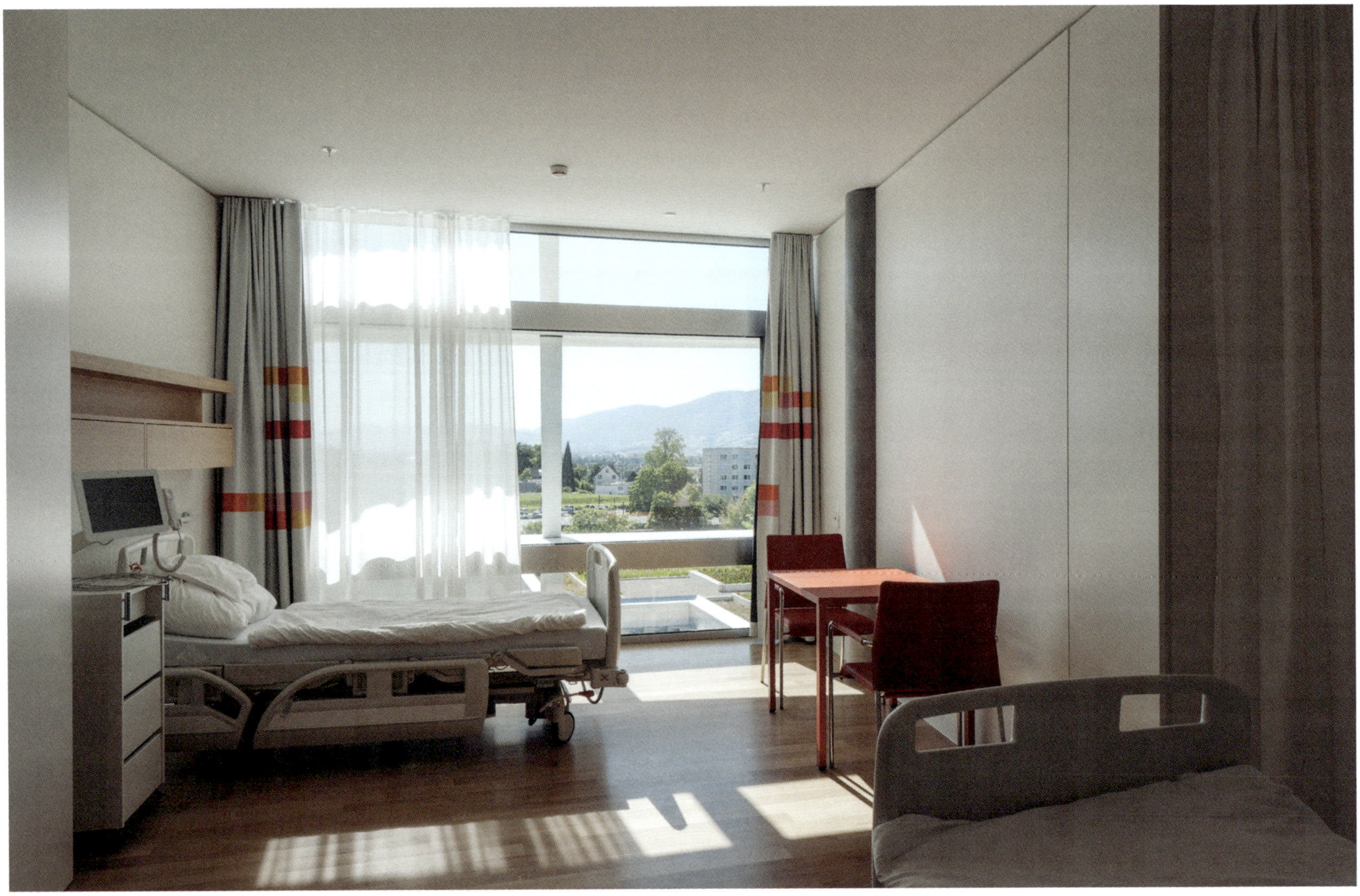

Spacious patient's room with ample natural light.

Section.

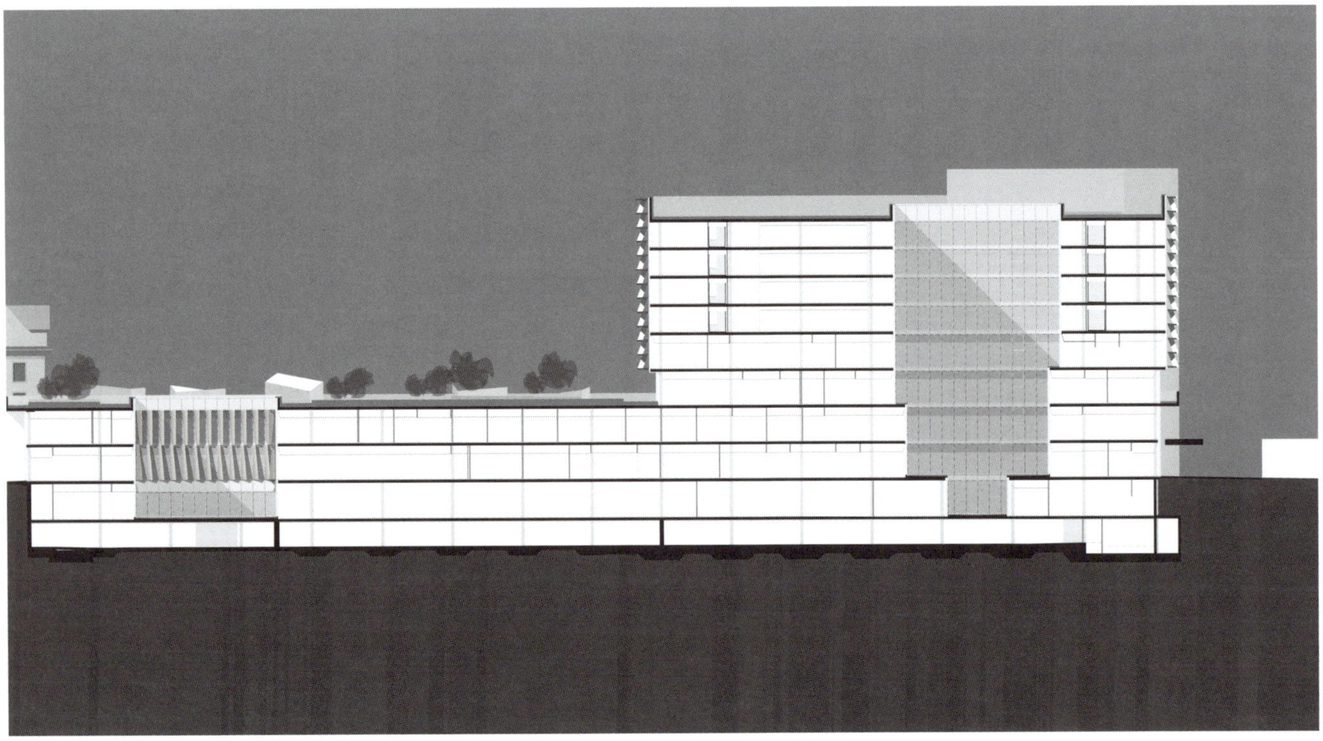

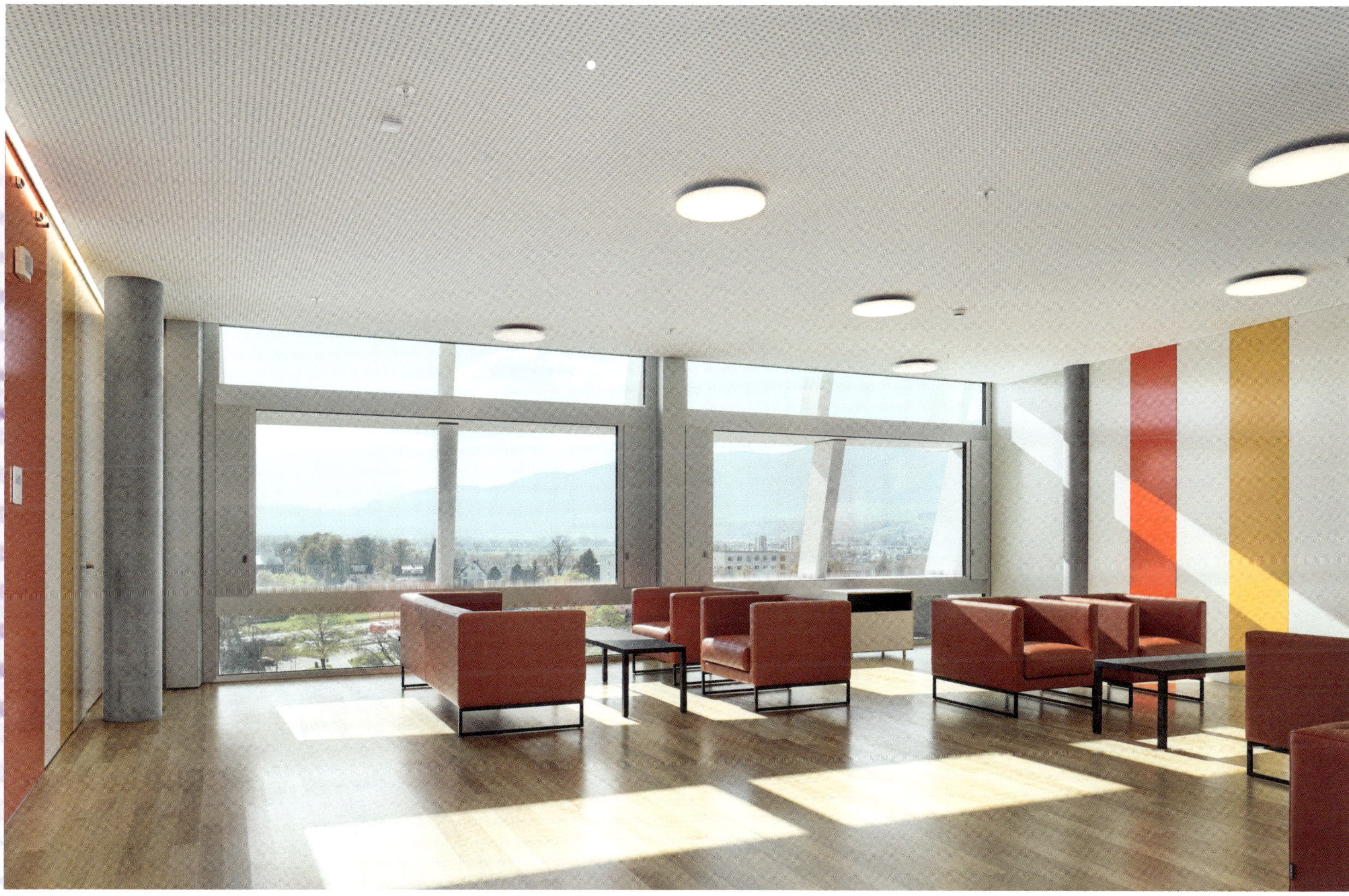

Nursing station's lounge room.

Patient room plan.

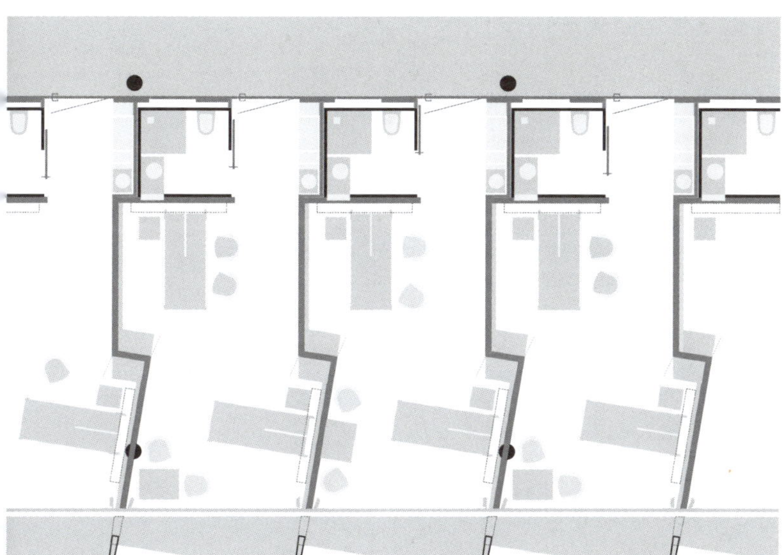

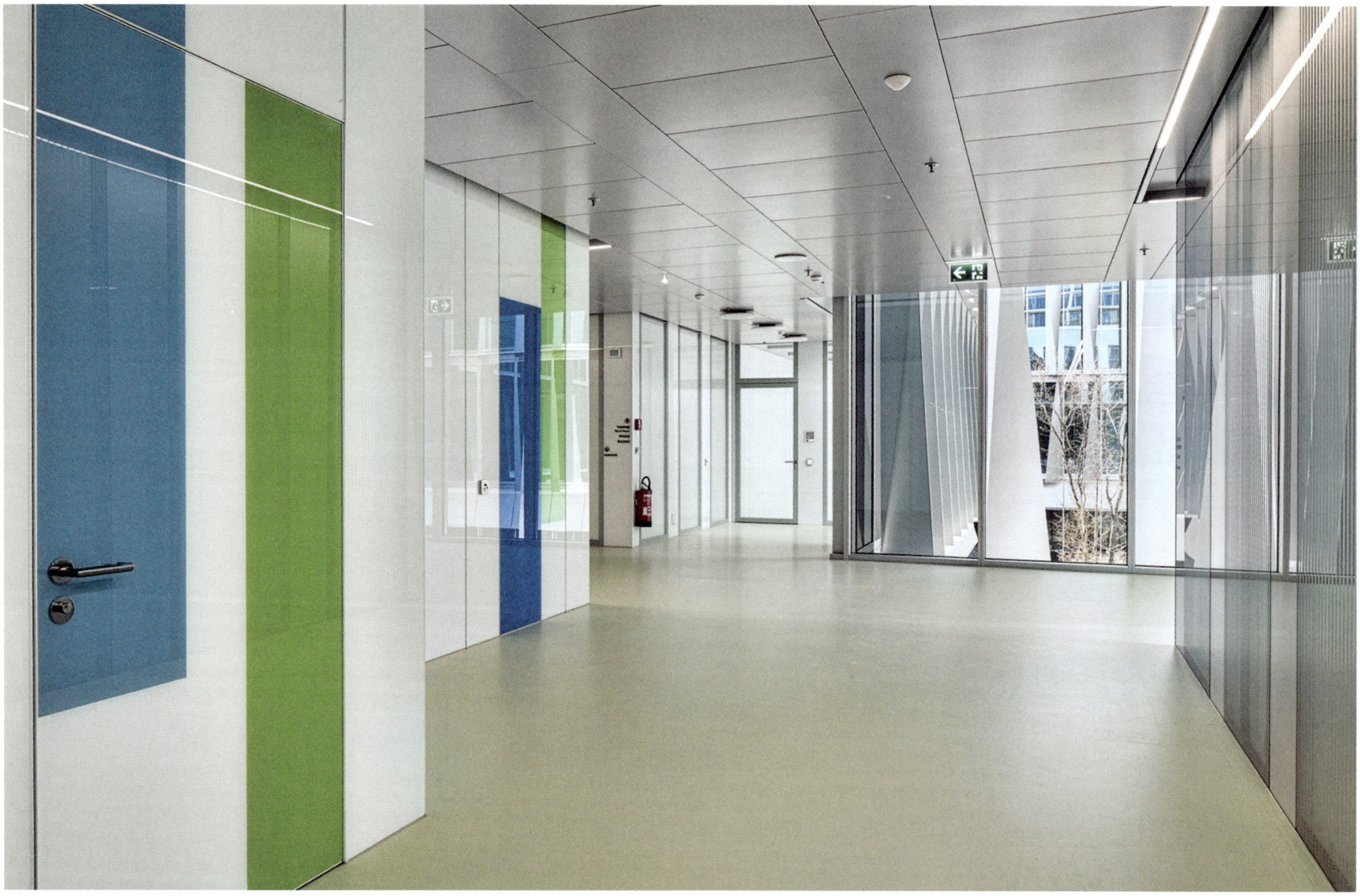

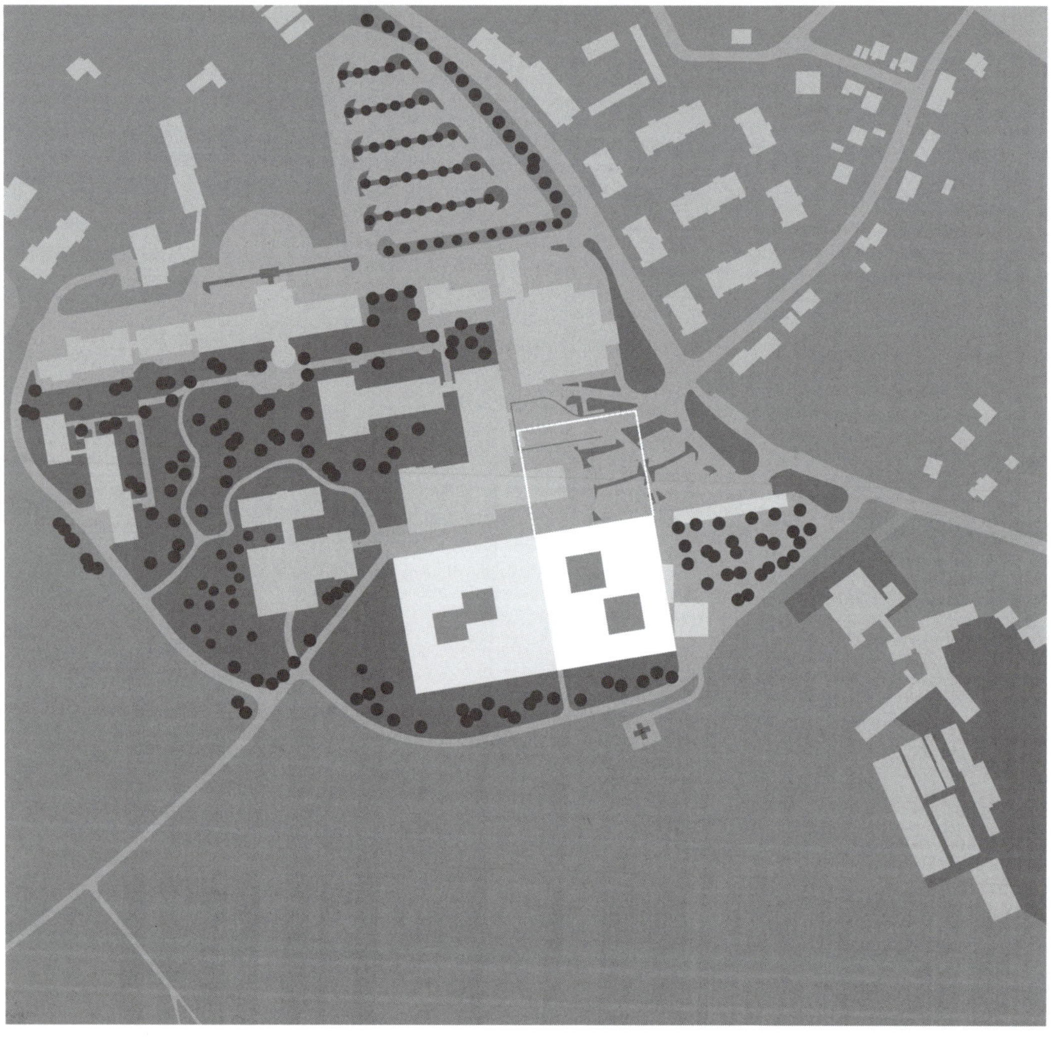

Radiology with orientation through natural daylight.

Site plan.

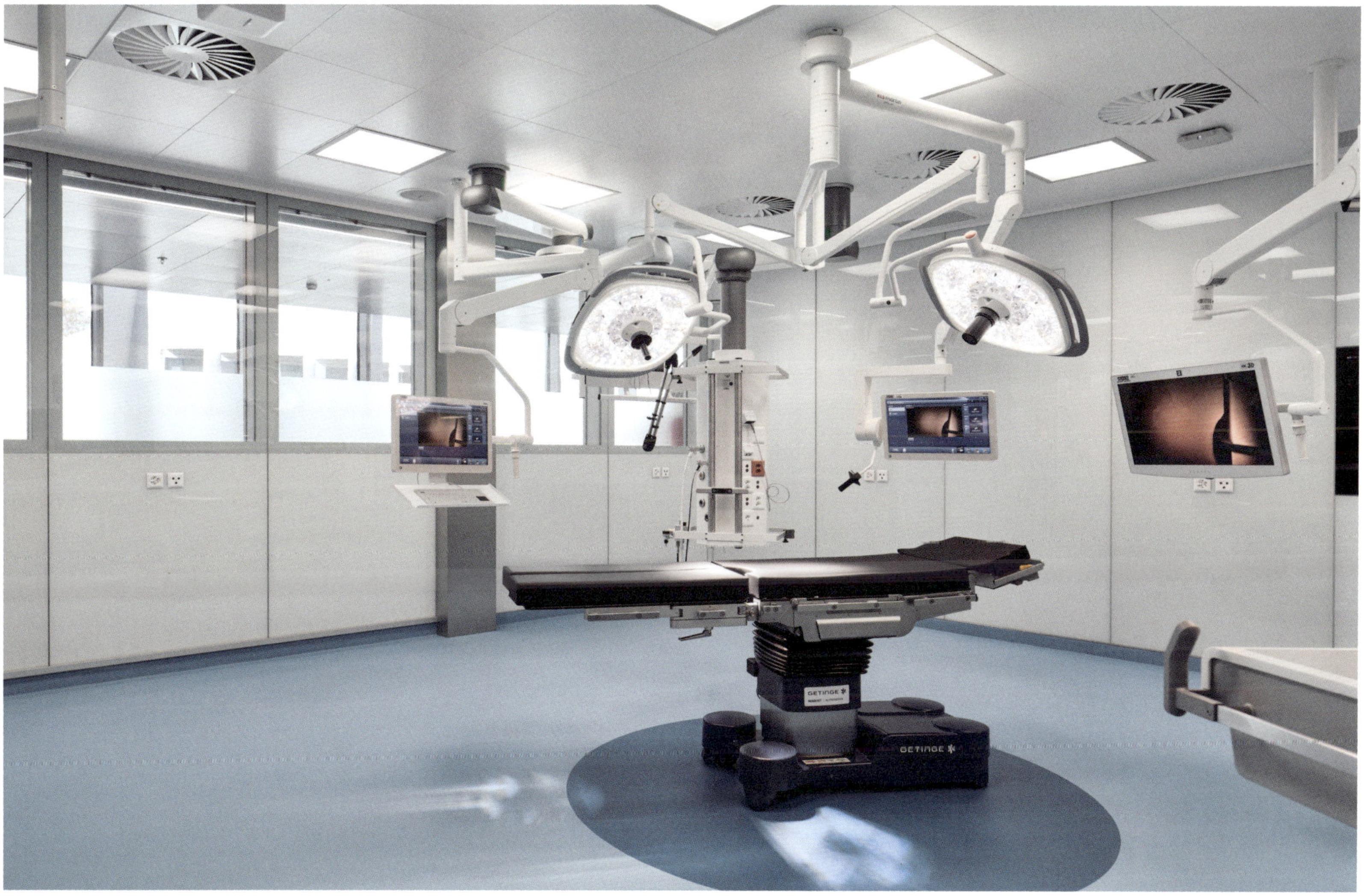

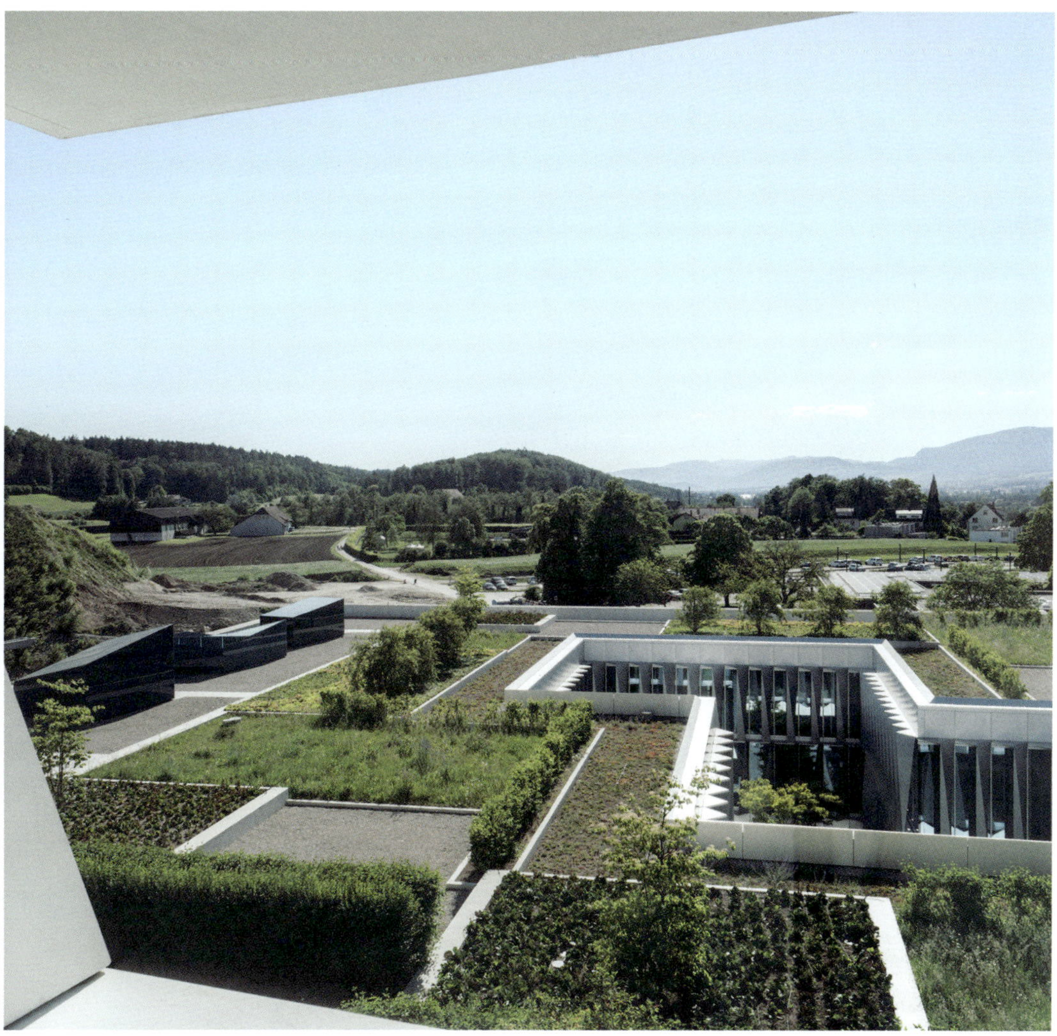

Operation theater with windows.

View of the roof garden from the bedroom.

Architekten BDA
RDS Partner

Wolfsburg
Germany

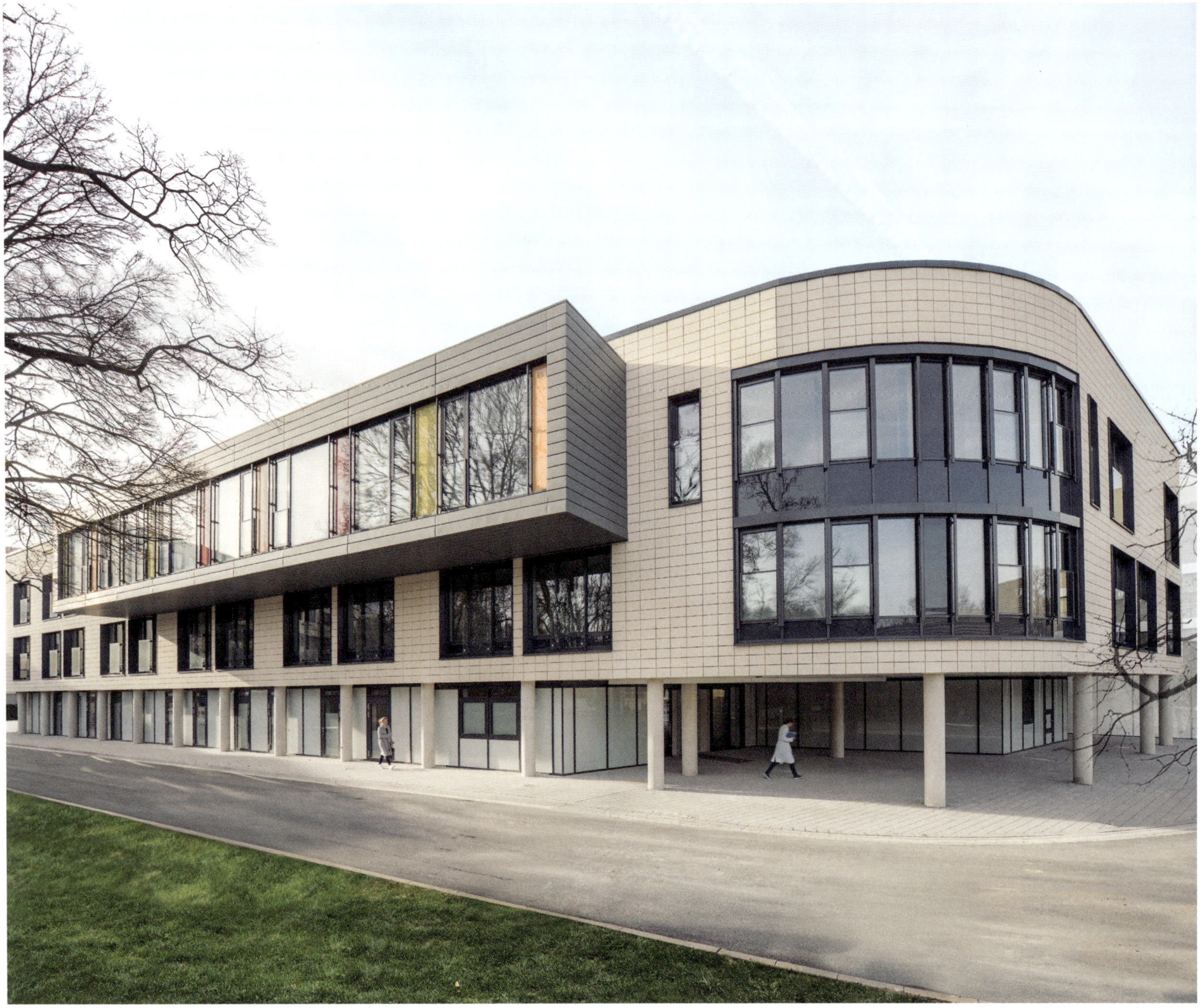

View of the Children's Hospital from the zoo.

West façade with access to the event area.

Building G with the main entrance.

Wolfsburg Hospital

The Wolfsburg Hospital campus was reorganized and strategically developed within the framework of a long-term master plan to meet future healthcare demands. A central circulation spine, conceived as the primary organizational axis, improves orientation, strengthens internal connectivity and creates clear functional relationships across the hospital. House G forms a key component of this development, accommodating eight general nursing wards (256 beds) together with a new main entrance and cafeteria that serve as the hospital's central public hub. As part of the overall transformation, the outpatient center including surgical facilities, the internal medicine ICU, and a central admissions unit were restructured. The addition of the new pediatric clinic, including intensive care facilities and a level 1 perinatal center, further strengthens the medical infrastructure and care for premature infants and high-risk births.

Address: Sauerbruchstraße 7, 38440 Wolfsburg, Germany | **Client:** City of Wolfsburg | **Completion:** 2021 | **Size:** 30,700 m² | **Original building:** Hospital, Titus Taescher, 1953 | **Sector:** state | **Specialization:** 20 clinical departments and institutes | **Number of beds:** 547

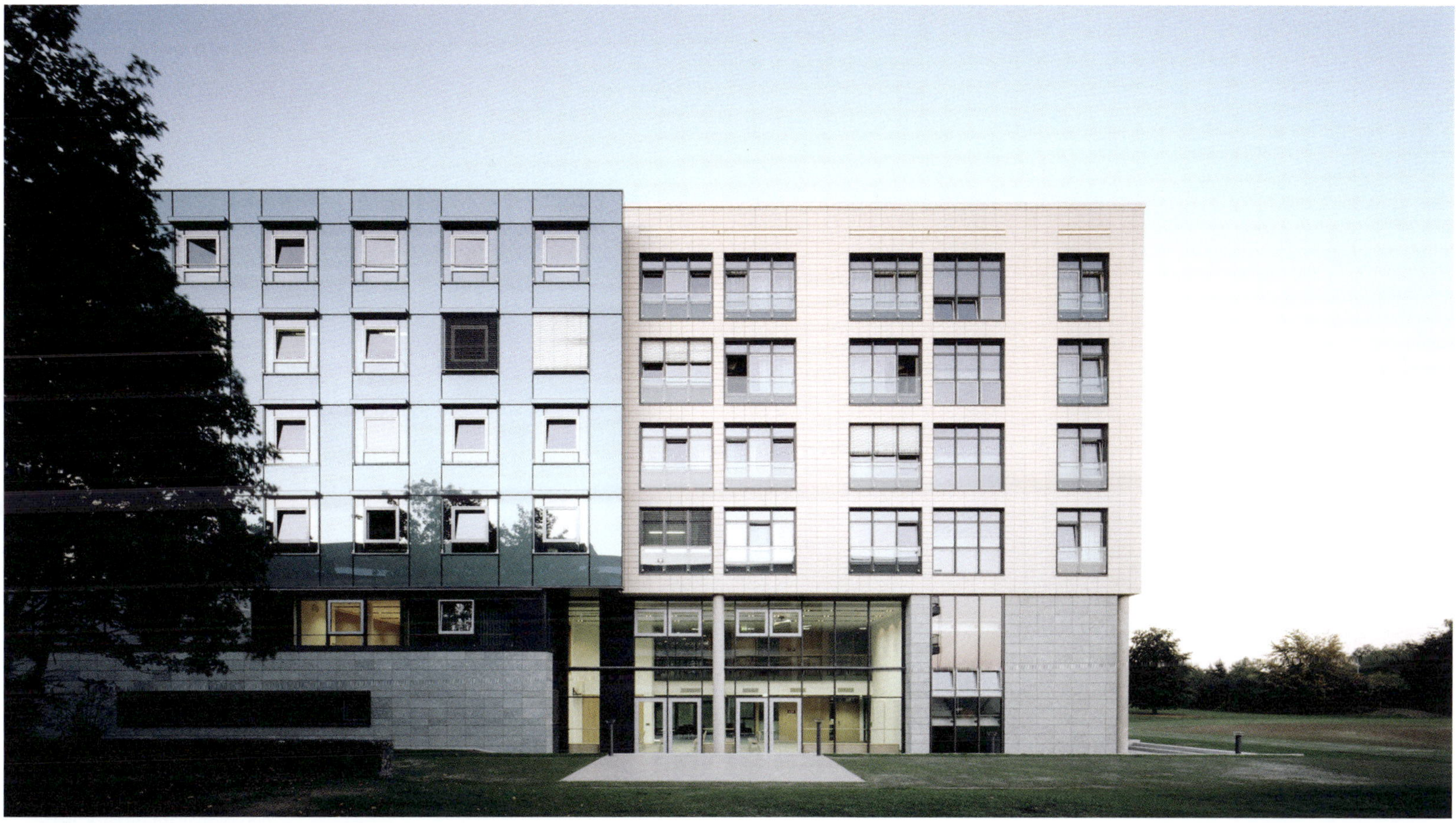

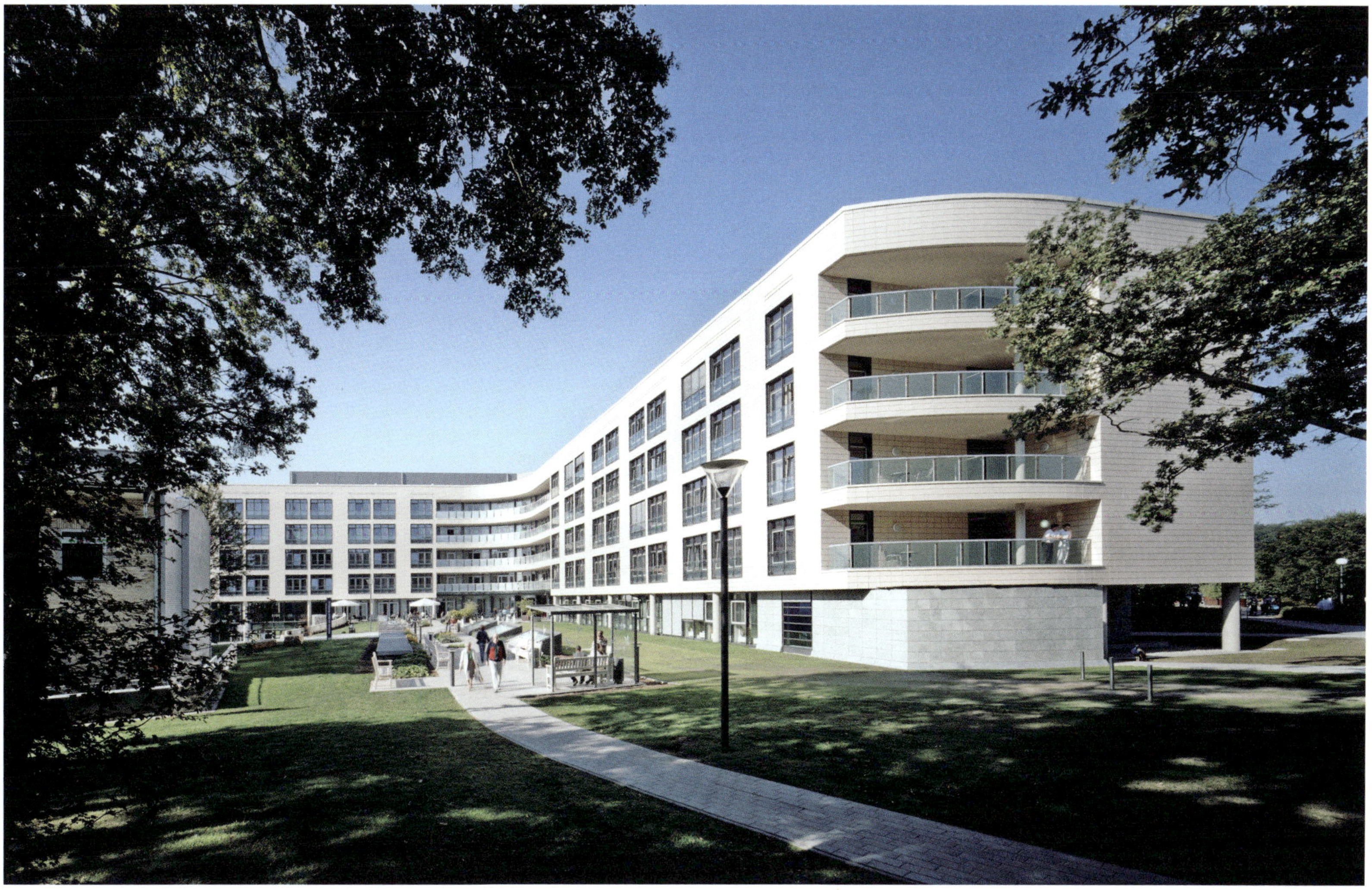

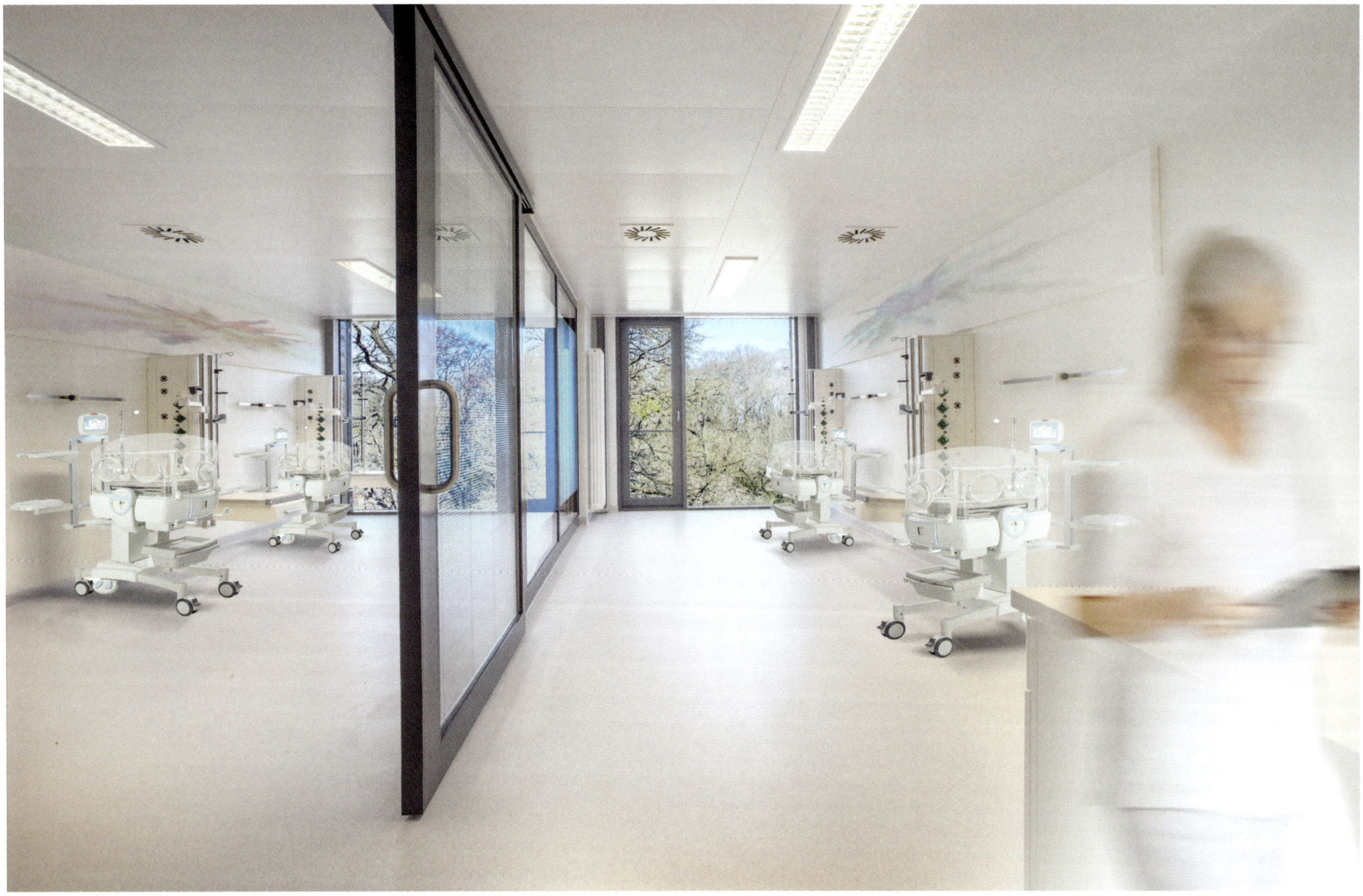

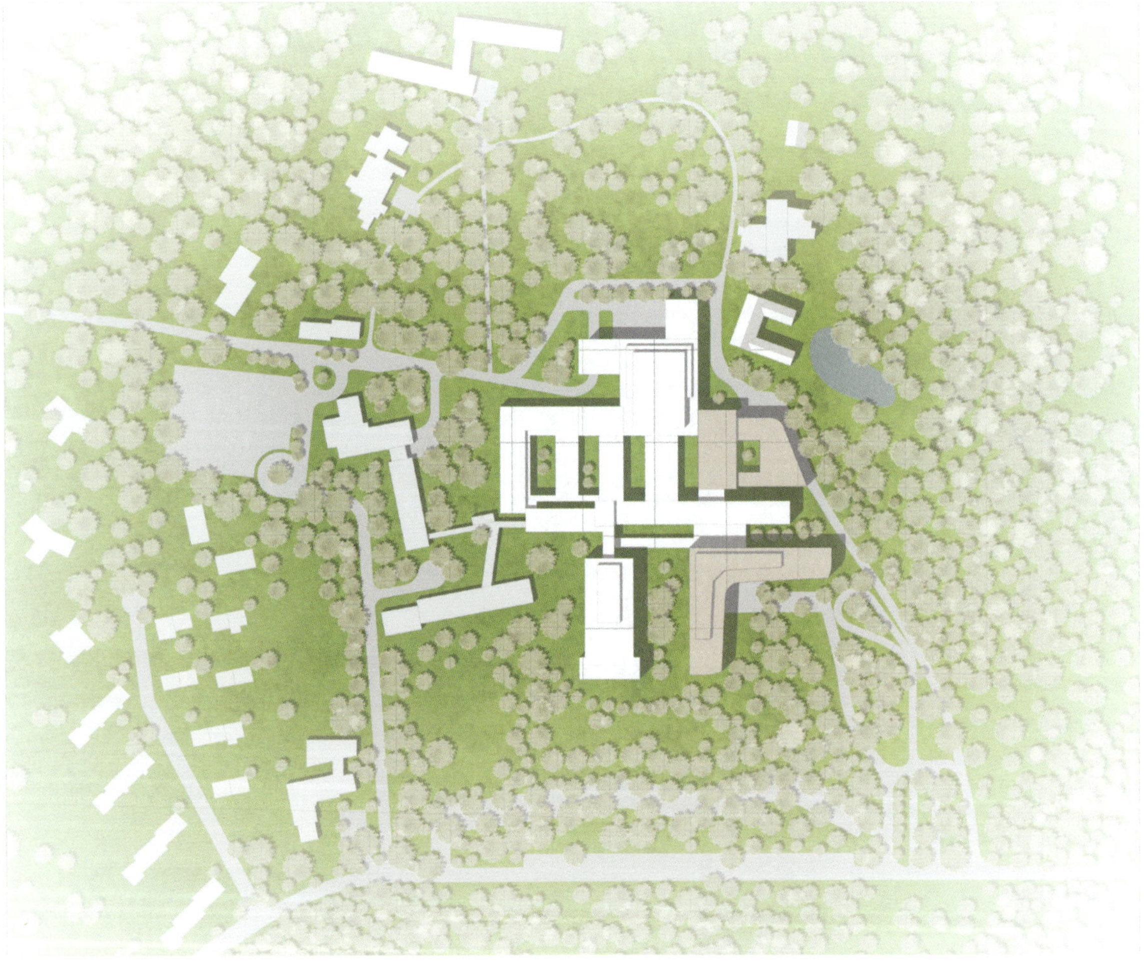

Hospital's child Intensive Care Unit.

Site plan.

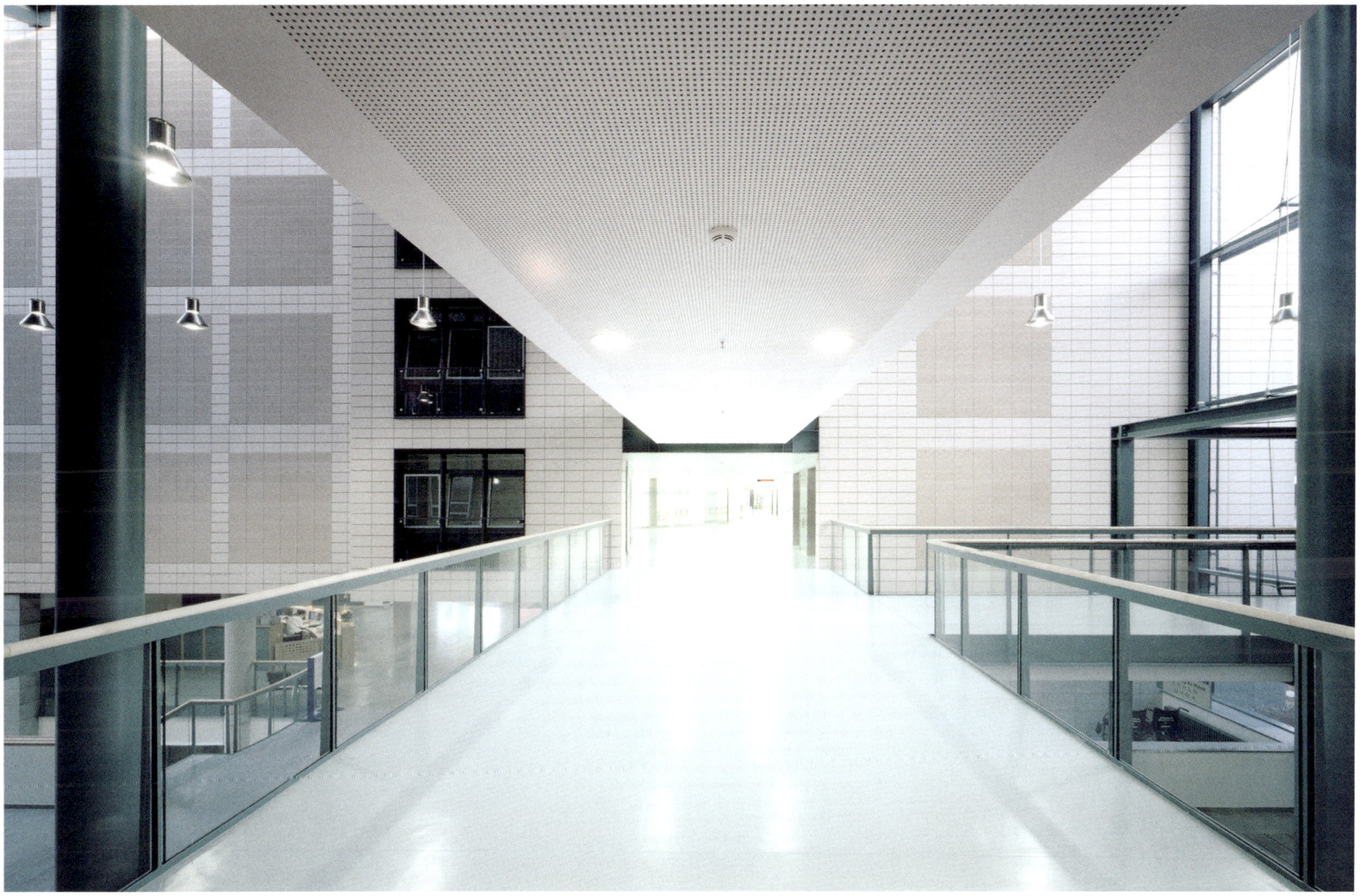

Hospital's main corridor.

Target planning.

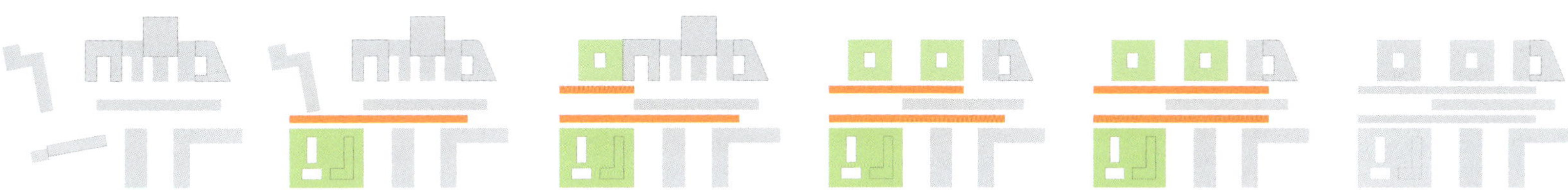

Saboia + Ruiz Arquitetos

Riacho Fundo II
Brazil

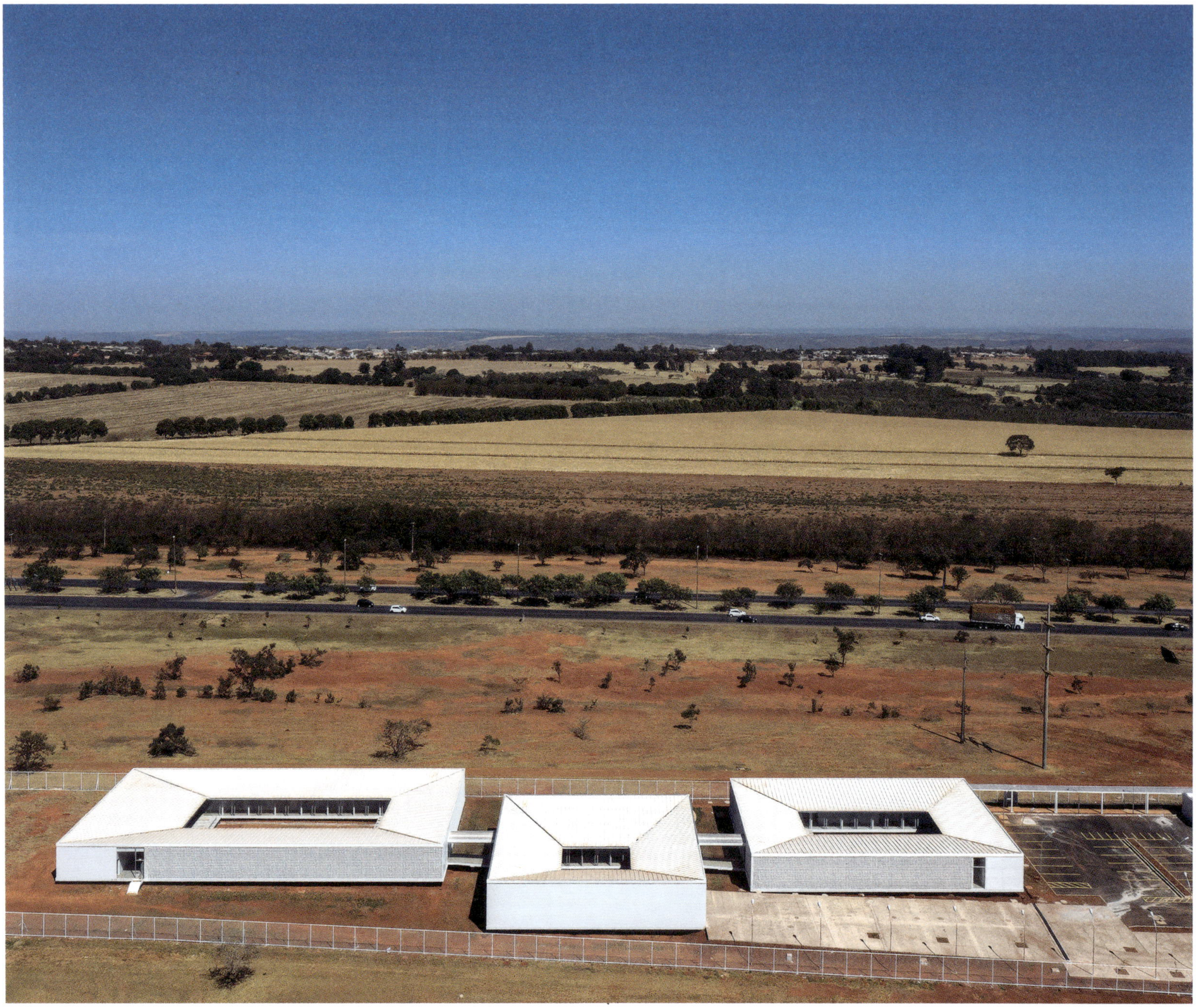

Aerial view of the healthcare complex and its courtyard structure.

Glazed passage linking the two building volumes.

Light-filled glazed corridor with a patio view, defined by soft white and gray tones.

UBS Primary Care Unit Parque do Riacho

Designed for a large, complex site marked by highways, power lines, and elongated terrain far exceeding the building footprint, the project is organized into three rectangular blocks with internal courtyards, balancing urban integration and humanized healthcare spaces. Externally, the blocks define open areas, connect nearby housing and agricultural zones, and provide visibility and identity to the public facility. Internally, the courtyards ensure natural light, ventilation, acoustic protection, and contact with nature, creating welcoming environments. The block division also enabled adaptation to the terrain through ramps and accessible circulation, while preserving free areas for future expansion and community use. The program is sectorized among the blocks, separating administration, medical care, and technical services. Passive strategies enhance thermal comfort and reduce reliance on artificial air conditioning.

Address: 3A Etapa QS 9 – Riacho Fundo II, 71884-376 Brasilia, Brazil | **Client:** Federal District Government | **Completion:** 2021 | **Size:** 2,150 m² | **Sector:** private and public | **Specialization:** primary health care unit | **Number of treatment rooms:** 33 | **Open space planning:** Raul Pereira Arquitetos Associados

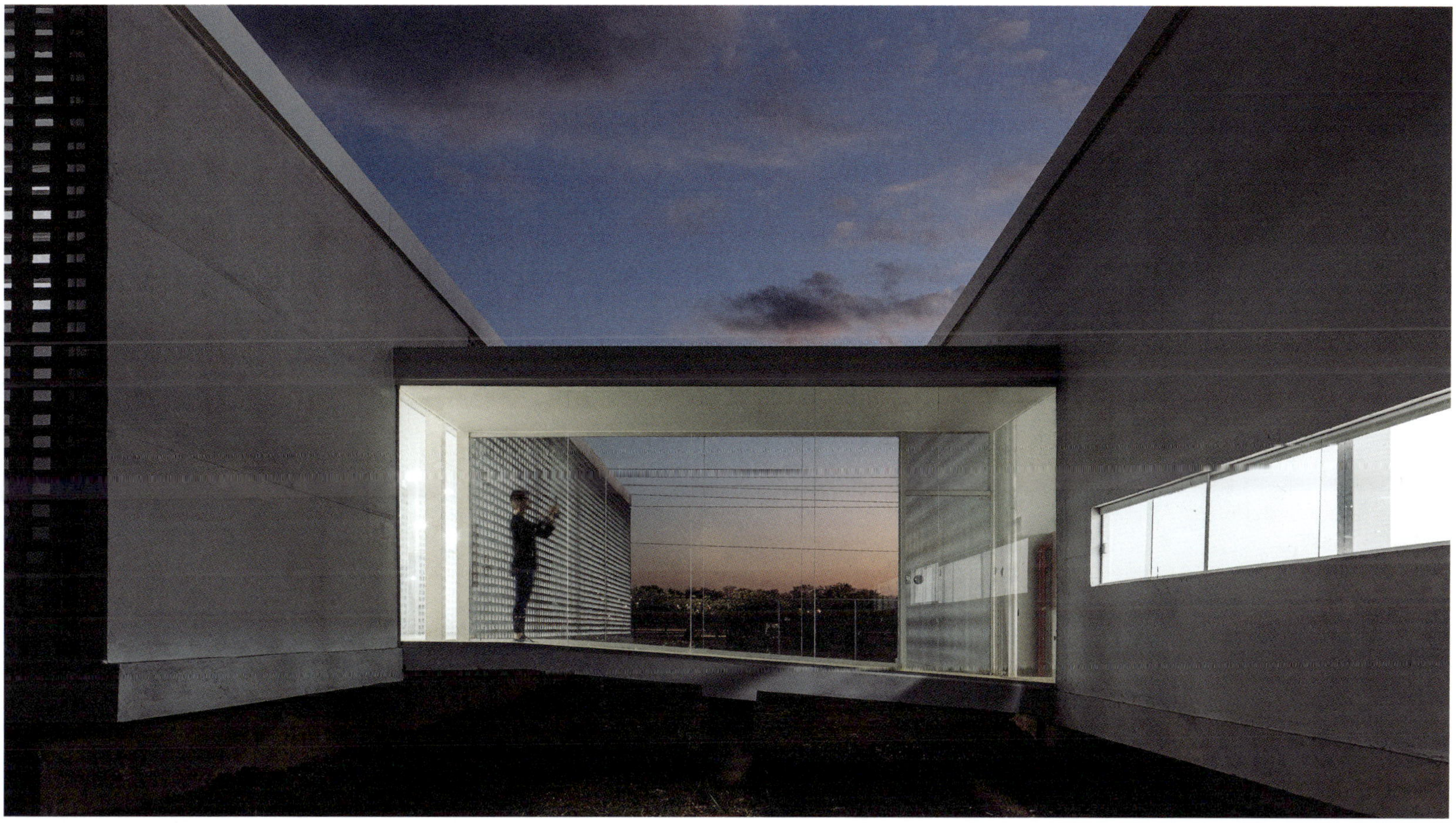

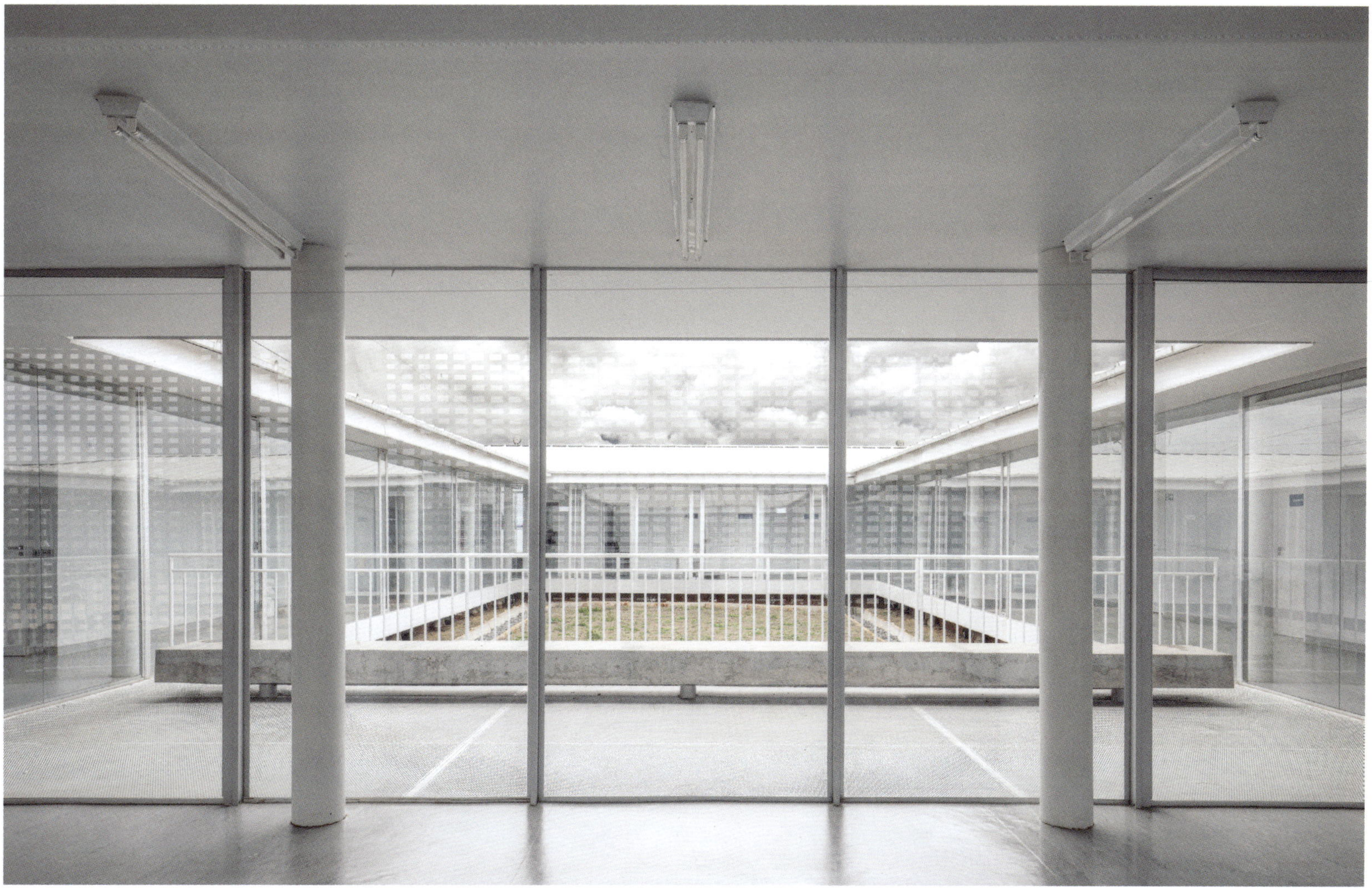

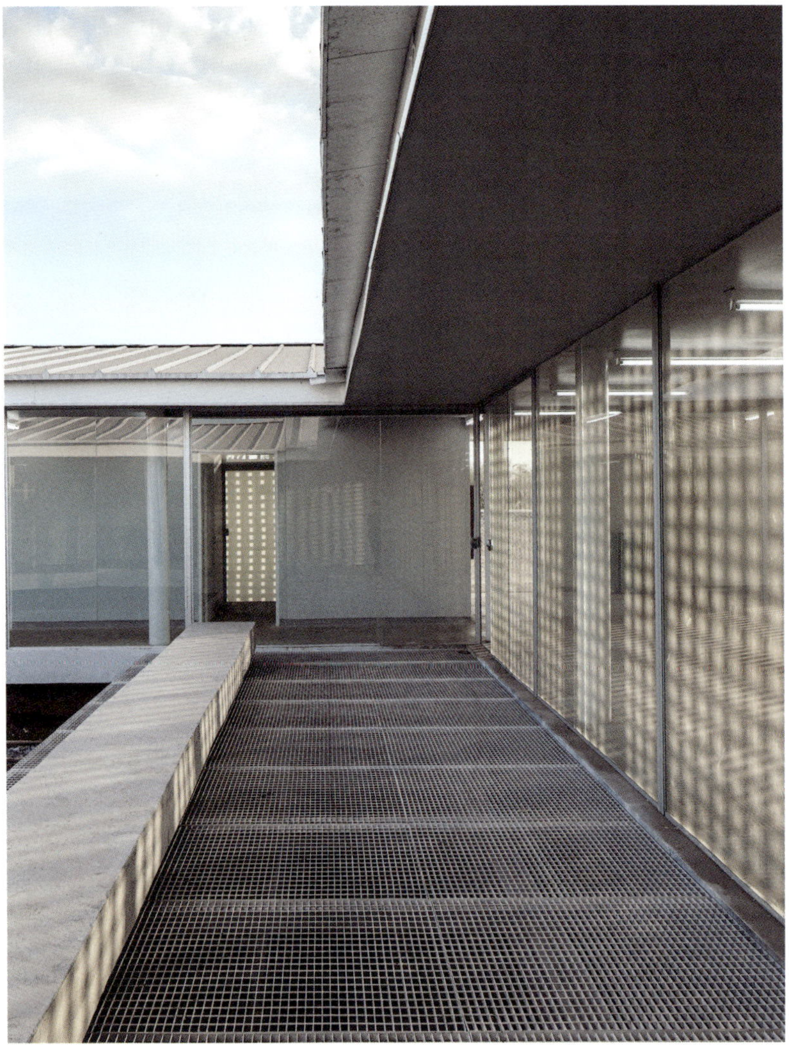

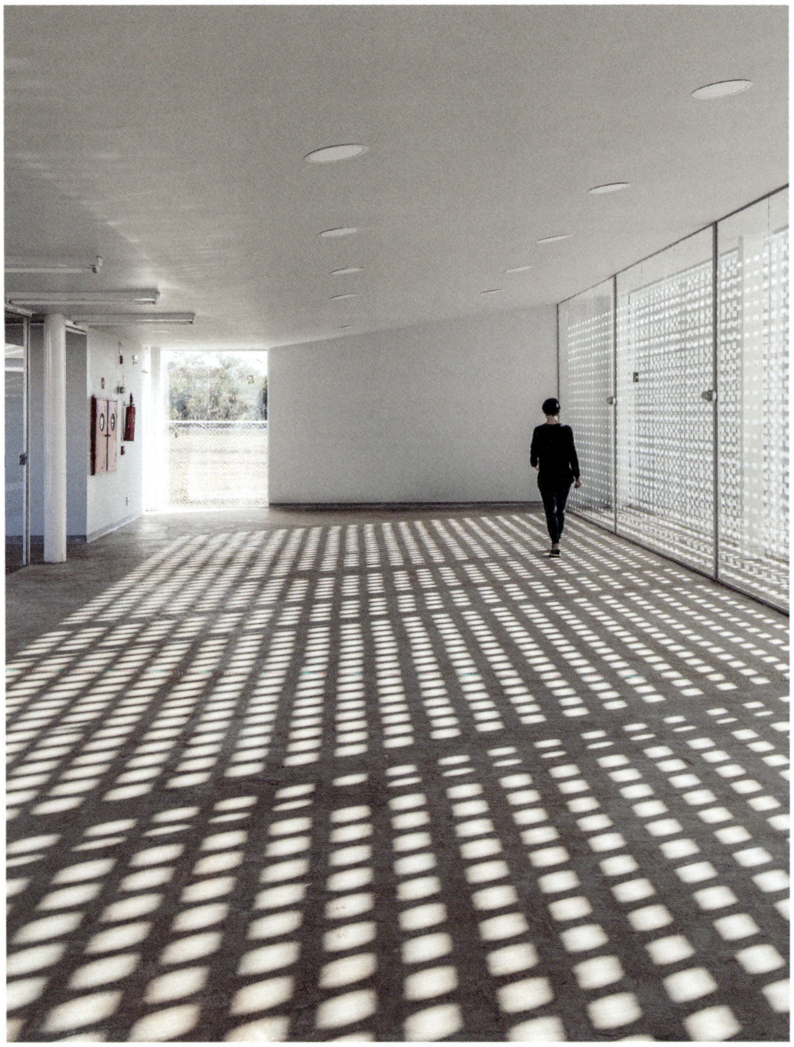

Textured paving along the circulation path.

Sunlight filtering through the perforated façade creates changing patterns of light and shadow.

Ground floor plan.

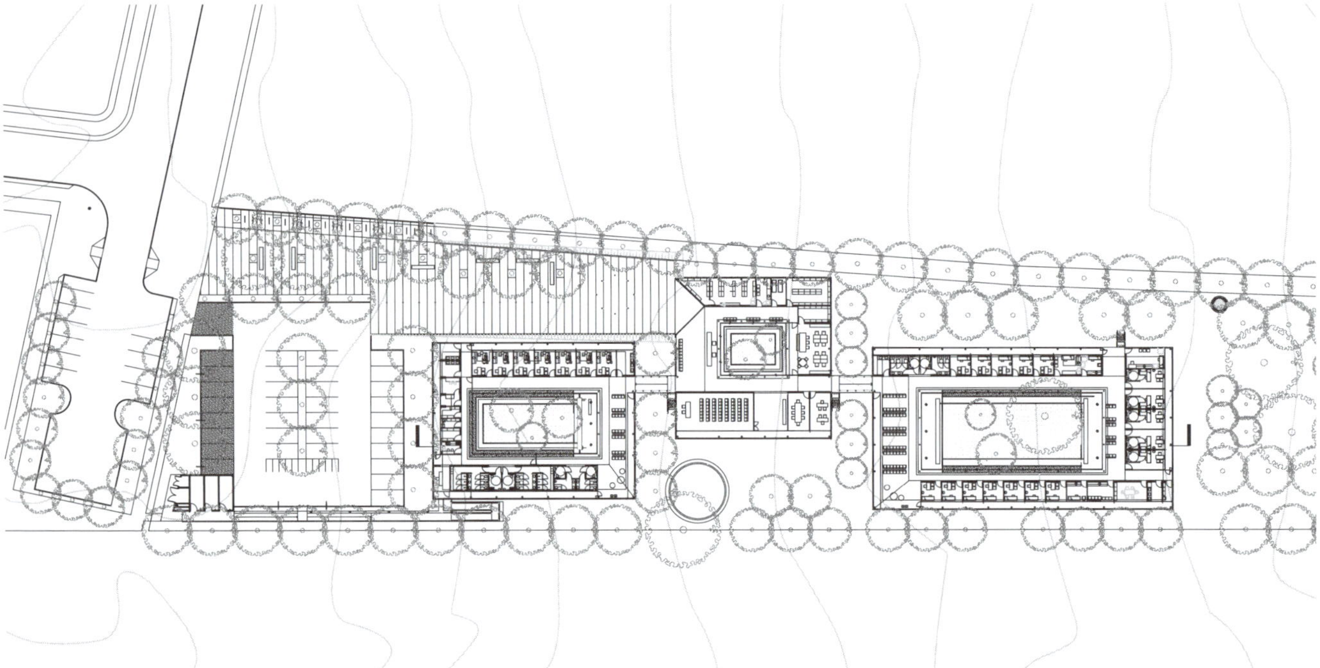

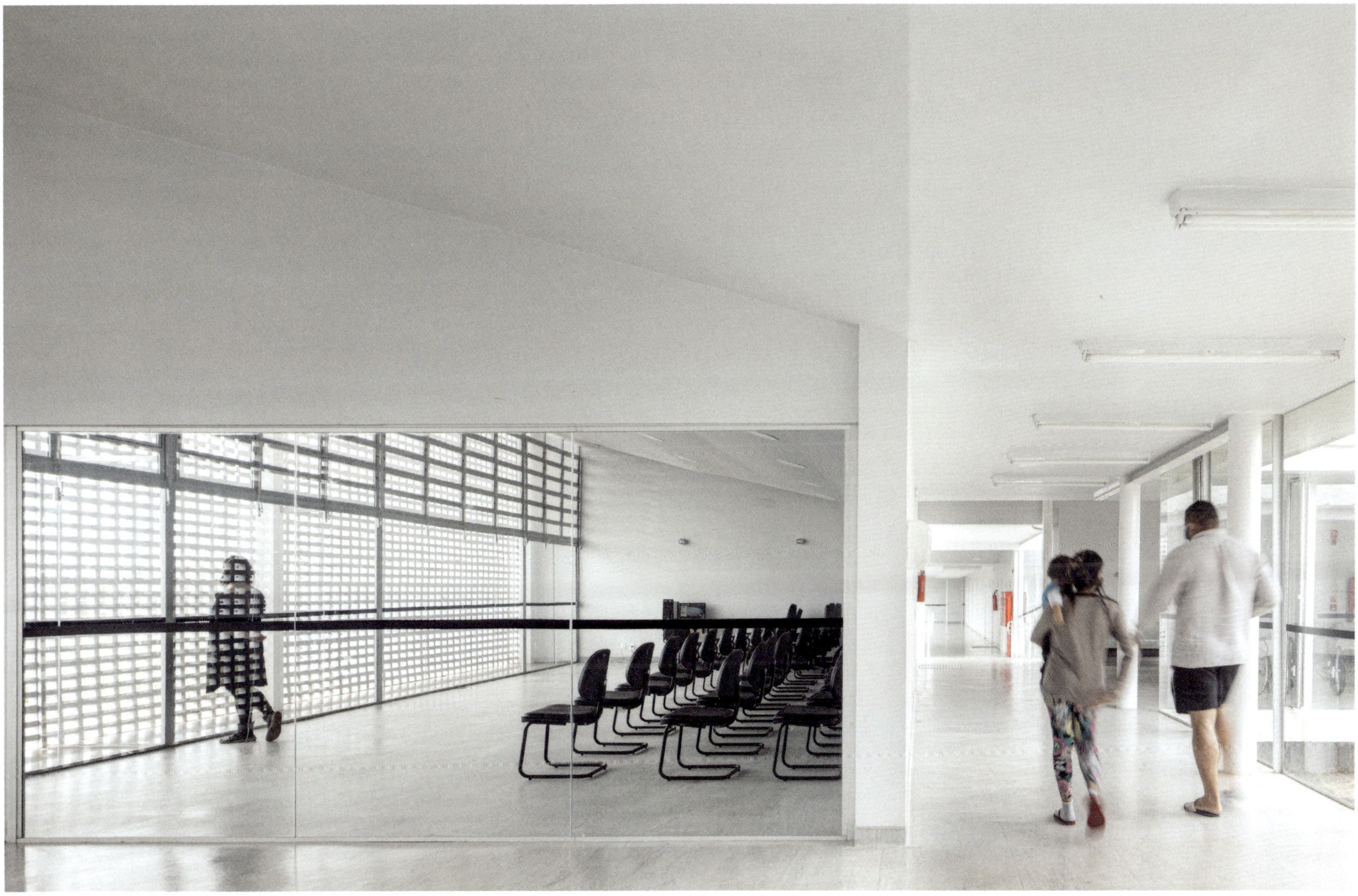

Light-filled waiting area and corridor, framed by large windows and perforated façade.

Section.

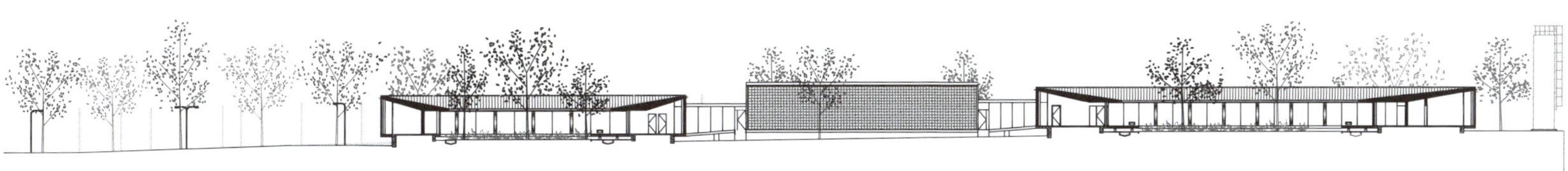

Scott Tallon Walker Architects with Cagni Williams

London
United Kingdom

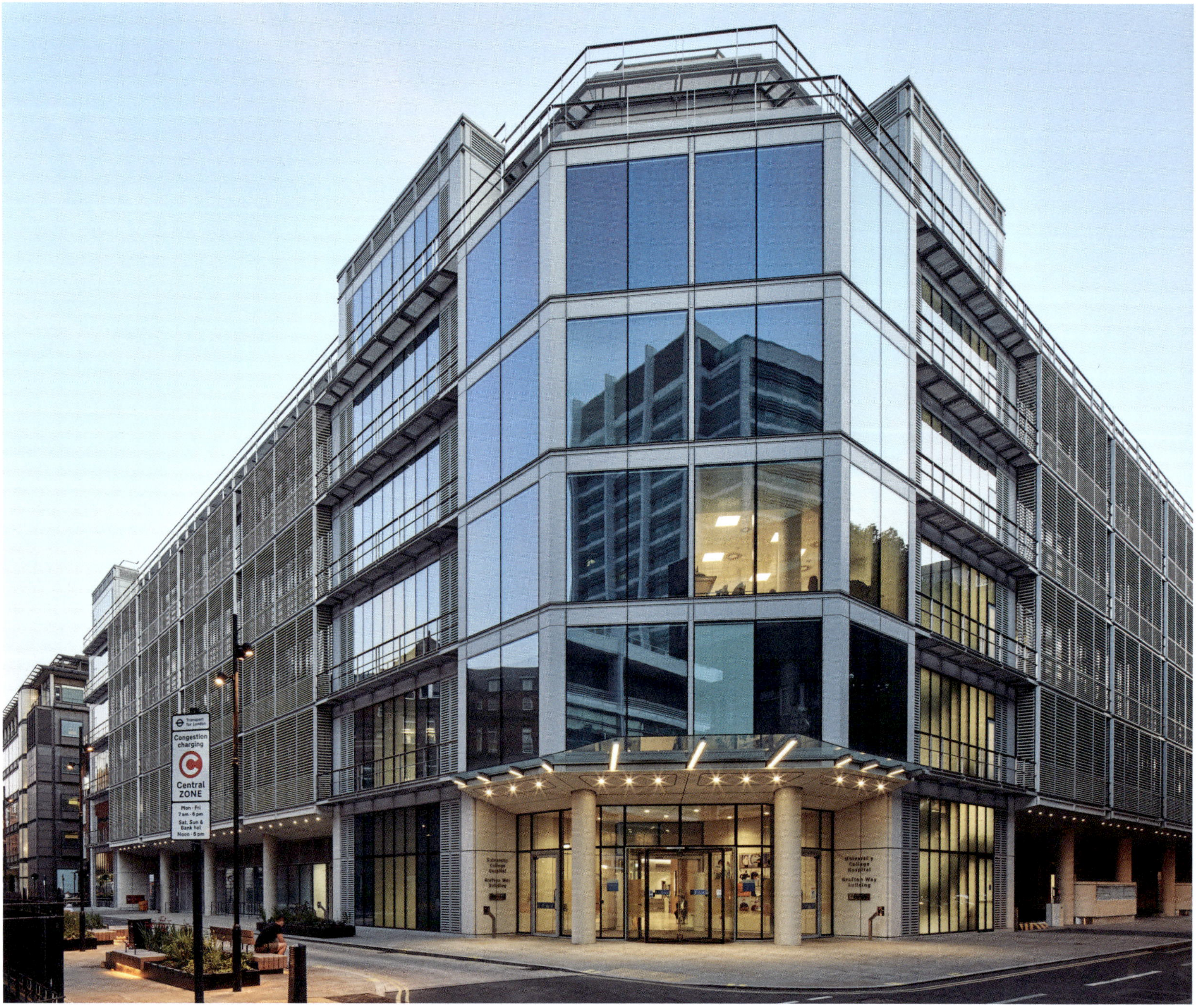

Main entrance with a restrained, glazed façade and a clearly articulated public threshold.

Reception area defined by an open, light-filled space.

Street view with veiled façade to bedrooms.

University College London Hospital Grafton Way Building

The Grafton Way Building is a highly specialized cancer hospital in the bustling city center. The building is vertically zoned to accommodate proton beam therapy and operating theaters below ground floor reception and imaging facilities, while the upper floors contain patient bedrooms, roof gardens, and support services. The external veil façade provides solar shading and layers of privacy, allowing more openness, connectivity, and visibility to the outside world. The hospital is characterized by operational clarity, daylight, transparency, and sensory rooftop gardens. A light-filled atrium aids orientation and brings daylight through the building and into all inpatient bedrooms. The building form is designed to have a positive impact on its urban setting, in plan and in section. Interiors are inspired by the color palate of an English country garden and selective artwork provide positive distraction from treatment.

Address: 1 Grafton Way, London WC1E 6AS, United Kingdom | **Client:** University College London Hospital | **Completion:** 2022 | **Size:** 34,500 m² | **Sector:** state | **Specialization:** specialist cancer hospital | **Number of treatment rooms:** 4 PBT gantries, 8 operating theaters | **Number of patient rooms:** 160

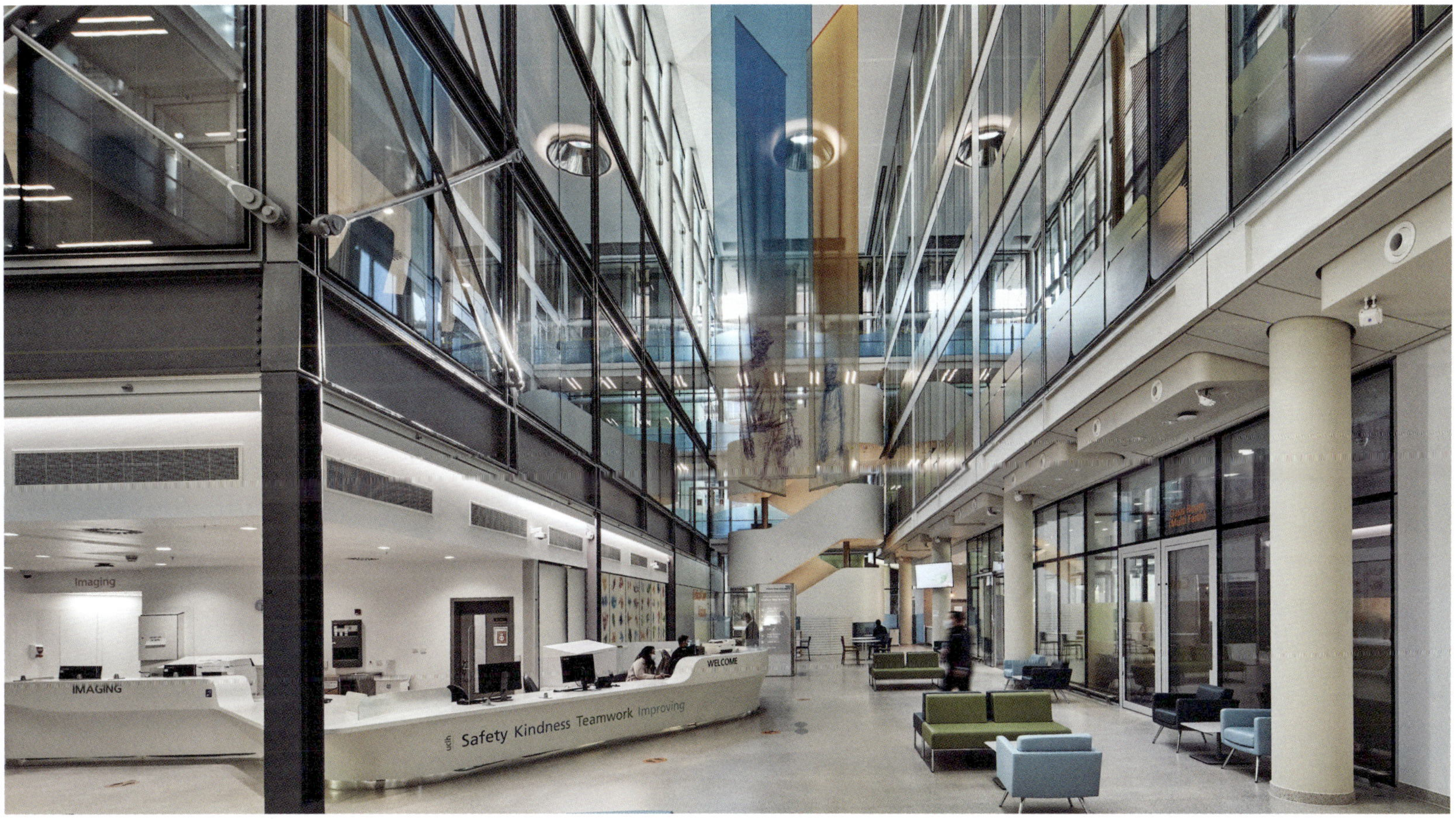

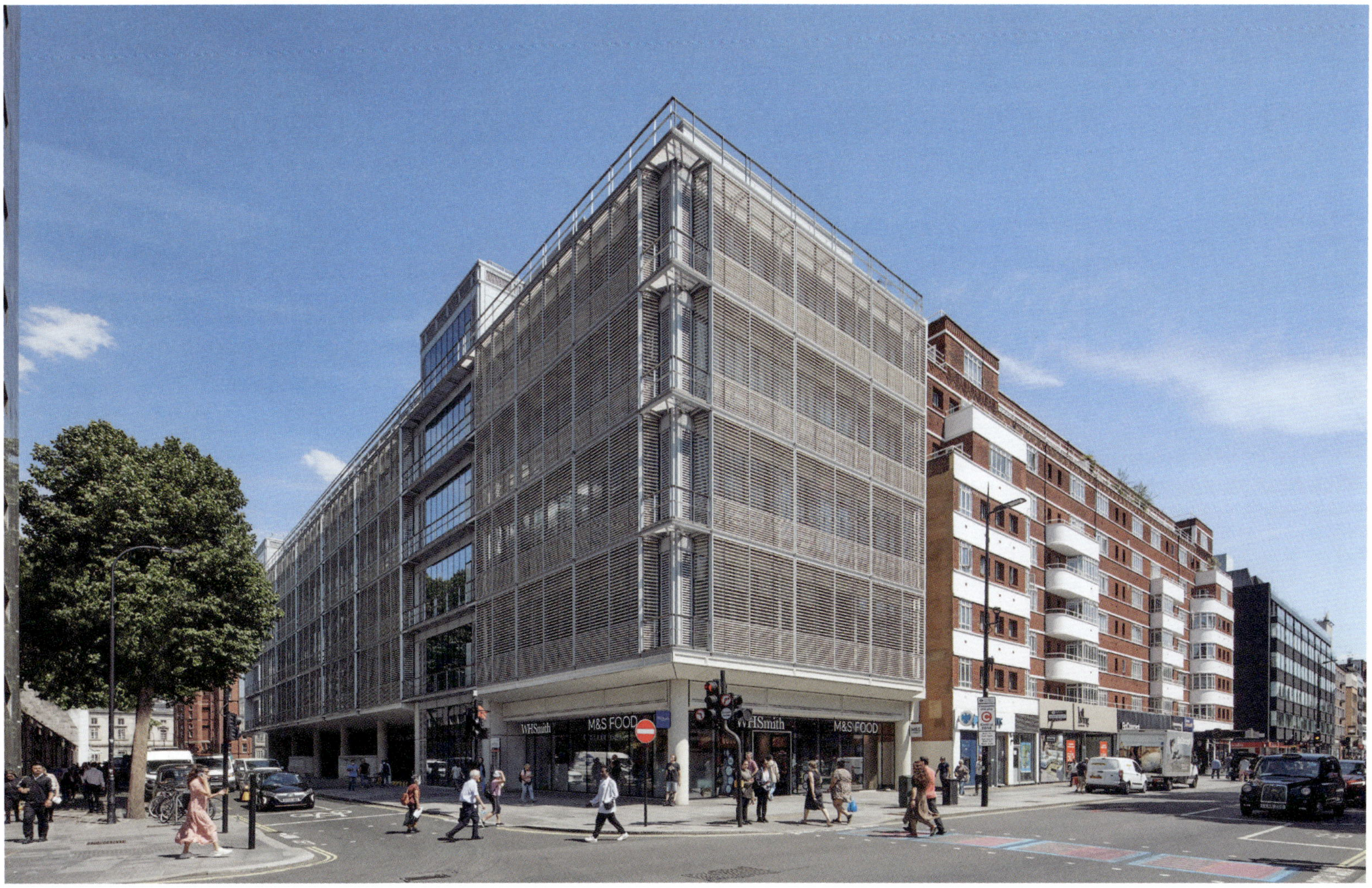

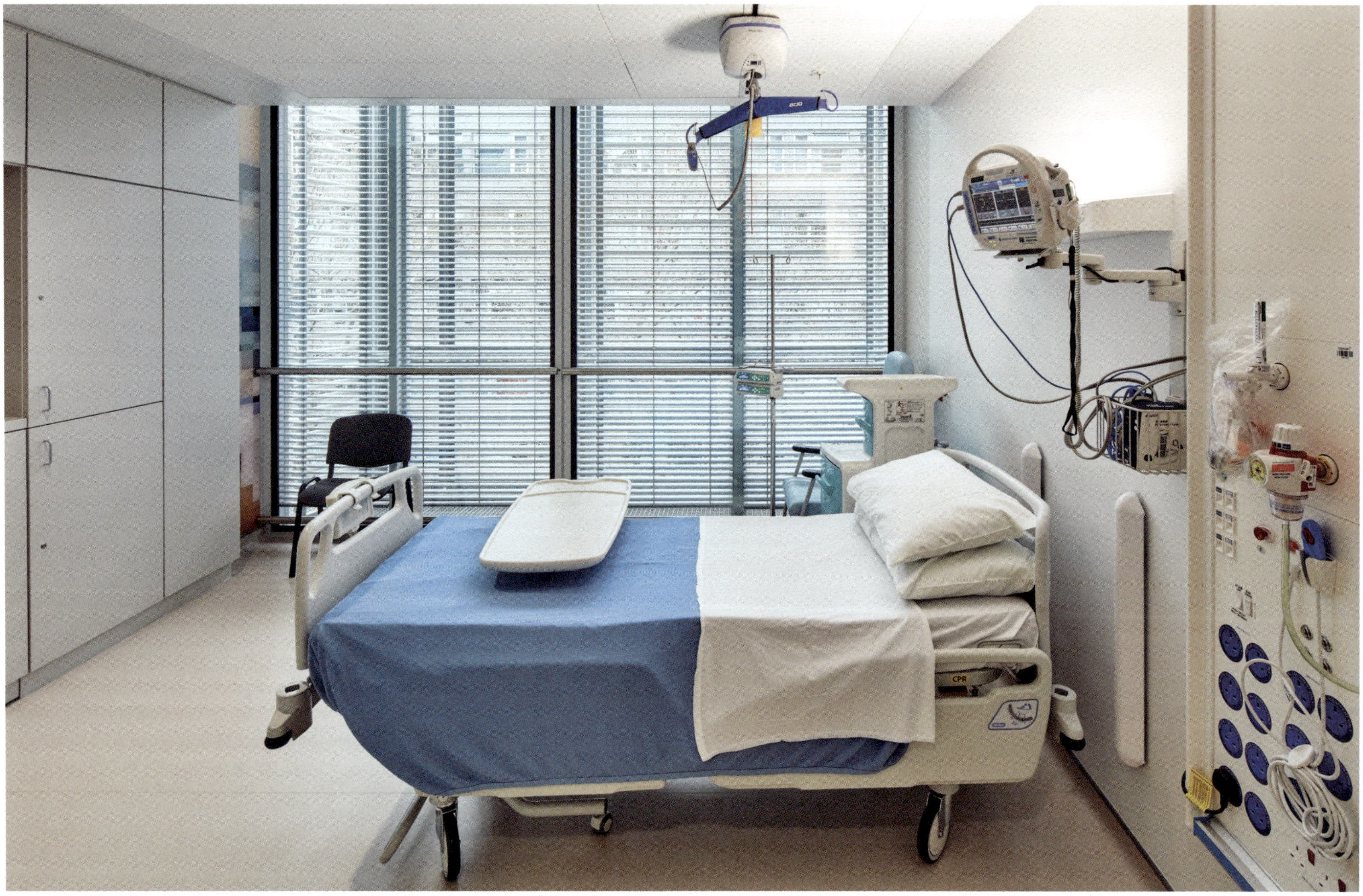

Multi-bed ward with floor to ceiling glazed façade.

Entrance level plan.

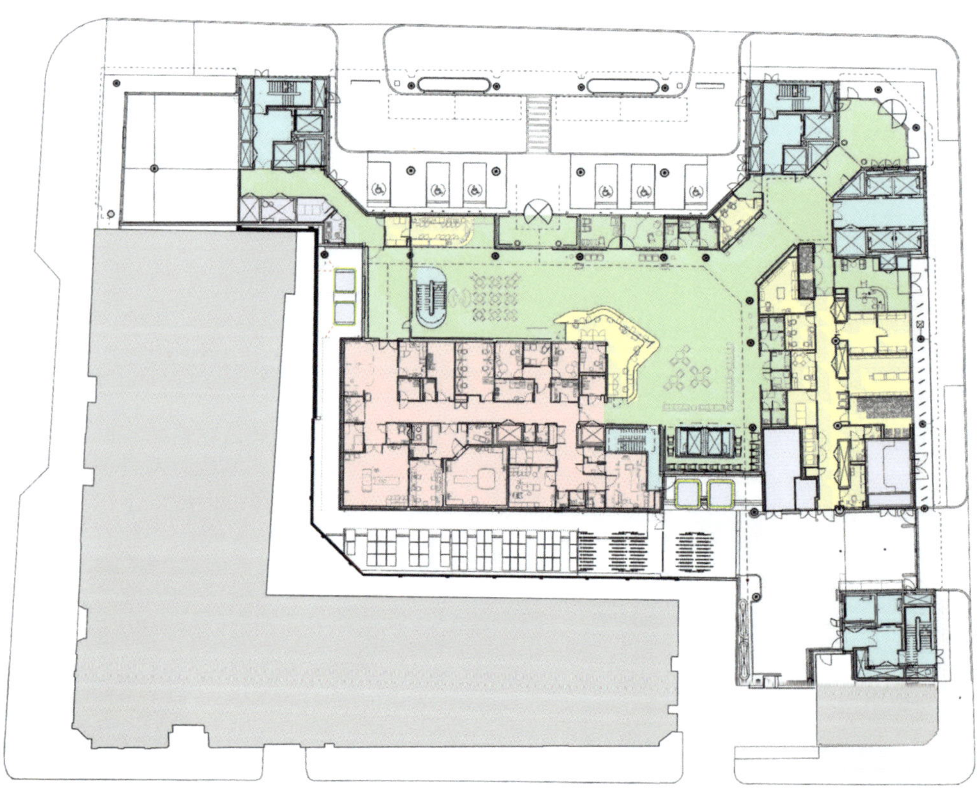

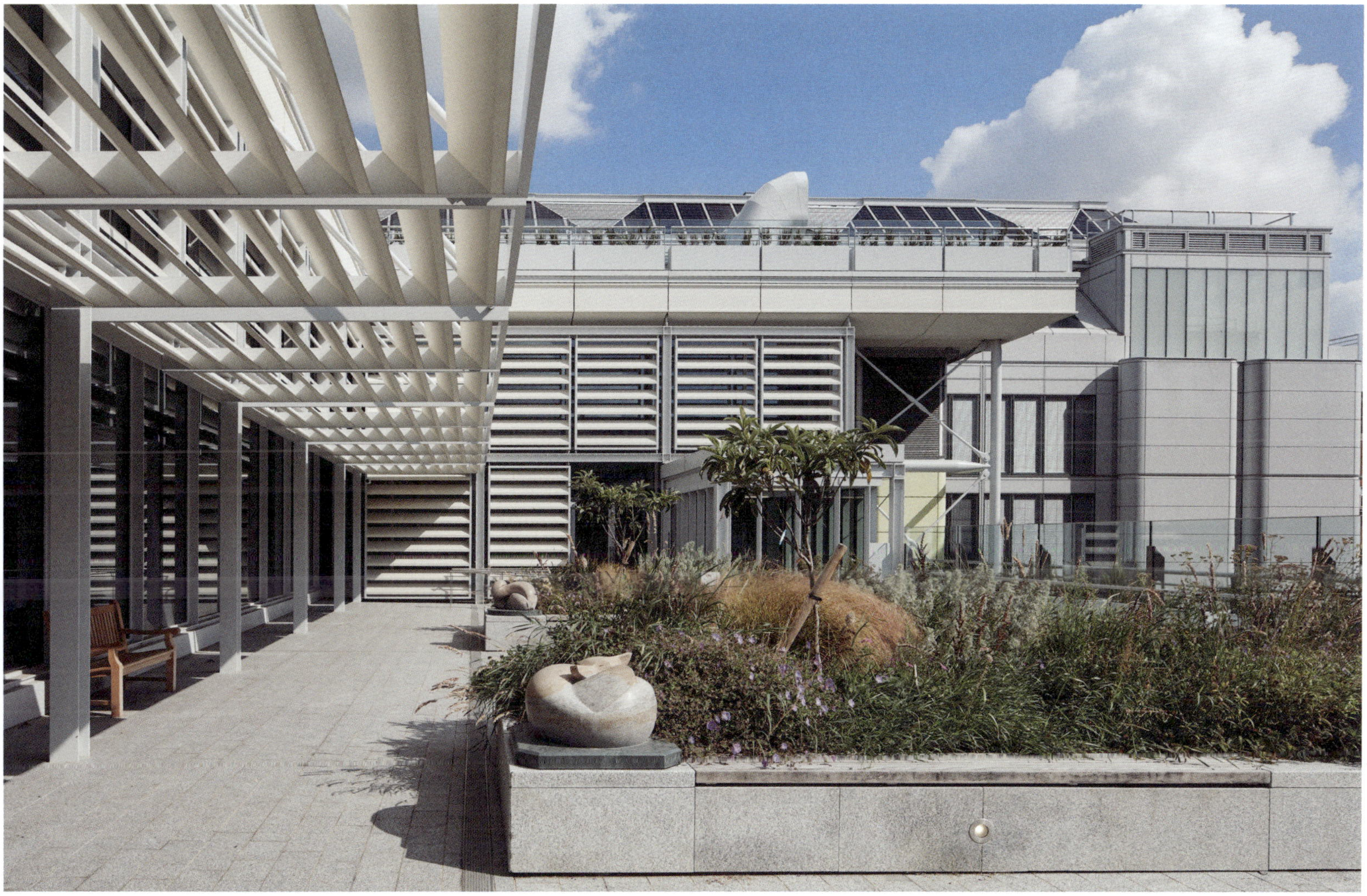

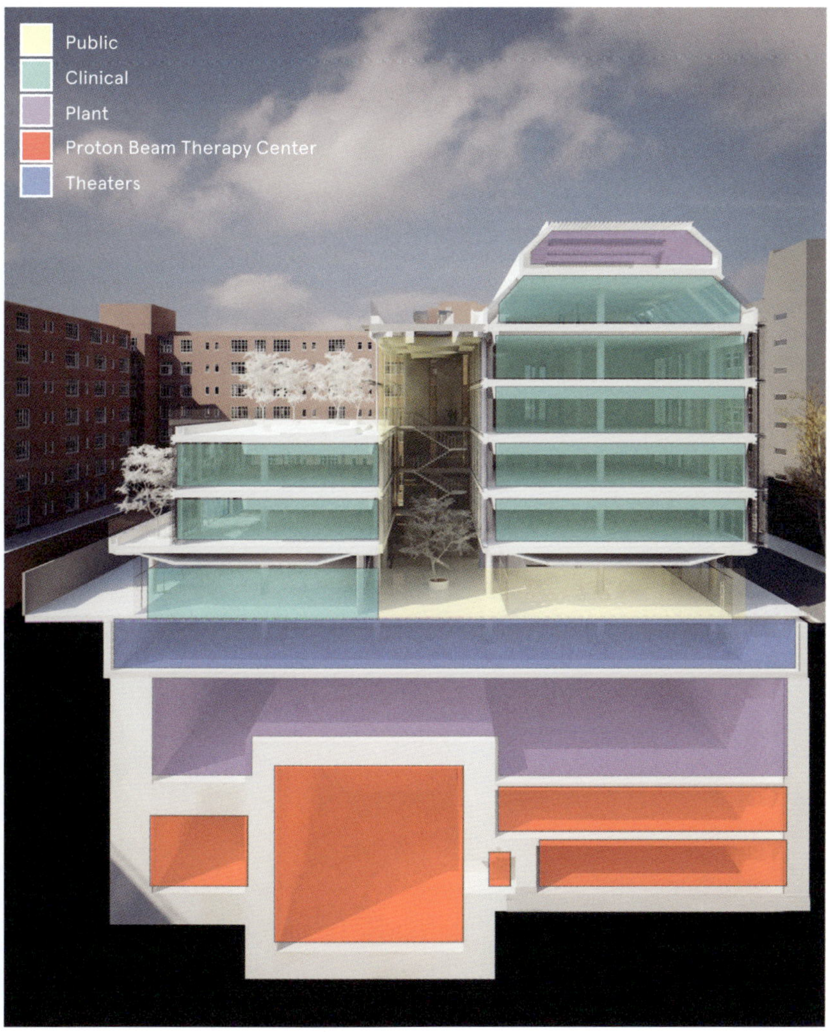

Rooftop with planted greenery and seating areas, supporting visual relief, rest, and the healing process.

Section of courtyard building, atrium, and main building.

P+HS Architect

Carlisle
United Kingdom

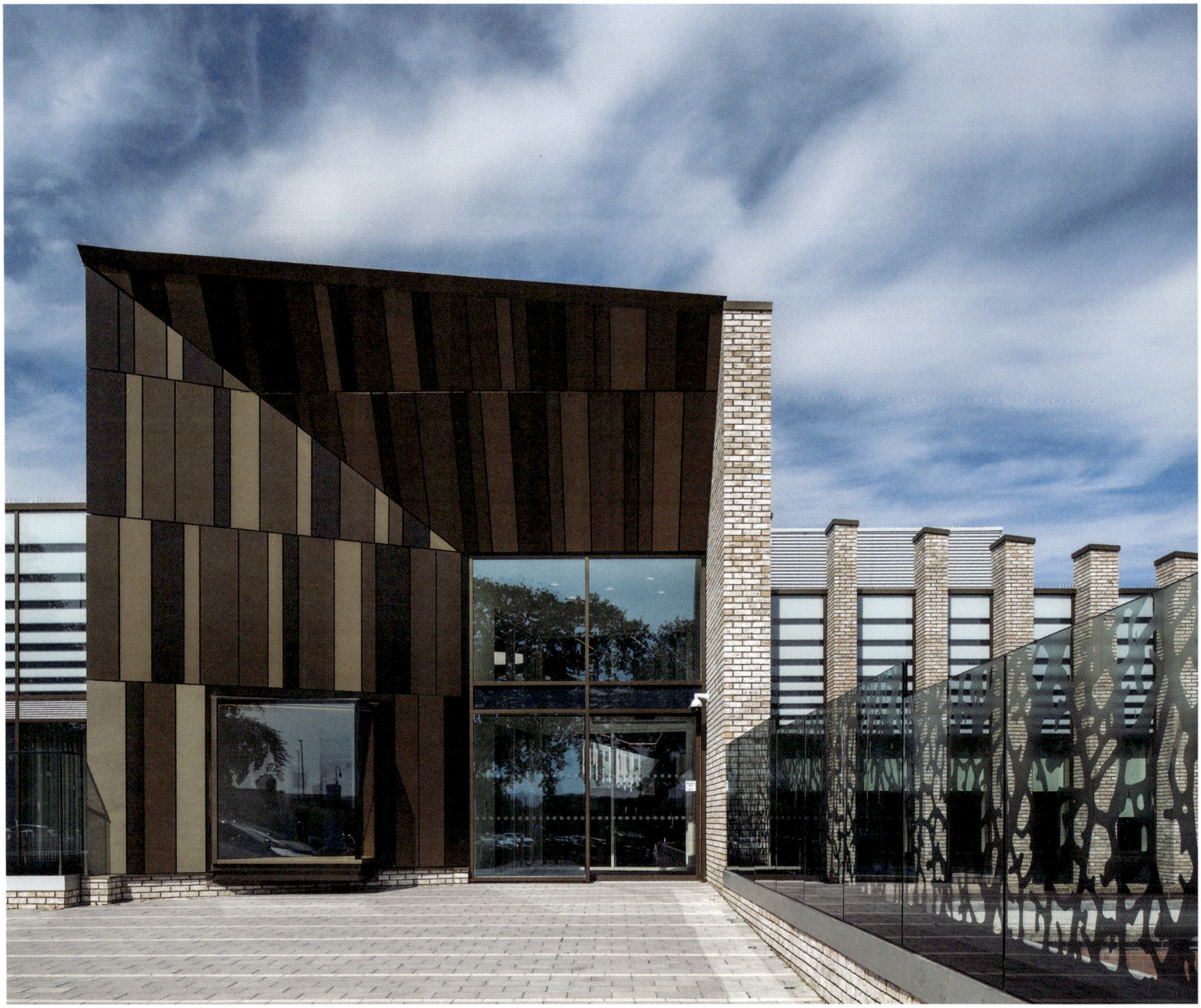

The main entrance has a large porch with a small window bay on the left.

The inside view shows the entrance, with the bay extending the waiting area on the right.

The Northern Centre for Cancer Care

The Northern Centre for Cancer Care at Cumberland Infirmary replaces outdated oncology facilities with a purpose-built environment that elevates patient and staff experience. Organized around clear clinical adjacencies and intuitive wayfinding, the design brings radiotherapy, chemotherapy, and outpatient services together to streamline patient journeys and reduce stress. A light-filled atrium creates a calm and welcoming arrival, while flexible, future-proofed spaces support evolving models of care. Prioritizing wellbeing, the Northern Centre for Cancer Care enhances staff recruitment and retention and delivers a BREEAM Excellent building that establishes a strong civic presence within the hospital campus.

Address: Cumberland Infirmary, Newtown Road, Carlisle CA2 7HY, United Kingdom | **Client:** North Cumbria Integrated Care NHS Foundation Trust | **Completion:** 2021 | **Size:** 3,900 m^2 | **Sector:** state | **Specialization:** cancer care, oncology | **Number of treatment rooms:** 19

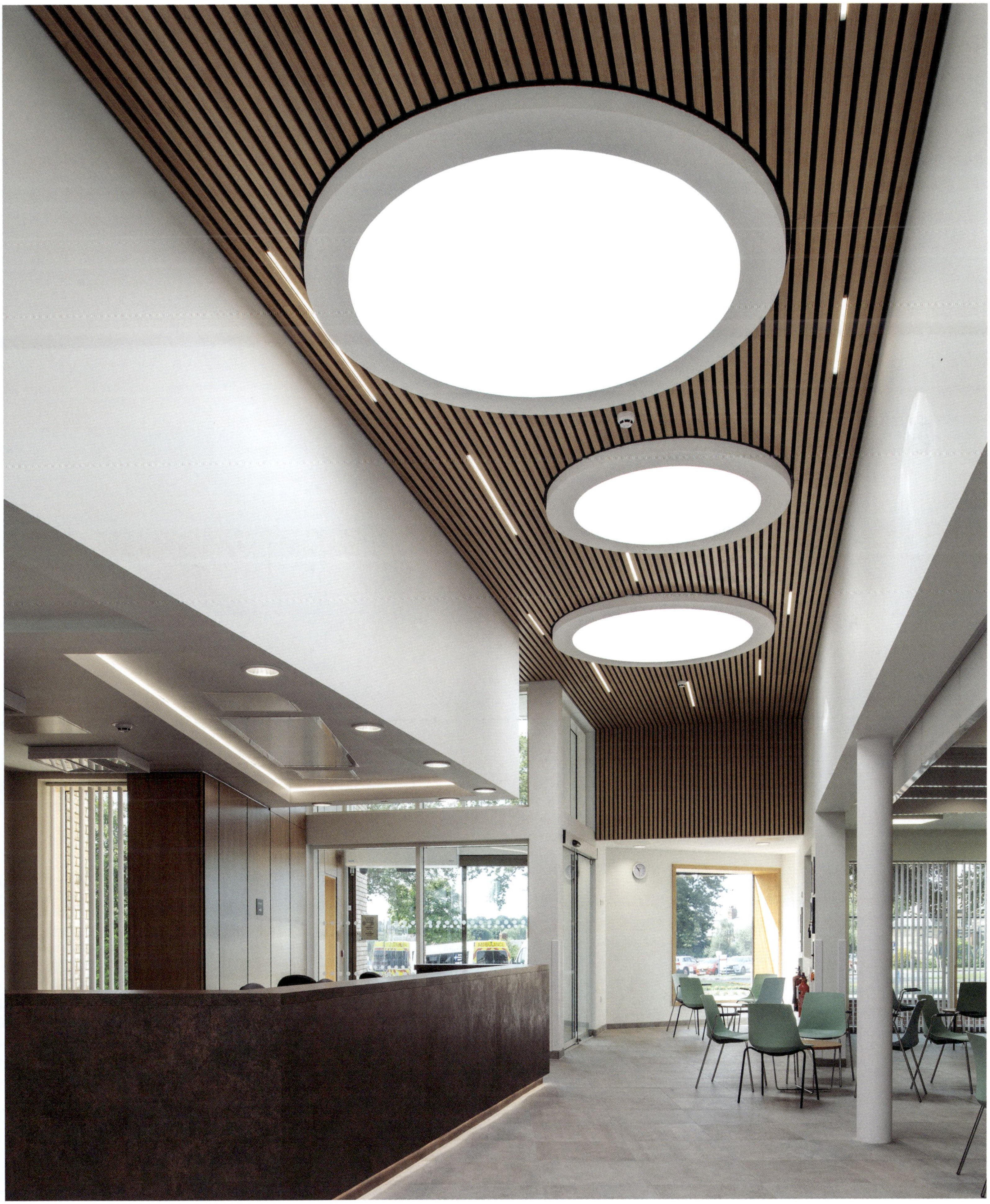

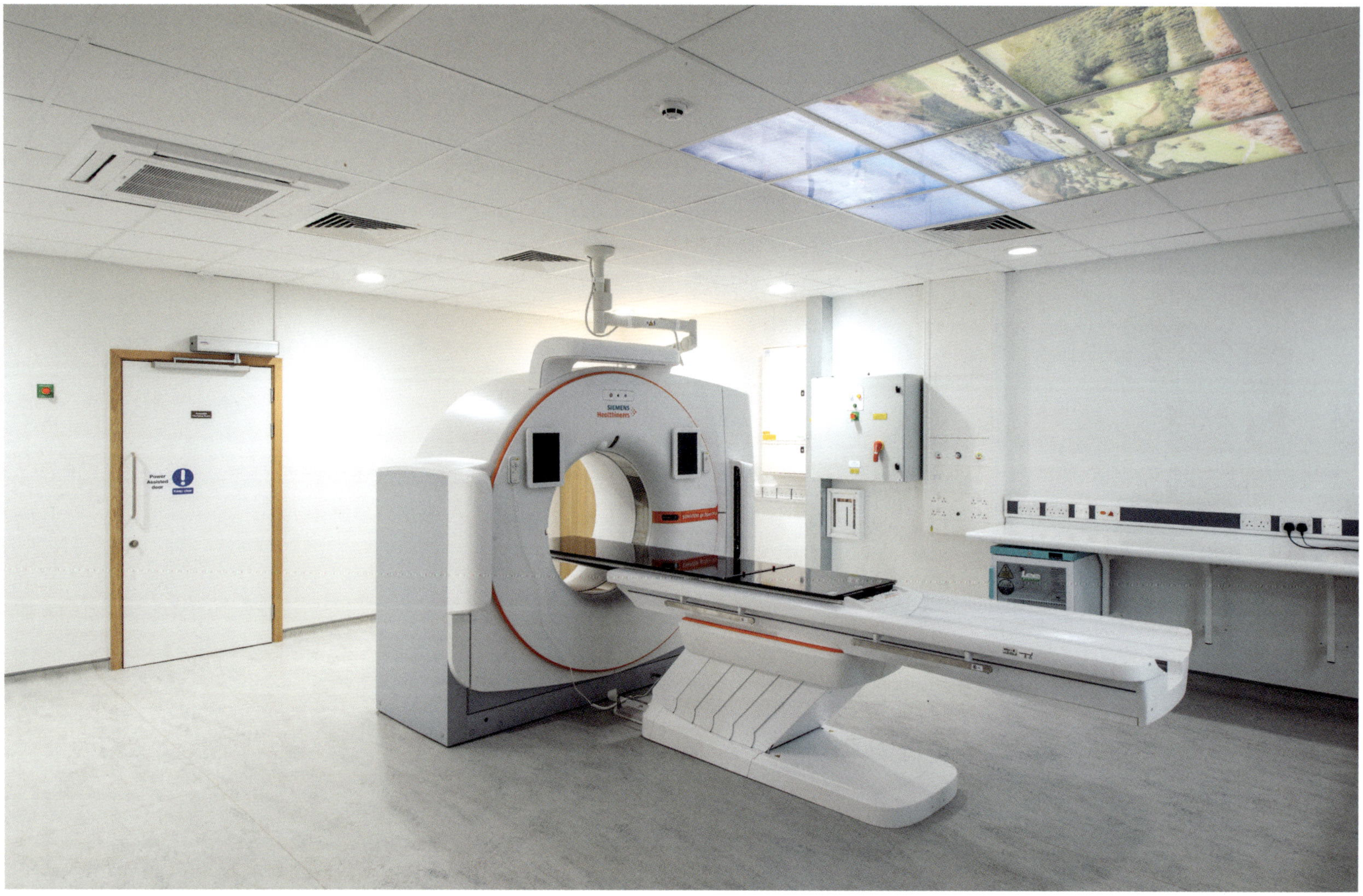

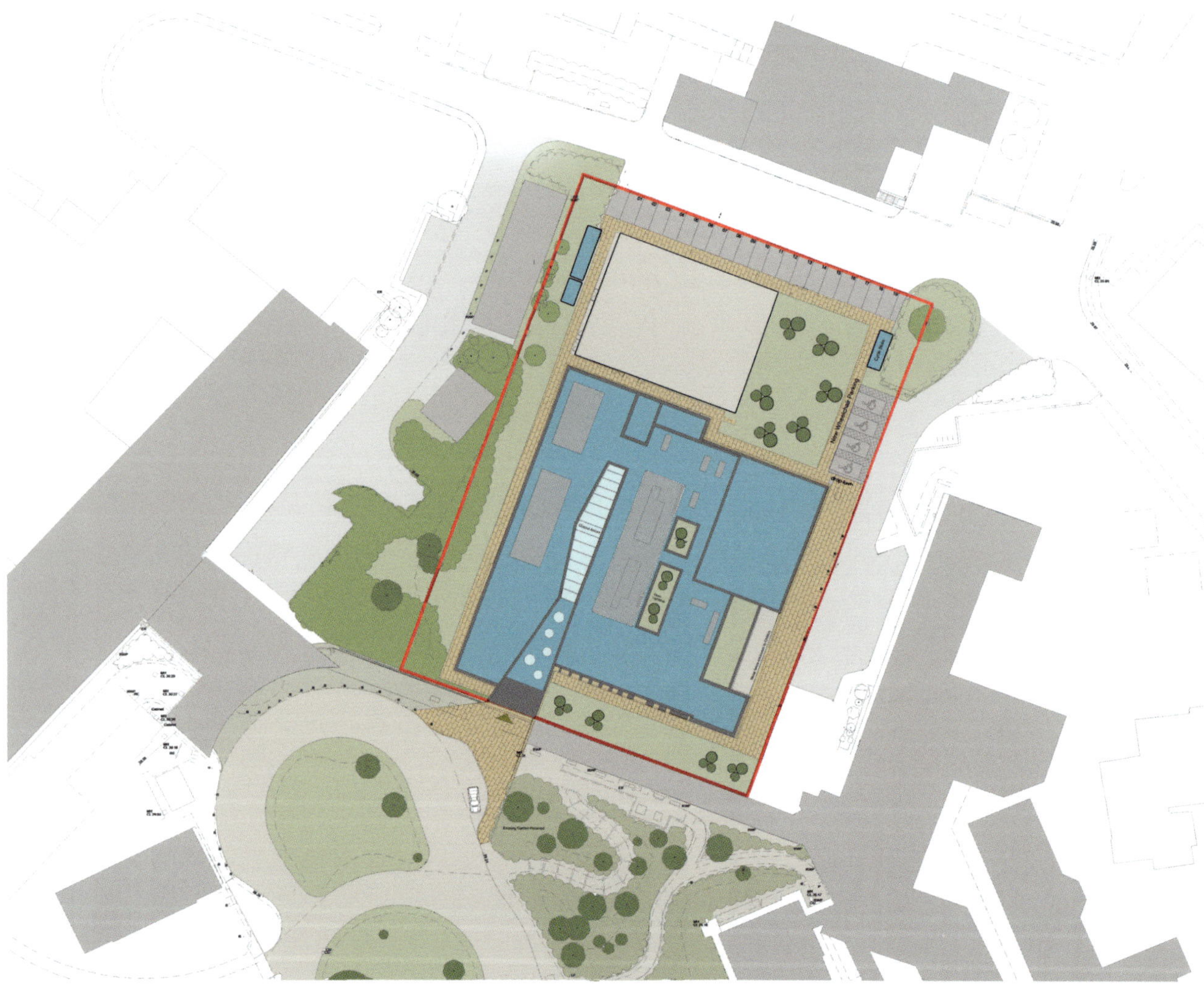

MRI with a soothing projection on the ceiling.

Situation.

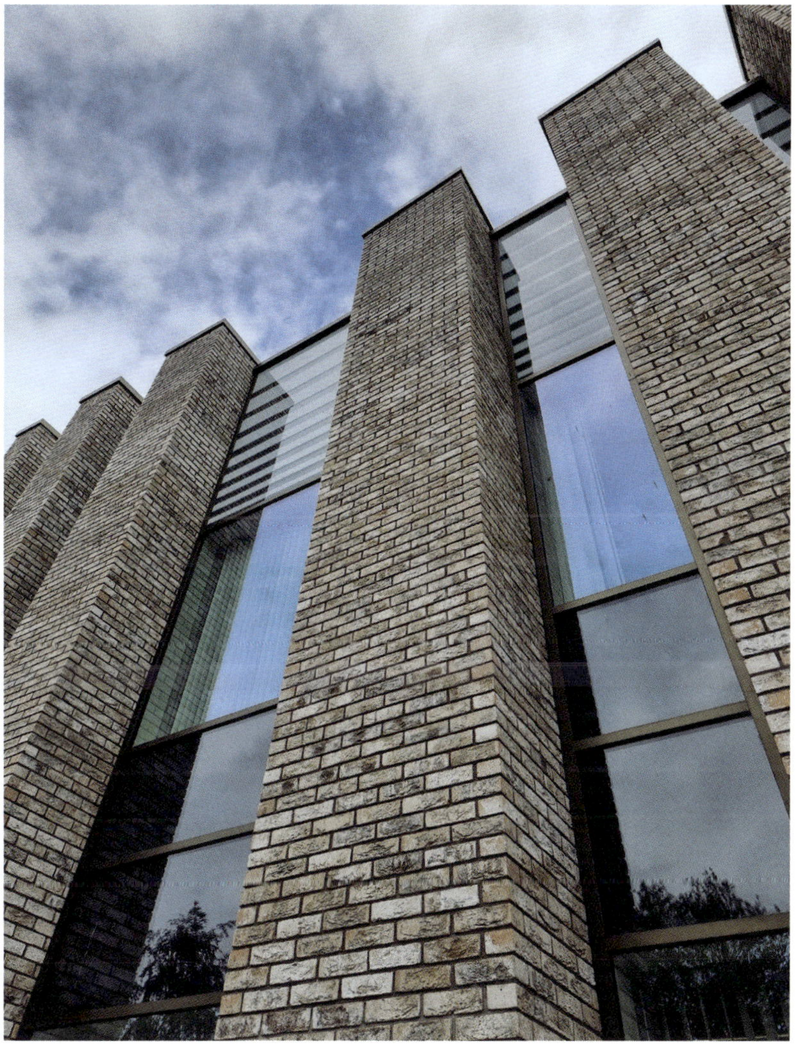

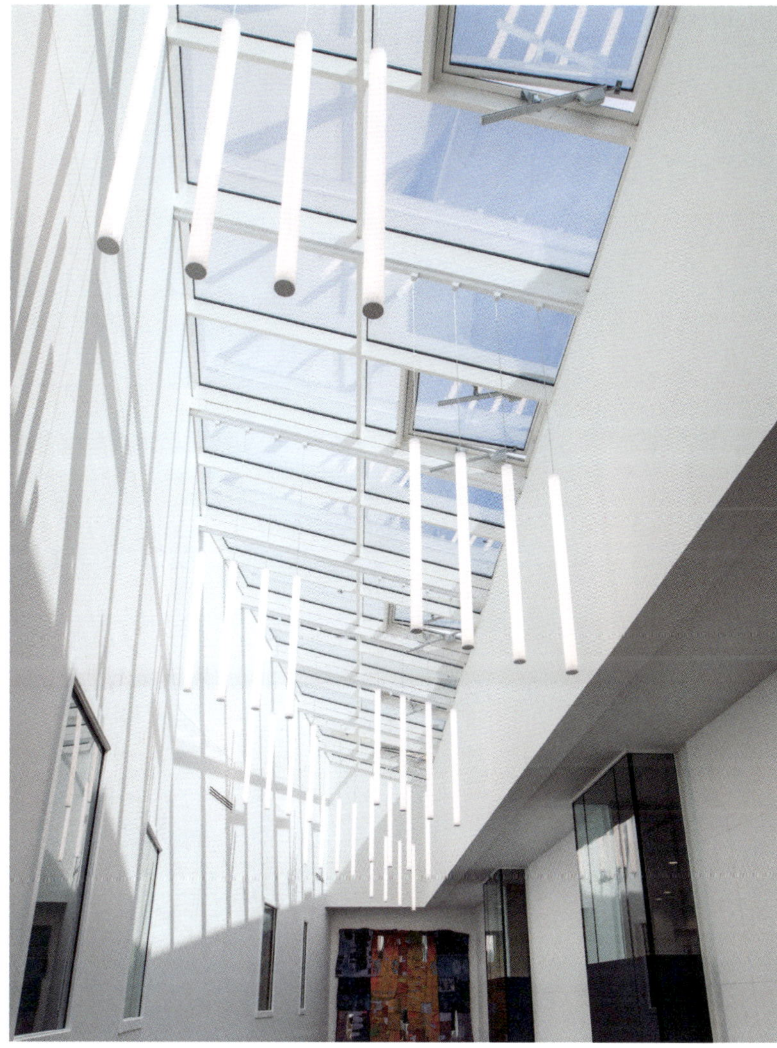

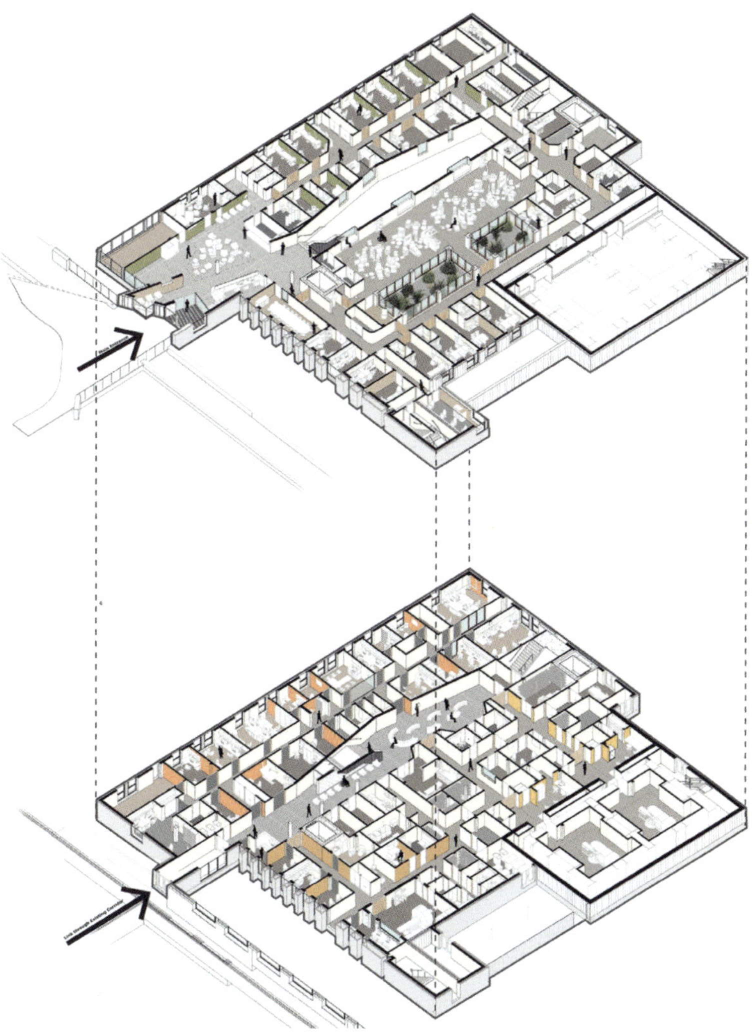

Old bricks, when used instead of newly manufactured ones, drastically cut down on embedded CO_2 and energy consumption.

Light-filled glazed atrium.

Floor plans upper and lower ground floor.

WAY Architecture
Architekten Maurer & Partner

Mauer
Austria

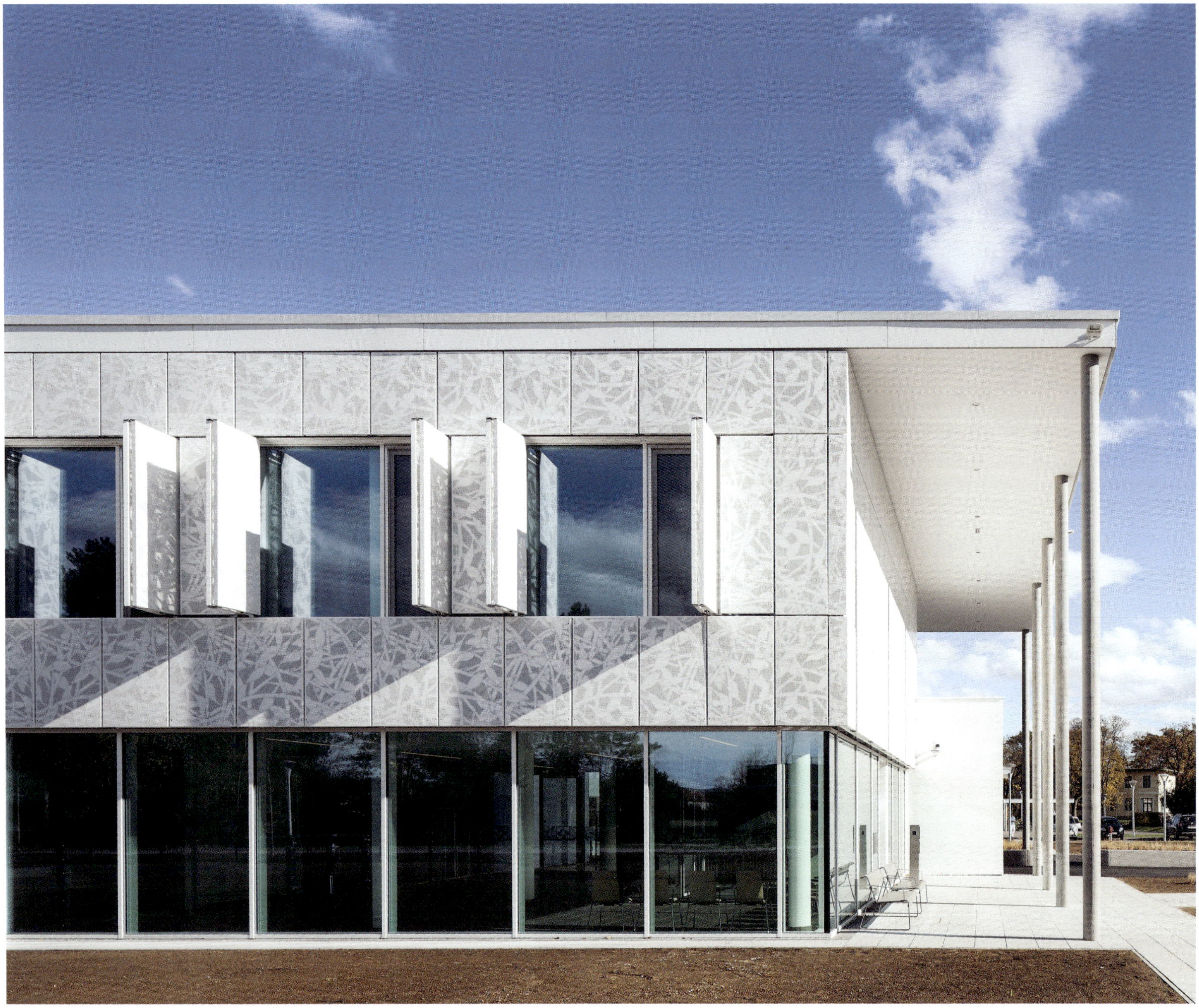

The southwest corner of the building, featuring round pillars that spans multiple floors.

Multi-story columns with a horizontally segmented, recessed façade.

Mauer Regional Hospital Building 49 – Adult Psychiatry

Founded in 1902 as the State Sanatorium and Nursing Home, the Mauer State Hospital symbolizes the shift toward a therapy-oriented approach to psychiatry. Carlo von Boog's Art Nouveau pavilion complex integrated architecture and landscape as part of the therapeutic concept – light, air, and movement were considered key factors in recovery. Over the past two decades, the complex has been carefully renovated and expanded. Building 49 continues this humanistic approach: A clearly structured building with 42 beds, plenty of natural light, views of the greenery, and direct access to the garden creates a sense of orientation, dignity, and a supportive atmosphere for people in exceptional mental health situations. The 24 patient rooms and seven treatment rooms are arranged along the length of the building, offering views of the surrounding greenery.

Address: Hausmeninger Straße 221, 3362 Mauer, Austria | **Client:** State of Lower Austria | **Completion:** 2018 | **Size:** 5,292.47 m^2 | **Sector:** public | **Specialization:** adult psychiatry | **Number of treatment rooms:** 7 | **Number of patient rooms:** 24

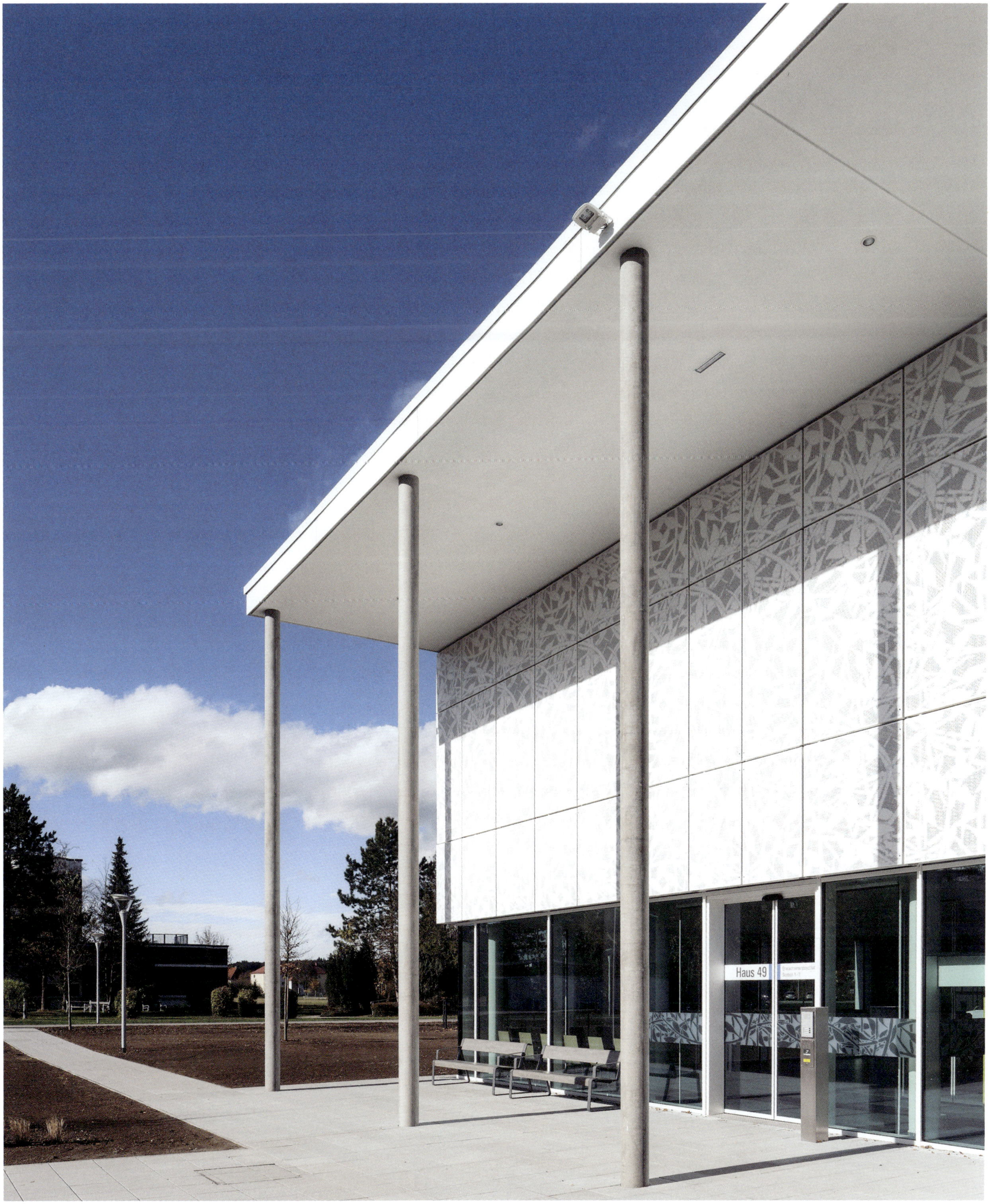

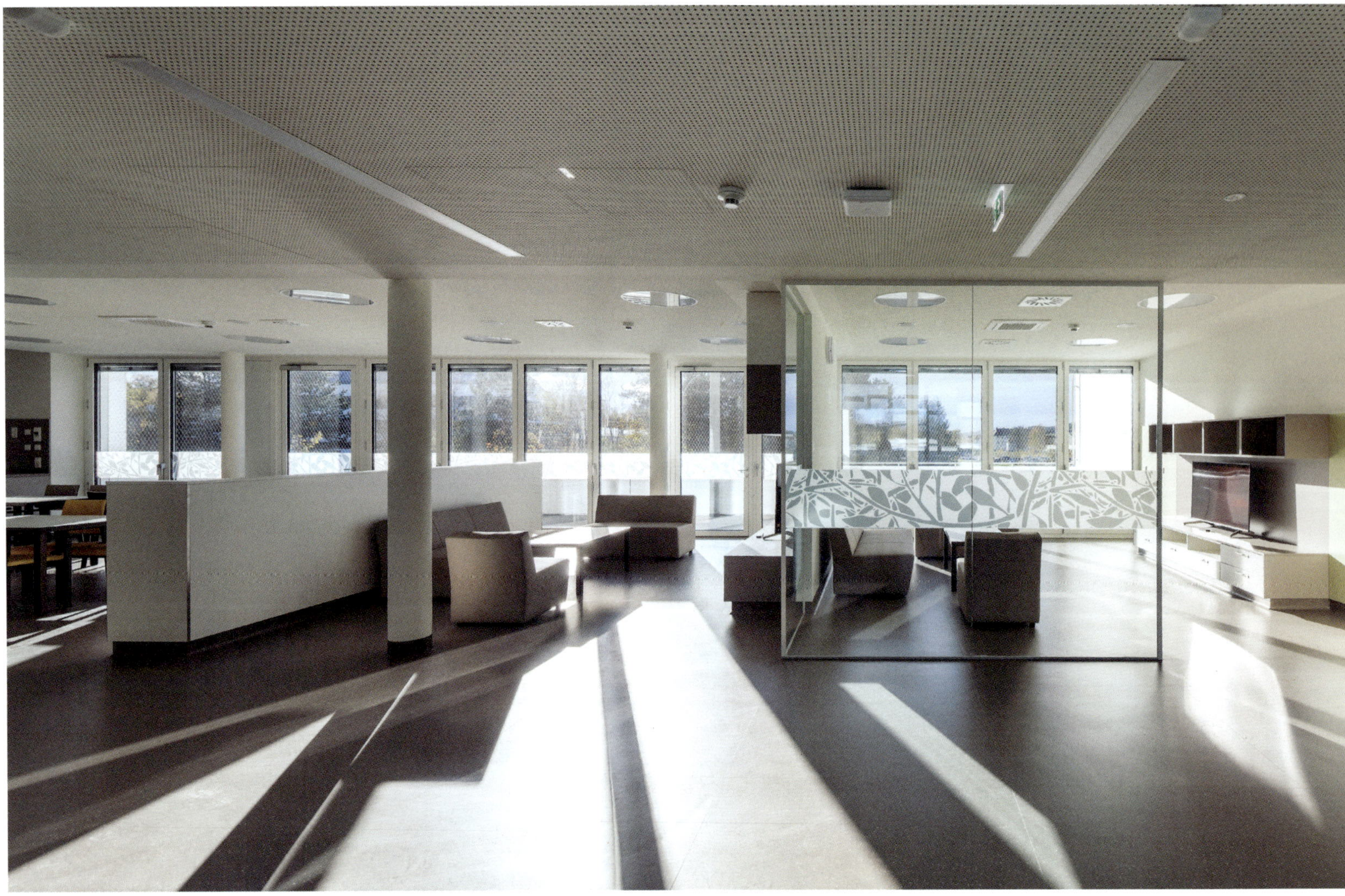

Brightly lit waiting area with glass walls and an acoustic ceiling.

Site plan.

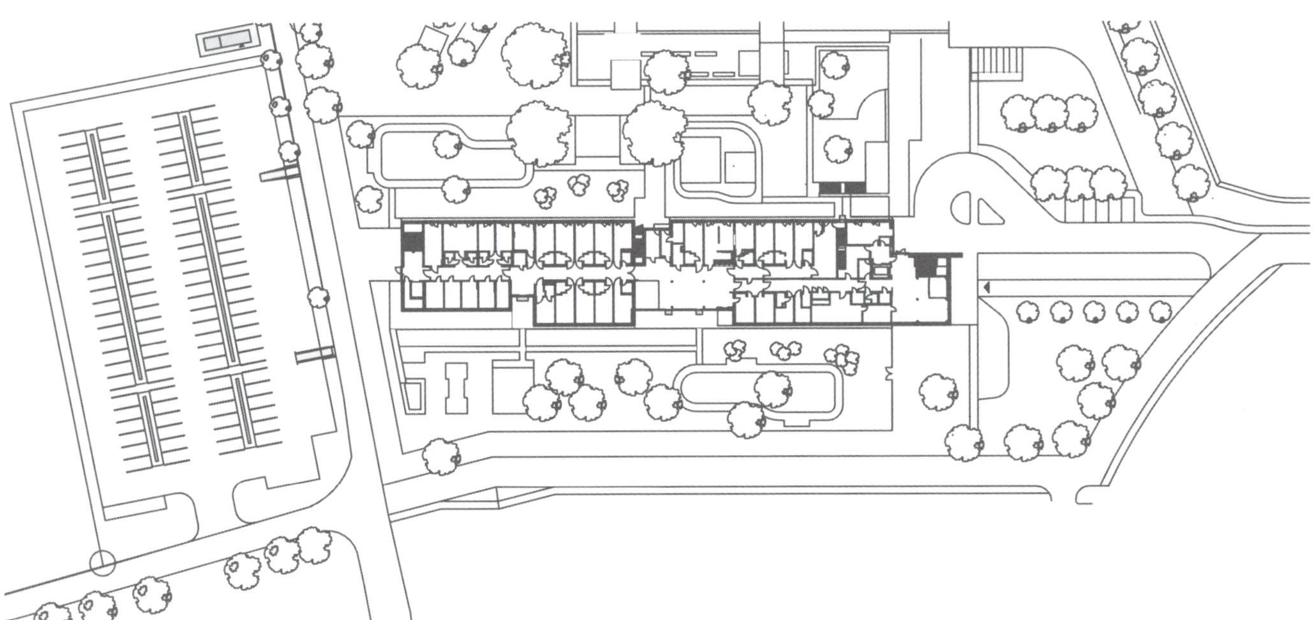

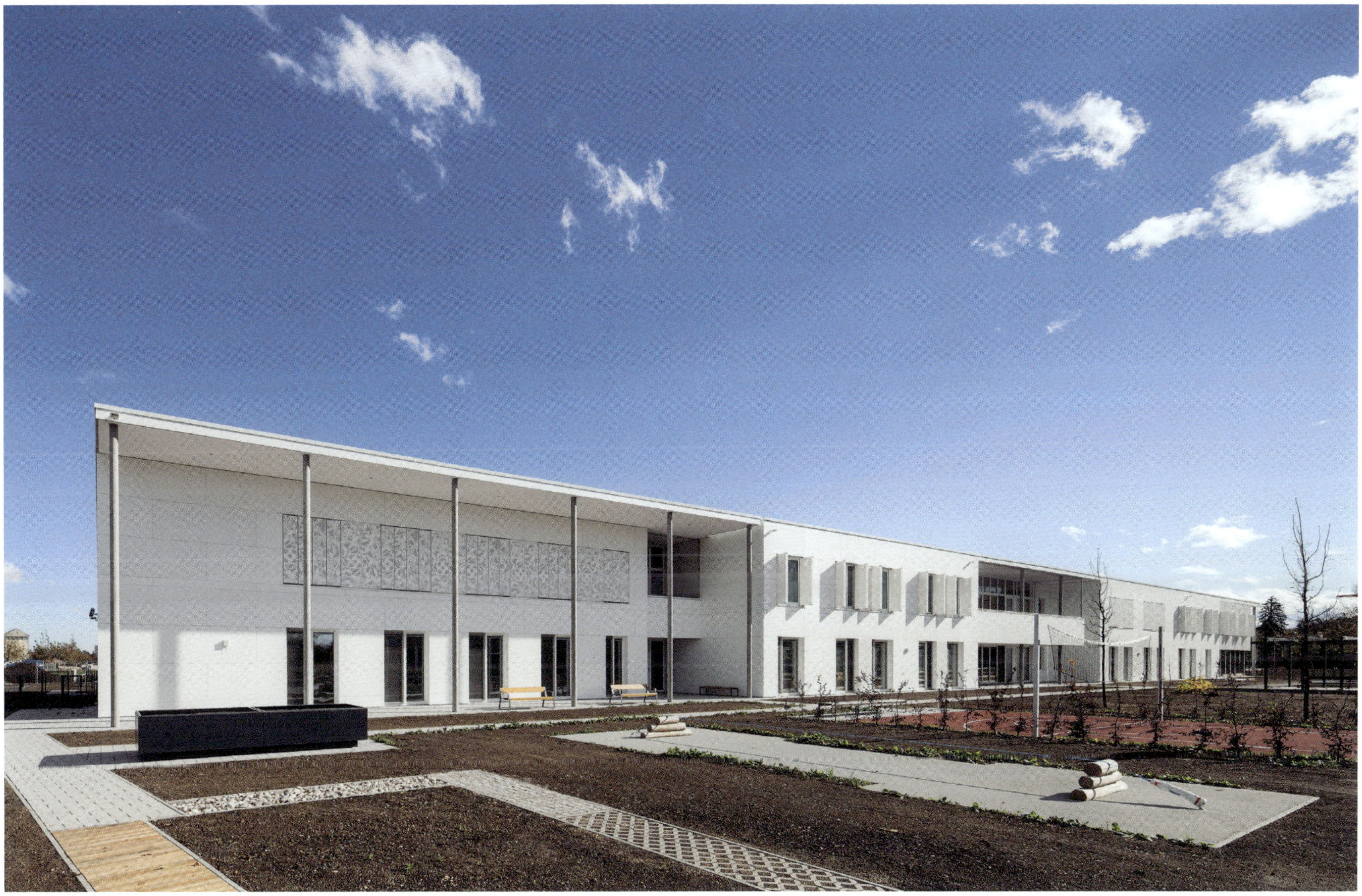

View of the west-facing façade with its green surroundings.

South and west elevation.

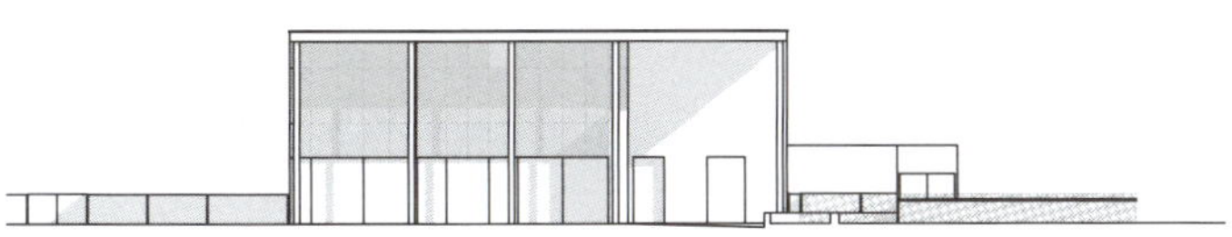

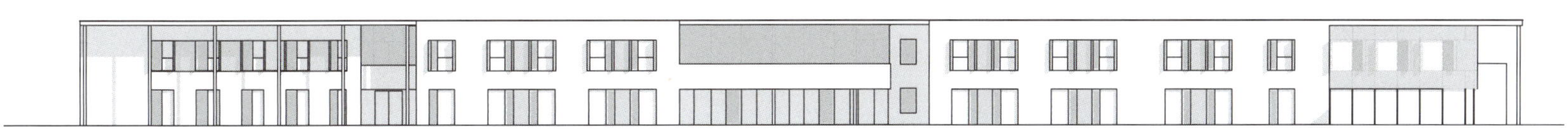

LIAG architecten en bouwadviseurs

Utrecht
The Netherlands

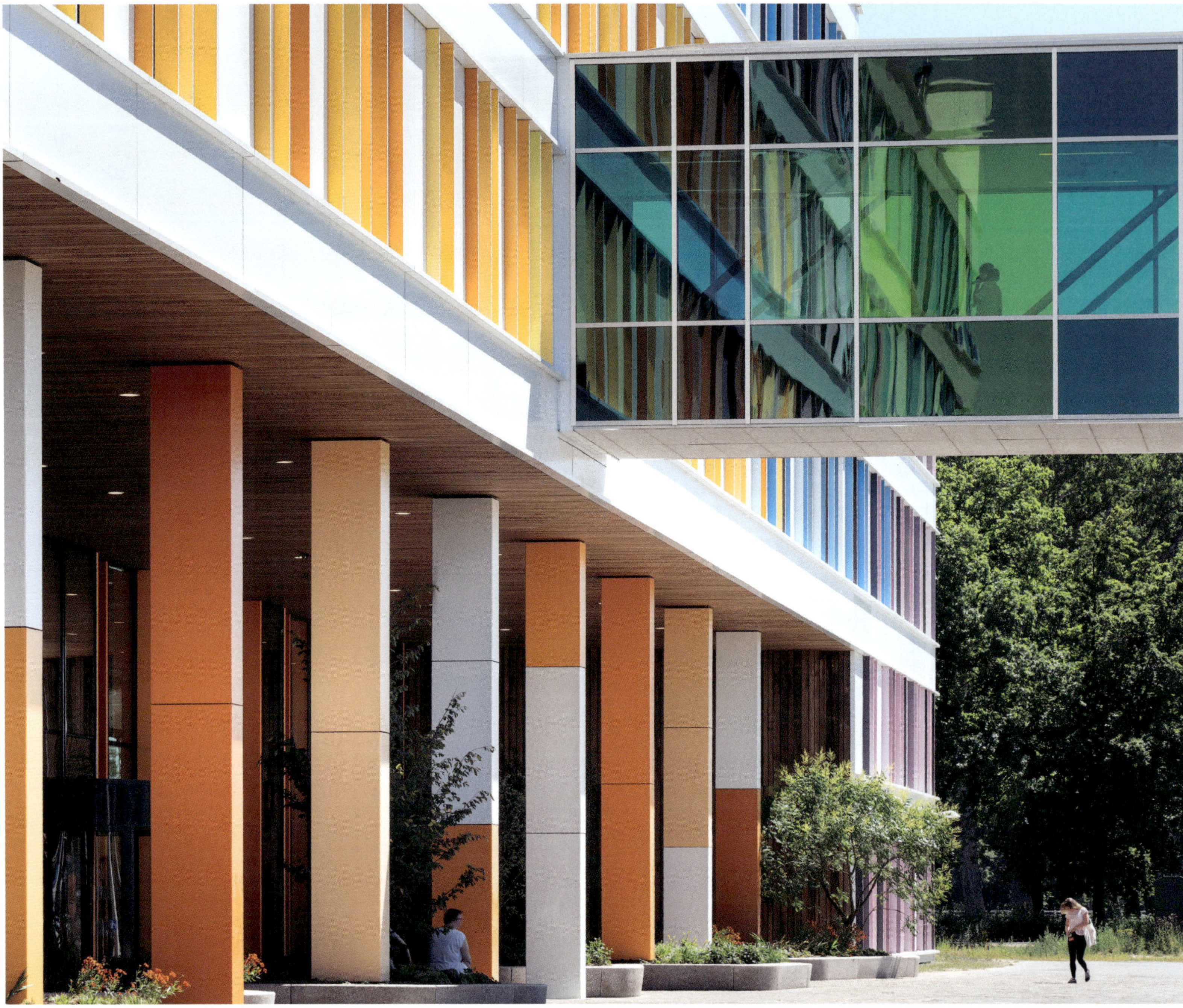

Entrance area with the bridge.

Central staircase.

The Princess Máxima Center for Pediatric Oncology

The Princess Máxima Center for Pediatric Oncology, a 45,000 square meter development in Utrecht, The Netherlands, opened its doors in May 2018. Here highly complex research, cure, and care came together in one building. The architecture was designed to support this goal. Extensive research into healing environments and evidence-based design informed the creation of a building that supports children's normal development despite their illness. The research was conducted by doctors, psychiatrist, engineers, and architects together closely with patients and parents. The terminology used for this approach was development-orientated care. Furthermore, particular attention was paid to the known aspects of a healing environment such as daylight, air, views, good acoustics, clear zoning, and so on in order to facilitate the healing process.

Address: Heidelberglaan 25, 3584 CS Utrecht, The Netherlands | **Client:** Board Princess Máxima Center, Utrecht, The Netherlands | **Completion:** 2018 | **Size:** 44,833 m² | **Sector:** private | **Specialization:** pediatric oncology | **Number of treatment rooms:** 20 | **Number of patient rooms:** 85 | **Landscape design:** BplusB | **Interior design:** LIAG / MMEK / Gispen

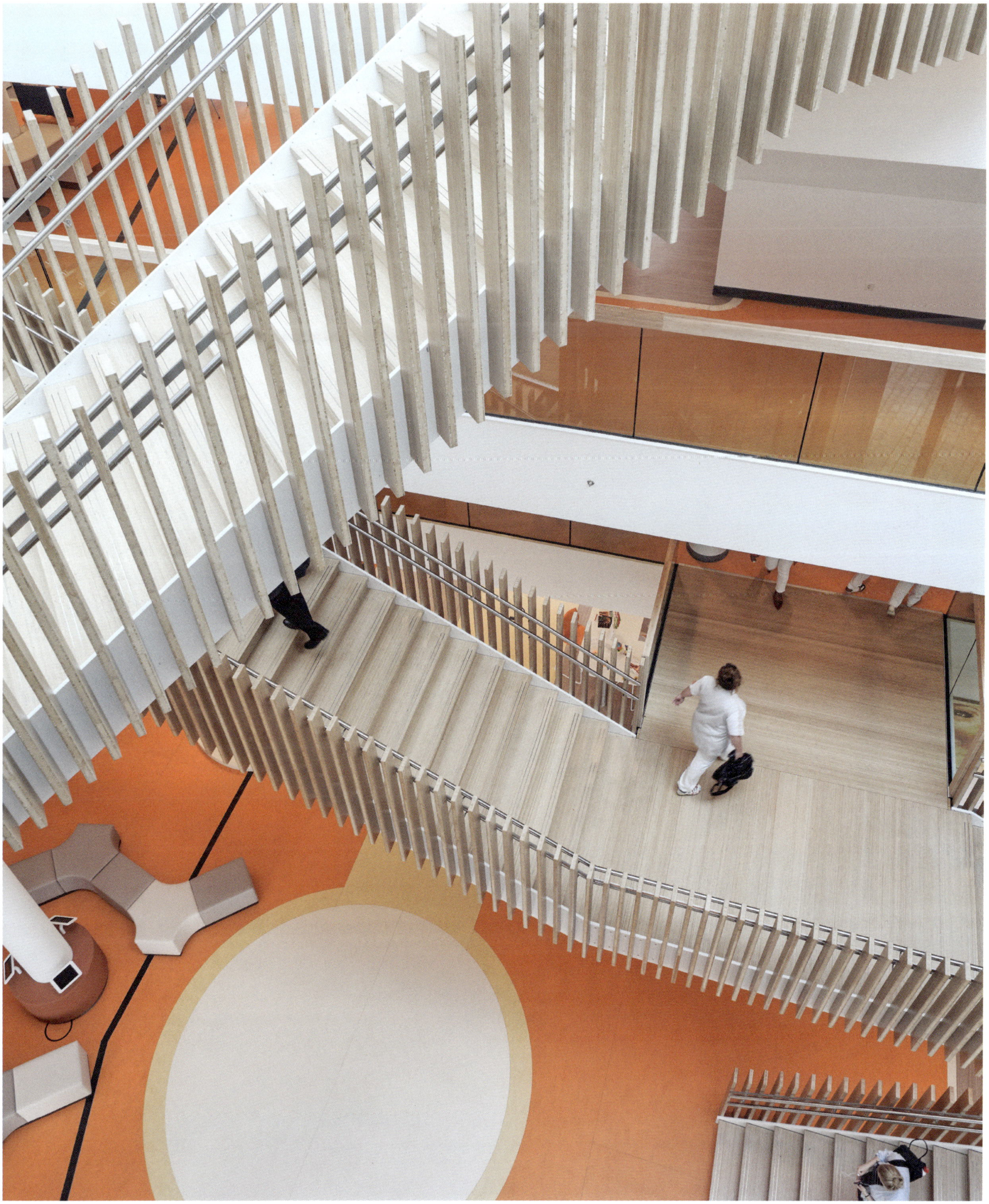

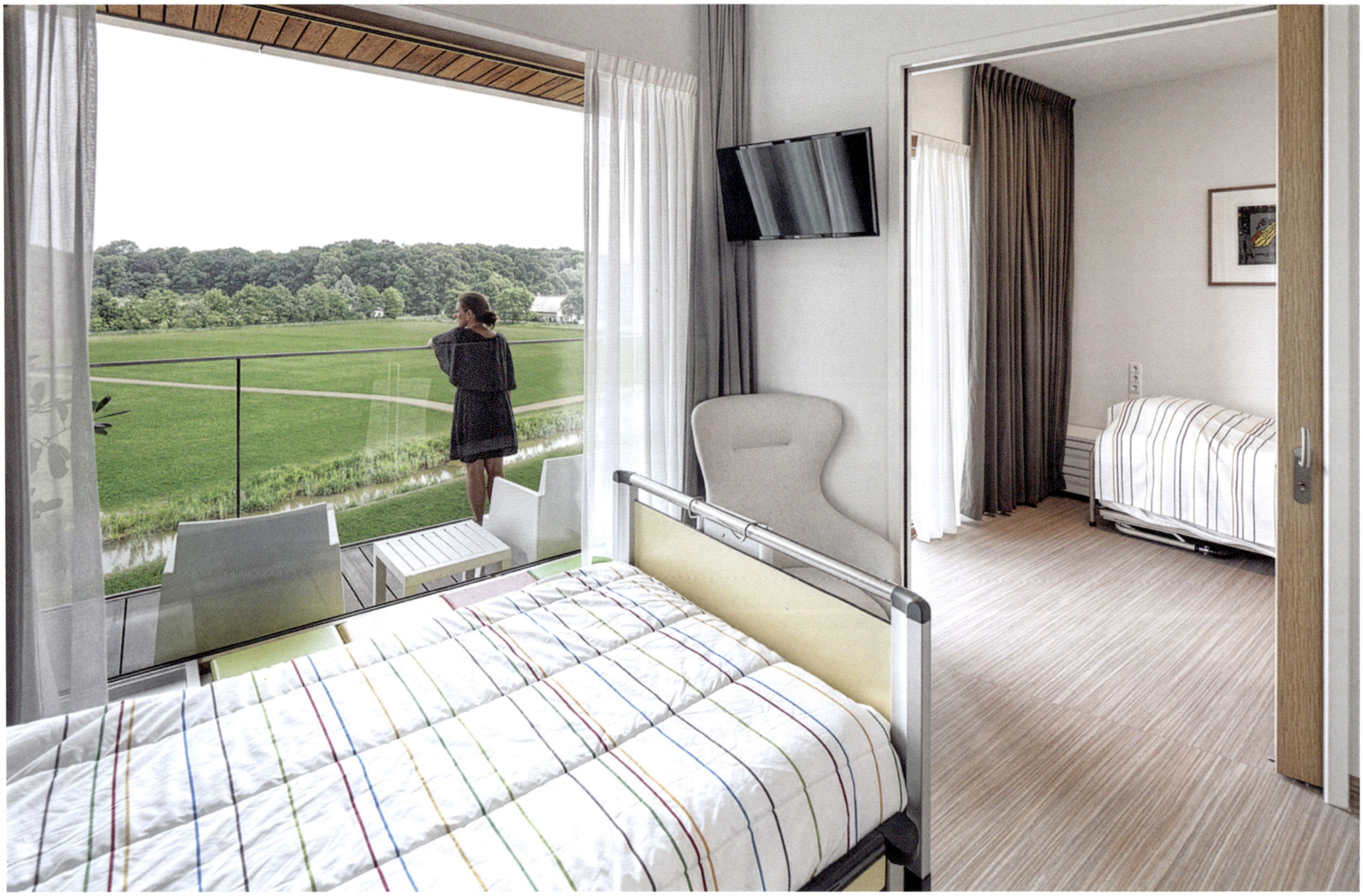

Patient room with a beautiful view in the nature.

Second floor plan.

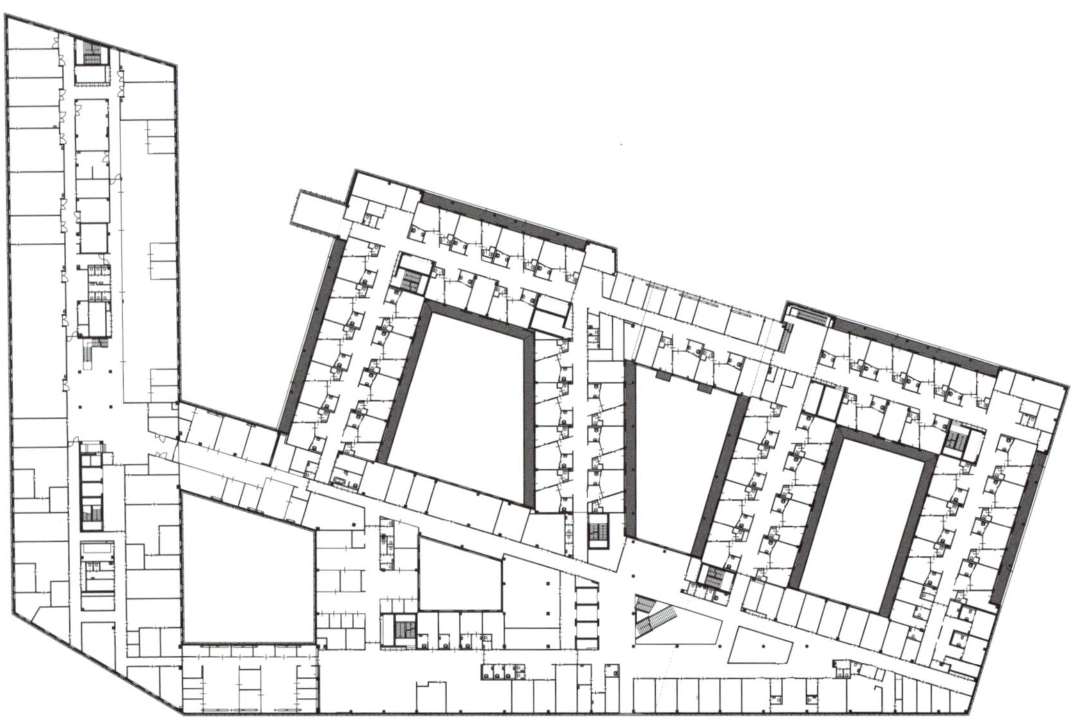

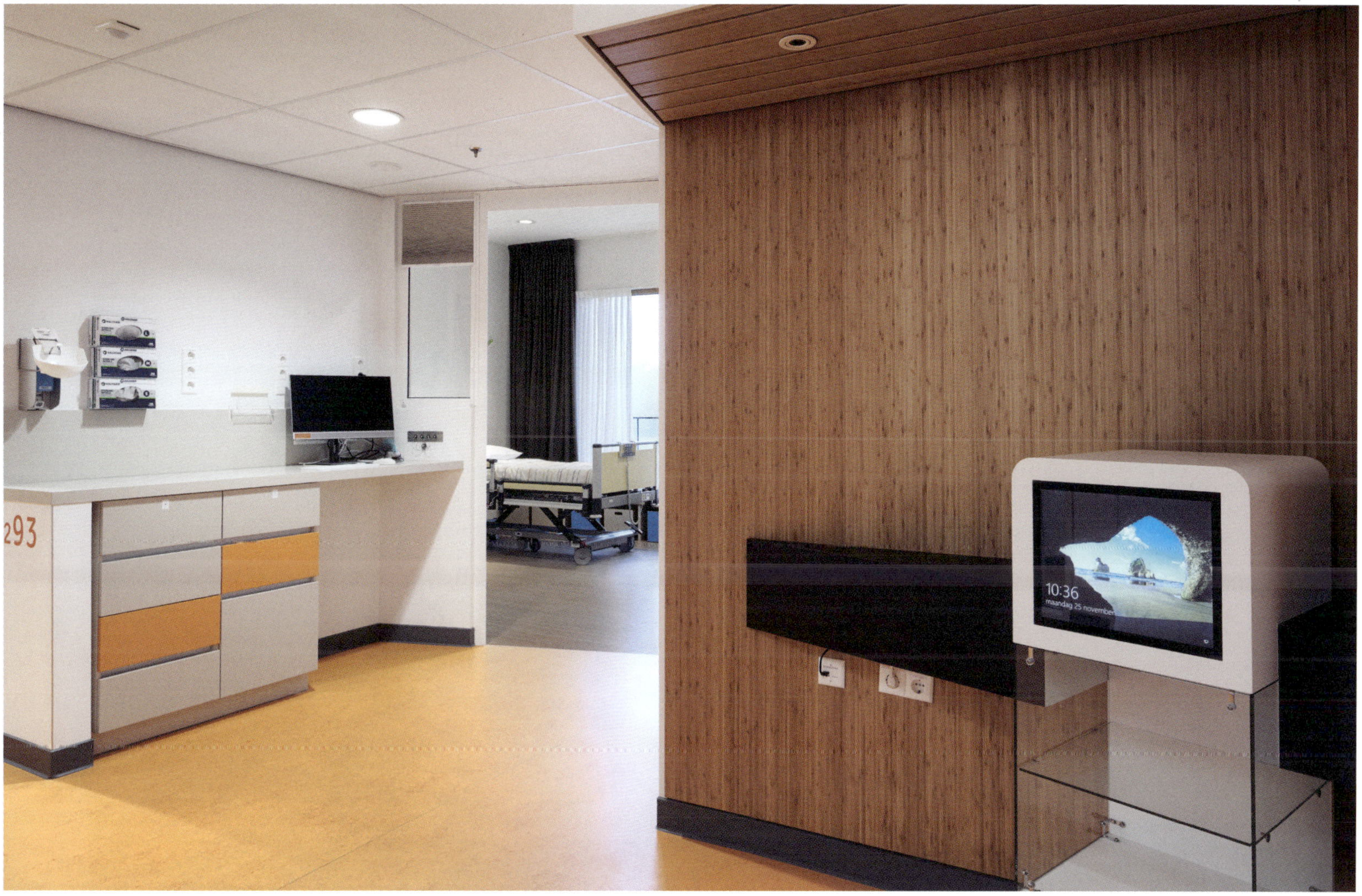

View towards a patient's room.

First floor plan.

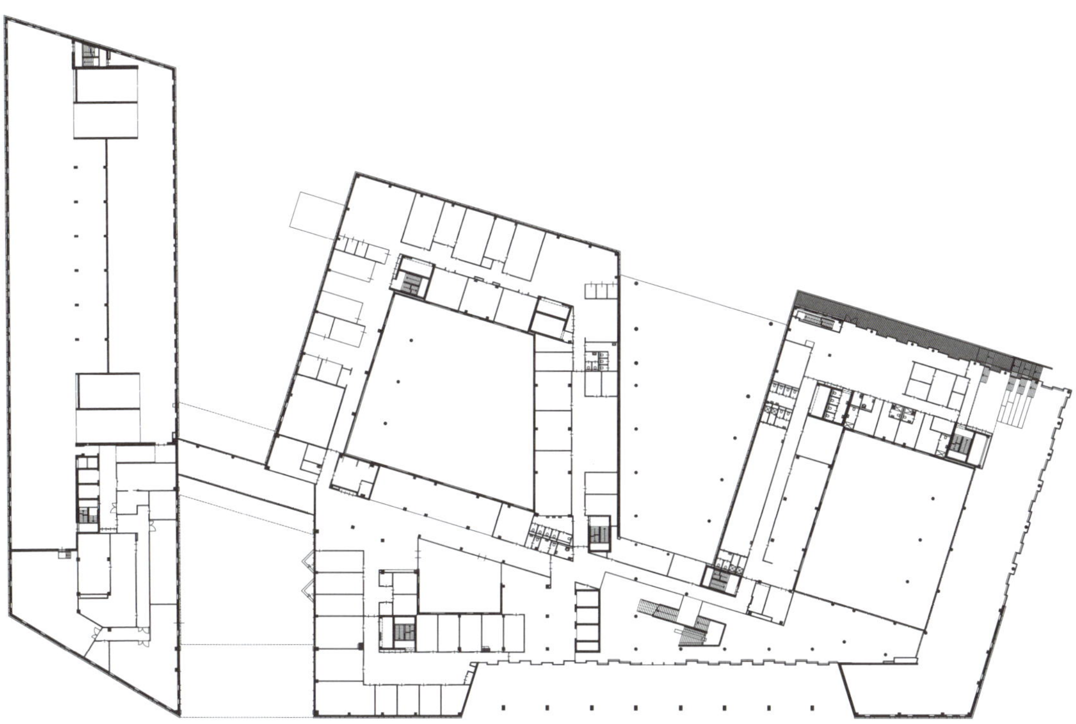

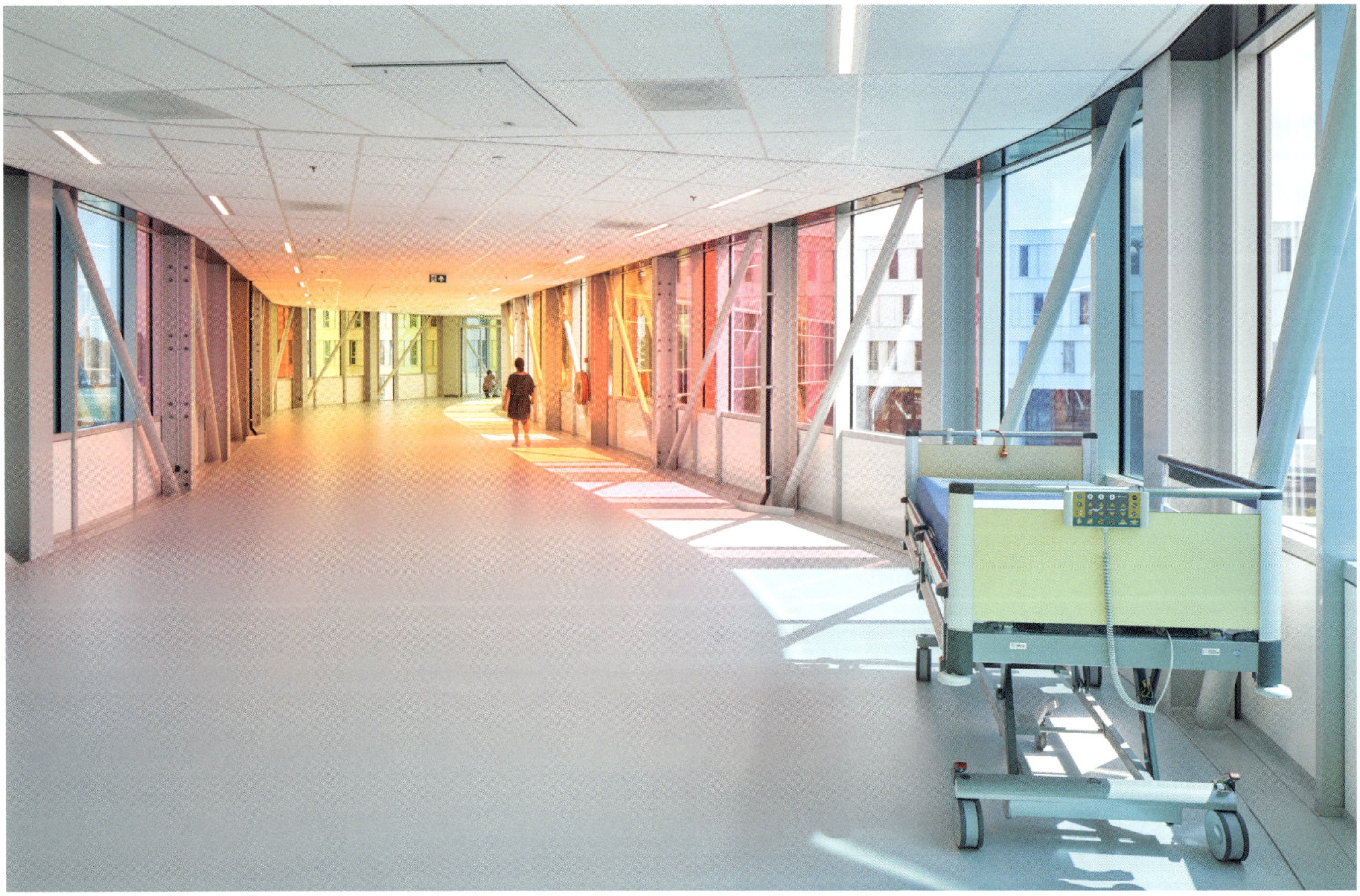

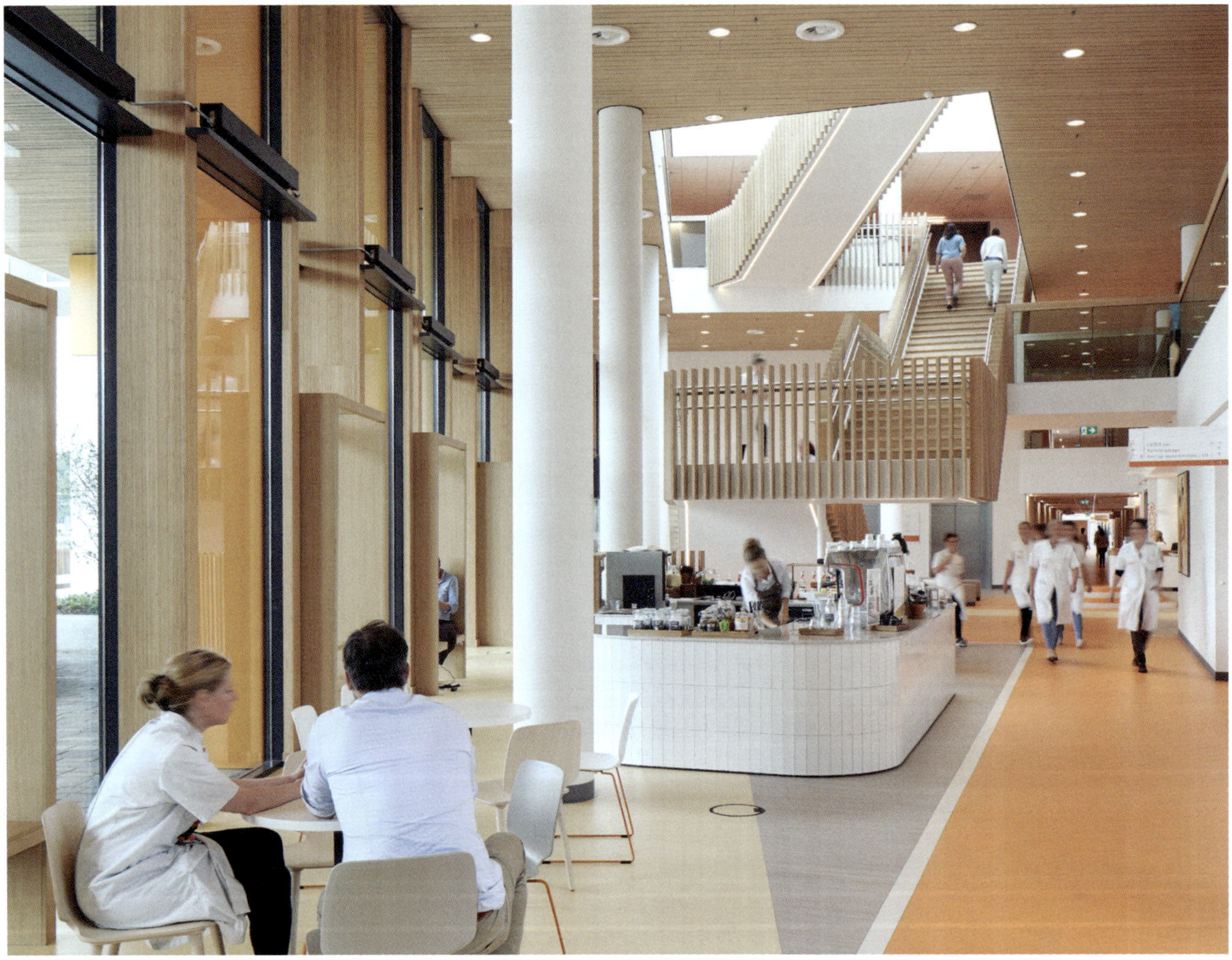

Colorful and brightly lit bridge connecting the center with the neighboring building.

Main axis that connects all parts of the center.

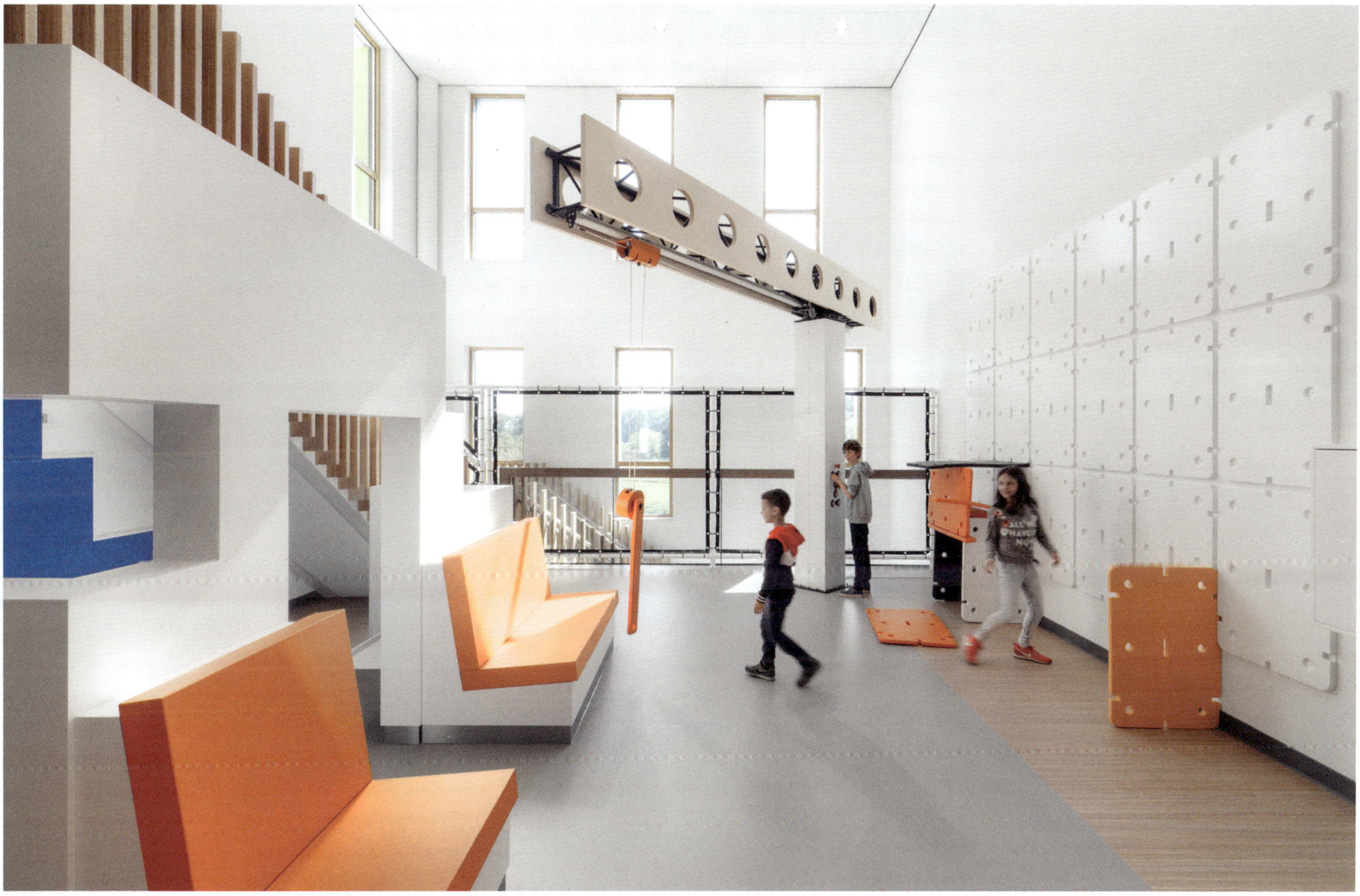

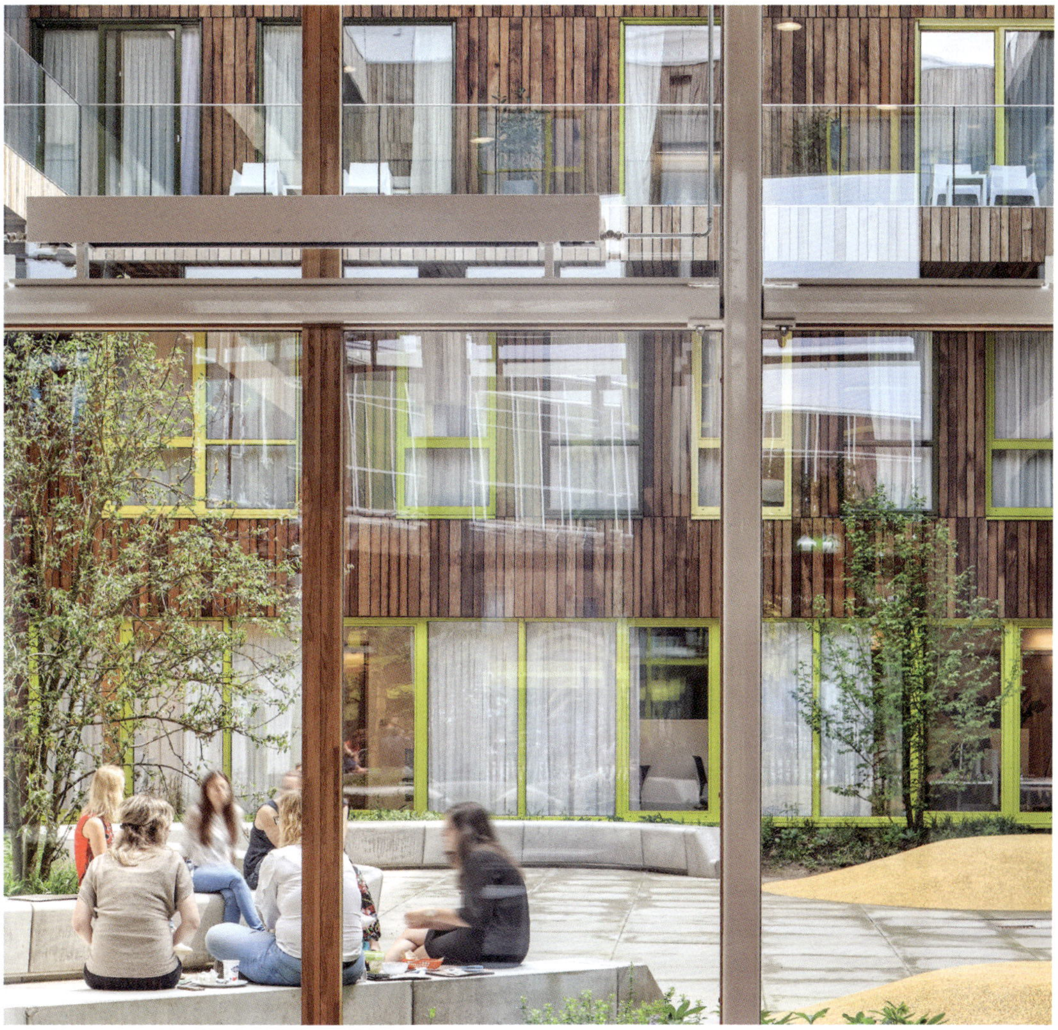

Play area for the children.

One of the two main courtyards.

Adam Rujbr Architects

Šternberk Czech Republic

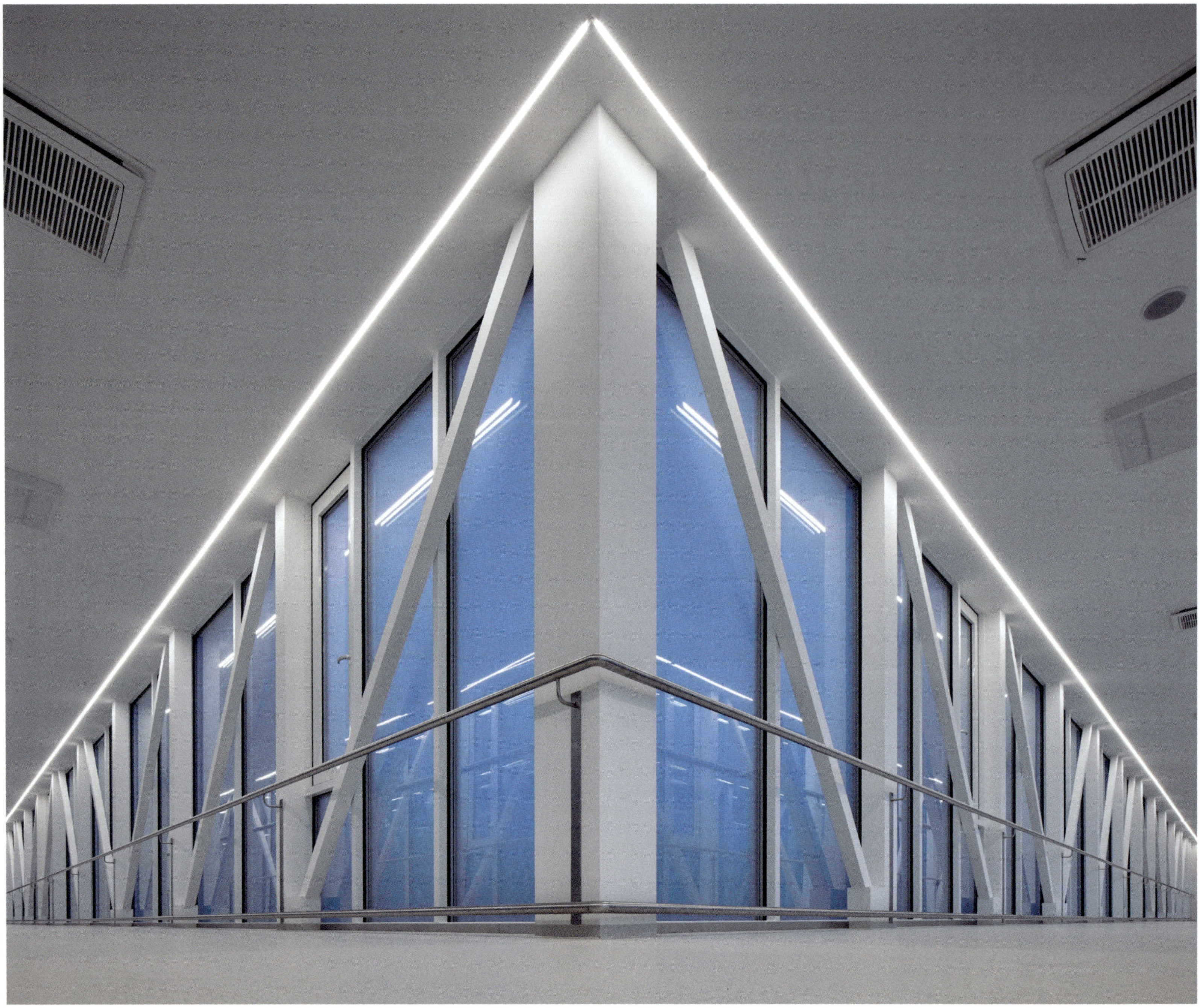

Two-way intersection leading to the old buildings.

The front façade is enlivened by vertical windows.

Connection of pavilion to the surrounding buildings.

Šternberk Hospital Internal Medicine Ward

The pavilion is a compact block with vertical windows that are not only an aesthetic element, but also functional. The architecture connects the pavilion with its surroundings and cleverly integrates the original substation into the new pavilion building. Glass tunnels connect the pavilion with the surrounding buildings and allow efficient movement through the hospital complex. The building has four above-ground floors and one underground floor, which house the technical facilities, an outpatient wing with specialized outpatient clinics, inpatient departments and an intensive care unit. Energy efficiency is a key element of the pavilion, which is classified as a passive building: The shape of the building minimizes heat loss and photovoltaics provide electricity. A retention roof and an underground rainwater tank contribute to the efficient use of water and promote sustainability and environmental responsibility.

Address: Jívavská 20, 785 01 Šternberk, Czech Republic | **Client:** Region of Olomouc | **Completion:** 2022 | **Size:** 5,445 m² | **Sector:** state | **Specialization:** internal medicine | **Number of treatment rooms:** 9 | **Number of patient rooms:** 28

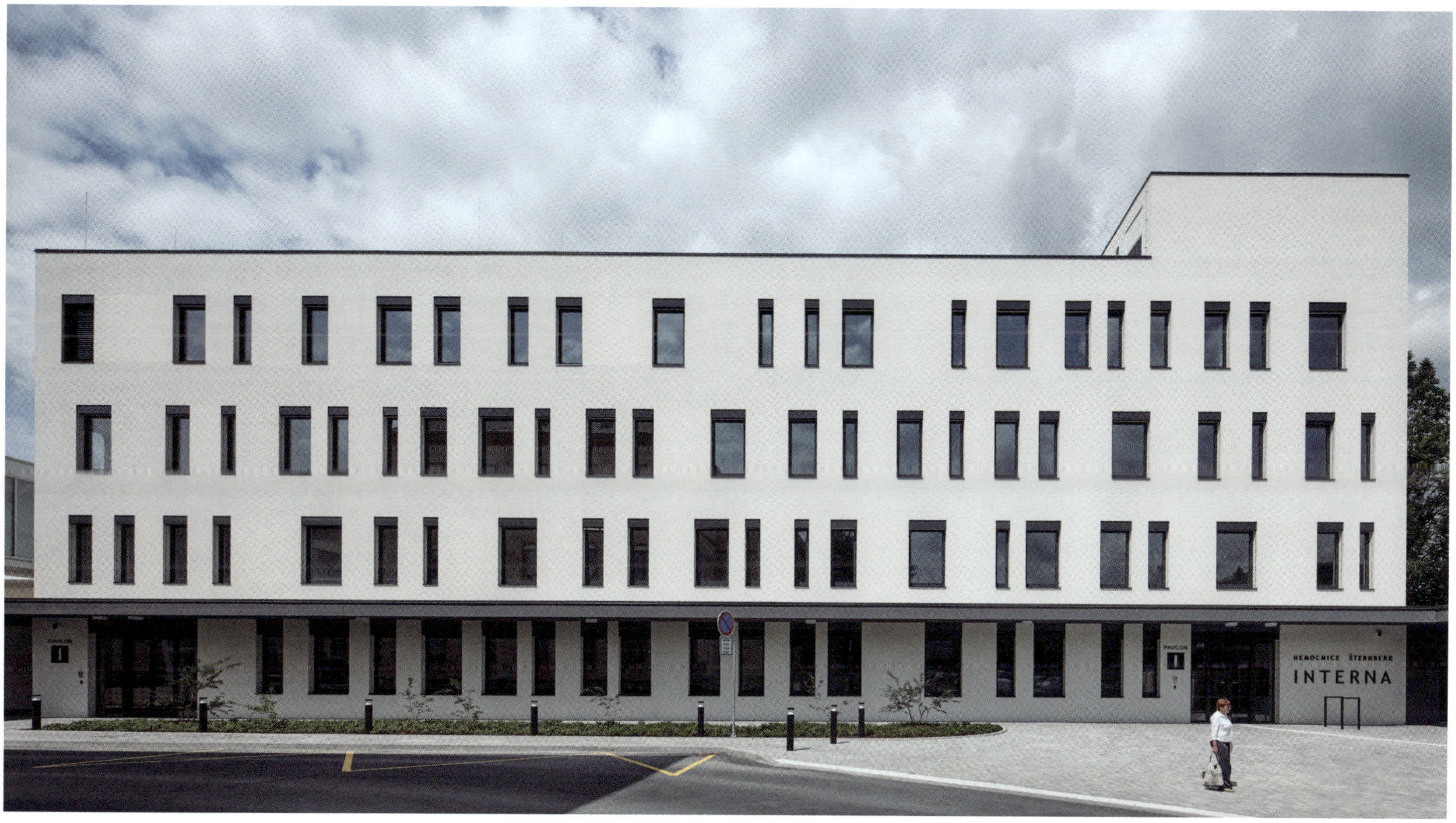

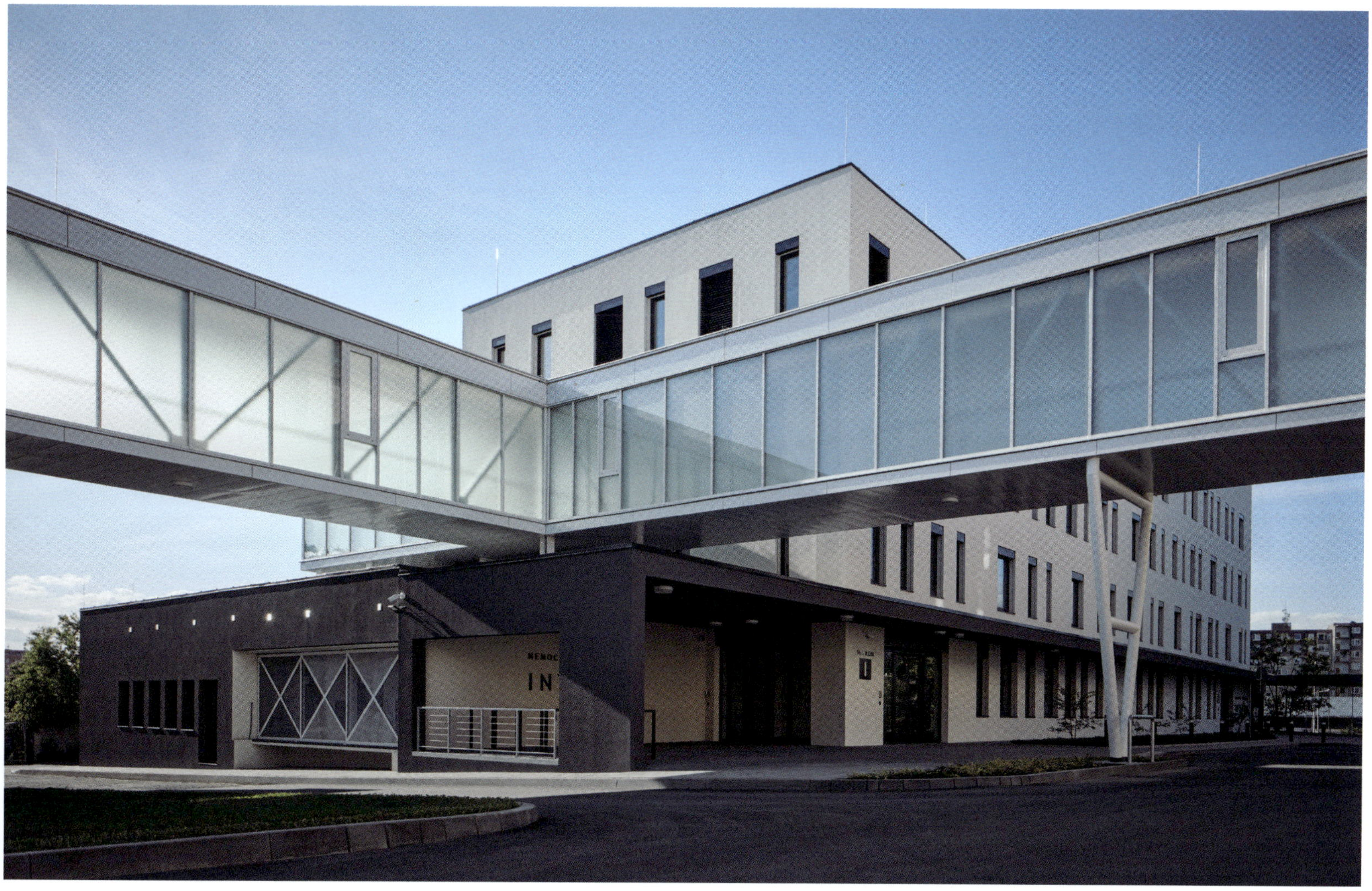

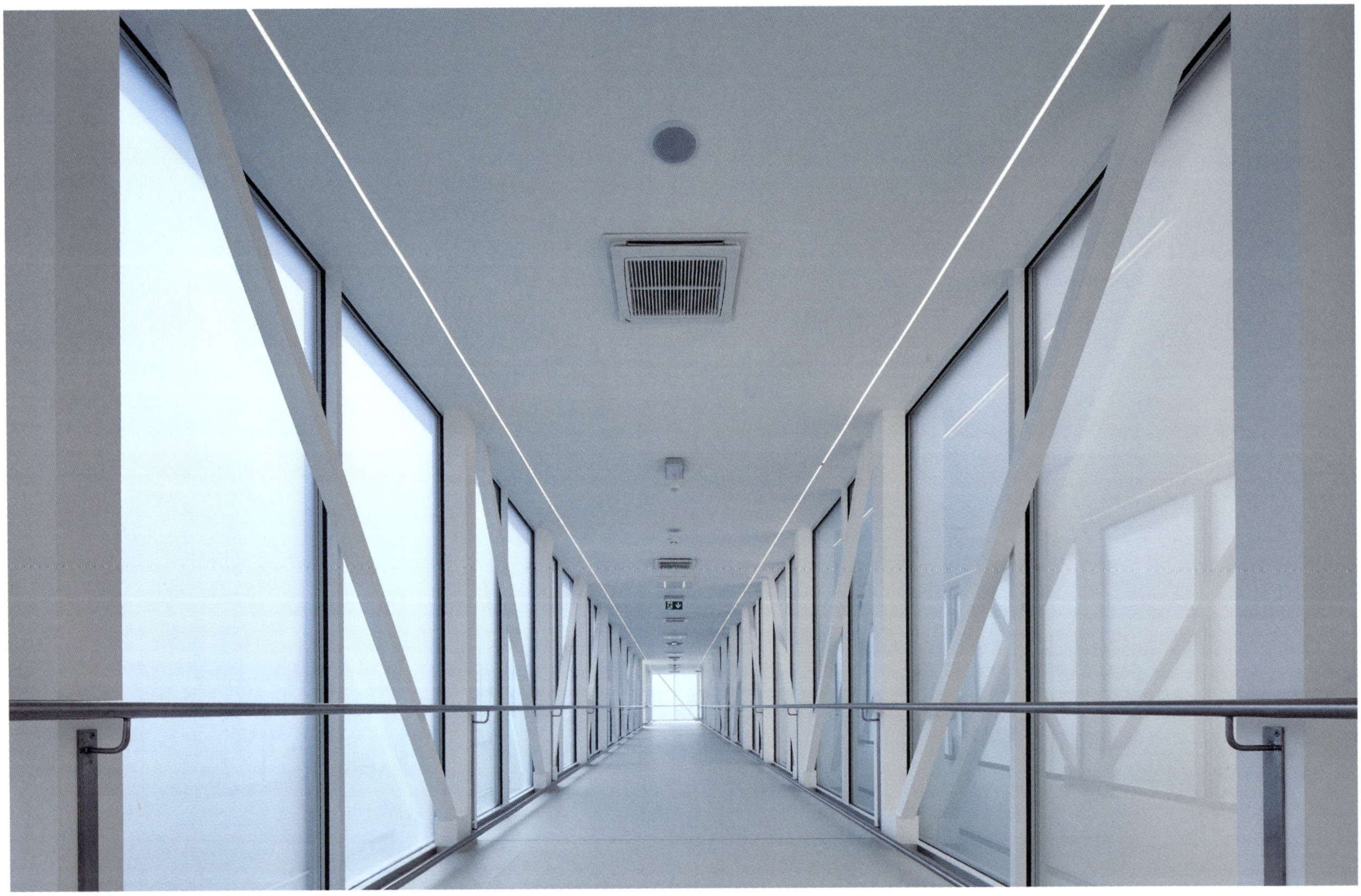

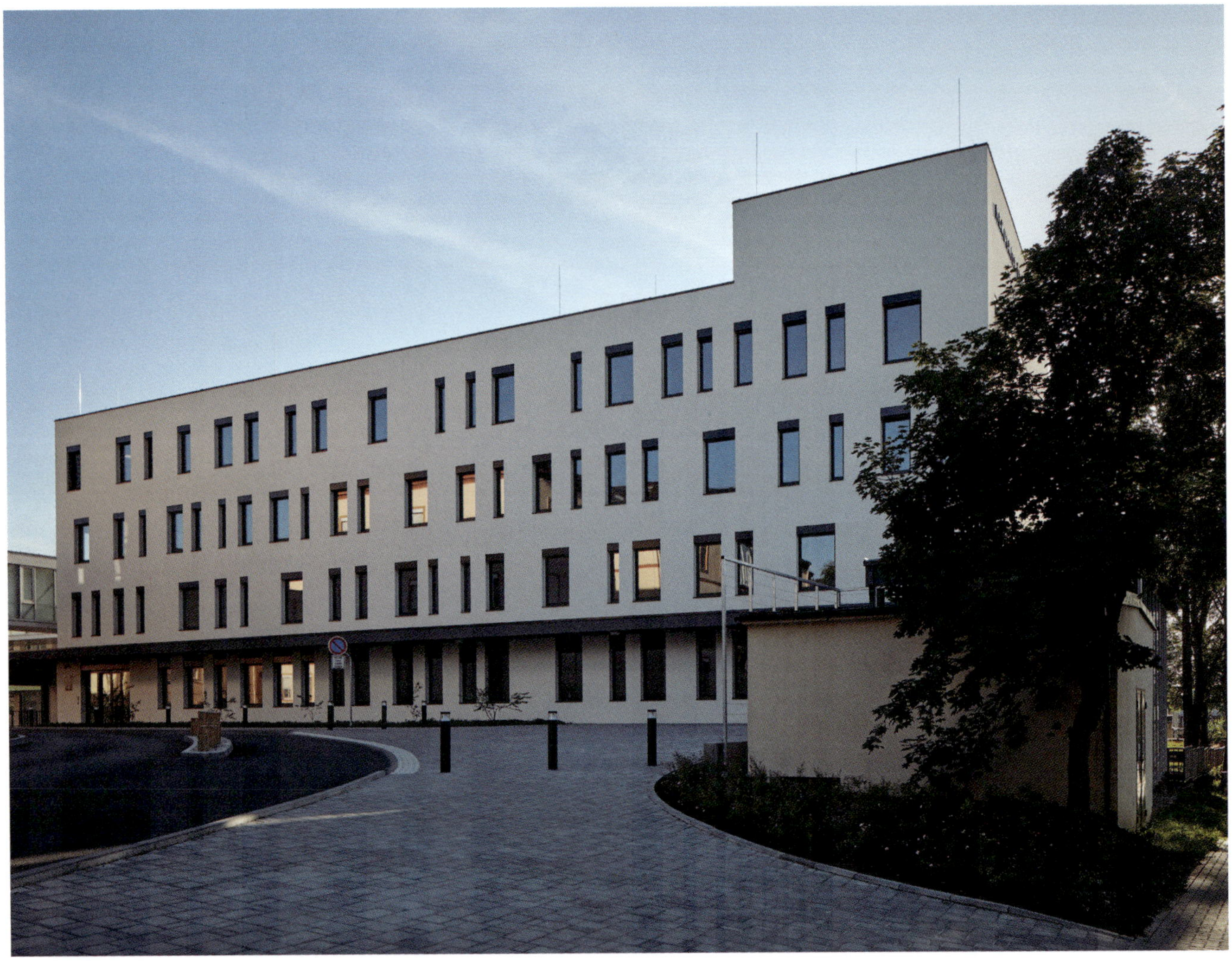

Structure and opaque windows of the connection.

Pavilion seen from the entrance to the hospital grounds.

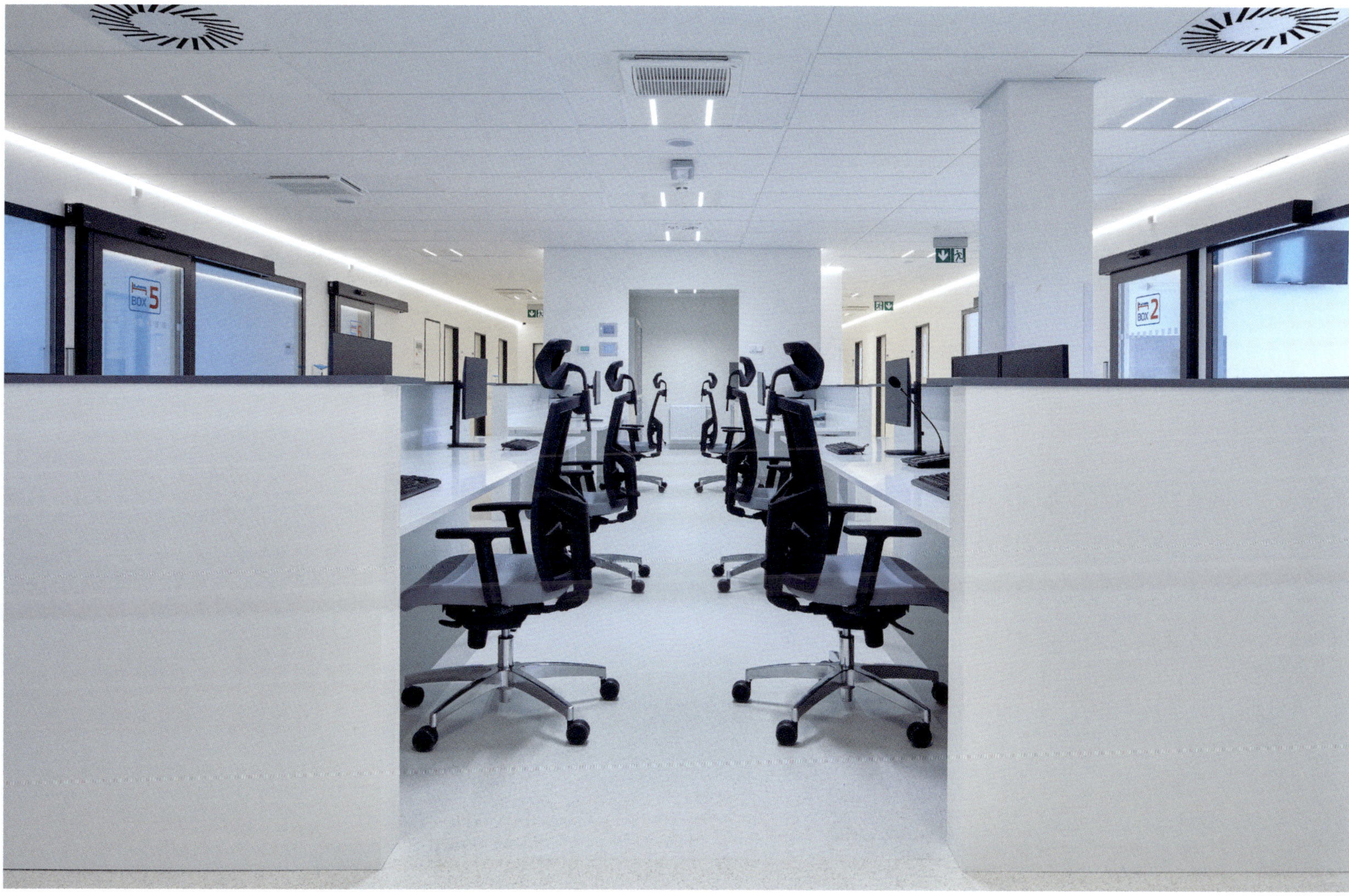

Department of intensive care unit.

Third floor, fourth floor, basement, and ground floor plan.

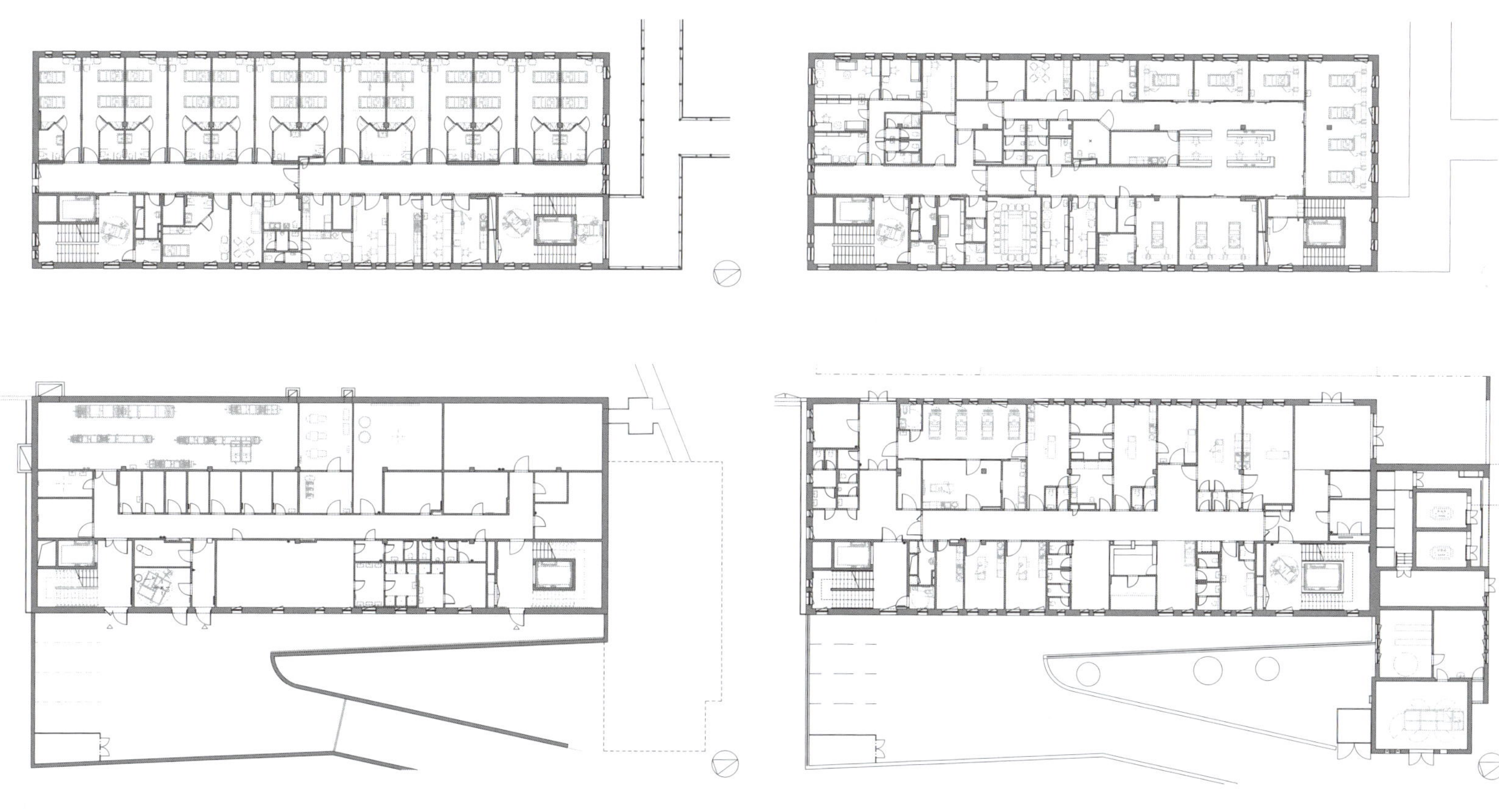

KHR Architecture
Henning Larsen
PKA Arkitekter

Bergen
Norway

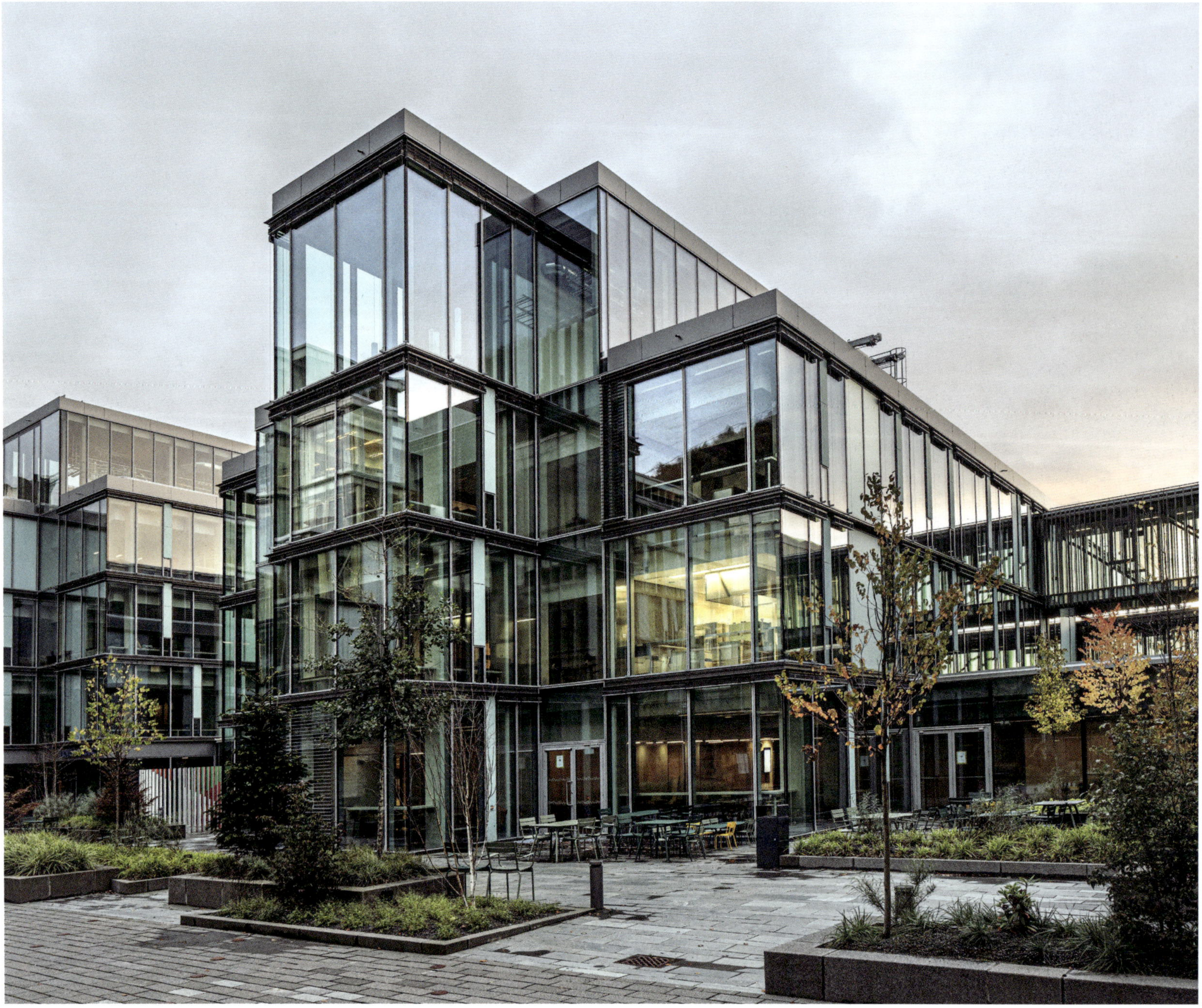

The entrance area is an urban and green square, with a welcoming atmosphere.

The placement of the blocks on a green slope enhances the connection between the exterior and interior.

Each garden has its own theme, based on natural types of landscape in Norwegian nature.

Glasblokkene – Haukeland Children's and Women's Hospital

Glasblokkene is designed to create a healthcare environment where children are children before they are patients. The architecture supports healing and wellbeing through a welcoming, playful setting for children, young people, women, families, and staff. Built into a sloping mountainside in Bergen, the hospital follows the natural terrain, breaking its large volume into smaller glass buildings that step down the hillside. This strengthens the connection between inside and outside, bringing daylight, views, gardens, and nature into everyday hospital life. Clear wayfinding, generous shared spaces, integrated art, and child-friendly details create an intuitive and engaging environment. By combining architecture, landscape, and sensory experiences, Glasblokkene transforms a complex healthcare facility into a place that supports care, comfort, and healing, while maintaining a sense of normality and everyday life.

Address: Haukelandsbakken 15, 5009 Bergen, Norway | **Client:** Helse Bergen | **Completion:** 2023 | **Size:** 79,000 m² | **Sector:** state | **Specialization:** children, youth, and women health | **Number of patient rooms:** 223 | **Landscape design:** Landskap Trondheim and Schønherr Landskab

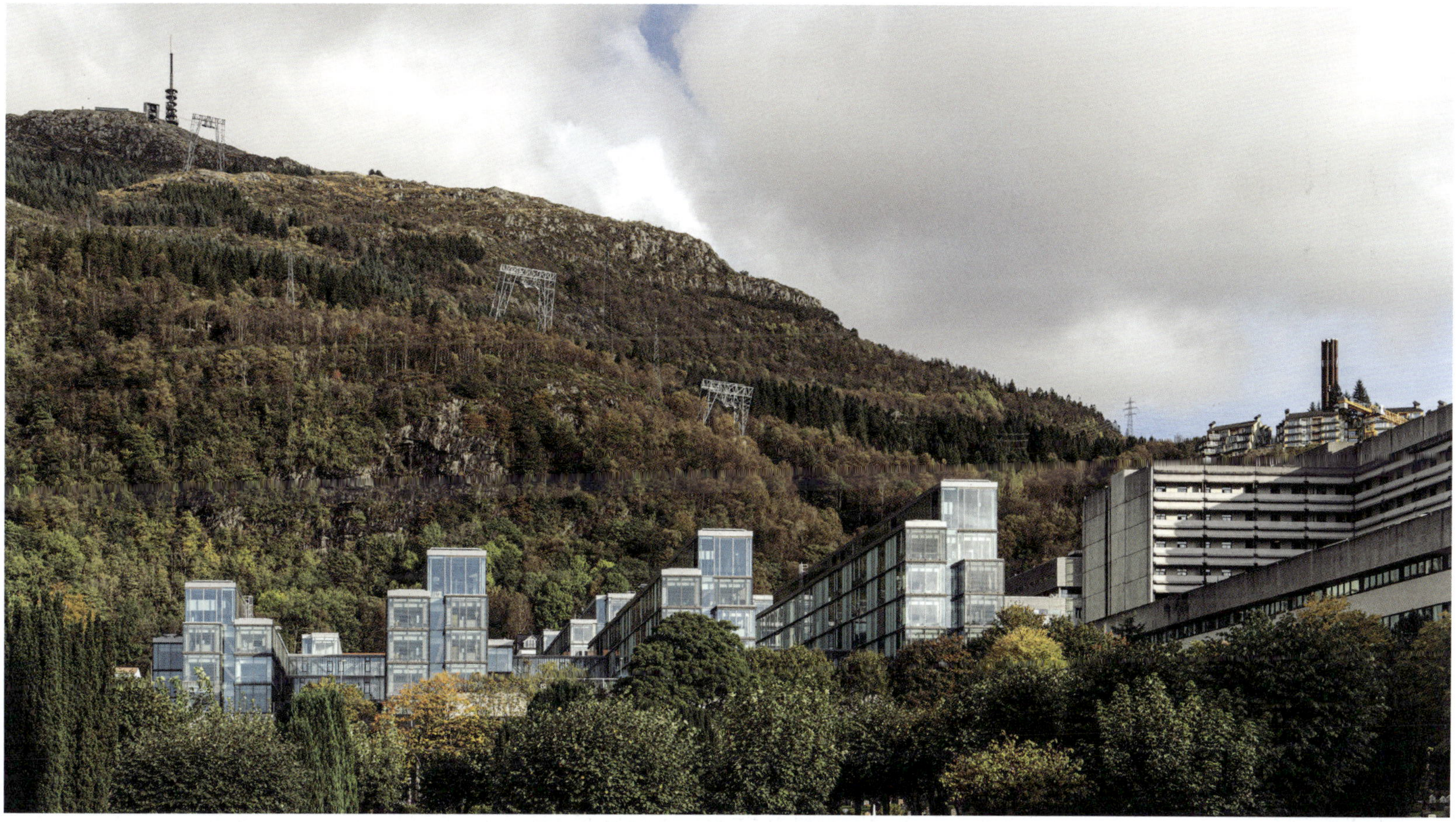

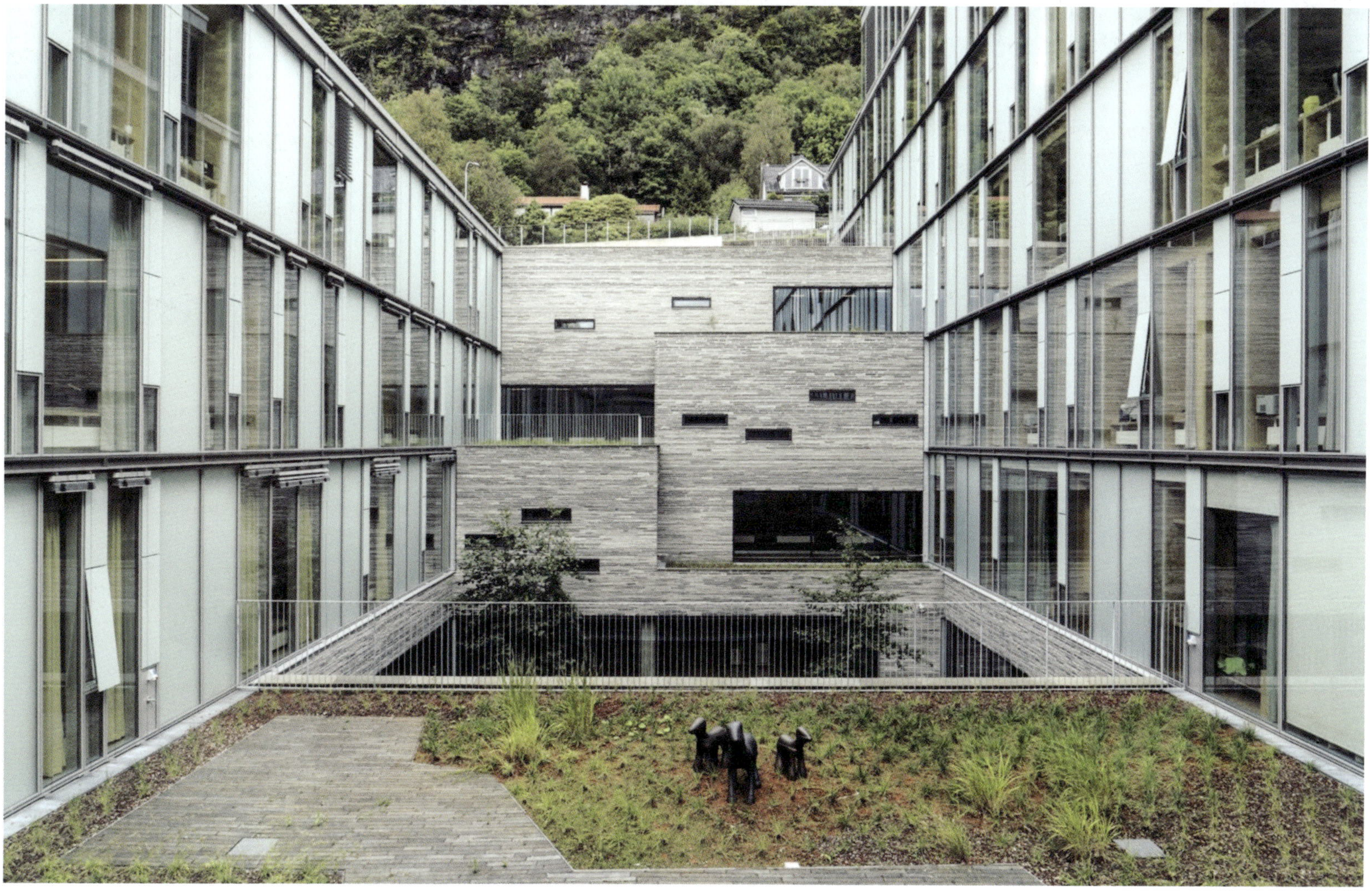

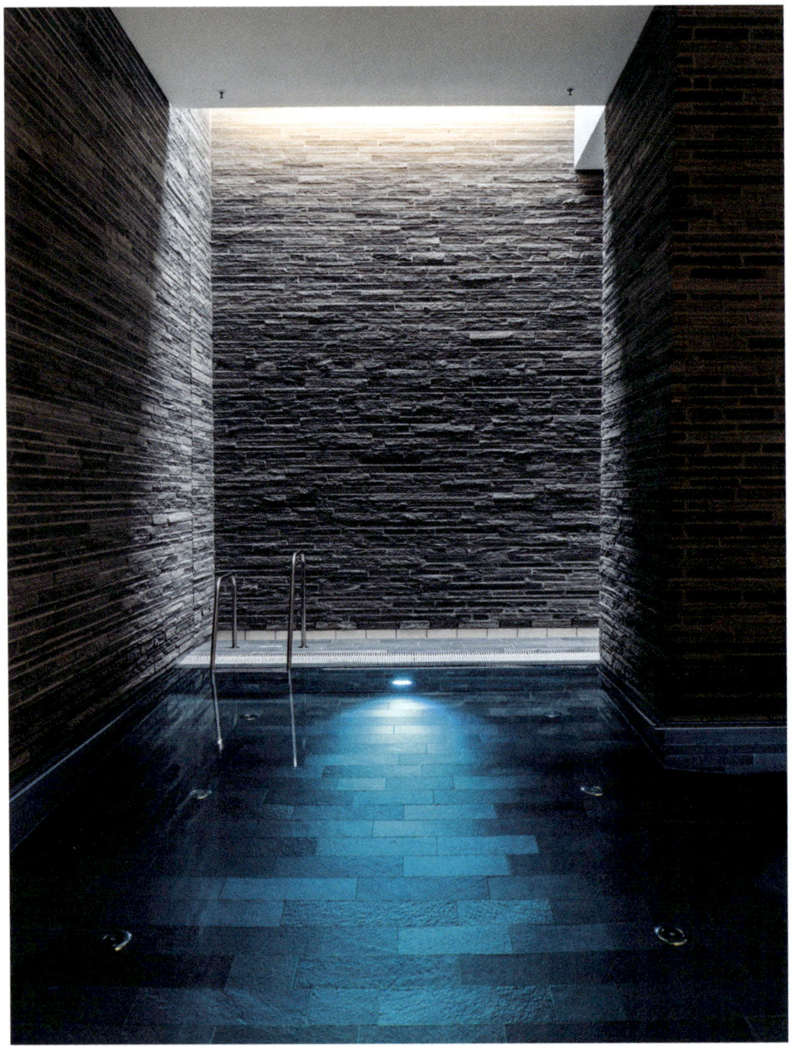

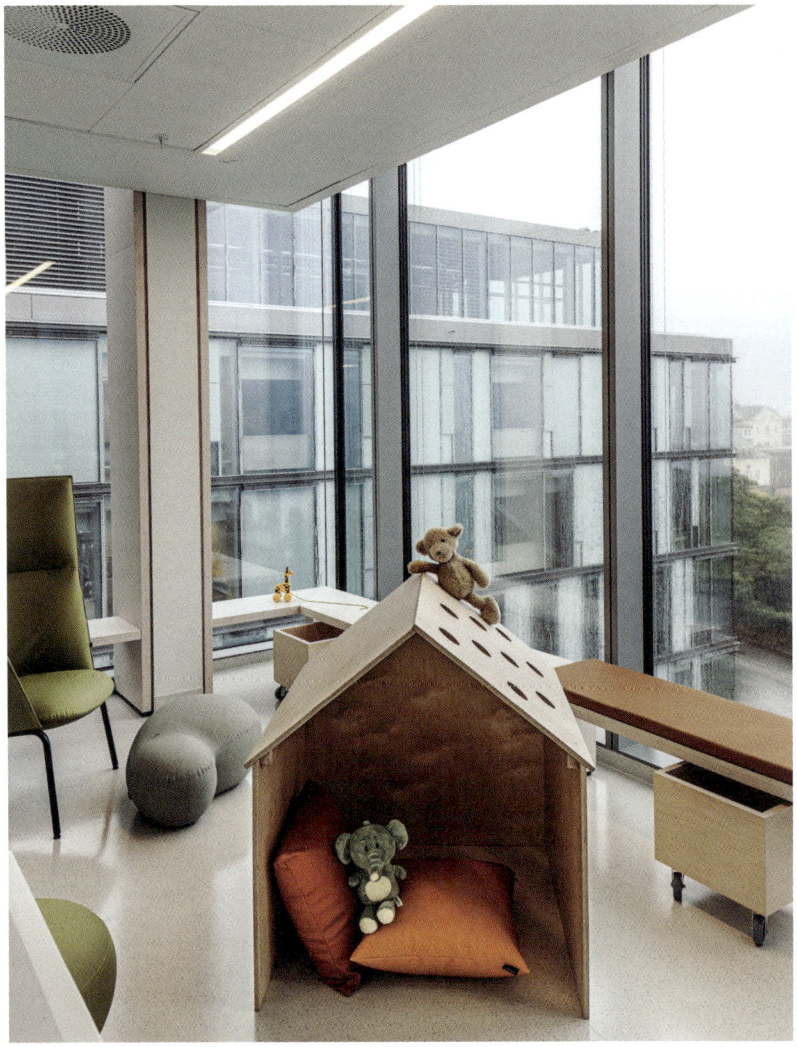

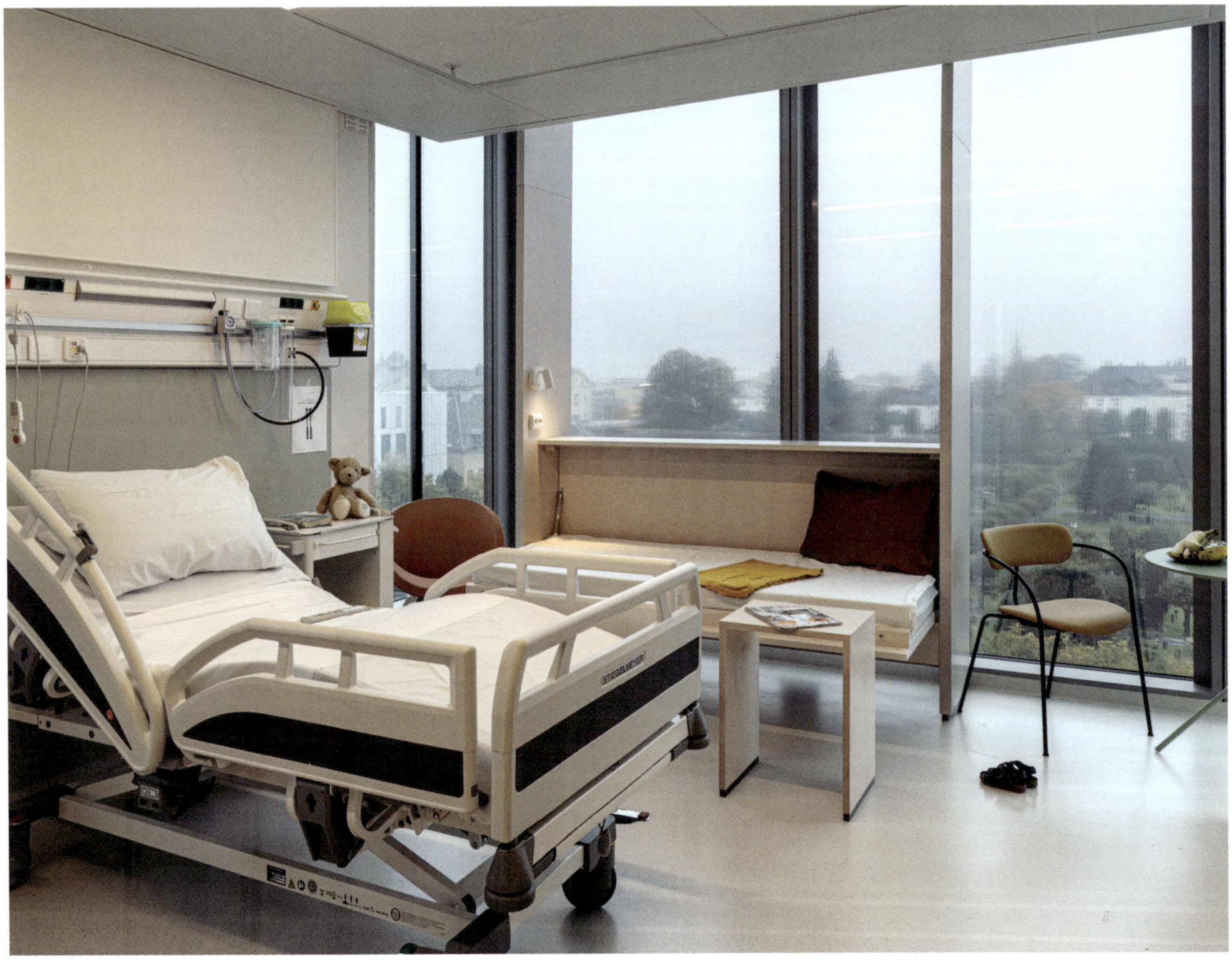

In the rehabilitation and well-being area, slate creates a clear reference to the surrounding landscape.

Each play area has its focus on different levels of activity and interaction.

The patient rooms provide integrated bed sofas for relatives.

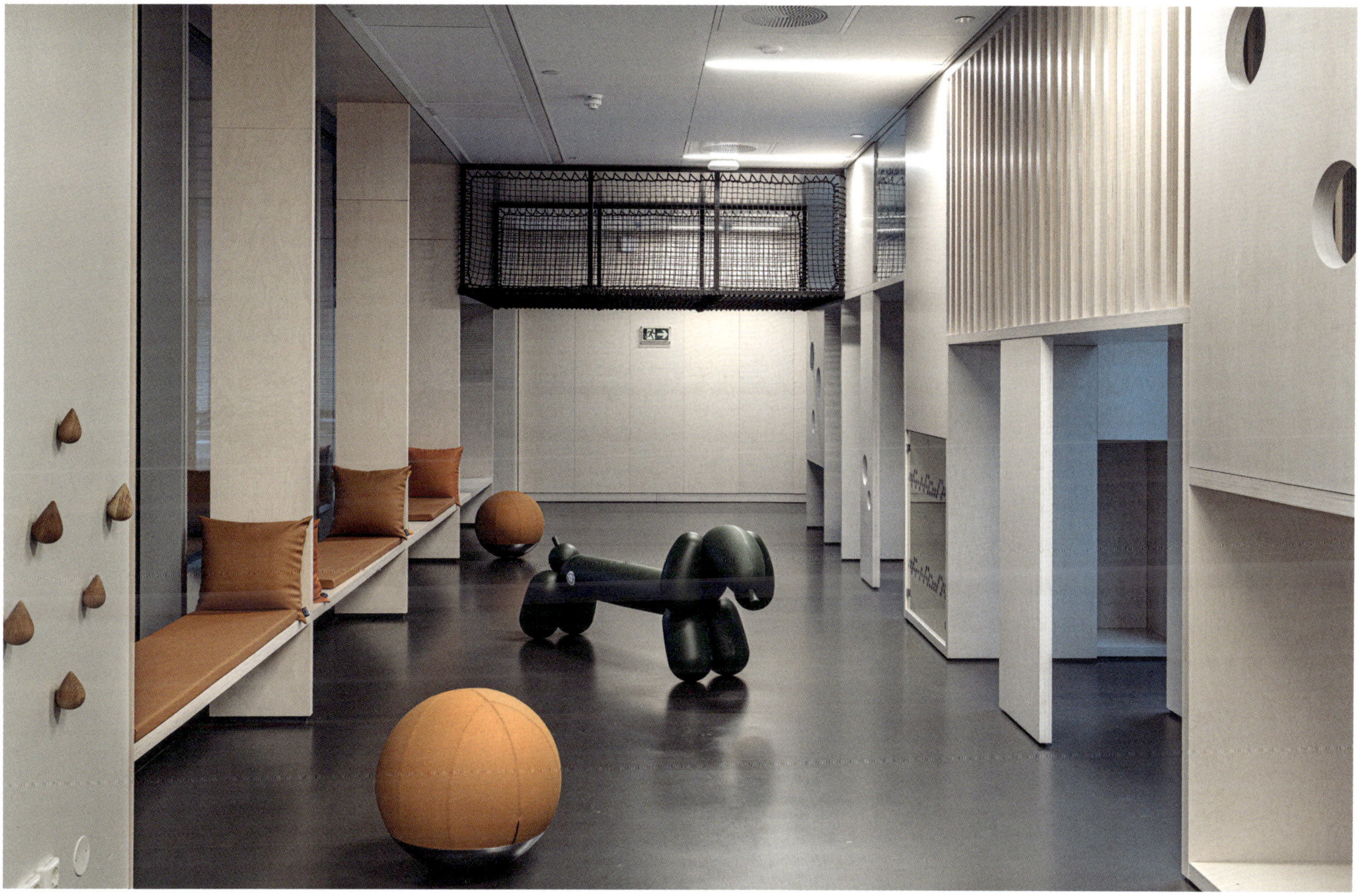

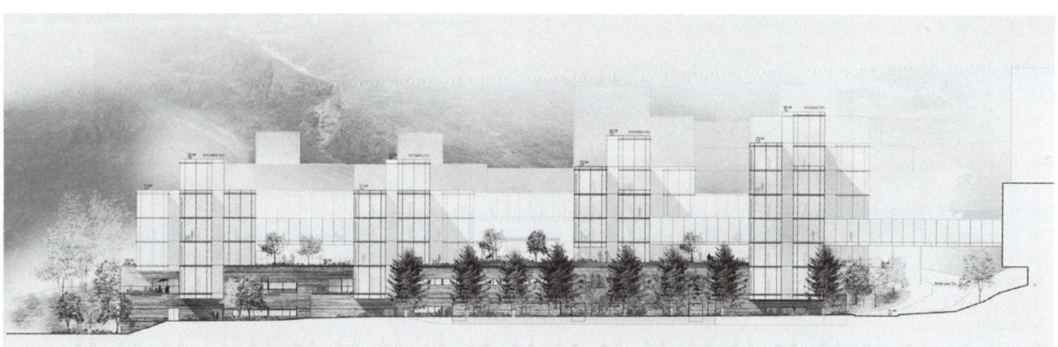

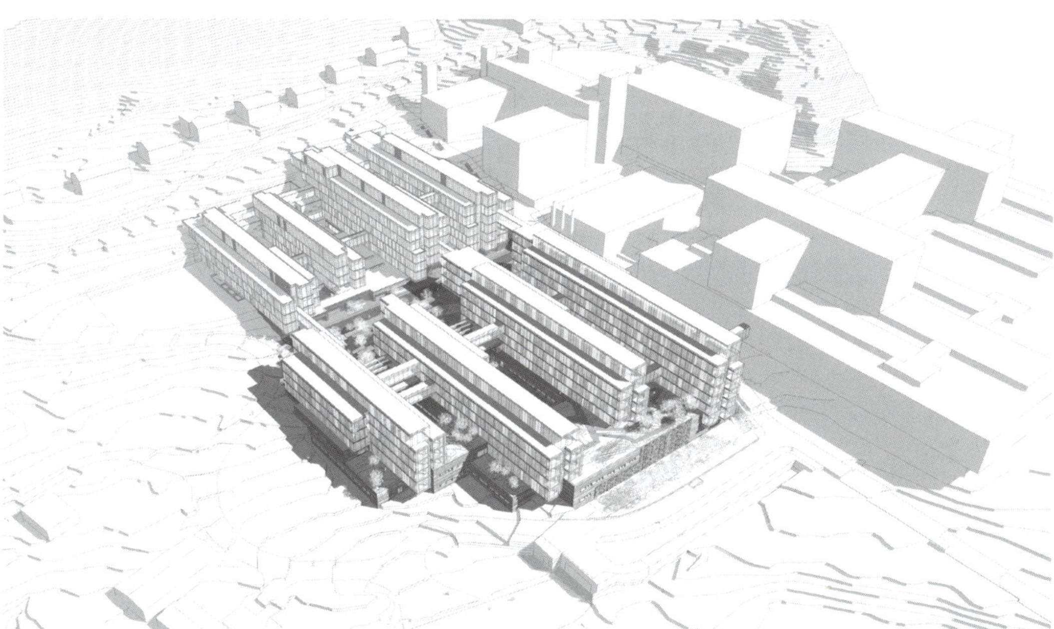

The playful entrance room provides a warm welcome.

West elevation.

3D drawing of Glasblokkene Haukeland Stage II and the existing volumes.

100% interior
Sylvia Leydecker

Erftstadt
Germany

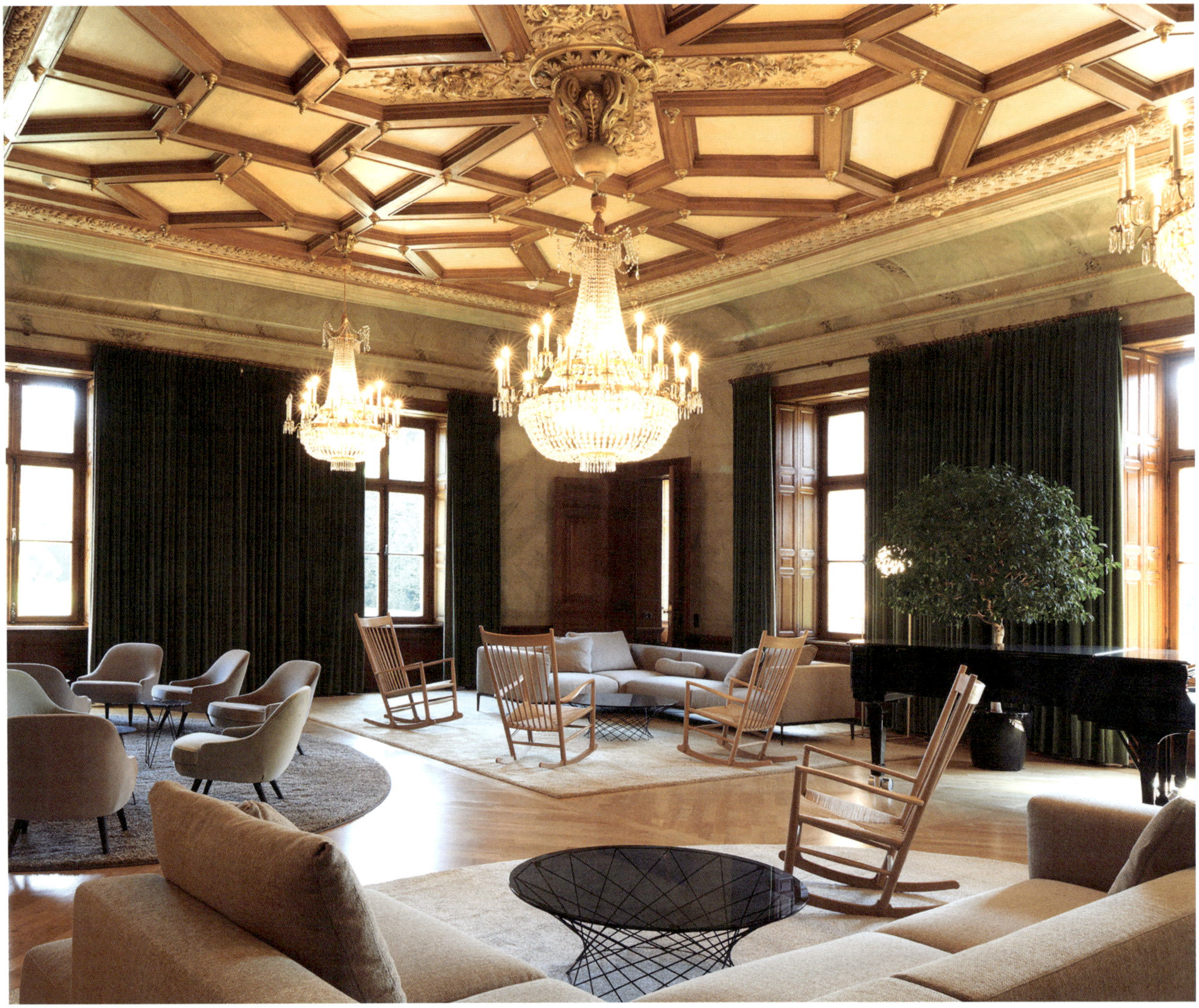

Harmoniously differentiated day lounge in the impressive knights hall.

The healing environment interior is enhanced by abundant daylight and views of the surrounding park.

Striking graphics, bold colors, and historic substance in perfect balance.

Libermenta Private Clinic Chateau Gracht

Chateau Gracht is a multi-award-winning private clinic for psychotherapy and psychosomatic medicine in Erftstadt. The interior architecture, designed by the interior architect Sylvia Leydecker, translates the historic fabric of the listed castle into a contemporary healing environment. Set in the highly unusual surroundings of a former castle, this clinic – which cares about approximately 80 private patients – combines a comfortable atmosphere with specialized therapy to heal the mind. Generous daylighting, circadian lighting, and multi-sensory, carefully coordinated materials create spaces of calm, protection, and comfort. The design combines emotional presence with a clear, modern formal language, subtly yet consistently supporting the therapeutic impact of the medical services. Tradition and contemporary healthcare design enter into a precise, forward-looking dialogue.

Address: Fritz-Erler-Straße 1, 50374 Erftstadt, Germany | **Client:** Dr. Karsten Wolf AG | **Completion:** 2019 | **Original building:** Manor house, Gottfried Laurenz Pictorius, 18th century | **Sector:** private | **Specialization:** psychodynamic psychiatry, psychotherapy and psychosomatic medicine | **Number of patient rooms:** 80

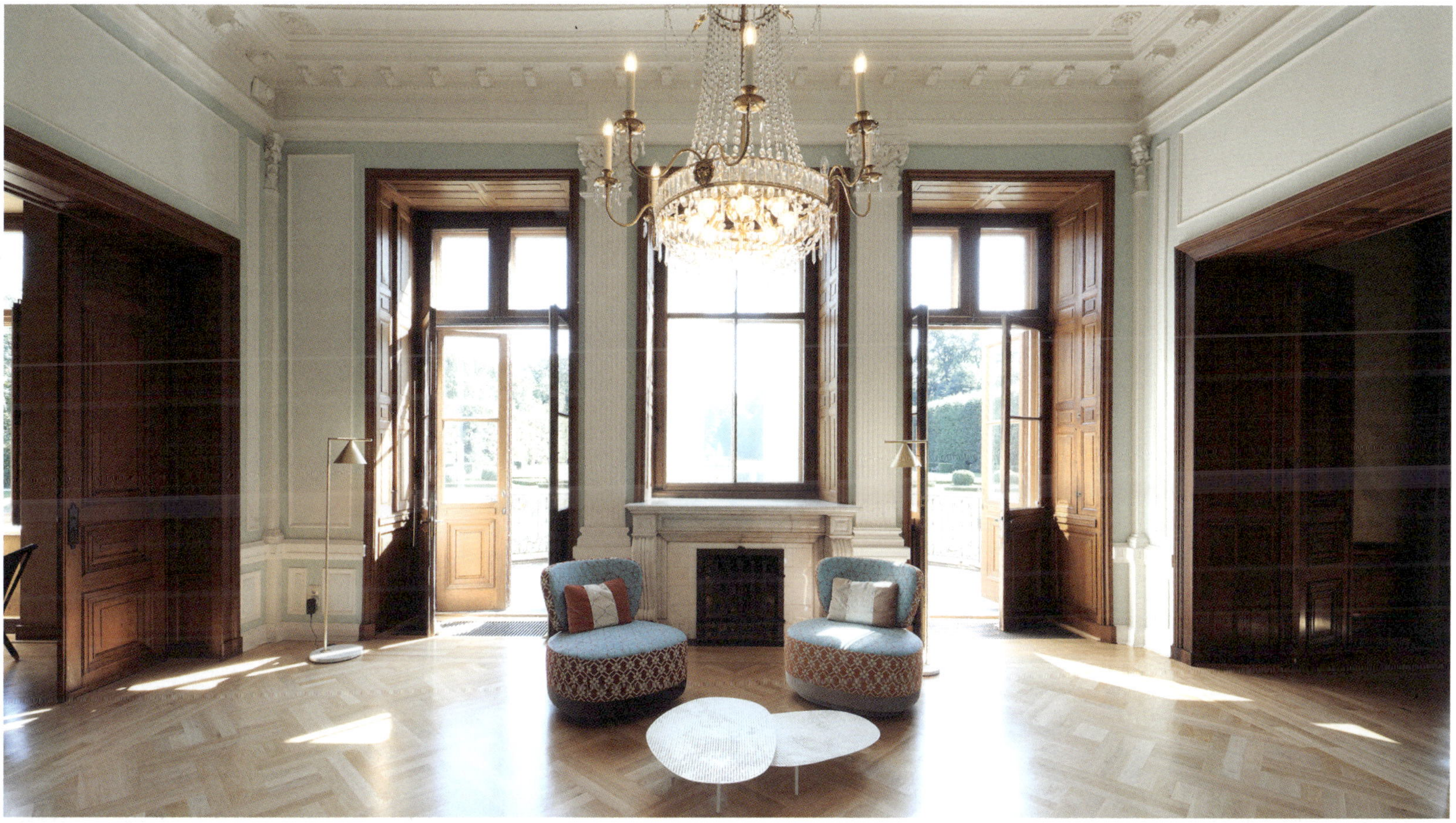

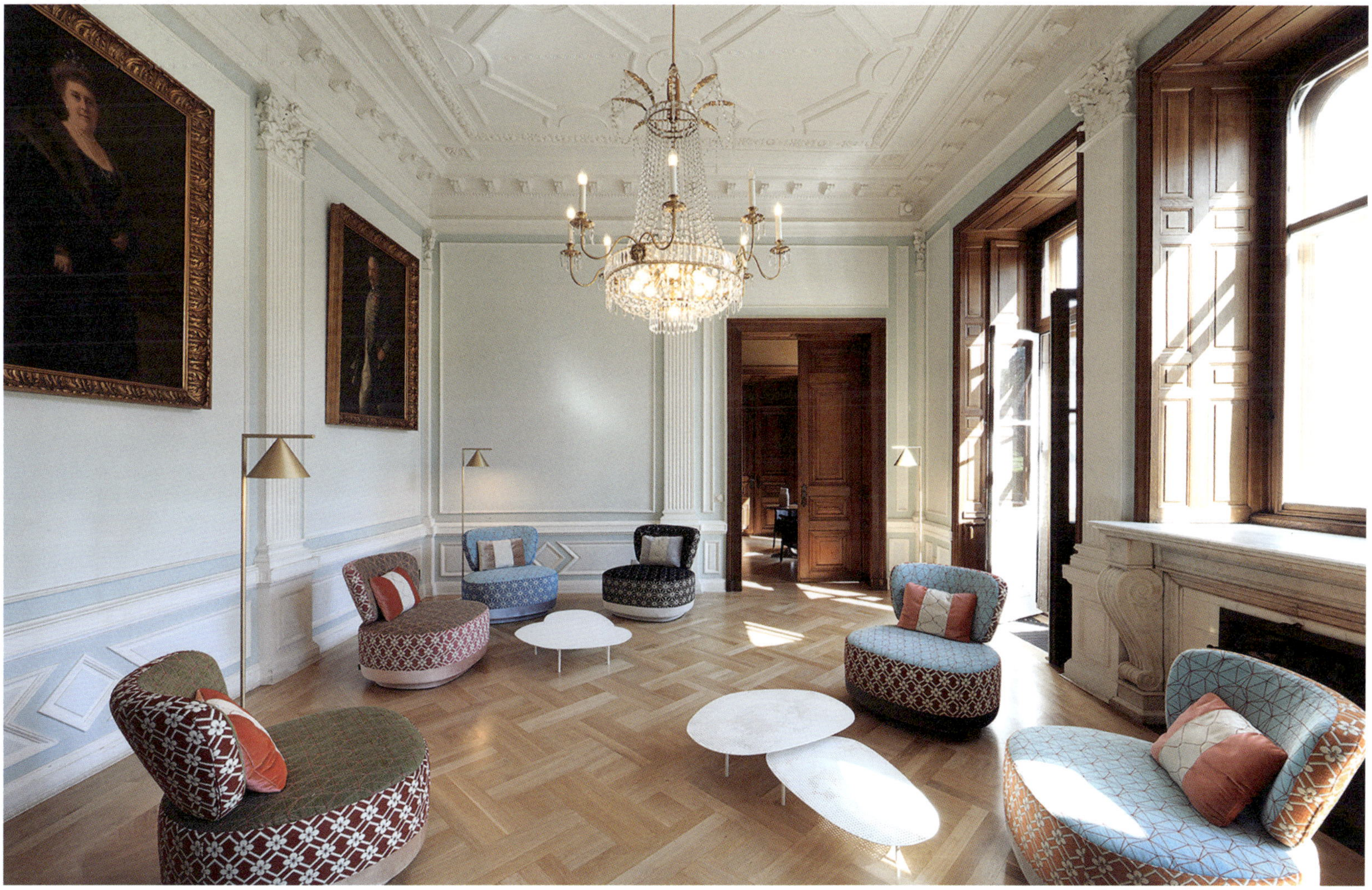

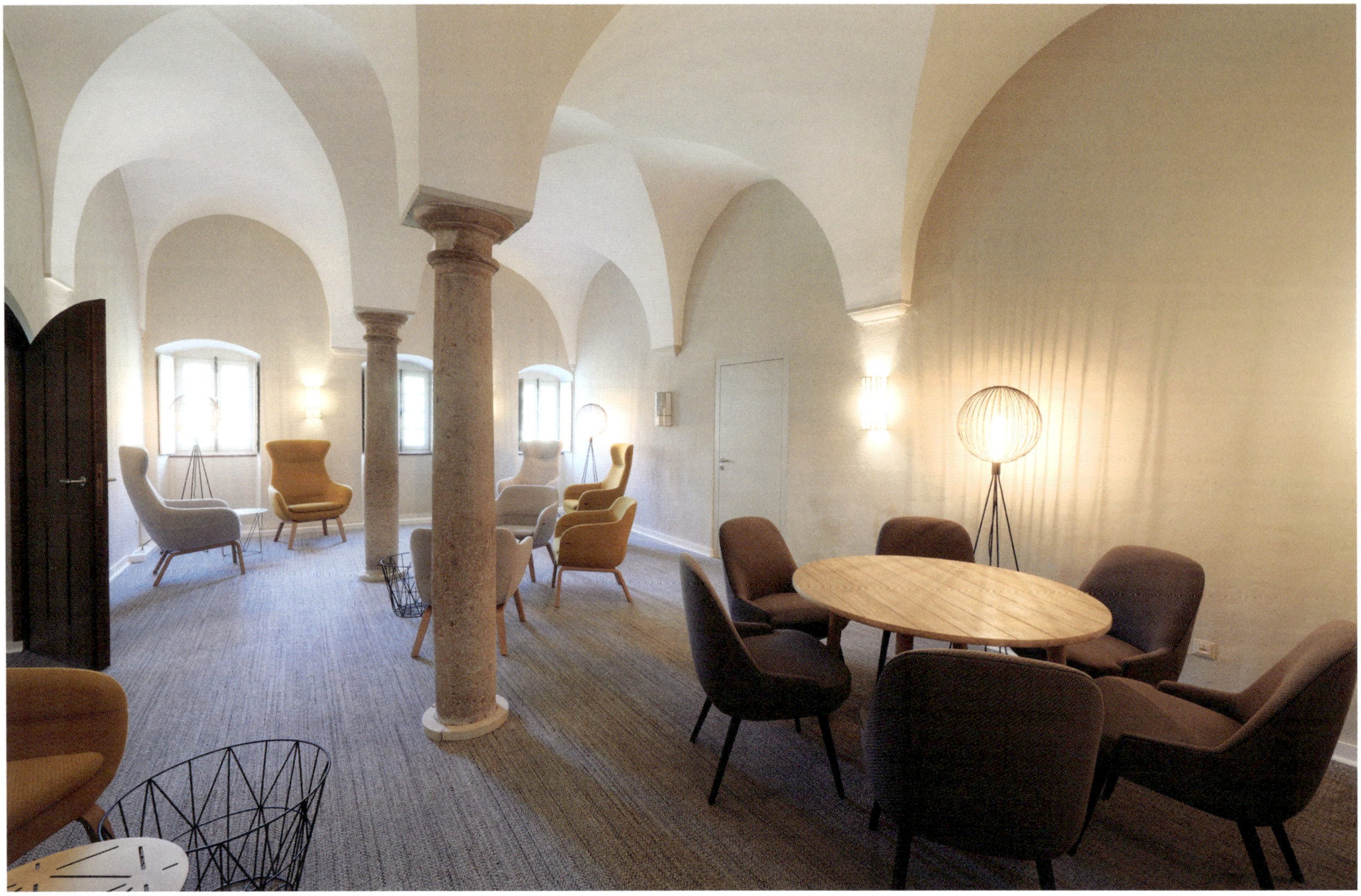

Comfortable club chairs and vaulted ceilings define the evening lounge.

Two-bed-room plan.

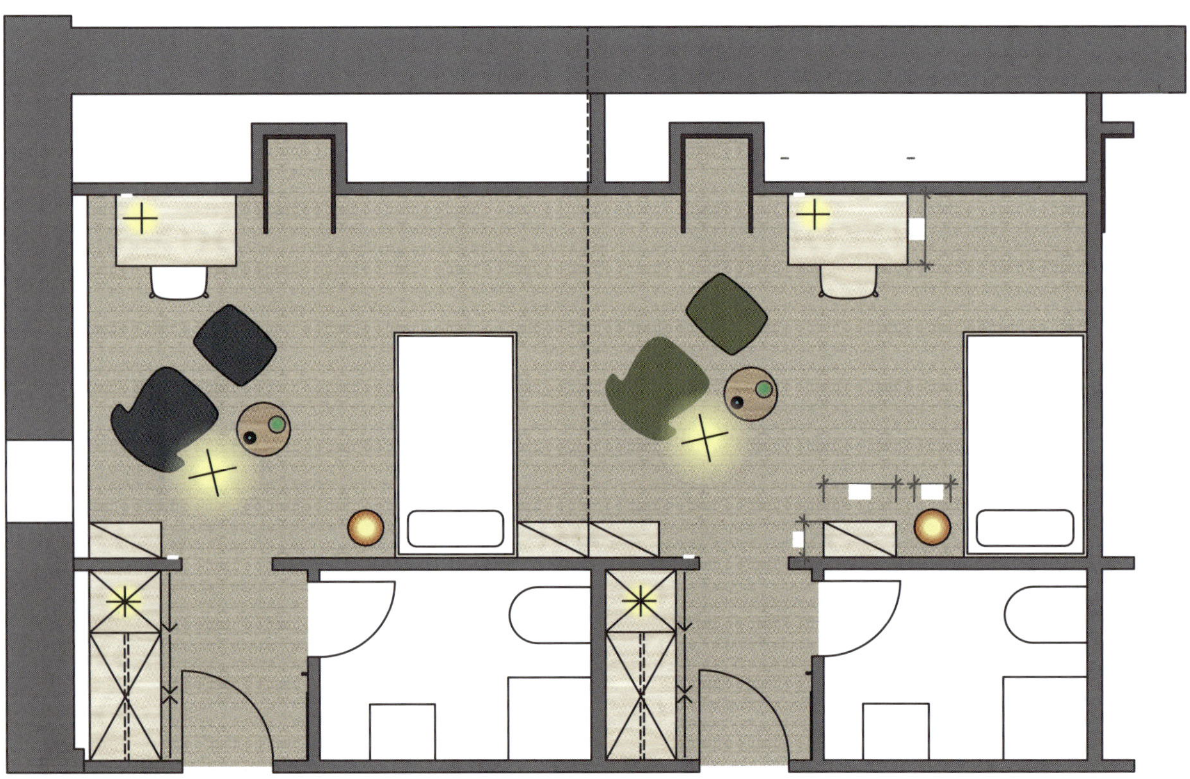

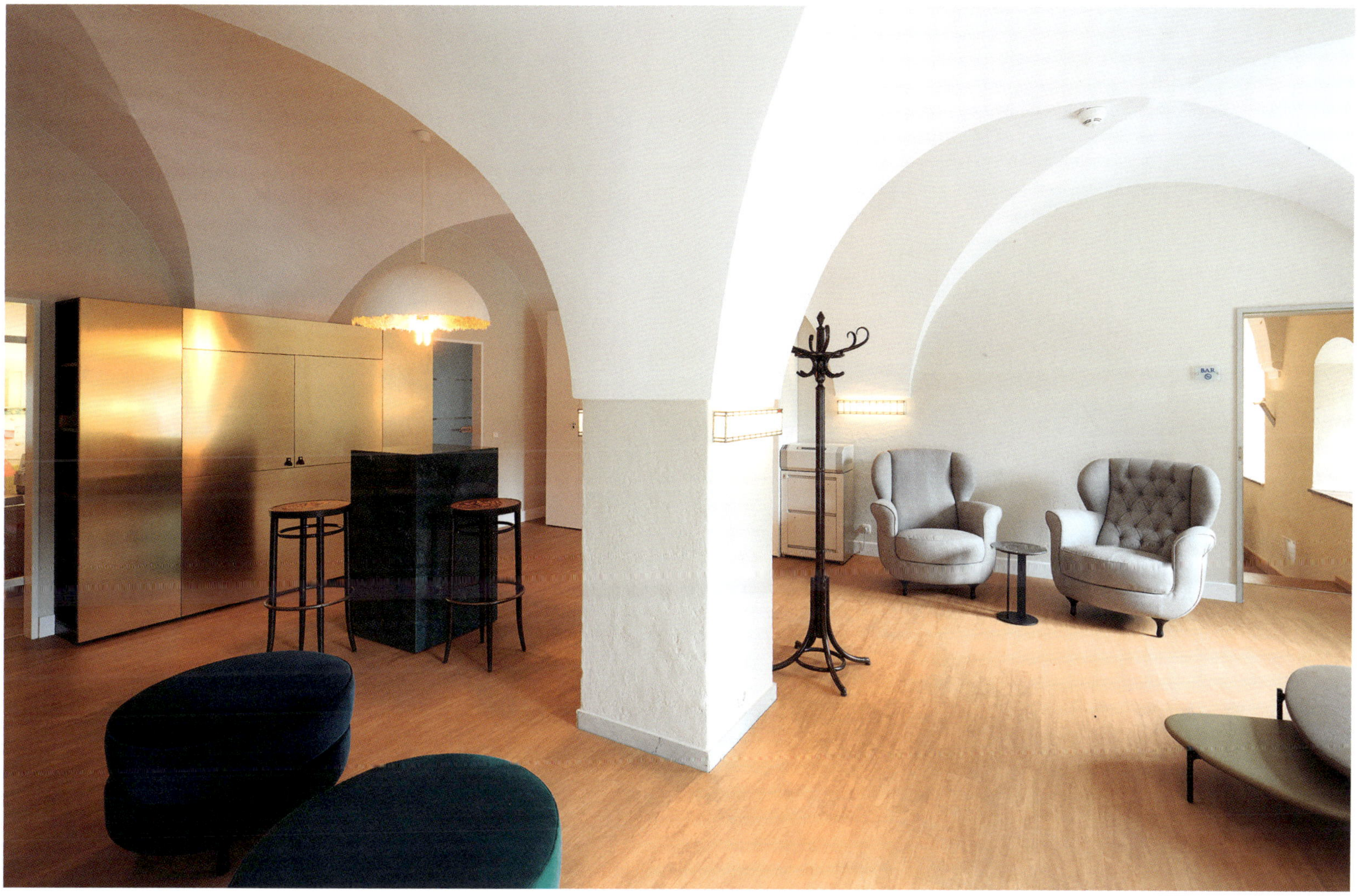

Charming entrance area, in which patients take a seat for an individual welcome-dialogue and receive their well-kept keys out of a golden shrine.

Single-bed-room plan.

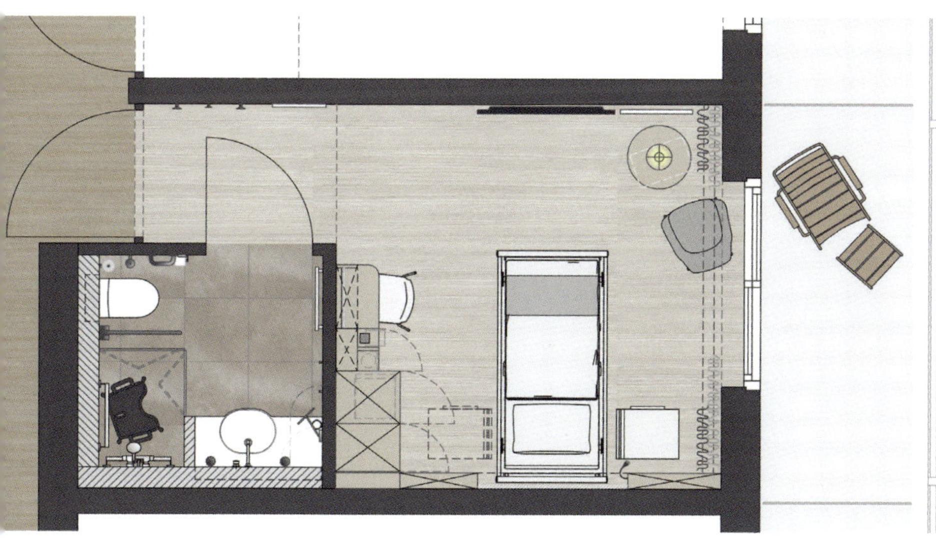

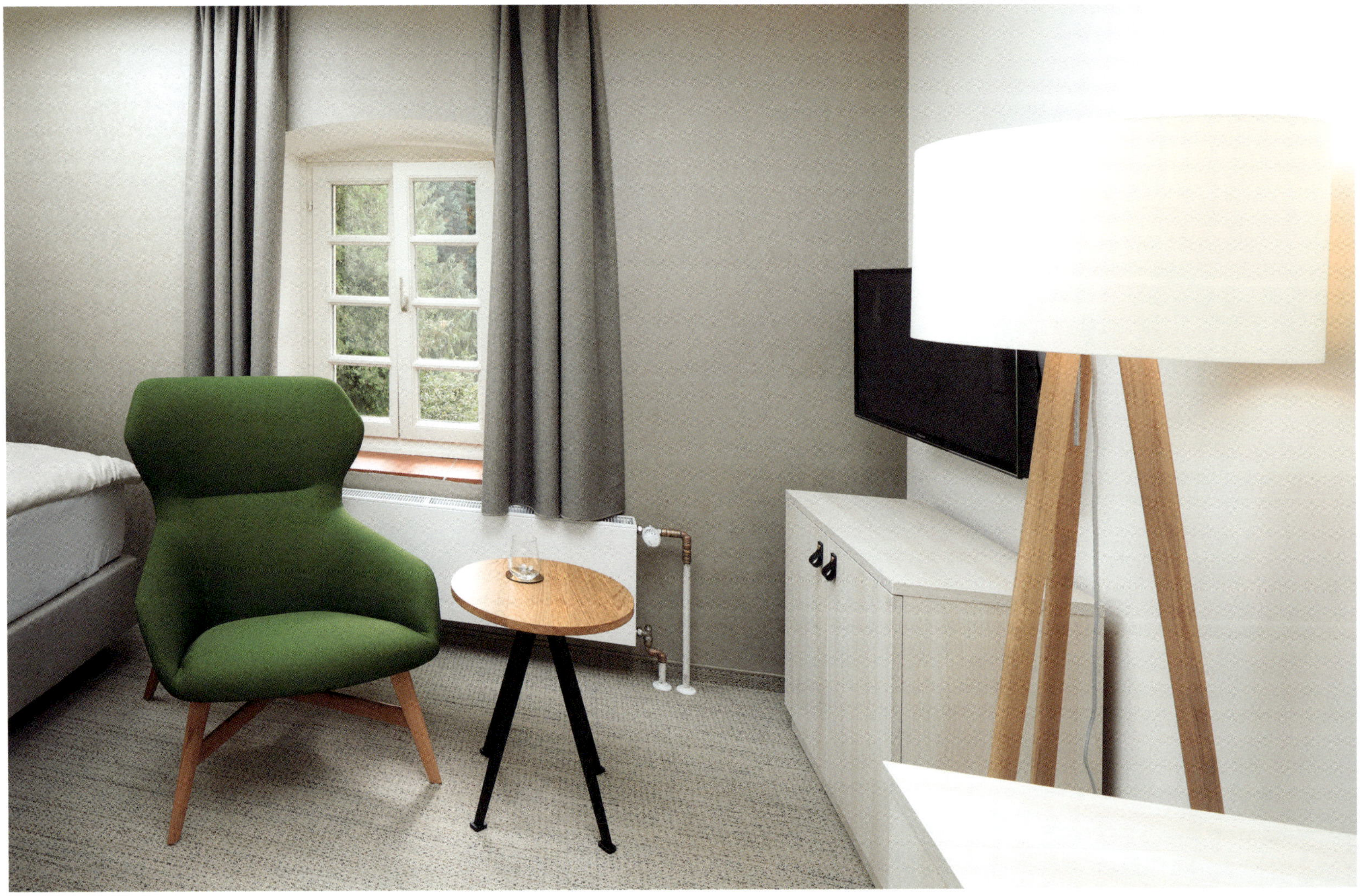

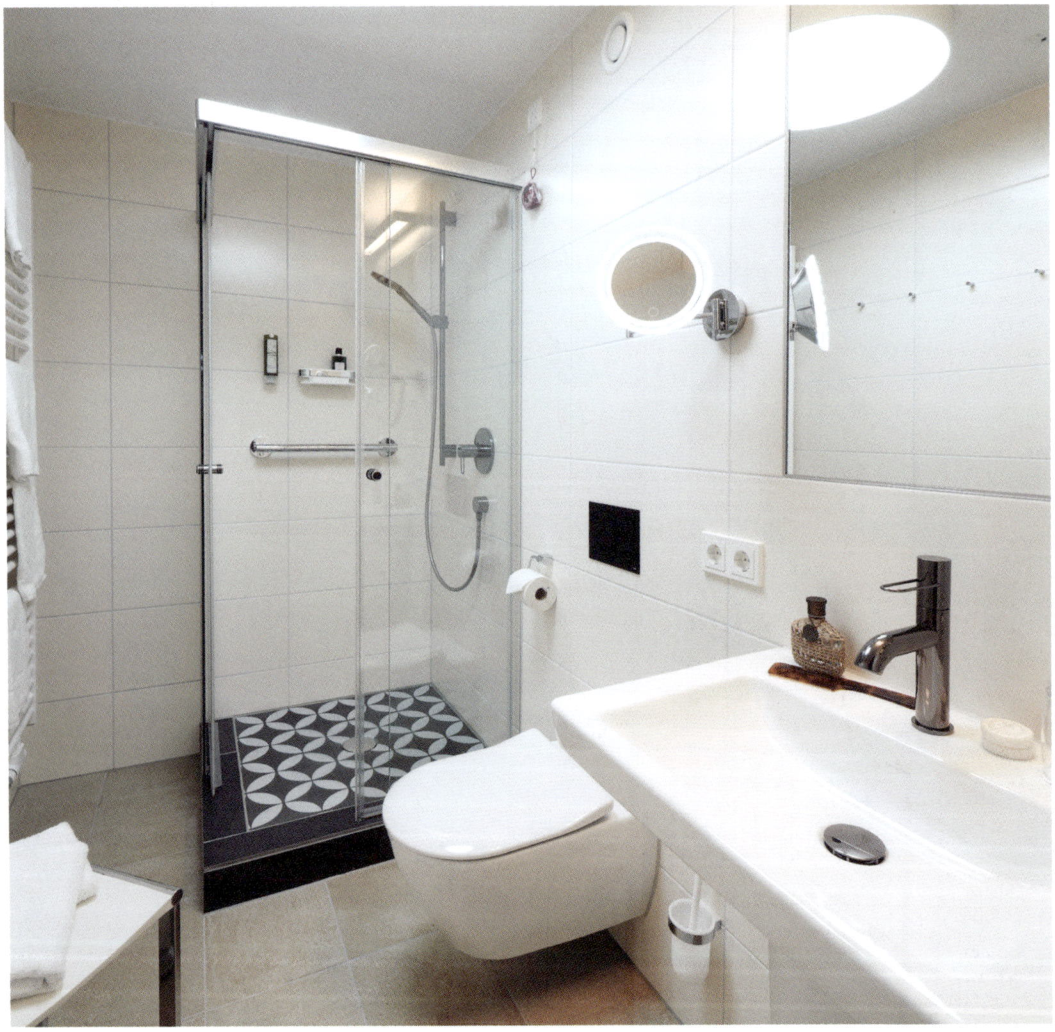

Circadian lighting also in the smallest patient room.

Bright patient bathroom culture in the 500-year-old moated castle.

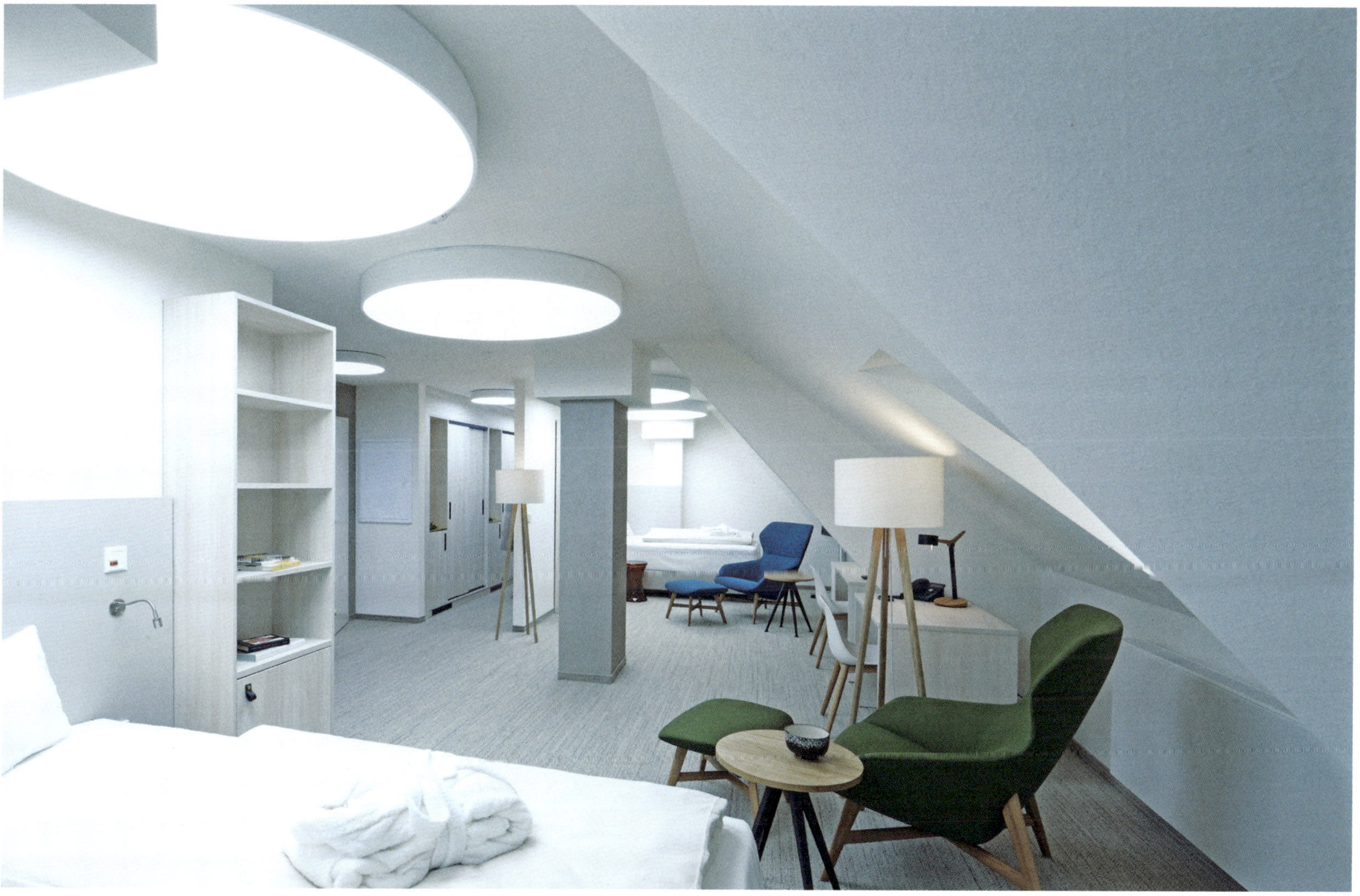

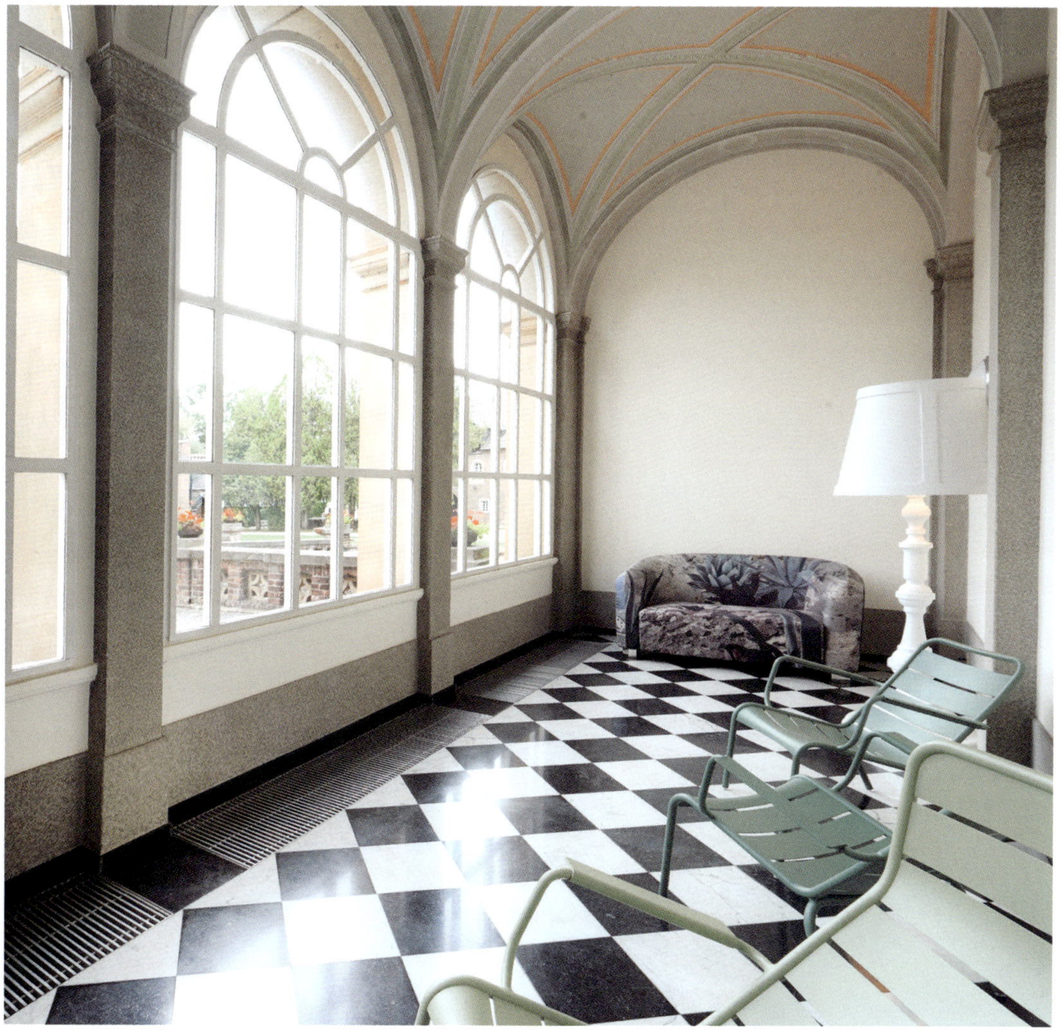

Patient room defined by circular skylights, soft natural materials, and a calm, residential healing atmosphere.

Large windows of the orangery overlooking the outside garden.

Architects Index

Photographers Index

IMPRINT

The Deutsche Nationalbibliothek lists this publication in the Deutsche Nationalbibliografie; detailed bibliographic data are available on the Internet at http://dnb.dnb.de

ISBN 978-3-03768-311-8

www.braun-publishing.ch

1st edition 2026

Texts and Layout: Lennart Melzer, Manjiri More, Emilia Luna Schöne, Klaudia Wojtczak
Graphic concept: Michaela Prinz, Berlin
Lithography: Paladin Design- und Werbemanufaktur

Product Safety
Publisher: Braun Publishing AG
Arenenbergstr. 2, 8268 Salenstein
Switzerland
publisher@braun-publishing.ch

EU-Representative: Bookwise GmbH
Zeppelinstr. 67, 81669 Munich
Germany
info@bookwise.de